HEMATOLOGIC PROBLEMS OF THE NEONATE

HEMATOLOGIC PROBLEMS OF THE NEONATE

Robert D. Christensen, M.D.
Professor of Pediatrics
Chief, Division of Neonatology
Vice Chairman for Research
Department of Pediatrics
University of Florida College of Medicine
Gainesville, Florida

W.B. SAUNDERS COMPANY
A Division of Harcourt Brace & Company
Philadelphia London Toronto Montreal Sydney Tokyo

W.B. SAUNDERS COMPANY
A Division of Harcourt Brace & Company

The Curtis Center
Independence Square West
Philadelphia, Pennsylvania 19106

Library of Congress Cataloging-in-Publication Data

Hematologic problems of the neonate / [edited by] Robert D. Christensen.—1st ed.

p. cm.

ISBN 0–7216–7727–4

1. Neonatal hematology. 2. Infants (Newborn)—Diseases. 3. Blood diseases in pregnancy. 4. Hematopoiesis. I. Christensen, Robert D., M.D. [DNLM: 1. Hematologic Diseases—in infancy & childhood. 2. Infant, Newborn, Diseases. 3. Fetal Diseases. 4. Hematopoiesis. WS 300 H4853 2000]

RJ269.5.H46 2000 618.92′15—dc21

DNLM/DLC 98–52044

HEMATOLOGIC PROBLEMS OF THE NEONATE ISBN 0–7216–7727–4

Printed in the United States of America.

Last digit is the print number: 9 8 7 6 5 4 3 2 1

Contributors

Maureen Andrew, M.D.
Professor of Pediatrics, Hamilton Civic Hospitals Research Center, McMaster University, Hamilton, Ontario, Canada
Developmental Aspects of Blood Hemostasis and Disorders of Coagulation and Fibrinolysis in the Neonatal Period

Harry Bard, M.D.
Professor of Pediatrics, Université de Montréal; Chief, Division of Neonatology, Ste. Justine's Hospital, Montréal, Quebec, Canada
Hemoglobin Synthesis and Metabolism During the Neonatal Period

Darlene A. Calhoun, D.O.
Assistant Professor, Division of Neonatology, Department of Pediatrics, University of Florida College of Medicine, Gainesville, Florida
Hematologic Aspects of the Maternal-Fetal Relationship

Robert D. Christensen, M.D.
Professor of Pediatrics, Chief, Division of Neonatology, and Vice Chairman for Research, Department of Pediatrics, University of Florida College of Medicine, Gainesville, Florida
Expected Hematologic Values for Term and Preterm Neonates; Developmental Aspects of Blood Hemostasis and Disorders of Coagulation and Fibrinolysis in the Neonatal Period; Developmental Aspects of Platelets and Disorders of Platelets in the Neonatal Period

D. Wade Clapp, M.D.
Associate Professor, Division of Neonatology, Department of Pediatrics, Indiana University School of Medicine, Indianapolis, Indiana
Bone Marrow Failure Syndromes in the Neonate and Infant

Karen M. Cost, B.S., M.S., Ph.D.
Associate Professor of Pediatrics and Associate Professor of Pathology, University of Louisville, School of Medicine; Chief of Immunology, Norton Healthcare, Louisville, Kentucky
Complement System Development and Disorders During the Neonatal Period

Cynthia S. Edstrom, M.D.
Instructor in Pediatrics, Division of Neonatology, Department of Pediatrics, University of Florida School of Medicine, Gainesville, Florida
Developmental Aspects of Blood Hemostasis and Disorders of Coagulation and Fibrinolysis in the Neonatal Period

Patrick G. Gallagher, M.D.
Assistant Professor, Division of Neonatology, Department of Pediatrics, Yale University School of Medicine; Attending Neonatologist, Yale–New Haven Hospital, New Haven, Connecticut
Disorders of Erythrocyte Metabolism and Shape

Per Hågå, M.D., Ph.D.
Assistant Professor, University of Oslo; Director of Pediatric Cardiology, Department of Pediatrics, Ullevål University Hospital, Oslo, Norway
Evaluation and Treatment of Polycythemia in the Neonate

Erzsebet Jung, M.D.
Attending Neonatologist, St. Louis Children's Hospital, Washington University Medical Center, St. Louis, Missouri
Complement System Development and Disorders During the Neonatal Period

Sandra E. Juul, M.D., Ph.D.
Assistant Professor, Division of Neonatology, Department of Pediatrics, University of Florida College of Medicine, Gainesville, Florida
Nonhematopoietic Actions of the Hematopoietic Growth Factors in the Fetus and Neonate

Joyce M. Koenig, M.D.
Assistant Professor, Division of Neonatology, Department of Pediatrics, University of Florida College of Medicine, Gainesville, Florida
Evaluation and Treatment of Erythroblastosis Fetalis in the Neonate

Herbert A. Lassiter, M.D.
Associate Professor of Pediatrics, University of Louisville School of Medicine; Director, Neonatal Immunology Laboratory, University of Louisville School of Medicine, Louisville, Kentucky
Complement System Development and Disorders During the Neonatal Period

Rolf Lindemann, M.D., Ph.D.
Assistant Professor, Division of Neonatology, Department of Pediatrics, University of Oslo; Director of Neonatology, Department of Pediatrics, Ullevål University Hospital, Oslo, Norway
Evaluation and Treatment of Polycythemia in the Neonate

Robin K. Ohls, M.D.
Associate Professor of Pediatrics, University of New Mexico; Attending Staff, Children's Hospital of New Mexico, Albuquerque, New Mexico
Evaluation and Treatment of Anemia in the Neonate

Paola Papoff, M.D.
Teaching Assistant, Division of Neonatology, Department of Pediatrics, La Sapienza University College of Medicine, Rome, Italy
Use of Hematologic Data to Evaluate Infections in Neonates

Kurt Schibler, M.D.
Associate Professor, Division of Neonatology, Department of Pediatrics, University of Utah School of Medicine, Salt Lake City, Utah
Leukocyte Development and Disorders During the Neonatal Period

William Slayton, M.D.
Instructor, Division of Pediatric Hematology/Oncology, Department of Pediatrics, University of Utah, Salt Lake City, Utah
Development of the Immune System in the Human Fetus

Martha C. Sola, M.D.
Instructor in Pediatrics, Division of Neonatology, Department of Pediatrics, University of Florida College of Medicine, Gainesville, Florida
Fetal Megakaryocytopoiesis; Developmental Aspects of Platelets and Disorders of Platelets in the Neonatal Period

Ronald G. Strauss, M.D.
Professor of Pathology and Pediatrics, University of Iowa College of Medicine; Medical Director, De Gowin Blood Center, University of Iowa Hospitals and Clinics, Iowa City, Iowa
Blood Banking and Transfusion Issues in Perinatal Medicine

Mervin C. Yoder, M.D.
Professor of Pediatrics and of Biochemistry and Molecular Biology, Division of Neonatology, Department of Pediatrics, Indiana University School of Medicine, Indianapolis, Indiana
Embryonic Hematopoiesis

Preface

This book is intended to be a single-source reference for the common and rare hematologic problems of neonates. I emphasize that this is a "neonatology book," not a "hematology book." Certainly, it is *about* hematologic problems, but its perspective is that of a neonatologist concerned with the hematologic abnormalities of the patients under her or his care. Each chapter (with two exceptions) was written by a physician who practices clinical neonatology. Each chapter author was selected because of his or her contributions to that particular field of neonatal hematology. For instance, I know of no neonatologist who has contributed more to developmental aspects of hemoglobin synthesis than has Harry Bard, no neonatologist who has contributed more to the understanding of the complement system than has Hal Lassiter. The same applies to erythrocyte structure for Pat Gallagher, to erythropoietin use in the Neonatal Intensive Care Unit for Robin Ohls, to embryonic hematopoiesis for Merve Yoder, to Fanconi anemia for Wade Clapp, and the list goes on . . . to include all 18 chapter authors.

Only two chapters were *not* written by neonatologists: Development of the Immune System in the Human Fetus was written by Bill Slayton, a pediatric hematologist who I tried repeatedly but unsuccessfully to convince to do a neonatology fellowship. Bill *had* to write this chapter because he understands more about this topic than anyone I know and he discovered much of the information firsthand. Blood Banking and Transfusion Issues in Perinatal Medicine was written by Ron Strauss, a pediatric hematologist and an international leader in perinatal blood banking, whose research, perhaps more than that of any other individual, has advanced the practical aspects of perinatal blood banking.

The older chapter authors were all trained by hematologists who were, in most instances, internists. To some of our neonatology colleagues these mentoring arrangements seemed odd, but they served the unique purpose of instilling in young neonatologists an interest in experimental hematology and an ability to apply methods of hematologic research to neonates who had perplexing hematologic findings. My mentor was Gerald Rothstein, who at the time of our first meeting (I was an undergraduate at the University of Utah), had just finished his hematology fellowship with Maxwell Wintrobe, George Cartwright, and Jack Athens—pioneers in the relatively new field of hematology. After completing medical school and pediatric residency, I returned to the Wintrobe/Cartwright/Athens laboratory (then the Rothstein laboratory) to combine clinical neonatology and experimental hematology training. The other hematologists who served as great mentors for young neonatologists included David Nathan, Frank Oski, Bernie Forget, and Stan Gerson. Indeed, these men were the fathers of modern neonatal hematology, since it is their work and the work of their fellows that constitute much of what has been learned about hematologic problems of the neonate over the past two decades. We dedicate this first edition of *Hematologic Problems of the Neonate* to these hematologists, our mentors.

ROBERT D. CHRISTENSEN, M.D.

NOTICE

Neonatology is an ever-changing field. Standard safety precautions must be followed, but as new research and clinical experience broaden our knowledge, changes in treatment and drug therapy become necessary or appropriate. Readers are advised to check the product information currently provided by the manufacturer of each drug to be administered to verify the recommended dose, the method and duration of administration, and the contraindications. It is the responsibility of the treating physician, relying on experience and knowledge of the patient, to determine dosages and the best treatment for the patient. Neither the publisher nor the editor assumes any responsibility for any injury and/or damage to persons or property.

THE PUBLISHER

Contents

SECTION 1

Hematopoiesis and Hematopoietic Growth Factors

CHAPTER 1

Embryonic Hematopoiesis

Mervin C. Yoder, M.D.

Hematopoiesis refers to the continuous production of circulating blood cells. From early in embryonic life to our final days on earth, newly formed cells enter the circulation while injured, senescent, and tissue-recruited cells are withdrawn. Nearly 200 billion red blood cells, 10 billion white blood cells, and 400 billion platelets are produced daily throughout a normal lifetime. In addition to the requirement for high cell production, the concentration of individual blood cell lineages is precisely regulated in the peripheral blood and tissues. The production and use of circulating blood cells increase during periods of altered homeostasis such as defense against infection or replenishment of circulating red cells after hemorrhage. When the tightly regulated production of blood cells fails, the host may encounter life-threatening anemia or other cytopenias or suffer from excessive neoplastic growth of blood cells manifesting as leukemia.

Blood cell production also is developmentally regulated and tissue specific. Blood cells are produced in several different tissues during human development, with each tissue having a characteristic pattern of the mature blood cell lineages formed. This important relationship between nonhematopoietic tissue stromal elements and hematopoietic cells in regulating tissue-specific cell proliferation and differentiation is most evident during the embryonic period.

This chapter briefly reviews the cellular model of hematopoiesis and describes the onset of hematopoiesis in the human embryo. Although the focus of this chapter is on *human* embryonic hematopoiesis, certain concepts gleaned from *murine* studies are presented to illustrate some basic hematopoietic principles.

OVERVIEW OF HEMATOPOIESIS

Early Blood Cell Investigations

Erythrocytes were the first blood cells identified with the aid of the microscope in the late 1600s, but the colorless white blood cells remained obscured from observation for many years.[1] In 1877, Paul Ehrlich, while a medical student, devised a triacid stain that permitted identification of hematopoietic precursor cells and specific white blood cell lineages based on size, nuclear shape, and cytoplasmic constituents.[1] With further improvements in microscopes and the use of the triacid stain, a new era in hematology was born in which changes in blood cell number or function were correlated with specific human diseases. Further progress in studying hematopoiesis was largely limited to conjecture and opinion derived from morphologic studies of blood cell–containing tissues until the middle of the 20th century, when hematologists began to examine the hematopoietic consequences of animal exposure to ionizing radiation.[1]

Methods of Identifying Hematopoietic Stem Cells and Progenitor Cells

Whole-body irradiation of animals was observed to depress hematopoiesis and cause life-threatening pancytopenia (i.e., all blood lineages diminished in number).[2] Mice were protected from radiation-induced hematopoietic impairment if their spleens were shielded from the radiation beam or if hematopoietic cells from another mouse were infused into the irradiated host.[3] Confirmation that hematopoietic cells, not plasma, conferred radiation protection was reported by Ford and colleagues[4] in 1956. In 1961, Till and McCulloch[5] provided evidence that single, multipotent hematopoietic precursors (i.e., cells giving rise to more than one lineage of blood cells) could be identified in vivo by injecting the donor marrow cells into the spleen of a lethally irradiated recipient animal and examining the recipient spleen for hematopoietic colonies 8 to 12 days later (Fig. 1–1). Each colony of hematopoietic cells in the spleen arose from a single precursor cell, the colony-forming unit in the spleen cell (CFU-S).[6] Although this method advanced the study of hematopoietic stem cell biology, little was known in the early 1960s of the mechanisms that caused or permitted stem cells to differentiate into mature cells.

In the mid-1960s, Pluznik and Sachs[7] and Bradley and Metcalf[8] reported that murine hematopoietic cells could be cultured in vitro and that addition of soluble fluid from several murine organs (e.g., urine or pregnant uterine extract) resulted in formation of myeloid colonies in vitro. This biologically active tissue fluid was called colony-stimulating activity (CSA). Each myeloid colony was derived from a single precursor cell, called a colony-forming unit in culture (CFU-C). Further work revealed that colonies were composed of granulocytes, macrophages, or both (CFU-GM) (Fig. 1–2) and that the type of colony formed was related to the type of CSA added. Later, using anemic mouse serum as a source of red blood cell CSA, Axelrad and coworkers[9] demonstrated that red blood cell colonies were clonally derived in vitro, and they called the most primitive red cell precursors the erythroid burst-forming unit (BFU-E) and the most committed erythroid precursors colony-forming unit–erythroid cells (CFU-E) (see Fig. 1–2). Multipotent progenitor cells were also identified and called colony-forming unit–mix. These assays, developed for studying murine hematopoiesis, were rapidly adapted for human studies and continue to be sensitive assays for detecting human hematopoietic progenitor cells.[10]

Because the frequency of human and murine hematopoietic stem cells is estimated to be 1 of 10^4 to 10^5 marrow cells,[11–14] the primary obstacle in studying human hematopoietic stem cell biology is that few methods can identify these rare cells. Great progress in the study of the human hematopoietic stem cell resulted from the study of murine hematopoietic stem cells. Murine bone marrow transplantation experiments provided the evidence to reliably identify hematopoietic stem cells. Hematopoietic stem cells are defined as cells that self-renew in vivo and that proliferate and differentiate into all lineages of circulating peripheral blood cells for more than 4 months after transplantation into recipient animals.[15] Because of ethical constraints, similar in vivo reconstitution assays are not possible in human patients, and several alternative in vitro

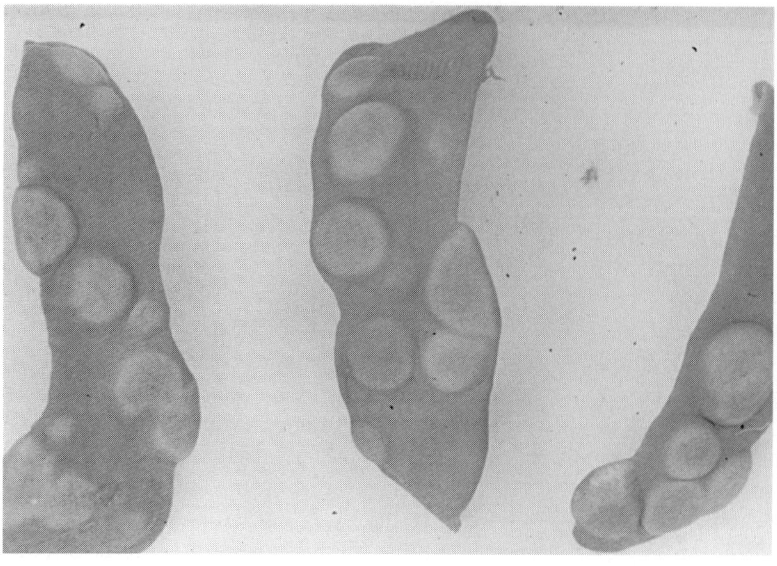

Figure 1–1. Colony-forming unit–spleen (CFU-S) assay. Transplantation of murine hematopoietic cells into lethally irradiated recipient mice results in the formation of donor hematopoietic colonies in the spleen of the recipients in 8 to 12 days. Each colony of hematopoiesis is the direct progeny of a single donor CFU-S progenitor cell. (From Hoffman R, Benz EJ, Shattil SJ, et al [eds]: Hematology: Basic Principles and Practice, 2nd ed. New York: Churchill Livingstone, 1995, p 181.)

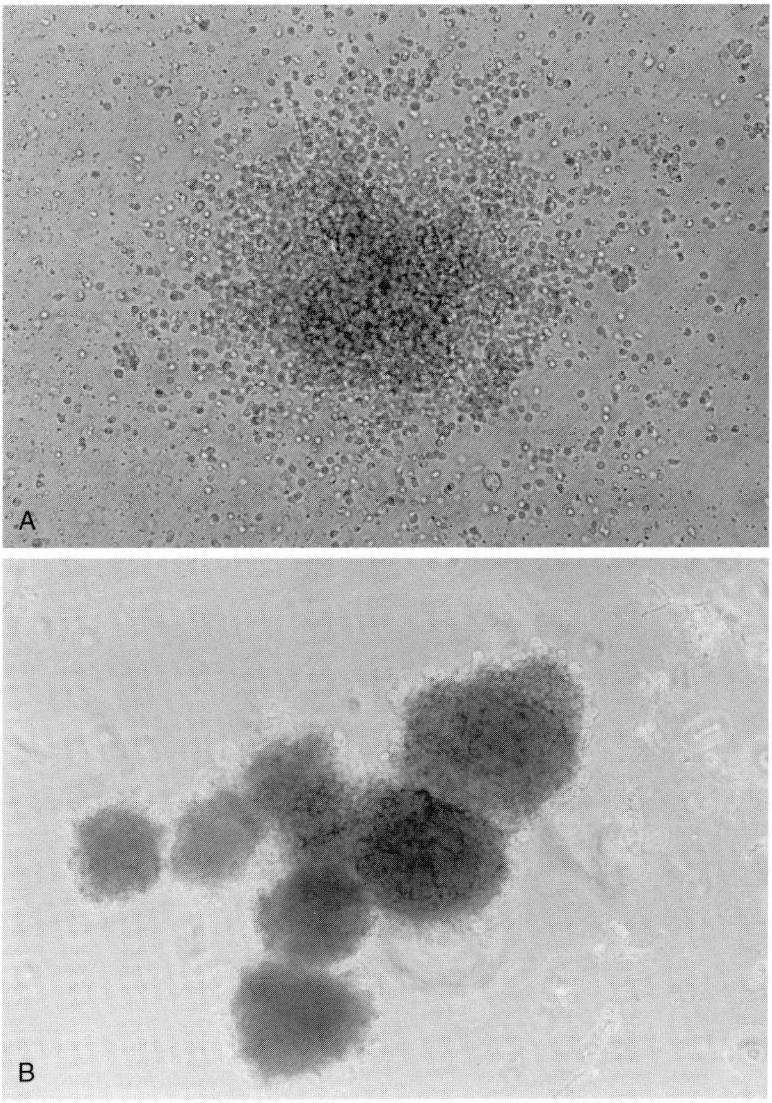

Figure 1–2. Hematopoietic colonies formed by colony-forming unit–granulocyte-macrophage (CFU-GM) and burst-forming unit–erythroid (BFU-E) progenitor cells. *A*, CFU-GM culture with hematopoietic growth factors results in formation of a colony of cells composed of macrophages and neutrophils, which migrate into the culture medium and give the colonies a dispersed appearance. *B*, BFU-E cells give rise to compact colonies with multiple foci that appear red (red blood cell hemoglobin) on microscopic examination. (From Hoffman R, Benz EJ, Shattil SJ, et al [eds]: Hematology: Basic Principles and Practice, 2nd ed. New York: Churchill Livingstone, 1995, p 182.)

and in vivo estimates of hematopoietic precursors have been developed.

Lineage-committed hematopoietic progenitor cells form colonies in vitro in response to one or two recombinant growth factors. In contrast, more primitive multipotent hematopoietic cells form in vitro colonies only when cultured with multiple recombinant growth factors. These results have been interpreted as evidence that the more primitive hematopoietic stem and progenitor cells require complex growth factor combinations to fuel or support lineage commitment and progenitor cell differentiation. Plating hematopoietic stem cells in special double-layer agar cultures with multiple recombinant cytokines permits identification of hematopoietic progenitors that are highly proliferative (i.e., high proliferative potential–colony-forming cells [HPP-CFC]), producing colonies containing more than 50,000 cells that are visible without magnification (most CFU-Cs are less than 50,000 and microscopic). HPP-CFCs are considered to be a more primitive cell than the multipotent hematopoietic progenitors (Fig. 1–3).

Complex in vitro cultures of hematopoietic stem cells with a monolayer of bone marrow or fetal liver nonhematopoietic tissue stromal cells (includes macrophages, endothelial cells, fibroblasts, and preadipocytes) result in sustained hematopoiesis for several months.[16] The most primitive hematopoietic cells (i.e., those giving

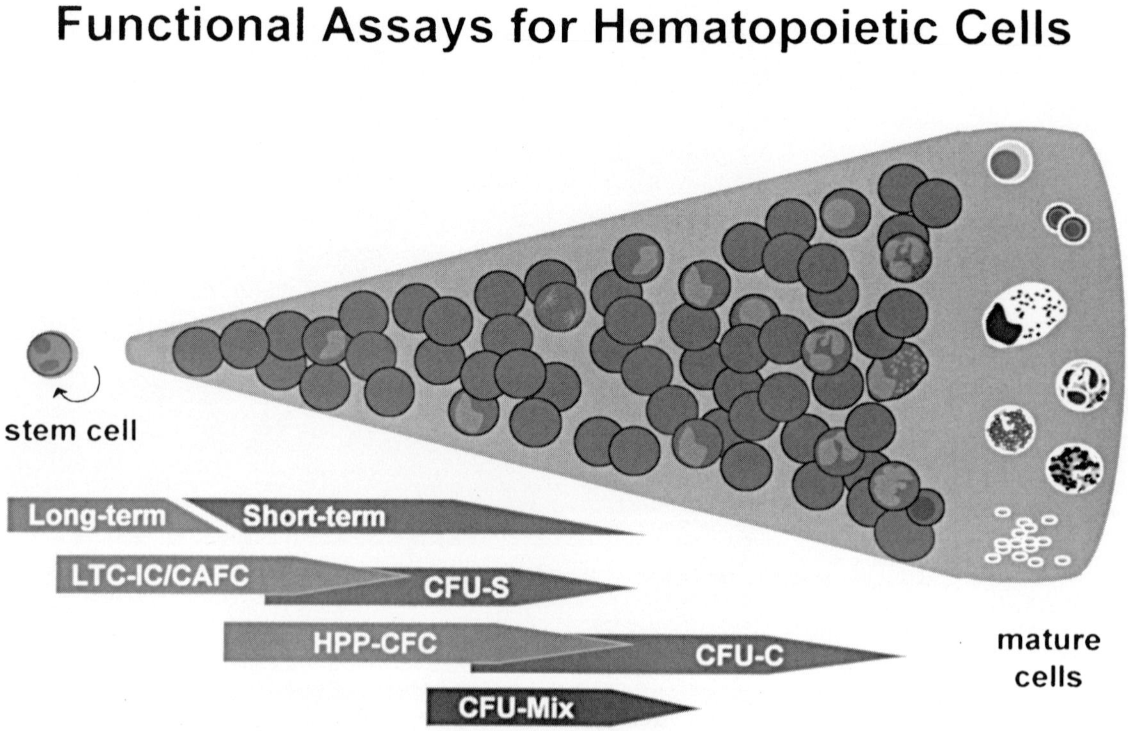

Figure 1–3. Hierarchy of hematopoietic stem and progenitor cell compartments as functionally assayed by in vitro assays. The hematopoietic stem cell self-renews *(arrow)* or commits to differentiation into primitive progenitor cells detectable as long-term culture–initiating cells (LTC-IC) or cobblestone area–forming cells (CAFC). As the progenitors differentiate, long-term repopulating ability is lost. High proliferative potential–colony-forming cells (HPP-CFC) and colony-forming unit–spleen (CFU-S) cells are multipotential progenitor cells that can provide short-term but not life-sparing hematopoietic recovery when transplanted into irradiated mice. Colony-forming unit–mix (CFU-Mix) cells are multipotential cells giving rise to erythroid, myeloid, and megakaryocytic cells within the same colony in vitro. The colony-forming unit–culture (CFU-C) cells are committed to produce single-lineage blood cells on in vitro culture.

rise to hematopoietic progenitors) reside beneath the stromal monolayers (cobblestone area–forming cells), whereas the mature blood cells produced are released into the tissue culture medium as nonadherent cells.[17] Using limiting dilution analysis, the number of such murine or human long-term culture–initiating cells (LTC-IC) that give rise to multipotent and committed progenitors for 3 to 4 weeks in vitro can be calculated.[18–20] LTC-ICs are considered to be the most primitive hematopoietic precursor detectable by means of in vitro assays (see Fig. 1–3).

In attempts to develop an in vivo system for detection of human hematopoietic stem cells, several groups developed xenotransplantation models. Enriched populations of human hematopoietic stem cells from human bone marrow, cord blood, or fetal liver have been observed to engraft in the preimmune sheep fetus (<60 days of gestation) with long-term evidence of multilineage peripheral human blood cell chimerism in the transplanted animals.[21–23] Nonobese diabetic (NOD) mice bred with severe combined immunodeficient (SCID) mice produce NOD/SCID mice that accept human hematopoietic grafts.[24] This NOD/SCID model permits calculation of the frequency of human repopulating cells in a donor sample,[25] but it remains unclear whether this assay is robust and can accurately identify the same hematopoietic stem cells that repopulate the blood system of transplanted human patients.

Stem Cell Model of Hematopoiesis

The stem cell theory of hematopoiesis posits that the hematopoietic system comprises a continuum of functionally distinct hematopoietic cell compartments. Stem cells are rare, self-renewing, relatively quiescent cells (see Fig. 1–3). In the mouse, hematopoietic stem cells have a half-life (i.e., time to 50% of stem cells cycled) of approximately 19 days.[26] Stem cells can divide to give rise to a daughter cell that retains all of the pluripotentiality of the parent (i.e., self-renewal) or can proliferate into daughter cells that have lost some multipotentiality and have become committed to producing progenitor cells.[27] After the commitment decision is made, the progenitor cell gives rise to progressively more lineage-committed hematopoietic progenitor cells and eventually to mature blood cells (see Fig. 1–3). It remains unclear whether the commitment process in hematopoietic stem cells occurs by chance (i.e., stochastic model) or is induced by tissue-specific growth factors, cytokines, metabolic products, oxygen levels, extracellular matrix molecules, or cell-cell interactions (i.e., inductive model).[28–31]

With the development of flow cytometry, monoclonal antibodies to cell-surface antigens, and in vivo and in vitro assays for primitive hematopoietic cells, investigators succeeded in identifying enriched populations of human hematopoietic stem cells and provided evidence that a single murine hematopoietic stem cell is sufficient to restore multilineage hematopoiesis in an irradiated host.[32] Purification of hematopoietic stem cells permitted investigators to pursue basic investigations of stem cell biology that translated into new methods for human hematopoietic transplantations and improved methods of somatic gene transfer.[33] Further studies to examine hematopoietic stem cell function in patients with bone marrow failure syndromes and hematologic malignancies will also probably translate into clinical therapies.

A significant challenge to the in vitro study of hematopoietic stem cells is the realization that many of the growth factors required to stimulate the in vitro proliferation and differentiation of hematopoietic progenitor cells are associated with measurable declines in the concentrations of functional hematopoietic stem cells. Although certain stromal cell lines and primary human or murine stromal cells can maintain hematopoietic stem cell function in vitro, only recently have tissue culture conditions been developed that permit expansion of murine hematopoietic cell numbers with retention of individual hematopoietic stem cell self-renewal and reconstituting ability.[34–36] The conditions to support in vitro expansion of adult human and murine bone marrow hematopoietic progenitor cells indicate that the proliferative potential and growth factor requirements for survival in vitro differ among hematopoietic cells during ontogeny.[35, 37–39]

EMBRYONIC HEMATOPOIESIS

Studies of Murine Embryonic Hematopoiesis

The murine visceral yolk sac is composed of visceral endoderm and mesoderm cells that proliferate, differentiate, migrate, and co-localize during gastrulation.[40, 41] The endoderm cells face the yolk sac cavity and are highly active in the absorption of material from the maternal circulation and in the biosynthesis and secretion of numerous nutrients.[42] In the mouse, yolk sac endoderm cells are also the primary route for transporting maternal immunoglobulins into the embryo. The mesoderm cells of the yolk sac give rise to blood islands containing blood cells and endothelial cells.[43–45] The simultaneous appearance of endothelial and hematopoietic cells in the blood islands, the apparent intimate cell-to-cell contact of the blood island endothelial and hematopoietic cells, and the shared requirements for certain growth factors and growth factor receptors support the idea that blood island endothelial cells and hematopoietic cells must be derived from a common precursor, called the hemangioblast.[45–48] Study of the hemangioblast remains elusive, although some reports have suggested that isolating the cell is feasible.[46, 47]

The precise temporal and spatial origins of the first hematopoietic stem cells in the murine embryo remain unknown. Studies using chicks and frogs indicate that the mesoderm cells that become committed to the formation of blood cells migrate from the posterior primitive streak and into the embryo and the extraembryonic yolk sac.[49] The mesoderm cells contributing to the formation of murine blood cells are also restricted to the posterior primitive streak at 6.75 days postconception (DPC). Some mesoderm cells fated to become blood cells migrate along the extraembryonic endoderm cells and participate in forming the extraembryonic yolk sac blood islands.[49] Presumably, certain mesoderm cells are acted on by local factors to undergo differentiation into endothelial and hematopoietic stem and progenitor cells. Although little is known about the factors that induce murine mesodermal cell commitment to blood and endothelial differentiation, some evidence suggests that certain transcription factors and growth factor receptors are required for this process.[31, 41, 50]

Because blood cells arise from different sites at different times during murine embryogenesis, the site of origin of hematopoietic stem cells remains a vital question in experimental hematology. Hematopoietic stem cells may arise de novo in each hematopoietic site during ontogeny.[51] Alternatively, all hematopoietic stem cells may arise in the embryonic yolk sac and migrate to all other sites during development.[52, 53] Several groups of investigators[54–56] have identified hematopoietic stem cell activity in the mouse that appears to originate from the ventral wall of the embryonic paired dorsal aorta and from the extravascular mesenchyme of the para-aortic splanchnopleura (PS). When murine hematopoietic cells from these sites are transplanted into lethally irradiated adult recipient mice, donor cell engraftment can be identified in tissue removed from murine embryos at 10 DPC. In contrast, engraftment of yolk sac hematopoietic cells in the adult recipients did not occur until 11 DPC, when hematopoietic stem cell activity was already present in the developing fetal liver, a site known to contain hematopoietic stem cells that engraft in the adult marrow. These results suggested that the first hematopoietic stem cells with the capacity to engraft in the adult marrow compartment are derived from the PS region within the embryo, not in the yolk sac.[55, 56] Investigators proposed that, although primitive hematopoietic progenitors may first appear in the yolk sac, no definitive reconstituting hematopoietic stem cell activity occurred at this site; rather, the PS at 10 DPC was the site of origin of hematopoietic stem cells that migrate to the fetal liver and establish hematopoiesis in that organ.[57]

Several groups have reported that yolk sac cells can engraft in fetal mice.[58, 59] We reexamined the repopulating ability of embryonic hematopoietic cells using myeloablated newborn mice as recipients. We used newborn mice as recipients because their livers, spleens, and bone marrow are hematopoietically active at birth, whereas adult mice generally produce blood cells only in the spleen and bone marrow.[60] We speculated that yolk sac and PS cells isolated at or before 10 DPC would engraft in the myeloablated newborn mice because the liver retained the ability to support hematopoietic cell growth and differentiation. When 9- or 10-DPC yolk sac cell suspensions were transplanted into conditioned newborn mice, long-term reconstitution in all lymphomyeloid blood cell lineages was evident.[61, 62] When fluorescence-activated cell sorted (FACS), highly enriched hematopoietic cells from the 9-DPC yolk sac and PS were transplanted into myeloablated newborn recipients, both cell populations had equivalent long-term (>6 months), multilineage repopulating ability.[63] Although these sites were equivalent in hematopoietic stem cell function, nearly 40-fold more FACS-enriched hematopoietic cells were isolated from the DPC yolk sac than the 9-DPC PS.[63] The observation that donor hematopoietic stem cells contributing to long-term hematopoiesis in recipients are concomitantly present in the yolk sac and PS calls for a reassessment of the role of yolk sac hematopoietic stem cells in the colonization of the liver during murine development. Additional studies are needed to determine the site of origin of hematopoietic stem cells in the murine embryo.

Because 9-DPC yolk sac and PS cells engraft in newborn recipients, functional changes must occur in hematopoietic cells in the PS at 10 DPC and in the yolk sac at 11 DPC that permit these cells to directly engraft in adult recipient mice. This gain of function may result from de novo expression and activation of expressed cell-surface molecules on the embryonic hematopoietic stem cells that interact with molecules on the luminal surface of bone marrow endothelial cells to permit engraftment. The mechanisms of yolk sac and PS hematopoietic stem cell mobilization into the circulation and engraftment in the fetal liver and other hematopoietic organs during fetal life remain unknown.

Differentiated blood cells are first recognizable in the murine yolk sac at 7 DPC. The primary cells observed are nucleated red blood cells expressing embryonic forms of hemoglobin.[64] Hematopoiesis peaks in the murine yolk sac at 11 DPC, and the liver becomes the predominant site of hematopoiesis at 12 DPC. The murine fetal liver remains the primary site of hematopoiesis until the time of birth, when the bone marrow and to some extent the spleen provide lifelong provision of circulating blood cells (Fig. 1–4). Although red blood cell production predominates in the liver and spleen, white blood cell production predominates in the bone marrow compartment.[64]

The pattern of hematopoietic cell differentiation also varies greatly in the yolk sac and PS. Only primitive red blood cells and macrophages are produced in the yolk sac. The red blood cells are called primitive because they are large, nucleated cells that contain hemoglobins expressed only during the embryonic phase of development. When cultured in vitro, hematopoietic progenitors of the yolk sac give rise to BFU-E (expressing primitive and adult-type hemoglobins) and CFU-GM (predominantly macrophages) that vary with the age of the donor embryo.[65] Identification of the primitive red blood cell progenitor in vitro diminishes after 9 to 10 DPC. Culture of hematopoietic progenitors from the PS gives rise to BFU-E and CFU-GM that are composed of cells with definitive features; red blood cells are enucleated and synthesize adult-type hemoglobins, and granulocytes predominate over macrophages in the CFU-GM. The mechanisms accounting for the highly restricted differentiation of hematopoietic cells in the yolk sac compared with the more definitive differentiation program of the PS cells remain unknown.[64]

Studies of Human Embryonic Hematopoiesis

The inability to use transplantation methods for identification of hematopoietic stem cells in human patients has limited the analysis of stem cell function during human embryonic hematopoiesis. However, much of the ontogeny of blood cell production in the human embryo has been described using morphologic approaches and some in vitro hematopoietic progenitor cell assays. This section reviews the formation and function of the human yolk sac, determination of the site and kinetics of blood cell appearance, and determination of the number and behavior of cultured human embryonic hematopoietic progenitor cells.

The human yolk sac develops in three stages: a formative period, a period of yolk sac function, and a period of yolk sac regression.[66] The first phase of yolk sac formation can be further subdivided into formation of the primary and secondary yolk sacs. The primary yolk sac is formed after implantation (7 to 8 DPC) by proliferation and differentiation of primitive endoderm cells into visceral endoderm adjacent to the developing embryonic disk and parietal endoderm projecting into the uterine lumen. This simple bilaminar structure has no identifiable

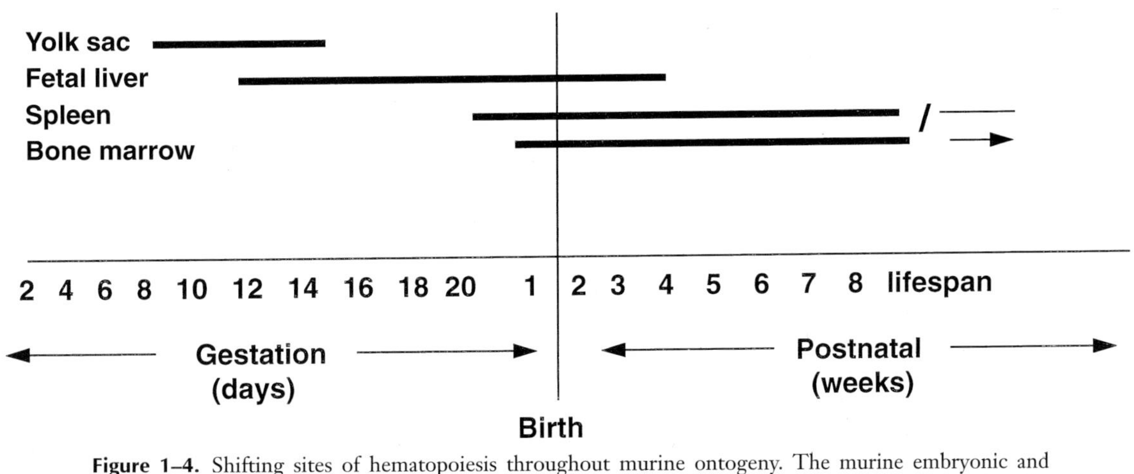

Figure 1–4. Shifting sites of hematopoiesis throughout murine ontogeny. The murine embryonic and fetal stages of hematopoiesis are transient. Blood cells are first produced in the murine yolk sac, but the liver becomes the predominant hematopoietic organ at day 12 of gestation. The spleen and bone marrow become hematopoietically active several days before birth and become the predominant sites of blood cell production for the life of the adult mouse. The liver of the newborn mouse continues as a hematopoietic organ until 2 to 3 weeks postnatally.

function, but the endoderm cells lining the primary yolk sac give rise to mesodermal precursors (i.e., intermediate cells) that colonize the space between the yolk sac cavity and the surrounding trophoblast cells (Fig. 1–5). The primary yolk sac then appears to collapse, with heterogenous foci of reexpansion breaking up the primary yolk sac into smaller vesicles (see Fig. 1–5). The secondary yolk sac is formed (12 to 15 DPC) from the remnants of the primary yolk sac (i.e., parietal endoderm and mesoderm) that are contiguous with the visceral endoderm underlying the embryonic disk (see Fig. 1–5).

The secondary yolk sac is an active site of protein biosynthesis, nutrient transport, and hematopoiesis. A variety of proteins are synthesized, including albumin, α-fetoprotein, prealbumin, apolipoproteins, insulin-like growth factor, transferrin, vascular endothelial growth factor, and colony-stimulating factor 1 (i.e., macrophage colony-stimulating factor).[66–69] The endodermal component of the primate secondary yolk sac is a transporter of proteins and vitamins.[70–72] Another primary function of the secondary yolk sac is to produce hematopoietic cells. The first primitive red blood cells in the yolk sac adhere to surrounding endothelial cells, and these hematopoietic-endothelial masses are called blood islands. Commensurate with blood island formation, the mesenchymal layer in the

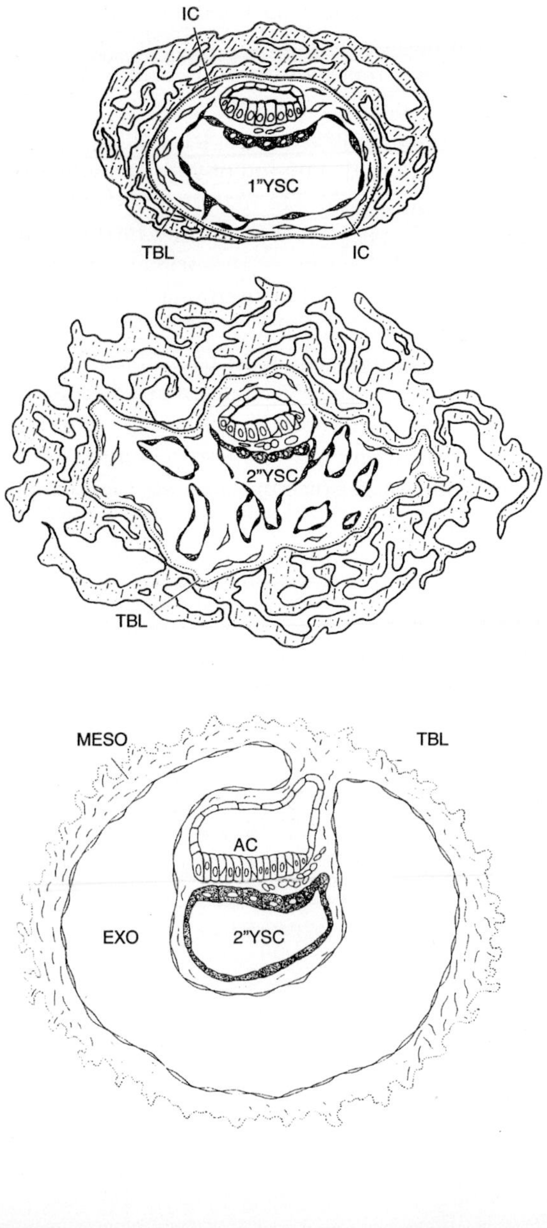

Figure 1–5. Stages of human yolk sac formation. *Top,* The primary yolk sac is formed 7 to 8 days after conception. Intermediate cells (IC, *white cells*) migrate from the endodermal layer *(dark cells)* of the primary yolk sac to fill in the space between the endoderm and trophoblastic basal lamina (TBL). *Middle,* The secondary yolk sac is formed by the remnants of the primary yolk sac that remain after the primary yolk sac has collapsed and fragmented into smaller vesicles. *Bottom,* By 12 days after conception, the secondary yolk sac has expanded to the edge of the embryonic disk, is lined by endoderm cells *(dark cells),* and protrudes into the exocelom (EXO), which surrounds the amniotic cavity (AC) of the embryonic disk. The mesoderm lying next to the TBL has differentiated into mesothelium (MESO). Hematopoietic activity occurs in yolk sac blood islands arising in the secondary yolk sac by week 3 of gestation. (From Nogales FF [ed]: The Human Yolk Sac and Yolk Sac Tumors. Berlin: Springer-Verlag, 1993, pp 35, 36. Copyright © 1993 Springer-Verlag.)

secondary yolk sac thickens, but the endoderm layer is not affected.

Macroscopically, the secondary yolk sac begins as a small structure (<0.4 mm) but steadily increases in size to 2 mm by day 19, 4 to 5 mm by 7 weeks, and 6 to 6.5 mm by the end of week 10. As the yolk sac matures, an extensive network of superficial capillaries is formed as the blood island endothelial cells migrate toward one another and form vascular channels. The secondary yolk sac circulation is fed and drained by the vitelline arteries and veins, which connect the embryonic to the extraembryonic circulation. Initially, the vitelline vessels empty into the sinus venosus of the liver, establishing a preportal-type circulation. Later in gestation, as the yolk sac regresses, new capillaries arising from the developing gut contribute to the vitelline circulation, and as the liver cords proliferate, the portal circulation is established.[73] Although evident until week 12 of development, the yolk sac begins regressing around week 10, with progressive evidence of tissue degeneration and with loss of blood flow through the yolk sac vascular network.[66]

Many 20th century investigators using microscopic analysis of tissue sections of human embryonic tissues described the sequence of hematopoietic development that occurs in the human embryo and fetus.[74–78] During human development in utero, blood cells first arise in the yolk sac between days 16 and 19, followed sequentially by fetal liver hematopoiesis by weeks 5 to 6 and engraftment and expansion of hematopoietic cells in developing long bones by weeks 8 to 19 (e.g., most bones become hematopoietic between weeks 11 and 12).[79, 80] The liver functions as the primary site of hematopoiesis from weeks 6 through 22 of gestation until the bone marrow becomes the lifelong predominant site of blood cell production. Distinct patterns of blood cell differentiation and proliferation occur in each specific site of hematopoiesis during ontogeny.[81–83]

The most extensive morphologic analysis of hematopoiesis in the developing human was reported in a 1979 monograph by Kelemen and colleagues.[79] These investigators studied tissue sections from 190 human embryos and fetuses between 3 and 28 weeks of gestation. These specimens were collected from 1971 through 1978 after surgical termination of pregnancies in normal, healthy women. Cells and tissues were stained using standard techniques, and a record of the cells identified was performed using a Zeiss photomicroscope.

Hematopoietic cells were first observed in the human embryo at day 18 in the mesenchymal layer of the secondary yolk sac. Most blood islands were composed of hematopoietic cells completely surrounded by endothelial cells, but some extravascular free aggregates of blood cells were present in the mesenchyme close to the visceral endoderm. The 3- to 4-week embryo had more defined vessels, many which were empty of hematopoietic cells. Frequently, small clusters of undifferentiated cells called hemocytoblasts (equivalent to the hemangioblast in the mouse) associated with the endothelium protruded into the vessel lumen. Concomitantly, clusters of primitive erythroblasts (≥20-μm cells with central to eccentric nucleus and orthochromatic cytoplasmic staining) began to fill capillaries and larger vessels (e.g., vitelline, umbilical, chorionic, and amniotic). Wherever the number of primitive erythroblasts predominated in vessels, few hemocytoblasts were detectable. This was a surprising finding, because the erythroblasts had previously been thought to originate from the hemocytoblasts.[51] At the sixth week of development, intraembryonic and extraembryonic blood vessels became macroscopically visible, and definitive erythroblasts (<20-μm cells with condensed nuclei and abundant hemoglobin cytoplasmic staining) and primitive erythroblasts could be identified in the yolk sac vessels. The only other mature blood cell in the yolk sac was the macrophage. In contrast to normal fetal liver and bone marrow patterns of differentiation, macrophages in the yolk sac arose without evidence of a monocytic precursor. An overall decline in hematopoiesis was observed in the human yolk sac after the eighth week of gestation.

Hematopoiesis occurred in the liver by the fifth to sixth week of gestation. The establishment of the systemic circulation (weeks 4 to 5) had just commenced before liver hematopoiesis at week 5. The predominant blood cell observed in the large vessels and in developing liver sinusoids was the primitive erythroblast. In the next 4 weeks, there was a shift away from the primitive to the definitive erythroblast and mature enucleated red blood cell production in the fetal liver (Fig. 1–6). During this period, there was also a 40-fold increase in the total liver mass,

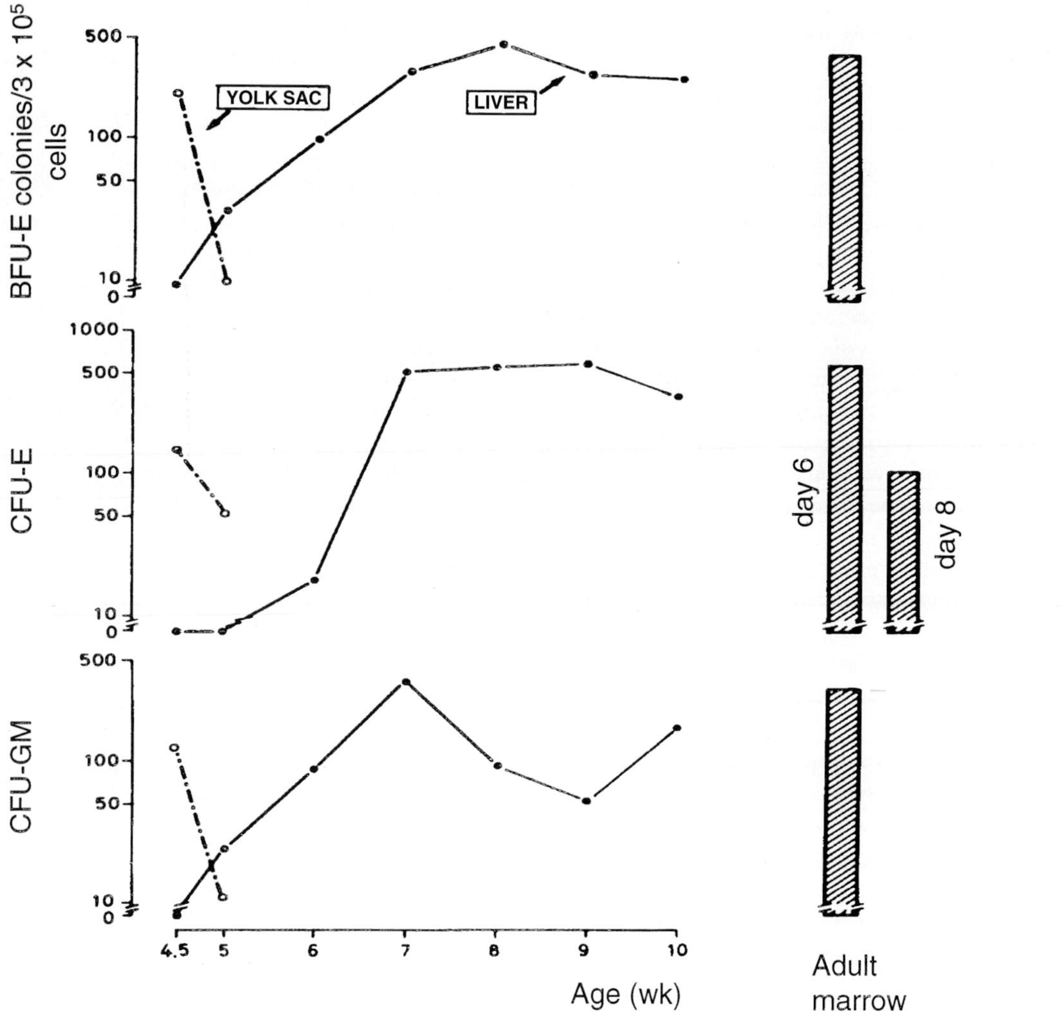

Figure 1–6. Concentration of hematopoietic progenitor cells in the yolk sac and liver of human embryos (4.5- to 10-week gestation samples) compared with adult bone marrow progenitor cell concentrations. A rapid increase in burst-forming unit–erythroid (BFU-E) and colony-forming unit–granulocyte-macrophage (CFU-GM) progenitor cells becomes evident in the liver between 5 and 6 weeks' gestation as the number of these progenitor cells in the yolk sac falls. The onset of CFU-E production lags behind the increasing BFU-E concentration in the liver, consistent with the derivation of CFU-E as more mature progeny of BFU-E. Near-adult concentrations of progenitor cells are achieved by 10 weeks of gestation. (From Migliaccio G, Migliaccio A, Petti S, et al: Human embryonic hematopoiesis: kinetics of progenitors and precursors underlying the yolk sac–liver transition. J Clin Invest 1986;78:53; reproduced from the Journal of Clinical Investigation by copyright permission of the American Society for Clinical Investigation.)

with hematopoietic cells comprising 60% of the total cell number (weeks 11 to 12). Macrophages, megakaryocytes, granulocytes, and lymphocytes also were identifiable during weeks 5 through 22. Macrophages were the predominant mature blood cell type identified early in liver hematopoiesis (weeks 5 to 6), but the concentration of macrophages diminished thereafter. Megakaryocytes were present throughout the liver phase of hematopoiesis, but a notable shift from megakaryocytes with one to two nuclei to megakaryocytes with four or more nuclei occurred as liver hematopoiesis diminished (weeks 18 to 21) and bone marrow hematopoiesis began to flourish. The few granulocytes were restricted to the connective tissue of the hepatic portal area from weeks 5 through 15. A significant increase in granulocytes was observed beyond week 21 of development, coinciding with enhanced hematopoiesis in the bone marrow.

Lymphocytes were sparse until week 7 of development, and even through week 13, they remained a minor population (1% of blood cells) in the liver. It was not evident whether these lymphocytes were of the B or T cell lineage, but the thymus did not have lymphocytes until week 9. The percentage of hemocytoblasts (presumed stem cells) was high (10% of blood cells) in the 5- to 6-week embryo liver but declined for the remainder of the liver phase of hematopoiesis.

The earliest bone marrow sample in which hematopoietic cells were present was taken from an embryo at week 8 of development. The predominant cell type at 8 to 9 weeks was the primitive erythroblast. Definitive erythroblast production increased greatly from weeks 11 through 14, and by 14 weeks, nearly all erythroblasts were definitive types. It was speculated that primitive erythroblasts were presented to the marrow by means of the systemic circulation and that only definitive erythroblasts were produced in the marrow. Erythrocytic cells constituted about 35% of total marrow cells by week 12 and 20% to 30% thereafter. At weeks 8 to 9 of embryonic development, granulocytes were observed in the marrow of long bones. Neutrophilic granulocytes composed 30% to 40% of total marrow cells between weeks 10 and 13. By 21 weeks, neutrophilic granulocytes were the major blood cell produced, and nearly 60% of hematopoietic cells in the marrow were proliferating or mature neutrophilic granulocytes. Eosinophilic granulocytes (1%) were present in the marrow of embryos at week 10 and gradually increased to nearly 5% of total marrow cells by week 21. Basophilic granulocytes were few in the 10-week embryo and remained low (0.3%) even in the 28-week embryo. Macrophages were most numerous in the embryonic marrow at weeks 10 through 16, whereas monocytes peaked between weeks 12 and 16. Lymphocytes increased from 12% of total marrow cells at week 12 to 20% to 30% in older embryos. Megakaryocytes were present in all samples examined. The percentage of immature "blast cells," which probably represented hematopoietic stem and progenitor cells, varied from 15% at weeks 12 through 13 to 1% to 4% at weeks 21 through 23. Whereas erythropoiesis exceeded granulopoiesis in the 10- to 11-week-old embryo (erythropoiesis/granulopoiesis ratio of 0.8), granulopoiesis predominated by week 12 and reached a nearly adult ratio of 3 (1.8 to 3.3) by the 21st week of human development.

Splenic hematopoiesis in the human embryo has been difficult to prove. At 8 weeks of gestation, the spleen is composed primarily of a meshwork of mesenchymal cells with some primitive erythroblasts contained in the blood vessels.[79] Few macrophage and neutrophil precursors were present in the spleen at 8 weeks. The hematopoietic cells in the spleen were dispersed throughout, but most erythroblasts were confined to the vascular system. This distribution of hematopoietic cells in the spleen contrasted with the same-stage embryo liver in which the developing blood cells were confined to focal sites of hematopoiesis. Similar observations were made by other investigators,[84–86] and these results raised the question of whether the hematopoietic cells observed in the embryonic spleen were circulating blood cells or were cells produced in the spleen.[84]

Calhoun and coworkers[87] used several methods to determine whether the human mid-gestation spleen (13 to 22 weeks' gestation) was an active site of hematopoiesis. Liver, spleen, and bone marrow samples were examined by histology, and cell suspensions from each site were prepared for enumeration of mature blood cells and their immediate precursors. Lymphocytes, macrophages, and erythroid cells predominated at 13 weeks' gestation. Neither mature nor immature neutrophils were identified in the spleen until 16 weeks' gestation. Throughout the study period, active foci of hematopoiesis were present in the liver and bone marrow but never in the spleen. Because the distribution of blood cells observed for the splenic suspensions was similar to the blood cell concentrations previously reported after fetal blood sampling,[88] these results in total suggest that the mid-gestation human spleen is not normally an active hematopoietic organ.[87]

Numerous investigators extended these morphologic observations by examining the onset of human hematopoiesis by means of functional assays of hematopoietic CFU-C formation and by using cell-surface antigen detection to identify specific hematopoietic lineages (i.e., monoclonal antibodies with immunohistochemical or FACS analysis). Although many studies have focused on human fetal liver and marrow hematopoiesis, little is known about the biology of hematopoietic stem and progenitor cells that arise in the human yolk sac. The data reviewed indicate that the transient population of yolk sac hematopoietic cells differs in many aspects from hematopoietic cells produced within the embryo proper or in the liver or bone marrow.

Migliaccio and colleagues[89] performed a careful examination of the kinetics of yolk sac CFU-C in human embryos from 4.5 to 10 weeks' gestation. This stage encompassed the period of yolk sac hematopoietic decline and initiation of liver hematopoiesis. CFU-E and BFU-E were abundant in the yolk sac of the 4.5-week embryos (see Fig. 1–6). CFU-GMs were also present in high concentration (see Fig. 1–6). At 5 weeks, the liver contained abundant primitive erythroblasts and some macrophages in the hepatic sinusoids. The concentrations of CFU-E, BFU-E, and CFU-GM in the liver rose rapidly over the next 3 weeks and reached a plateau by 8 to 9 weeks of gestation (see Fig. 1–6). Although definitive erythropoiesis (i.e., CFU-E and BFU-E) predominated for the remainder of the fetal liver phase of hematopoiesis, CFU-GMs increased from week 8 through 12 and remained stable until almost 20 weeks, when the number of myeloid progenitor cells declined.[90–92] Concomitant with the changes in progenitor cell concentrations, the percentage of circulating and tissue-restricted mature blood cells of the myeloerythroid lineages changed (Fig. 1–7) as hematopoiesis shifted from the yolk sac to the liver. A gradual shift from primarily embryonic to primarily fetal and adult hemoglobin molecules also occurred in yolk sac and liver BFU-E–derived red blood cells,[82, 93] respectively, during the fifth through eighth weeks of gestation.

Investigators have focused on isolating enriched populations of hematopoietic stem and progenitor cells from the developing human embryo. Through the use of monoclonal antibodies and FACS, a stem cell–surface "phenotype" has emerged that is useful in isolating hematopoietic progenitor and putative hematopoietic stem cells. Because numerous monoclonal antibodies may recognize the same cell-surface antigen, an international classification is assigned to each monoclonal antibody; all monoclonal antibodies reacting with a single blood cell–surface antigen are given a cluster of differentiation (CD) number designation.[94]

CD34 is an antigen that has been used extensively in the positive selection of human adult hematopoietic stem and progenitor cells.[95]

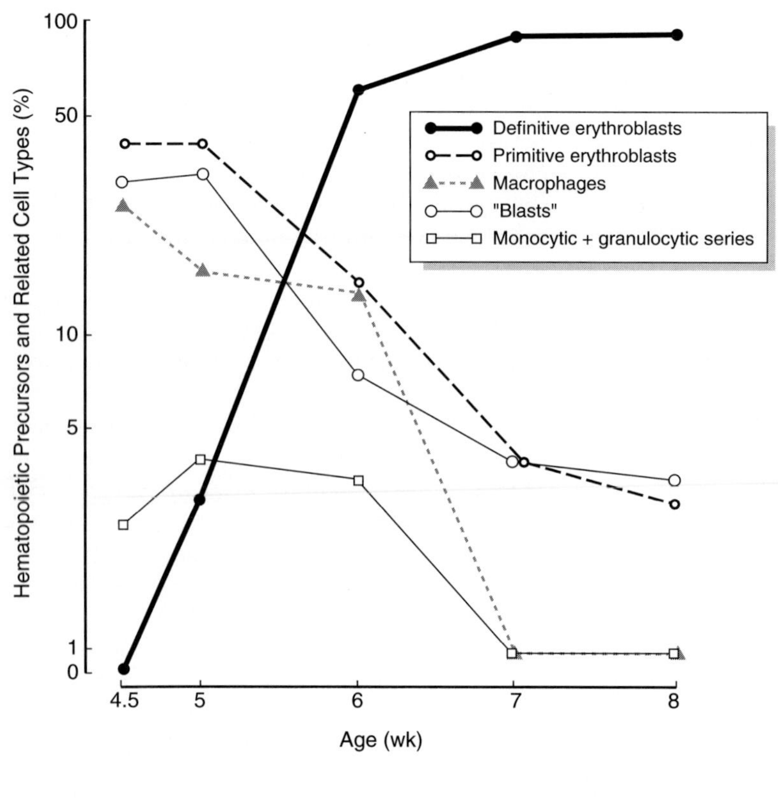

Figure 1–7. Changes in the total percentage of embryonic liver hematopoietic cells comprising each mature lineage or progenitor cells during human ontogeny. Primitive erythroblasts, macrophages, and "blast" cells (presumed stem cells) predominate in the liver at 4.5 to 5 weeks of gestation. By 8 weeks of gestation, the liver hematopoietic tissue is composed predominantly of definitive erythroblasts with small populations of primitive erythroblasts and few blast cells. (From Migliaccio G, Migliaccio A, Petti S, et al: Human embryonic hematopoiesis: kinetics of progenitors and precursors underlying the yolk sac–liver transition. J Clin Invest 1986;78:55; reproduced from the Journal of Clinical Investigation by copyright permission of the American Society for Clinical Investigation.)

CD34, a cell-surface sialomucin, is also expressed on human fetal liver hematopoietic cells; more CD34 is expressed on the fetal hematopoietic progenitor cells than on adult hematopoietic progenitor cells.[96–98] The cell-surface phenotype that permits the highest enrichment of committed and primitive hematopoietic progenitor cells is found in embryonic and fetal hematopoietic cells that do not express any mature blood cell lineage antigens (lin^-), CD38 (a transmembrane glycoprotein), or CD71 (transferrin receptor) but express CD4, CD34, CD117 (*KIT* tyrosine kinase receptor), and CD90 (antigen not characterized).[96–102] Other antigens that are more controversial with regard to enriching for hematopoietic stem and progenitor cell activity in the embryo and fetus include expression of CD15 (3-fucosyl-*N*-acetyl-lactosamine), CD33 (transmembrane glycoprotein), and human major histocompatibility complex class II antigen (HLA-DR).[99]

$CD34^+$ hematopoietic progenitor cells have been identified as early as day 23 of human gestation in the yolk sac and within the embryo proper.[103] The intraembryonic $CD34^+$ cells were localized to the ventral aspect of the dorsal aorta around the preumbilical region. The hematopoietic clusters were in the luminal side in tight association with the endothelial cells.[103] When tissue explants of the preumbilical aortic region, liver, heart, limbs, blood, and umbilical cord of embryos at days 30 through 40 of gestation were co-cultured in vitro with a murine bone marrow stromal cell line, fivefold more hematopoietic progenitors were derived from the preumbilical aortic region than from all other sites combined.[103] These results confirmed the presence of hematopoietic progenitor cells in the human embryo at sites distinct from the yolk sac and liver.[104] Huyhn and coworkers[104] had isolated yolk sac, liver, and embryonic tissues from 25- to 40-day-gestation embryos and plated the enzyme-disaggregated samples in methylcellulose culture for detection of hematopoietic progenitor cells. Although the concentration of BFU-E in the yolk sacs and embryo proper were similar, 7- to 12-fold higher numbers of CFU-GM were present in the embryo proper than in the yolk sac. Huyhn and colleagues[104] isolated $CD34^+$ cells from embryonic (35 to 40 days' gestation) yolk sac, liver, and embryo proper and cultured these cells in the hematopoietic progenitor assay. Hematopoietic progenitor cells were more numerous in the embryo than in the liver and yolk sac. These results were interpreted as evidence that intraembryonic hematopoietic precursors occur in high concentrations when the liver is initiating hematopoiesis, and they support murine studies suggesting that definitive liver hematopoiesis follows seeding of the liver with hematopoietic cells from within the embryo.[57]

In addition to differences in progenitor cell concentration in the 25- to 50-day yolk sac, liver, and embryo samples, distinct differences in the biology of the hematopoietic progenitors were also observed. Yolk sac BFU-Es were distinct from liver- and embryo proper–derived BFU-Es by being larger and containing dispersed myeloid cells on microscopic examination. It appeared that the yolk sac BFU-Es were more primitive (i.e., containing erythroid and myeloid progenitor activity) than typical adult marrow-derived BFU-Es. Although this finding has been observed when plating human umbilical cord–derived hematopoietic progenitors,[105] BFU-Es from adult marrow do not contain any myeloid elements. Dose-response curves analyzing the in vitro growth of progenitor cells (i.e., yolk sac, liver, and embryo proper) after addition of recombinant growth factors did not indicate any difference in the growth factor sensitivity of progenitors from these sites.[104] CFU-E concentrations were low in the yolk sac and embryo proper but were abundant in the liver. These CFU-E results contrast with the findings of Migliaccio and coworkers,[89] who observed high numbers of yolk sac CFU-Es in the 4.5- to 5-week human embryonic yolk sac. No apparent technical error explained this discrepancy.

The yolk sac and embryo proper were composed of hematopoietic cells demonstrating HPP-CFC activity. $CD34^+$ hematopoietic cells recovered from the yolk sac and embryo yielded 45 HPP-CFC and 20 HPP-CFC, respectively, when 10,000 $CD34^+$ cells were plated with the growth factors recombinant human stem cell factor (rhSCF) and interleukin-3 (IL-3). Addition of recombinant human granulocyte (rhGCSF) or granulocyte-macrophage (rhGM-CSF) colony-stimulating factors failed to influence the number or size of the HPP-CFC grown in rhSCF or rhIL-3.[104] All $CD34^+$ progenitors and HPP-CFC in the yolk sac and embryo proper failed to express CD38 or

CD33, consistent with the pattern of expression observed for adult marrow hematopoietic stem cells.

Comparison of CFC formation in vitro in cells isolated from human fetal liver (7 to 14 weeks' gestation) and adult marrow $CD34^+CD38^-$ cells reveals that the fetal liver has a fourfold higher percentage of BFU-E. Each fetal liver BFU-E colony also is composed of at least twofold more blood cells per colony. The time for blood cells to differentiate in vitro into mature forms is diminished in the fetal liver $CD34^+CD38^-$–derived CFC compared with adult marrow $CD34^+CD38^-$–derived CFC. The LTC-IC concentration was higher in fetal liver $CD34^+CD38^-$ cells than in phenotypically similar adult marrow cells, and the number of secondary colonies derived from cultured LTC-IC was sevenfold higher in fetal liver compared with adult marrow $CD34^+CD38^-$ cells.[98] Further studies are required to determine whether the highly enriched fetal liver hematopoietic cell populations contain hematopoietic stem cells. Hematopoietic stem cells from the livers of 12- to 15-week-gestation human fetuses can engraft and produce circulating blood cell progeny for more than 2 years after in utero transplantation into preimmune fetal sheep.[21, 106] Human fetal liver can also engraft and repopulate blood cell lineages in human patients with a variety of hematopoietic disorders.[107–111]

No published reports characterize the biology of hematopoietic stem and progenitor cells in the human late embryonic and early fetal bone marrow. Several groups have isolated enriched populations of hematopoietic cells from the bone marrow (e.g., tibias and femurs) of human fetuses at 12 to 24 weeks' gestation. Turner and colleagues[112] compared in vivo repopulating ability of $CD34^+$ cells isolated from fetal bone marrow, adult bone marrow, and mobilized peripheral blood cells (e.g., patients treated for 5 to 7 days with rhG-CSF and cells collected by apheresis). The fetal marrow cells expanded to constitute 23% of the total number of marrow and spleen cells in 15% of the recipient mice, whereas adult marrow cells only engrafted in 2% of the recipients. Human peripheral blood cells engrafted in 3% of the mice but only in the T lymphocyte lineage. The investigators concluded that fetal marrow appears superior to adult marrow and mobilized peripheral blood in engrafting in this xenograft model and that human hematopoiesis can occur in this model without the administration of human cytokines to recipient mice. One factor that may have contributed to the high level of fetal marrow engraftment in the mice was that 18- and 9-fold more $CD34^+$ cells were recovered in the fetal marrow than in the mobilized peripheral blood and adult bone marrow, respectively.

Huang and Terstappen[113] reported that human fetal bone marrow hematopoietic cells expressing CD34 could be further enriched by analyzing cells for CD38 and HLA-DR expression. Of the $CD34^+$ fetal marrow population, 3% expressed HLA-DR but not CD38, and 4% did not express HLA-DR or CD38. In contrast, almost 90% of $CD34^+$ cells expressed both HLA-DR and CD38. When these subpopulations were individually plated with recombinant growth factors, only single $CD34^+$ cells that lacked CD38 gave rise to multiple hematopoietic lineages. Only $CD34^+CD38^-HLA\text{-}DR^+$ fetal marrow cells gave rise to all hematopoietic lineages tested (i.e., B lymphocytes, neutrophils, monocytes, macrophages, osteoclasts, basophil or mast cells, eosinophils, erythrocytes, megakaryocytes, and platelets). Because only 9% of the $CD34^+CD38^-HLA\text{-}DR^+$ fetal marrow cells produced blood cells in vitro, these investigators postulated that this small subpopulation of cells could be further enriched. Other investigators demonstrated that expression of CD4 on $CD34^+lin^-$ hematopoietic cells enriches the fetal bone marrow cells for HPP-CFC and for cells that engraft and repopulate the bone marrow of SCID mice.[99] $CD4^+CD34^+lin^-$ fetal marrow cells demonstrated greater proliferative potential in the reconstituted mice than $CD4^-CD34^+lin^-$ cells. The $CD4^+CD34^+lin^-$ were also enriched for CD90, CD117, CD123, and HLA-DR and did not express CD38 or CD71.[99] The higher proliferative potential of the fetal liver and marrow hematopoietic stem cells suggests these cells may be excellent targets of gene therapy for congenital or acquired hematopoietic disorders.[33, 37]

References

1. Wintrobe M: Milestones on the path of progress. In Wintrobe M (ed): Blood, Pure and Eloquent. New York: McGraw-Hill, 1980, p 1.

2. Jacobson L, Simmons E, Marks E, et al: Further studies on recovery from radiation injury. J Lab Clin Med 1951;37:683.
3. Jacobson L, Marks E, Robson M, et al: The effect of spleen protection on mortality following X-irradiation. J Lab Clin Med 1949;34:1538.
4. Ford C, Hamerton J, Barnes W, et al: Cytological identification of radiation-chimaeras. Nature 1956;177:452.
5. Till J, McCulloch E: A direct measurement of the radiation sensitivity of normal mouse bone marrow cells. Radiat Res 1961;14:213.
6. Becker A, McCulloch E, Till J: Cytological demonstration of the clonal nature of spleen colonies derived from transplanted mouse marrow cells. Nature 1963;197:452.
7. Pluznik D, Sachs L: The cloning of normal "mast" cells in tissue culture. J Cell Comp Physiol 1965;66:319.
8. Bradley T, Metcalf D: The growth of mouse bone marrow cells in vitro. Aust J Exp Biol Med Sci 1966;44:287.
9. Axelrad A, McLeod D, Shreeve M, et al (eds): Properties of Cells that Produce Erythrocytic Colonies in Vitro. Washington, DC: National Institutes of Health, 1974.
10. Spangrude G: Biological and clinical aspects of hematopoietic stem cells. Annu Rev Med 1994;45:93.
11. Harrison D, Astle C, Stone M: Numbers and functions of transplantable primitive immunohematopoietic stem cells. J Immunol 1989;142:3833.
12. Harrison D: Competitive repopulation in unirradiated normal recipients. Blood 1993;81:2473.
13. Szilvassy S, Hoffman R: Enriched hematopoietic stem cells: basic biology and clinical utility. Biol Blood Marrow Transplant 1995;1:3.
14. Sutherland H, Eaves C, Eaves A: Characterization and partial purification of human marrow cells capable of initiating long-term hematopoiesis in vitro. Blood 1989;74:1563.
15. Orlic D, Bodine D: What defines a pluripotent hematopoietic stem cell (PHSC): will the real PHSC please stand up! Blood 1994;84:3991.
16. Dexter T, Allen T, Lajtha L: Conditions controlling the proliferation of haemopoietic stem cells in vitro. J Cell Physiol 1976;91:335.
17. Ploemacher R, vanderSluijs J, Voerman J, et al: An in vitro limiting-dilution assay of long-term repopulating hematopoietic stem cells in the mouse. Blood 1989;74:2755.
18. Verfaillie C, Miller J: A novel single-cell proliferation assay shows that long-term culture-initiating cell (LTC-IC) maintenance over time results from the extensive proliferation of a small fraction of LTC-IC. Blood 1995;86:2137.
19. Ponchio L, Conneally E, Eaves C: Quantitation of the quiescent fraction of long-term culture-initiating cells in normal human blood and marrow and the kinetics of their growth factor-stimulated entry into S-phase in vitro. Blood 1995;86:3314.
20. Leemhuis T, Yoder MC, Grigsby S, et al: Isolation of primitive human bone marrow hematopoietic progenitor cells using Hoechst 33342 and Rhodamine 123. Exp Hematol 1996;24:1215.
21. Zanjani E, Pallavicini M, Ascensao J, et al: Engraftment and long-term expression of human fetal hematopoietic stem cells in sheep following transplantation in utero. J Clin Invest 1992;89:1178.
22. Civin C, Porada G, Lee M-Ä, et al: Sustained, retransplantable, multilineage engraftment of highly purified adult human bone marrow stem cells in vivo. Blood 1996;88:4102.
23. Srour E, Zanjani E, Cornetta K, et al: Persistence of human multilineage, self-renewing lymphohematopoietic stem cells in chimeric sheep. Blood 1993;82:3333.
24. Schultz L, Schweitzer P, Christianson S, et al: Multiple defects in innate and adaptive immunologic function in NOD/LtSz-SCID mice. J Immunol 1995;154:180.
25. Dick J, Bhatia M, Gan O, et al: Assay of human cells by repopulation of NOD/SCID mice. Stem Cells 1997;15(Suppl 1):199.
26. Bradford G, Williams B, Rossi R, et al: Quiescence, cycling, and turnover in the primitive hematopoietic stem cell compartment. Exp Hematol 1997;25:445.
27. Ogawa M: Differentiation and proliferation of hematopoietic stem cells. Blood 1993;81:2844.
28. Hu M, Drause D, Greaves M, et al: Multilineage gene expression precedes commitment in the hematopoietic system. Genes Dev 1997;11:774.
29. Metcalf D: Hematopoietic regulators: redundancy or subtlety? Blood 1993;82:3515.
30. Yoder M, Williams D: Matrix molecule interactions with hematopoietic stem cells. Exp Hematol 1995;23:961.
31. Watowich S, Wu H, Socolovsky M, et al: Cytokine receptor signal transduction and the control of hematopoietic cell development. Annu Rev Cell Dev Biol 1996;12:91.
32. Osawa M, Hanada K, Hamada H, et al: Long-term lymphohematopoietic reconstitution by a single CD34-low/negative hematopoietic stem cell. Science 1996;273:242.
33. Fraser C, Hoffman R: Hematopoietic stem cell behavior: potential implications for gene therapy. J Lab Clin Med 1995;125:692.
34. Fraser C, Eaves C, Szilvassy S, et al: Expansion in vitro of retrovirally marked totipotent hematopoietic stem cells. Blood 1990;76:1071.
35. Miller C, Eaves C: Expansion in vitro of adult murine hematopoietic stem cells with transplantable lymphomyeloid reconstituting ability. Proc Natl Acad Sci U S A 1997;94:13648.
36. Wineman J, Moore K, Lemischka I, et al: Functional heterogeneity of the hematopoietic microenvironment: rare stromal elements maintain long-term repopulating stem cells. Blood 1996;87:4082.
37. Lansdorp P: Developmental changes in the function of hematopoietic stem cells. Exp Hematol 1995;23:187.
38. Lansdorp P, Dragowska W, Thomas T, et al: Age-related decline in proliferative potential of purified stem cell candidates. Blood Cells 1994;20:376.
39. Lansdorp P, Dragowska W, Mayani H: Ontogeny-related changes in proliferative potential of human hematopoietic cells. J Exp Med 1993;178:787.
40. Jollie W: Development, morphology, and function of the yolk-sac placenta of laboratory rodents. Teratology 1990;41:361.
41. Rossant J: Development of the extraembryonic lineages. Semin Dev Biol 1995;6:237.
42. Jollie W: Ultrastructural studies of protein transfer across rodent yolk sac. Placenta 1986;7:263.
43. Zon L: Developmental biology of hematopoiesis. Blood 1995;86:2876.
44. Shalaby F, Rossant J, Yamaguchi T, et al: Failure of blood-island formation and vasculogenesis in Flk-1–deficient mice. Nature 1995;376:62.
45. Shalaby F, Ho J, Stanford W, et al: A requirement for Flk1 in primitive and definitive hematopoiesis and vasculogenesis. Cell 1997;89:981.

46. Choi K, Kennedy M, Kazarov A, et al: A common precursor for hematopoietic and endothelial cells. Development 1998;125:725.
47. Eichmann A, Corbel C, Nataf V, et al: Ligand-dependent development of the endothelial and hemopoietic lineages from embryonic mesodermal cells expressing vascular endothelial growth factor receptor 2. Proc Natl Acad Sci U S A 1997;94:5141.
48. Kabrun N, Buhring H, Choi K, et al: Flk-1 expression defines a population of early embryonic hematopoietic precursors. Development 1997;124:2039.
49. Zon LI: Development biology of hematopoiesis. Blood 1995;86:2876.
50. Shivdasani R, Orkin S: The transcriptional control of hematopoiesis. Blood 1996;87:4025.
51. Maximow AA: Relation of blood cells to connective tissues and endothelium. Physiol Rev 1924;4:533.
52. Moore M, Owen J: Stem-cell migration in developing myeloid and lymphoid systems. Lancet 1967;2:658.
53. Moore M, Metcalf D: Ontogeny of the haemopoietic system: yolk sac origin of in vivo and in vitro colony forming cells in the developing mouse embryo. Br J Haematol 1970;18:279.
54. Muller A, Medvinsky A, Strouboulis J, et al: Development of hematopoietic stem cell activity in the mouse embryo. Immunity 1994;1:291.
55. Medvinsky A, Dzierzak E: Definitive hematopoiesis is autonomously initiated by the AGM region. Cell 1996;86:897.
56. Cumano A, Dieterlen-Lievre F, Godin I: Lymphoid potential, probed before circulation in mouse, is restricted to caudal intraembryonic splanchnopleura. Cell 1996;86:907.
57. Dzierzak E, Medvinsky A: Mouse embryonic hematopoiesis. Trends Genet 1995;11:359.
58. Weissman I, Papaioannou V, Gardner R: Fetal hematopoietic origins of the adult hematolymphoid system. In Clarkson B, Marks, PA, Till, JE (ed): Differentiation of Normal and Neoplastic Hematopoietic Cells. Cold Spring Harbor, NY: Cold Spring Harbor Laboratory, 1978, p 33.
59. Toles JF, Chui DHK, Belbeck LW, et al: Hemopoietic stem cells in murine embryonic yolk sac and peripheral blood. Proc Natl Acad Sci U S A 1989;86:7456.
60. Wolf N, Bertoncello I, Jiang D, et al: Developmental hematopoiesis from prenatal to young-adult life in the mouse model. Exp Hematol 1995;23:142.
61. Yoder M, Hiatt K: Engraftment of embryonic hematopoietic cells in conditioned newborn recipients. Blood 1997; 89:2176.
62. Yoder M, Hiatt K, Mukherjee P: In vivo repopulating hematopoietic stem cells are present in the murine yolk sac at day 9.0 postcoitus. Proc Natl Acad Sci U S A 1997; 94:6776.
63. Yoder MC, Hiatt K, Dutt P, et al: Characterization of definitive lymphohematopoietic stem cells in the day 9 murine yolk sac. Immunity 1997;7:335.
64. Tavassoli M: Embryonic and fetal hemopoiesis: an overview. Blood Cells 1991;1:269.
65. Rich I: The developmental biology of hemopoiesis: effect of growth factors on the colony formation by embryonic cells. Exp Hematol 1992;20:368.
66. Enders A, King B: Development of the human yolk sac. In Nogales F (ed): The Human Yolk Sac and Yolk Sac Tumors. Berlin: Springer-Verlag, 1993, p 33.
67. Breier G, Albrecht U, Sterrer S, et al: Expression of vascular endothelial growth factor during embryonic angiogenesis and endothelial cell differentiation. Development 1992;114:521.
68. Regenstreif L, Rossant J: Expression of the c-fms proto-oncogene and of the cytokine, CSF-1, during mouse embryogenesis. Dev Biol 1989;133:284.
69. Azoulay M, Webb C, Sachs L: Control of hematopoietic cell growth regulators during mouse fetal development. Mol Cell Biol 1987;7:3361.
70. Brent R, Beckman D, Jensen M, et al: Experimental yolk sac dysfunction as a model for studying the nutritional disturbances in the embryo during early organogenesis. Teratology 1990;41:405.
71. Wilson J, King B: Transport of horseradish peroxidase across monkey trophoblastic epithelium in coated and uncoated vesicles. Anat Rec 1985;211:174.
72. Brent R, Fawcett L: Nutritional studies of the embryo during early organogenesis with normal embryos and embryos exhibiting yolk sac dysfunction. J Pediatr 1998;132:S6.
73. Bremer J: The earliest blood vessels in man. Am J Anat 1914;16:447.
74. Gilmour J: Normal hematopoiesis in intra-uterine and neonatal life. J Pathol 1941;52:25.
75. Yoffey J: The stem cell problem in the fetus. Isr J Med Sci 1971;7:825.
76. Luckett W: Origin and differentiation of the yolk sac and extraembryonic mesoderm in presomite human and rhesus monkey embryos. Am J Anat 1978;152:59.
77. Thomas D, Yoffey J: Human foetal haematopoiesis. II. Hepatic haematopoiesis in the human foetus. Br J Haematol 1964;10:193.
78. Thomas DB, Yoffey JM: Human foetal haemoposiesis. I. The cellular composition of foetal blood. Br J Haematol 1962;8:290.
79. Kelemen E, Calvo W, Fleidner TM: Atlas of Human Hemopoietic Development. New York: Springer-Verlag, 1979.
80. Charbord P, Tavian M, Humeau L, et al: Early ontogeny of the human marrow from long bones: an immunohistochemical study of hematopoiesis and its microenvironment. Blood 1996;87:4109.
81. Tavassoli M: Ontogeny of hemopoiesis. In Meisami E, Timiras P (eds): Handbook of Human Growth and Developmental Biology. Boca Raton: CRC Press, 1988, p 101.
82. Stamatoyannopoulos G, Constantoulakis P, Brice M, et al: Coexpression of embryonic, fetal, and adult globins in erythroid cells of human embryos: relevance to the cell-lineage models of globin switching. Dev Biol 1987;123:191.
83. Kelemen E, Gulya E, Vass K: Ontogeny of human neutrophil granulocyte alkaline phosphatase. J Cell Physiol 1978;95:353.
84. Wolf B, Luevano E, Neiman R: Evidence to suggest that the human fetal spleen is not a hematopoietic organ. Am J Clin Pathol 1983;80:140.
85. Wilkins B, Green A, Wild A, et al: Extramedullary hematopoiesis in fetal and adult human spleen: a quantitative immunohistological study. Histopathology 1994;24:241.
86. Rosenthal P, Rimm I, Umiel T, et al: Ontogeny of human hematopoietic cells: analysis utilizing monoclonal antibodies. J Immunol 1983;131:232.
87. Calhoun D, Li Y, Braylan R, et al: Assessment of the contribution of the spleen to granulocytopoiesis and erythropoiesis of the mid-gestation human fetus. Early Hum Dev 1996;46:217.
88. Forestier F, Daffos F, Galacteros F: Hematological values of 163 normal fetuses between 18 and 30 weeks of gestation. Pediatr Res 1986;20:342.
89. Migliaccio G, Migliaccio A, Petti S, et al: Human embryonic hemopoiesis: kinetics of progenitors and precursors underlying the yolk sac–liver transition. J Clin Invest 1986;78:51.

90. Porcellini A, Manna A, Manna M, et al: Ontogeny of granulocyte-macrophage progenitor cells in the human fetus. Int J Cell Cloning 1983;1:92.
91. Hann I, Bodger M, Hoffbrand A: Development of pluripotent hematopoietic progenitor cells in the human fetus. Blood 1983;62:118.
92. Kitazawa M, Ohnishi Y: Granulocyte-macrophage progenitor cells in the liver of human embryo and fetus. Acta Haematol 1985;48:1341.
93. Peschle C, Migliaccio A, Migliaccio G, et al: Embryonic-fetal Hb switch in humans: studies on erythroid bursts generated by embryonic progenitors from yolk sac and liver. Proc Natl Acad Sci U S A 1984;81:2416.
94. Barclay A, Birkeland M, Brown M, et al: The Leucocyte Antigen Facts Book. London: Academic Press, 1993.
95. Krause D, Fackler M, Civin C, et al: CD34: structure, biology, and clinical utility. Blood 1996;87:1.
96. Gilles J, Divon M, Bentolila E, et al: Immunophenotypic characterization of human fetal liver hematopoietic stem cells during the midtrimester of gestation. Am J Obstet Gynecol 1997;177:619.
97. Muench M, Roncarolo M, Menon S, et al: FLK-2/FLT-3 ligand regulates the growth of early myeloid progenitors lisolated from human fetal liver. Blood 1995;85:963.
98. Roy V, Miller J, Verfaillie C: Phenotypic and functional characterization of committed and primitive myeloid and lymphoid hematopoietic precursors in human fetal liver. Exp Hematol 1997;25:387.
99. Muench M, Roncarlo M, Namikawa R: Phenotypic and functional evidence for the expression of CD4 by hematopoietic stem cells isolated from human fetal liver. Blood 1997;89:1364.
100. Craig W, Kay R, Cutler R, et al: Expression of Thy-1 on human hematopoietic progenitor cells. J Exp Med 1993;177:267.
101. Gabbianelli M, Pelosi E, Montesoro E, et al: Multilevel effects of FLT3 ligand on human hematopoiesis: expansion of putative stem cells and proliferation of granulomonocytic progenitors/monocytic precursors. Blood 1995;86:1661.
102. Emerson S: The regulation of hematopoiesis in the human fetal liver. Biol Hemato 1990;1:21.
103. Tavian M, Coulombel L, Luton D, et al: Aorta-associated CD34+ hematopoietic cells in the early human embryo. Blood 1996;87:67.
104. Huyhn A, Dommergues M, Izac B, et al: Characterization of hematopoietic progenitors from human yolk sacs and embryos. Blood 1995;86:4474.
105. Broxmeyer H, Hangoc G, Cooper S, et al: Growth characteristics and expansion of human umbilical cord blood and estimation of its potential for transplantation in adults. Proc Natl Acad Sci U S A 1992;89:4109.
106. Zanjani E, Flake A, Rice H, et al: Long-term repopulating ability of xenogenic transplanted human fetal liver hematopoietic stem cells in sheep. J Clin Invest 1994;93:1051.
107. Touraine J: In utero transplantation of fetal liver stem cells in humans. Blood 1991;17:379.
108. Touraine J: In-utero transplantation of fetal liver stem cells into human fetuses. Hum Reprod 1992;7:44.
109. Touraine J, Bacchetta R, De Vries J, et al: Transplantation of mismatched human fetal liver cells: tolerance induction via clonal delection and clonal anergy. Transplant Proc 1995;27:622.
110. Kochupillai V, Sharma S, Sundaram K, et al: Hematopoietic improvement following fetal liver infusion in aplastic anemia. Eur J Haematol 1991;47:319.
111. Touraine J: Transplantation of fetal hematopoietic and lymphopoietic cells in humans, with special reference to in utero transplantation. In Edwards R (ed): Fetal Tissue Transplants in Medicine. Cambridge: Cambridge University Press, 1992, p 155.
112. Turner C, Yeager A, Waller E, et al: Engraftment potential of different sources of human hematopoietic progenitor cells in BNX mice. Blood 1996;87:3237.
113. Huang S, Terstappen L: Lymphoid and myeloid differentiation of single human $CD34^+$, $HLA\text{-}DR^+$, $CD38^-$ hematopoietic stem cells. Blood 1994;83:1515.

CHAPTER 2

Development of the Immune System in the Human Fetus

William Slayton, M.D.

Infection is a significant cause of morbidity and mortality in the premature and term neonate. The susceptibility of the neonate to infection can be understood in relation to immaturity of the immune system. The development of a defense system that recognizes and protects against myriad pathogens is one of the wonders of development.

Only recently has attention been focused on developmental aspects of immunity. The use of stem cell sources, such as the fetal liver and umbilical cord blood, and the advent of fetal bone marrow transplantation spurred interest in T cell ontogeny and immunotolerance. There has been less experimental activity in the developmental aspects of macrophages and neutrophils. Knowledge of the development of the immune system provides an understanding of the specific immune deficiencies in the premature and term neonate.

We are only beginning to apply advances in molecular biology and hematopoietic progenitor cell culture techniques to increase our understanding of how the immune system develops. Much of what we know comes from animal studies. However, knowledge derived from animal systems is not always relevant to humans. For instance, the fetal lamb has a placental system that, unlike the human system, does not allow the passage of IgG.[1] In humans, placental passage of maternal IgG is thought to provide humoral immunity before the maturity of the fetal system. Interleukin (IL)-13, which is a potent stimulator of B cells in humans, does not stimulate B cells in the mouse.[2] Ideally, all questions about the development of the human immune system could be answered best by using human tissue. However, there are obvious and important limits on our ability to perform experiments using human fetal tissue.

EVOLUTION OF IMMUNITY

Self-recognition and elimination of potentially harmful pathogens are basic immunologic characteristics in all organisms. The most primitive immune systems involve interactions that are not antigen specific; these are systems of "natural" or "innate" immunity. Such nonspecific mechanisms include specialized cells such as macrophages, and humoral factors such as C-reactive protein. The innate immune response is not amplified with repeat exposure to a given pathogen.[3]

Antigen-specific "adaptive" immune mechanisms exist in more complex organisms. Adaptive immunity improves on natural systems by providing greater specificity and the ability to respond more quickly and effectively to pathogens to which the organism has previously been exposed. One element of adaptive immunity is the specificity provided by rearrangements in the genes that produce T cell receptors (TCRs) and antibodies that specifically recognize antigens. Gene rearrangements result in an immune repertoire that provides the ability to recognize and respond to almost any foreign antigen.[3] Another adaptive ability is memory, which allows lymphocytes to proliferate quickly after repeated antigen exposure. This proliferation is achieved through clonal expansion of lymphocytes that have receptors specific to the pathogen.[4]

To understand the evolution of the immune system, scientists have studied organisms from the most primitive invertebrates to humans. Recognition of self is a necessary corollary to immune reactions. The most primitive chordates lack the major histocompatibility complex (MHC) proteins that are critical to self-recognition. The MHC is found in some fish, amphibians, birds, and mammals.[5] Although systems of natural immunity exist in primitive invertebrates, adaptive mechanisms first appear in the vertebrates. Phagocytic cells first appear in invertebrate animals and perform many of the functions that macrophages perform in humans. For instance, phagocytic cells in the starfish produce IL-1.[6] Invertebrate phagocytic cells kill bacteria by producing superoxide through an enzyme homologous to cytochrome *b* in humans. The absence or reduced function of this cytochrome is the cause of X-linked chronic granulomatous disease in humans.[7, 8]

Aggregates of immune tissue that are directly associated with epithelial tissues, such as the skin, gill regions, and gut, form in echinoderms and tunicates and are similar to the location of lymphatic tissue in mammals.[5] Lymphocytes are thought to have appeared first in the jawless fishes, ancestors to the lamprey, and the more specialized T and B cells may have evolved in the ancestors of the sharks.[9]

The order in which different cells of the immune system appear as development progresses may be related to when these cells appeared during evolution. At the very earliest stages of embryonic development, the embryos of the most primitive to the most advanced vertebrates look remarkably similar. This led to the theory that "ontogeny recapitulates phylogeny," meaning that the embryo passes through the physical form of its evolutionary ancestors as it develops. However, although humans have gill rudiments in the form of branchial arches, they never develop true gills. For this and other reasons, this theory was rejected. In the late 1800s, Karl von Baer observed that the common features of vertebrates appear early in fetal development, with specialized features appearing later.[10] This observation can be applied to the ontogeny of blood, in which the first red blood cells produced in the developing human embryo are nucleated, similar to red cells in reptiles and amphibians. Similarly, the first immunocytes to appear in the human fetus are macrophages, followed by the more elaborate natural killer (NK) cells and neutrophils (Table 2–1). Lymphocytes appear late and become fully functional months after birth. It is as if the more primitive components of the immune system were not lost, but rather, the more elaborate adaptive systems were superimposed and integrated with the natural systems to provide greater efficacy and specificity.[11]

LEUKOCYTE PRODUCTION AND DEVELOPMENT OF THE ORGANS OF IMMUNITY

Although the traditional view is that the onset of hematopoiesis occurs extraembryonically, in the yolk sac, modern studies indicate a simultaneous embryonic origin of mammalian hematopoiesis. Avian studies suggest that the yolk sac contributes primarily to primitive erythroid lineages, whereas definitive hematopoiesis has an intraembryonic origin.[12] Investigators have identified hematopoietic stem cells in the periaortic tissue in mice and humans.[13, 14]

Few leukocytes are produced at the earliest stages of hematopoiesis in the human fetus. Hematopoiesis begins in the yolk sac (weeks 2 through 5), moves to the liver (weeks 5 through 24), and then moves to the bone marrow (week 11 through adulthood).[15] The phases of fetal hematopoiesis overlap significantly, and it is not known what mechanisms trigger the movement

Table 2–1. **Location of Immunocytes During Development**

Cell Type	Fetal Age (weeks)	Organ
Macrophage	2–3	Yolk sac; few cells
	5	Liver, lung, brain; more cells
Natural killer cells	8	Liver
Neutrophils	5	Liver; few cells
	11	Bone marrow; many cells
B cells	8	Liver, omentum
T cells	8–9	Thymus

of hematopoiesis from one organ to the next. Yolk sac hematopoiesis is restricted almost entirely to erythropoiesis, although some macrophages are produced there.[16] Yolk sac stem cells are multipotent when studied in vitro and in transplantation experiments, but they produce only a narrow spectrum of hematopoietic cells in vivo. Tavasolli speculates that this is an example of embryologic "impermissiveness" and hypothesizes that the yolk sac does not produce the growth factors that support the development of neutrophils and lymphocytes.[15]

Circulation begins in the human fetus by the four to fifth week after conception.[17] During this time, macrophages appear in the liver, brain, and lungs. During the fifth week, hematopoiesis begins in the liver, and the first hematopoietic cells to appear are macrophages.[18] These Kupffer cells line the sinusoidal spaces and account for approximately 70% of the hematopoietic cells in the liver when hematopoiesis begins at 5 weeks postconception, but erythropoiesis outpaces the production of other cell types, and red blood cells outnumber Kupffer cells by 6 to 7 weeks postconception. Whether Kupffer cells originate in the yolk sac and migrate to the liver or are the product of hematopoiesis in the liver is unknown. Similar to the yolk sac, stem cells in the fetal liver are multipotent when studied in vitro, but the products of hematopoiesis are restricted mainly to red blood cells in vivo.[15]

The marrow space begins to develop around the eighth week after conception, and hematopoiesis begins in the bone marrow between the 10th and 11th week.[17, 19, 20] Similar to the liver, the first hematopoietic cells to appear in the bones are phagocytic osteoclasts (Fig. 2–1). These cells are present at approximately 8 weeks postconception and seem to core out the marrow space. When hematopoiesis begins in the marrow, primarily neutrophils are produced, in contrast to the liver, where primarily macrophages are present.[19]

The thymus appears around 8 weeks postconception. The function of the thymus is to support the differentiation of T lymphocytes. Progenitors of T cells are thought to migrate from the fetal liver to the thymus at 8 to 9 weeks postconception.[21, 22] By the 10th week, lymphoid cells constitute 95% of the cells present in the thymus. Granulocyte precursors and

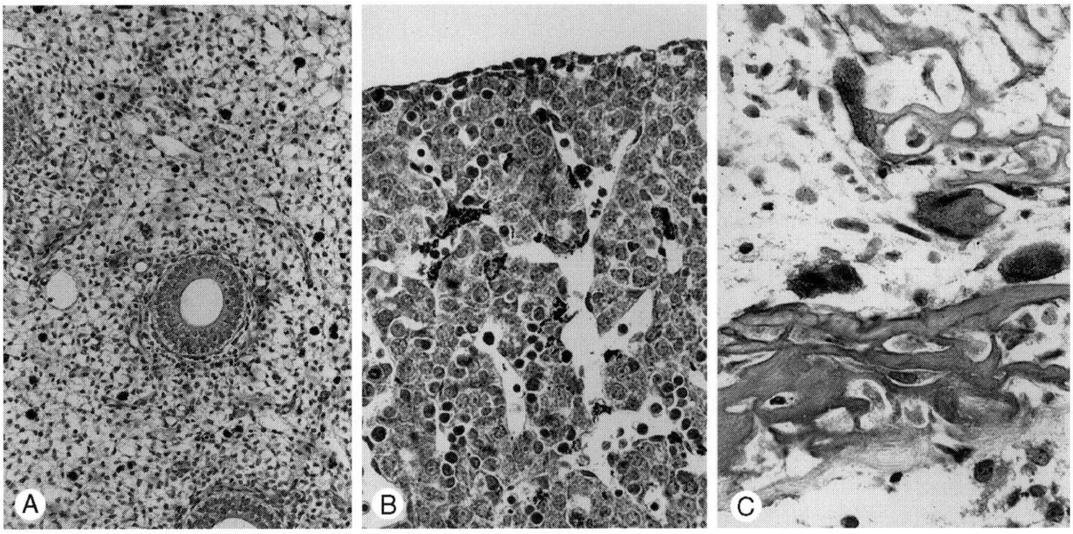

Figure 2–1. Phagocytic cells are the first hematopoietic cells to appear in a variety of organs. The panels demonstrate phagocytic cells that have been treated with monoclonal antibodies to KP-1, an enzyme in the lysosomes of macrophages (darkest stain). *A*, Human lung at 5 weeks after conception (original magnification ×40). Multiple macrophages are scattered within the developing lung, and they will later lie within the alveoli. (From Slayton WB, Juul SE, Calhoun DA, et al: Hematopoiesis in the liver and marrow. Pediatr Res 43, 774; © 1998, The Williams & Wilkins Company, Baltimore.) *B*, Human embryonic liver at 5 weeks after conception (original magnification ×100), demonstrating the presence of mainly empty sinusoids, with Kupffer cells lining the edges of these spaces. A few erythrocytes are present within the developing sinusoids. *C*, Human fetal bone at 8 weeks after conception (original magnification ×400) before the onset of hematopoiesis, demonstrating osteoclasts lining and coring out the marrow space.

macrophages are also present in the developing thymus. Precursors to B cells first appear in the omentum and the fetal liver at 8 weeks postconception. B cell production in the omentum occurs transiently from 8 to 10 weeks, while production continues in the fetal liver.

The spleen probably does not contribute significantly to hematopoiesis in the human fetus, although it is a hematopoietic organ in other mammals such as mice.[23] However, the spleen is an important secondary lymphatic organ in humans, and it plays a role in the protection of infants from infection caused by encapsulated organisms. Lymphocytes begin to appear in the spleen around 11 weeks postconception. By the 22nd week, 70% of the cells are lymphocytes.[17] Lymph nodes first appear around 11 weeks postconception, and lymphocytes appear within the lymph nodes approximately 1 week later.[17] At the same time, gut-associated lymphatic tissue begins to develop. By 19 weeks postconception, Peyer's patches that are structurally mature but immunologically naive are present in the intestines.[24] Although all the major lymphatic organs and cell types of the immune system are present by 11 weeks postconception, little is known about how these cells function and interact in utero as the immune system develops.

NATURAL IMMUNITY

At the earliest stages of human development, the immune system consists of cells and molecules that are nonspecific in their actions. The cellular component of the immune system during the embryonic stage (first 8 weeks) consists of macrophages, granulocytes, and NK cells. The humoral component consists of the complement system and passively acquired maternal immunoglobulin.

Monocytes and Macrophages

Recent observations have cast into doubt long-held theories about the origins of macrophages. Scientists believed that all macrophages were formed from precursor cells in the bone marrow, maturing through a progression of cell types from monoblast to promonocyte to monocyte. Monocytes then migrated to various tissues where they differentiated into macrophages.[25] Monocytes and tissue macrophages were thought to have little proliferative potential. Several observations in fetuses have challenged this theory. First, macrophages appear in the yolk sac, liver, lung, and brain long before the development of bone.[16, 18, 19] Second, promonocytes and monocytes are absent in the yolk sac and liver in the fetal mouse. Third, fetal liver and lung macrophages are capable of proliferation.[26, 27] Early fetal macrophages may develop directly from stem cells in the yolk sac, never passing through a monocyte stage. These primitive macrophages may then migrate from the yolk sac to populate the lung, liver, brain, and other organs.[27]

Macrophages are critical to the morphogenesis of the fetus. In addition to their role in immunity, macrophages shape organs and scavenge debris from apoptotic cells during embryogenesis.[28] Macrophages devour debris as one embryonic tissue replaces another.[29] For instance, they are present in the urogenital ridges, where they engulf degenerated cells of the müllerian duct in the male and the wolffian duct in the female.[30] They play a similar role in the retina and brain.[31, 32] Macrophages are closely associated with the areas of apoptosis in the fetal mouse footplate.[33] They have been implicated in triggering apoptosis in the developing eye.[34] In the human yolk sac, macrophages engulf primitive erythroblasts.[16]

In addition to their role in morphogenesis of organs, macrophages are capable of immune protection of the fetus. When macrophages appear in the fetal liver at the onset of hepatic hematopoiesis in the rat, they express Fc receptors and are capable of immune-mediated phagocytosis.[35] Macrophages are highly mobile, even in their most primitive form. Latex particles injected into the yolk sac of the mouse fetus were ingested by primitive macrophages and carried to the mesenchymal stroma and loose connective tissue. Fetal Kupffer cells may detoxify circulating endotoxin. Endotoxin that reaches the amniotic cavity is swallowed by the fetus and flows to the liver through the portal circulation.[36] Macrophages engulf endotoxin through the lipopolysaccharide (LPS) receptor. This receptor is present on human fetal Kupffer cells and can be up-regulated as early as 8 weeks postconception by IL-3.[19] Later, macrophages contribute to the adaptive immune system by acting as antigen-presenting cells and producing lymphokines such as IL-6, tumor necrosis factor (TNF), and IL-1, which enhance lymphocyte production and function.

Neutrophils

Neutrophils appear after macrophages in the human fetus. They cluster in small nests in mesenchymal areas in the neck and upper thorax before the onset of hematopoiesis in the liver.[17] Scattered neutrophil precursors appear in the liver as early as 5 weeks, but macrophages are the predominant white blood cell.[17–19, 37] In the bone marrow, neutrophils first appear in scattered clusters at the onset of hematopoiesis (10 to 11 weeks) and quickly multiply, composing approximately 40% of the hematopoietic cells by 14 weeks postconception (Fig. 2–2).[17, 38]

Compared with macrophages and lymphocytes, little is known about the function of neutrophils in the fetus. At the time of their appearance in the bone marrow, neutrophils contain myeloperoxidase, an enzyme produced by promyelocytes and present within the azurophilic granules of neutrophils.[39] They also have the surface markers CD11b, a protein that binds to complement, and CD15, a receptor that binds to the endothelial wall and causes extravasation of neutrophils from blood vessels.[38] During the fetal period, a time of rapid growth, the progenitor cells producing neutrophils and macrophages are already rapidly cycling, and increased proliferation in response to infection may therefore be restricted.[40, 41] Neutrophil function has been studied in more depth during the newborn period and is of interest to neonatologists because of the vulnerability of the neonate to bacterial sepsis.

Natural Killer Cells

NK cells are phylogenetically primitive lymphocytes that lack specific TCRs, and they have been referred to as large granular lymphocytes because of their numerous cytoplasmic granules. NK cells can kill tumors and virus-infected cells, but unlike cytotoxic lymphocytes, they can do so in the absence of MHC class I antigen. The molecular basis for NK cell target recognition is unknown. Theories posit that NK cells respond to the surface expression of a molecule induced by certain viruses or to the absence of a molecule that should be present on healthy cells.[42] NK cells kill by releasing granules containing esterase and perforin onto the plasma membrane of target cells.[43] Cells similar to NK cells have been described in invertebrates.[43]

NK cells do not undergo thymic maturation. They produce the regulatory cytokines interferon-γ (IFN-γ), granulocyte-macrophage colony-stimulating factor (GM-CSF), and TNF-α. These cells do not rearrange TCR genes.

NK cells appear in the human fetal liver 5 weeks postconception. As early as 6 weeks, 5% to 8% of cells in the fetal liver are NK cells, and by 18 weeks, they increase to 15% to 25% of cells. Approximately 10% to 15% of cord blood lymphocytes are NK cells. These cells are capable of antibody-dependent, cell-mediated cytotoxicity.[44] NK function increases as development progresses. However, even at birth, neonatal NK function is low compared with that of adults, which is why the neonate is particularly susceptible to certain viral infections such as herpes simplex.[45]

Complement

As detailed in Chapter 15, the complement system protects against a variety of fungal, bacterial, and viral organisms. The complement cascade consists of nine regulatory proteins.[3] The alternate pathway is believed to have evolved before the classic pathway. The alternative pathway is activated by nonspecific components of bacteria such as endotoxin or other polysaccharides and does not require antibody. The classic pathway is initiated by antibody binding to antigens and therefore requires the evolution of adaptive immunity. The proteins of this pathway are believed to have evolved as a result of duplication of genes encoding the components of the alternative pathway.[4] Each pathway activates C3, which causes the terminal cascade to form the *membrane attack complex* (C5b6789), which lyses invading cells by inserting itself into the cell membrane. Through a process called *opsonization*, C3b can coat antigen, resulting in more efficient phagocytosis and destruction by macrophages.[3]

There have been few studies of the complement system in early fetal development. Components of the complement cascade appear early

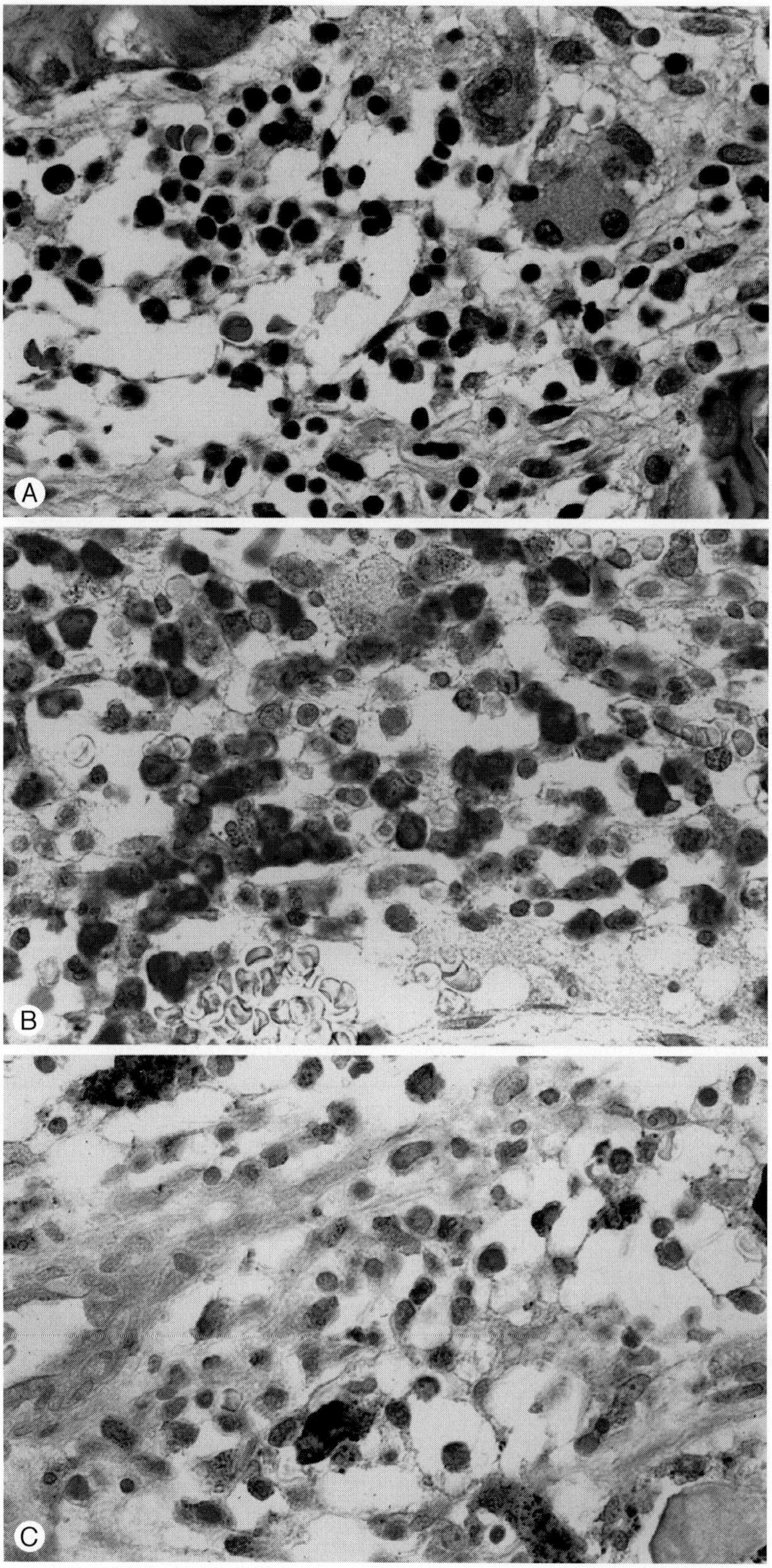

Figure 2–2. Marrow space at 14 weeks after conception. The marrow produces predominantly neutrophils at this gestational age. *A*, Hematoxylin and eosin stain reveals multiple nucleated cells within the marrow space. *B*, Myeloperoxidase (MPO) antibody reveals multiple MPO-positive cells (i.e., neutrophils and their precursors) within the marrow space. *C*, Less staining occurs with KP-1, a marker for macrophages. (*A* and *B* from Slayton WB, Juul SE, Calhoun DA, et al: Hematopoiesis in the liver and marrow. Pediatr Res 43, 774; © 1998, The Williams & Wilkins Company, Baltimore.)

in fetal development. C4 and C2, components of the classic system, are synthesized in the fetal liver as early as 8 weeks after conception.[46] By 13 weeks, C3, C1, and C5 appear. By 18 weeks, C7 and C9 are present in the fetal liver. At 11 weeks postconception, the receptor for C3B is present on macrophages and neutrophils in the bone marrow, suggesting that these cells have the ability to respond to C3, a chemoattractant mediator of the alternative pathway.[38] Serum complement levels are low until the third trimester, when they begin to rise and correlate with birth weight and gestational age. At term, levels of most of the complement enzymes are approximately 50% of their adult levels.[47]

ADAPTIVE IMMUNITY

The lymphocytic system is the last to develop and mature. The cellular immune system begins to function, although not at full capacity, by the second trimester. The fetus does not typically produce humoral immunity until after birth, although B cells are capable of making small amounts of IgM, IgG, and IgA as early as the second trimester. Passive acquisition of maternally produced IgG provides immune defense against microbial invasion that persists several months after birth. The natural system interacts with the adaptive system in many ways; most importantly, macrophages activate lymphocytes by processing and presenting antigen. Macrophages also produce cytokines such as TNF, IL-1, and IL-6 that activate lymphocytes.[3]

T Lymphocytes

Precursors of T cells are thought to migrate from the fetal liver to the thymus, where they mature, undergo gene rearrangements, and are selected for expansion based on expression of receptors that are not reactive with self antigens. Haynes described the presence of CD7-positive ($CD7^+$) T cell precursors that are negative for all other T cell markers in the yolk sac, liver, and thoracic mesenchyme in a fetus 7 weeks postconception. These $CD7^+$ cells are multipotent, producing colonies containing granulocytes, monocytes, erythrocytes, and megakaryocytes in tissue culture. By 8.5 weeks, cells coexpressing CD7 and CD2, which are progenitors committed to the T lymphocyte lineage, are present within the thymus. One week later, cells that express CD4 and CD8 are present.[22]

T cell maturation depends on the expression of an antigen recognition molecule, the TCR. Two types of TCR exist, one composed of a heterodimer made up of gamma and delta ($\gamma\delta$) polypeptides and the other of alpha and beta ($\alpha\beta$) polypeptides. The δ chain is rearranged before the β chain,[48, 49] and $\gamma\delta$ T cells appear before the $\alpha\beta$ T cells during development. The $\gamma\delta$ receptor is thought to be the first rearranging TCR to have arisen during evolution.[4] Human fetal and neonatal $\gamma\delta$ T cells produced IL-4 and IL-5, cytokines involved in the activation of B cells, after stimulation in culture, whereas adult $\gamma\delta$ cells did not.[50] The $\gamma\delta$ T cells have been associated with autoimmune disorders such as multiple sclerosis.[51] These early T cells may play an active role in the early development of the immune system and later become quiescent, only to become active again in autoimmune diseases. Most mature T cells express the $\alpha\beta$ receptor. The antigen-specific TCR is complexed to a signal transduction complex called CD3, and this complex, when stimulated with specific antigen, causes the activation and clonal proliferation of T cells bearing that receptor.[42]

As T cells mature, they progress through three developmental stages.[3] Stage I thymocytes are located in the subcapsular cortical zone of the thymus. These cells do not express CD4 or CD8 antigen and are therefore called *double negative*. This population contains the precursors of the major subsets of T cells.[52] Cells then enter stage II, in which they are *double positive*, expressing CD4 and CD8 antigens. These cells are located primarily in the inner cortical zone of the thymus. Double-positive cells exhibit low-level surface expression of the TCR-CD3 complex and are positively selected for rearranged TCRs that recognize MHC molecules expressed by thymic stromal cells. Stage III thymocytes are located in the thymic medulla, with small numbers located within the inner cortex. These cells express CD4 or CD8.

Cells expressing receptors that recognize “self” MHC or other endogenous antigens with high affinity undergo apoptosis within the thymus through a process called *negative selection*. Only a small proportion of cells that pass positive and negative selection are released into the circulation.[53] One result of positive selection is that T cells require antigen to be presented in the context of the MHC. $CD8^+$ T cells recognize antigen presented in the context of MHC class I. MHC class I molecules are expressed by most cells and are complexed to viral associated peptides that are displayed to $CD8^+$ T cells when a cell becomes infected. MHC class II molecules are expressed on B lymphocytes, macrophages, and other antigen-presenting cells. Foreign antigens presented by these cells are recognized by the $CD4^+$ T cells.[54]

After completing thymic differentiation, mature T cells enter the bloodstream and migrate to secondary lymphoid organs, including the spleen, peripheral lymph nodes, and mucosa-associated lymphoid tissue. Within the parenchyma of the secondary lymphoid organ, they can be activated after encountering processed antigen.

At birth, T cell immunity is weak compared with that of the adult, in part because of the lack of exposure of the fetal immune system to foreign antigens. Compared with adults, most of the T cells in the fetus express CD45RA, indicating an immunologically naive state.[55] These fetal T cells are able to respond to infection, although not at the levels of the T cells of a newborn or adult. T cells in congenitally infected fetuses express CD45RO, a phenotype consistent with antigenic activation, as early as 20 weeks postconception.[56, 57] They also express the IL-2 receptor-α (IL-2Rα), another marker of activation. The activation marker CD25 is expressed on 9% to 16% of fetal lymphocytes.[56] Peripheral blood lymphocytes are capable of cell-mediated lympholysis from 18 weeks on, but cells from the thymus and spleen are not.[58, 59] Antibody-dependent, cell-mediated cytotoxicity in response to herpes simplex infection has been demonstrated in fetal lymphocytes from 17 to 24 weeks of gestation, although at a lower level than in adults.

Another reason for relatively weak T cell immunity in the neonate is decreased cytokine production. In mice, the most immature T cells are capable of producing IL-2 only, but as they develop into $CD4^+$ cells, they can produce IL-4, IL-5, IL-10, and IFN-γ.[60] Compared with adults, neonates have decreased production of certain cytokines, such as IFN-γ, IL-4, and IL-5.[61]

In some ways, fetal T cells have abilities similar to their adult counterparts'. CD4:CD8 ratios and αβ:γδ T cell ratios in cord blood of fetuses from 18 to 34 weeks are similar to newborn and adult levels.[56] Common thymocytes, such as $CD1a^+$ or double-positive CD4CD8 cells are absent from the cord blood during this period, demonstrating that these immature T cells are not released from the fetal thymus until they complete maturation.

T cells also express CD40 ligand, which is necessary for B cell activation and class switching during the second trimester. Durandy found CD40 ligand expression in fetuses from 19 through 28 weeks, although not from 31 weeks' gestation to 10 days after birth. CD40 ligand was again detectable 3 weeks after birth. Presence of this antigen on T cells is necessary for the development of humoral immunity.[62]

B Lymphocytes

Humoral immunity begins to develop around the same time as cellular immunity. Pre-B cells appear in the fetal liver at approximately 8 weeks postconception. Mature B cells expressing surface immunoglobulin appear at 10 weeks.[63] By the 18th week, the absolute number of circulating and splenic B cells nears adult levels.[63, 64] Although B cells begin to differentiate in the fetal liver and bone marrow, independent of T cells, the final developmental step of becoming plasma cells requires functional T cells.[65] In response to T cell activation, mature B cells initially secrete IgM with the same specificity as their surface immunoglobulin, but they can give rise to a plasma cell that produces IgG, IgA, or IgE by changing the constant region gene sequences. These antibodies have different functions because of different constant domains.[3]

Fetal B cells have a phenotype different from adult B cells. The first B cells produced are primarily $CD5^+$ B-1 cells and are localized predominantly in the omentum and later in the intestine. B-1 cells have properties similar to those of B lymphocytes in fish, and B-1 cells might have preceded the more elaborate antigen-specific B cells during evolution.[11] The γδ T cells, also present in the intestine, may interact with B-1 cells and cause them to produce antibody. This interaction may be how "helper" activity evolved in vertebrates.[11] In the fetus,

B-1 cells produce IgM in response to various common bacterial products, including phosphatidyl choline, LPS, 1,3-dextran, and phosphocholine. Rather than being antigen specific, these antibodies are broadly reactive and can react to host tissue.[66] In adults, increased numbers of B-1 cells are associated with autoimmunity, particularly rheumatoid arthritis.[67] These cells are thought to be the source of antibody to single-stranded DNA and rheumatoid factor.[68] These broadly reactive immunoglobulins that constitute an early, nonspecific defense in the fetus are implicated in producing disease in the adult.

Immunoglobulin production in the fetus and neonate is normally low, and the defect in humoral immunity has been attributed to immature B cell function. Adult levels of IgG, IgA, and IgE are reached several months to years after birth.[69, 70] However, B cells from a human fetal spleen at 12 weeks postconception can be stimulated with IL-4 to produce IgM, IgG, and IgE, but not IgA. Infected fetuses can produce IgG and IgA.[69] IgA antibody specific to polio viruses and *Escherichia coli* are present in the meconium and saliva of neonates, which may be an anti-idiotypic response to maternal immunoglobulin specific to polio.[71] IgA is absent in plasma cells in the neonatal intestine. After birth, the infant intestine becomes colonized with bacteria, and the mucosa is exposed to a large number of antigens for the first time. Newborn infants are relatively IgA deficient unless supplied with IgA from mother's milk.[24]

CYTOKINES AND DEVELOPMENT

Little is known about the molecular events that control development of the immune system. The appearance and activation of the various components of the immune system probably are controlled in part by the fetal expression of cytokines. Despite advances in molecular biology and genetics that have provided tools to study how cytokines affect fetal development, cytokine production and function in the fetus is relatively unknown.

In addition to supporting hematopoiesis in the fetus, cytokines are involved in maternal-fetal homeostasis. Cytokine production from the placenta is thought to modulate maternal immunity so that the fetus is not rejected. The mouse placenta produces an excess of the cytokines IL-4 and IL-10, which promote humoral immunity and suppress cellular immunity.[72, 73] In addition to its role in preventing rejection, the placenta produces cytokines in response to infection. For instance, levels of the cytokines granulocyte colony-stimulating factor (G-CSF), GM-CSF, TNF-α, IL-1, IL-6, and IL-8 are increased 100-fold in the amniotic fluid of mothers with chorioamnionitis.[74]

Although the specifics of the evolution of cytokines have yet to be worked out, the lack of patients genetically deficient in cytokines suggests that these molecules have been highly conserved throughout evolution.[75] IL-1 and TNF have been demonstrated in invertebrates, and multiple unique invertebrate molecules that activate or modulate inflammation have been described.[75] Many vertebrate cytokines have receptors that share common chains, including IL-2, IL-4, IL-7, IL-9, and IL-15, which all share the IL-2R common gamma chain C.[76] Similarities in DNA sequence suggest a common evolutionary origin of IL-6, IL-11, IL-12, G-CSF, leukemia inhibitory factor, oncostatin M, and ciliary neurotrophic factor.[77]

Transgenic mouse models that are deficient or overexpress particular cytokines have been produced. These models elucidate the roles of these cytokines in hematopoietic and general development. The roles of various cytokines in the development of the immune system are given in Table 2–2.

Cytokines Modulating Natural Immunity

Type 1 Interferons

Production of type 1 interferons (IFN-α and IFN-β) represents a primitive mechanism of resistance against viruses. Many cell types produce both forms of interferon in response to viral infection, and they are produced by macrophages after stimulation by antigen-activated T cells. Both of these substances activate NK cells and inhibit viral replication.[42] Type 1 IFN is produced by the placenta and is thought to inhibit maternal T cell immunity and promote

Table 2–2. **Cytokines and Their Contribution to Development of Immunity**

Cytokine	Cell Source	Target Cells	Primary Effect	Fetal Studies	Maternofetal Unit	Deficient Mice
Type I interferon	Mononuclear cells and other cell types	All cells, especially NK cells	Antiviral, antiproliferative		Produced by placenta	Receptor-deficient mice susceptible to some viral infections
Tumor necrosis factor-α	T cells	Neutrophils Endothelial cells NK cells	Activation Activation Activation	TNF produced by fetal Kupffer cells exposed to LPS Produced by fetal adrenal	Low levels of TNF-α produced by monocytes within placenta	Increased susceptibility to *Listeria;* resistant to endotoxic shock Abnormal splenic follicles
Interleukin-1	Mononuclear cells, macrophages	Thymocytes Endothelium Hypothalamus Liver Muscle and fat	Costimulator Activation Fever Acute-phase response Cachexia	Produced by thymus (mouse) Stimulates production of G-CSF from fetal monocytes	Present in amniotic fluid; increases with premature rupture of membranes	Decreased inflammatory response; no fever or anorexia
Interleukin-6	Macrophages Endothelial cells T cells	Thymocytes Mature B cells Liver	Stimulation Growth Acute-phase response	Produced by fetal Kupffer cells 13–19 wk postconception	Present in amniotic fluid; increases with infection	Increased susceptibility to *Listeria;* no fever, cachexia, or anorexia
Interleukin-8	Thymic epithelium	Neutrophils Cervix	Chemotaxis Dilitation and softening	Produced constitutively by thymic epithelium; increased in cord blood with chorioamnionitis		
Interleukin-16 (soluble CD4 receptor)	$CD8^+$ T cells	Macrophages Eosinophils $CD4^+$ T cells	Chemotaxis Chemotaxis Chemotaxis, activation			
Interleukin-2	T cells	T cells NK cells B cells	Growth Growth, activation Growth, activation	Promotes expansion of NK cells from fetal liver (mice)		
Interleukin-4	$CD4^+$ T cells Mast cells	B cells Macrophages T cells	Isotype switch to IgE Inhibit activation Growth	Increased levels in cord blood in areas endemic for schistosomiasis, filariasis, and tuberculosis	Placental production may promote antibody production and inhibit rejection	
Transforming growth factor-β	T cells Macrophages	T cells Macrophages	Inhibition Inhibition	Fetal wounds heal without scarring (because of lack of TGF-β?)		Multiorgan system inflammation
Interferon-γ	T cells NK cells	Neutrophils Endothelium NK cells	Activation Activation Activation	In cord blood in endemic areas for schistosomiasis, filariasis, and tuberculosis	Produced by placenta during first trimester (mice)	Receptor-deficient mice susceptible to *Listeria* infection
Lymphotoxin	T cells	Neutrophils Endothelium	Activation Cytokine production			Lack lymph nodes, Peyer's patches, abnormal splenic follicles
Interleukin-5	T cells	Eosinophils B cells	Activation Growth, activation			Decreased activation and mobilization of eosinophils

Interleukin-10	T cells	Macrophages B cells	Inhibits activation		Placental production	Spontaneous enteritis
Interleukin-12	T cells B cells NK cells	Macrophages $CD8^+$ T cells	Immobilization Increased cytotoxicity			
Interleukin-13	T cells	B cells	Increased proliferation and differentiation, production of IgE			
Interleukin-15	Macrophages	T cells NK cells B cells	Activation Activation Stimulates immunoglobulins			
Interleukin-17	$CD4^+$ T cells	Bone marrow stroma	Stimulates IL-6 secretion			
Interleukin-18	Hepatocytes Osteoblasts Keratinocytes	$CD4^+$ T cells NK cells T cells	IFN-γ production Activation Activation			
Stem cell factor	Bone marrow stroma	Stem cells Progenitor cells	Activation Enhances effects of other CSFs	Increased during transition from yolk sac to hepatic to marrow hematopoiesis		Macrocytic anemia, death
Interleukin-3	$CD4^+$ T cells	B cells Macrophages T cells	Expands all lineages Mast cell expansion	Present in yolk sac (rat) Increased erythropoiesis from hepatic stem cells		
G-CSF	Monocytes Endothelial cells Fibroblasts	Committed progenitors	Differentiation to granulocytes	Present in fetal bone rudiment at 6 wk postconception and liver at 8 wk		Neutropenia
GM-CSF	T cells Monocytes Endothelial cells Fibroblasts	Progenitors Monocytes	Differentiation to granulocytes and monocytes	Present in yolk sac (rat)	In amniotic fluid; increases with gestation	
M-CSF	Monocytes Endothelial cells Fibroblasts	Progenitors	Differentiation to macrophages	In fetal liver and bone marrow at 6 wk postconception		Deficient in osteoclasts; osteopetrosis
Interleukin-7	Fibroblasts Bone marrow stroma	Progenitors	Differentiation of B cells	Increased B cell precursors and γβ receptor expression from fetal thymocytes (mice)		
Interleukin-11	Bone marrow stroma	Megakaryocytes	Increased megakaryopoiesis Increased macrophage production			

CSF, colony-stimulating factor; G-CSF, granulocyte colony-stimulating factor; GM-CSF, granulocyte-macrophage colony-stimulating factor; IFN, interferon; IgE, immunoglobulin E; LPS, lipopolysaccharide; M-CSF, macrophage colony-stimulating factor; NK, natural killer; TGF, transforming growth factor; TNF, tumor necrosis factor.

Adapted from Abbas AK, Lichtman AH, Prober JS (eds): Cellular and Molecular Immunology, 2nd ed. Philadelphia: WB Saunders, 1994, p 243.

fetal NK cell immunity to infections by viruses such as herpes simplex.[78, 79] Type 1 IFN-receptor–deficient mice have a threefold increase in circulating monocytes and neutrophils and are extremely susceptible to certain viral infections.[80]

Tumor Necrosis Factor-α

TNF-α is the cytokine responsible for the host response to gram-negative bacterial infection and specifically to LPS. TNF-α is produced by LPS-activated macrophages but can also be produced by activated T cells, NK cells, and mast cells. In mice, TNF stimulates macrophages and is an activator of B cells. This cytokine is a principal mediator of septic shock.[42] TNF-α is produced by human fetal Kupffer cells in response to LPS.[81] TNF is produced by placental mononuclear cells,[82] is present in the amniotic fluid during the second and third trimesters,[83] and increases with premature rupture of membranes.[84] A mouse strain lacking TNF-α is resistant to shock induced by endotoxin, has increased susceptibility to *Listeria monocytogenes*, and lacks splenic primary B cell follicle production.[85]

Interleukin-1

IL-1 is a proinflammatory cytokine that is produced by macrophages and functions as a mediator of host inflammatory responses in natural immunity.[42] This cytokine is produced by human fetal Kupffer cells in response to LPS[81] and up-regulates production of G-CSF by monocytes from the bone marrow and liver of human fetuses.[86] IL-1 is produced by the interdigitating reticulum cells in the fetal thymic medulla. It increases the proliferative responses of fetal thymocyte progenitors to IL-2.[87] IL-1 is present in amniotic fluid and increases in response to premature rupture of membranes.[88] In this setting, it is thought to up-regulate production of GM-CSF by tracheal and bronchial epithelial cells[89] and to increase antibody production induced by IL-2.[11] A natural IL-1 receptor antagonist binds to the IL-1 receptor without signal transduction. This antagonist is present in high levels in amniotic fluid and may play a role in modulating the maternal immune response to the fetus.[90] IL-1–deficient mice have an impaired acute-phase inflammatory response and do not develop fever or anorexia, suggesting that IL-1 is an endogenous pyrogen and a mediator of inflammation.[91]

Interleukin-6

IL-6 supports hematopoietic progenitor growth, promotes T and B cell function, and mediates the acute-phase response of hepatocytes to inflammation. This cytokine is produced by lymphoid cells, monocytes, fibroblasts, keratinocytes, endothelial cells, and mesangium cells.[92] IL-6 promotes the differentiation of plasma cells,[93] causes growth of T cells,[94] and induces hepatocytes to produce acute-phase reactants.[95] IL-6 is produced in response to inflammatory cytokines, including IL-1, TNF, and IFN-β. Human fetal Kupffer cells produce IL-6 as early as 13 weeks postconception after stimulation with LPS.[36] IL-6 concentration increases in amniotic fluid in response to infection.[96] IL-6–deficient mice have increased mortality associated with infection by *L. monocytogenes* and *Candida albicans* because of severe impairment of neutrophil and macrophage responses.[97] These animals do not develop cachexia, fever, or anorexia in response to inflammation from a sterile turpentine abscess. They also have a blunted febrile response to influenza infection.[98]

Chemokines

Chemokines are a large family of structurally related cytokines that cause leukocytes to move specifically. Little is known about the expression and function of the various chemokines in the fetus. RANTES (i.e., regulated on activation, normally T cell expressed and secreted), a chemokine that acts on $CD4^+$ T cells and monocytes, is expressed in various fetal tissues, but in adults it is uniformly absent except in disease states.[99] Mice lacking the chemokine receptor 1 had disrupted trafficking and proliferation of myeloid progenitor cells, failure of neutrophil chemotaxis, and disruption of inflammatory responses.[100]

Interleukin-8

IL-8 is a chemokine that attracts neutrophils to inflammatory sites. IL-8 is produced constitutively by fetal thymic epithelial cells, and production is increased in the presence of IL-1 in tissue culture.[101] IL-8 is present in the cord blood sera of babies born with chorioamnionitis and increases with gestation. Its expression is decreased, however, in babies of mothers receiving steroids to induce fetal maturation.[102] Whereas many cytokines are elevated in the maternal blood, amniotic cavity, and fetus during chorioamnionitis, IL-8 is elevated only in the fetal blood.[74]

Interleukin-16

IL-16 is produced by activated CD8$^+$ lymphocytes and eosinophils, and it acts on monocytes, eosinophils, and CD4$^+$ lymphocytes.[103, 104] IL-16 is a soluble CD4 ligand and binds to CD4 to activate helper T cells. It is also a strong chemoattractant for lymphocytes and eosinophils. This cytokine is an inhibitor of replication of human immunodeficiency virus.[105] The role of IL-16 in the development of the immune system has not been established.

Cytokines that Modulate Adaptive Immunity

Interleukin-2

IL-2, also called T cell growth factor, stimulates the proliferation of T cells and is a pleiotropic activator of T and B lymphocytes and NK cells.[106] IL-2 is produced by CD4$^+$ (helper) T cells. It stimulates CD8$^+$ cell-mediated cytotoxicity and delayed hypersensitivity. IL-2 promotes proliferation of mature B cells but not B-1 cells, the predominant B cell type in early human development. [107] IL-2 promotes immunoglobulin production by B-1 and mature B cells.[11] It is unknown when IL-2 is first produced in human fetal development. In mice, IL-2 promotes the expansion of NK cells in tissue culture from fetal liver cells.[108] When the IL-2 receptor-β is blocked with a neutralizing monoclonal antibody, mice fail to develop dendritic cells in the skin.[109]

Interleukin-4

IL-4 is a major regulator of allergic responses.[110] IL-4 is produced by helper T cells, mast cells, and basophils.[42] IL-4 stimulates the proliferation and differentiation of B cells and induces production of IgM, IgG, and IgE, but not IgA, by pre-B cells from the liver, spleen, and bone marrow as early as 12 weeks postconception.[111] Production of IL-4 by the mouse placenta is thought to promote antibody production and inhibit fetal rejection.[72] Excess IL-4 production has been associated with allergy, hyper-IgE syndrome, and Omen's syndrome.[61] Increased levels of IL-4 have been demonstrated in cord blood of neonates living in areas endemic for schistosomiasis, filariasis, and tuberculosis.[112]

Transforming Growth Factor-β

This cytokine family contains a number of genetically distinct but similar molecules that have pleiotropic effects on numerous tissue types and are important in normal development. Transforming growth factor-β (TGF-β) is produced by macrophages and T lymphocytes and is thought to inhibit the effects of inflammatory cytokines on their target cells.[42] It is present in large quantities in the extracellular matrix of the decidua and inhibits the proliferation of trophoblast cells in tissue culture.[113] Lack of TGF-β may explain why fetal skin does not scar when wounded, because production of this cytokine in the skin is thought to be necessary for the inflammatory reaction that results in scar in adult skin.[114] Deficient mice die from spontaneous multi-organ inflammatory reactions.[115, 116]

Cytokines that Regulate Immune-Mediated Inflammation

Interferon-γ

IFN-γ is produced by T cells and NK cells and is an activator of macrophages.[117] This cytokine has pleiotropic activity, including direct antiviral activity, stimulation of macrophages and NK cells, and increased expression of MHC antigens. Increased levels of IFN-γ have been demonstrated in cord blood of neonates living in areas endemic for schistosomiasis, filariasis, and tuberculosis.[112] In mice, IFN-γ is produced at low levels by the placenta in the first trimester but is not detectable during the rest of pregnancy.[72] Mice deficient in IFN-γ or its receptor have increased susceptibility to infection by intracellular organisms such as *L. monocytogenes* and certain viruses.[117, 118]

Lymphotoxin

Lymphotoxin, also called TNF-β, is produced by activated T lymphocytes and is approximately 30% homologous with TNF. In contrast to TNF, little lymphotoxin can be detected in the circulation, and it is thought to act in a paracrine fashion. Lymphotoxin activates neutrophils, stimulates vascular endothelial cells to produce cytokines, and promotes extravasation of leukocytes from blood vessels.[42] The expression of lymphotoxin in the human fetus is unknown. Lymphotoxin-deficient mice fail to form lymph nodes and Peyer's patches, and they have abnormal splenic follicular structure.[119] These animals produce high levels of antigen-specific IgM but are unable to class switch to IgG. This is thought to be caused by abnormal spleen follicle structure.[120]

Interleukin-5

IL-5 promotes the growth of activated B cells and eosinophils.[121] Like IL-4, increased levels of IL-5 have been demonstrated in cord blood of neonates living in areas endemic for schistosomiasis, filariasis, and tuberculosis.[112] This interleukin is produced by the placenta throughout pregnancy in mice.[72] IL-5–deficient mice are unable to mobilize eosinophils during allergic responses[122] and fail to develop eosinophilia when infected with the parasite *Toxocara canis*.[123]

Interleukin-10

IL-10 is an anti-inflammatory cytokine produced by activated CD4+ T cells,[124] B cells,[125] and monocytes.[126] IL-10 prevents antigen-specific T cell activation, causing a secondary decrease in antigen presentation by monocytes, macrophages, Langerhans cells, and dendritic cells. IL-10 inhibits T cell proliferation by inhibiting IL-2 production, and in mice it prevents the development of shock in response to LPS.[127] In contrast to its effects on T cells, IL-10 causes plasma cells to proliferate and enhances immunoglobulin production. Production by the placenta may prevent immune rejection of the fetus.[128] Mice deficient in IL-10 spontaneously develop enteritis, which resolves with administration of IL-10.[129–131]

Interleukin-12

IL-12 stimulates cell-mediated immunity after certain infections. It is produced by monocytes and macrophages, and it acts on T and B lymphocytes and NK cells. IL-12 is thought to connect innate immunity with acquired immunity. It stimulates CD8+ cells to become cytotoxic lymphocytes.[42] IL-12 is a potent inducer of IFN-γ production, conveys resistance to bacterial and parasitic infections, promotes antitumor immunity, and influences antiviral responses.[132] IL-12 is produced in active lesions in multiple sclerosis and may be a mediator of autoimmunity.[133] Little is known about its function in the fetus.

Interleukin-13

IL-13 is produce by activated T cells. It inhibits production of proinflammatory cytokines and chemokines by monocytes and promotes B cell proliferation and differentiation. Whereas IL-4 acts on T and B cells, IL-13 activity is limited to B cells.[134] This cytokine induces expression of IgE by pre-B cells from the marrow and spleen, although not to the same extent as IL-4.[135] Its expression and function in the fetus is unknown.

Interleukin-17

IL-17 is produced by CD4+ T cells and is a proinflammatory cytokine.[136] IL-17 induces IL-6 secretion from mouse stromal cells.[137] It is not known what influence IL-17 has on the development of immunity.

Interleukin-18

The cytokine IL-18 is a potent inducer of IFN-γ production by helper T cells.[138] IL-18 also increases the production of GM-CSF and decreases production of IL-10. This molecule was discovered in mouse hepatocytes,[139] but it is produced by multiple cell types, including osteoblasts, keratinocytes, and cells in the adrenal cortex.[140–142] IL-18 activates NK cells and cytotoxic T lymphocytes.[143] How this cytokine affects the development of the immune system is unknown.

Cytokines that Stimulate Hematopoiesis

Stem Cell Factor

Stem cell factor (SCF) acts on hematopoietic stem cells, progenitor cells, precursors, and mature forms of some cell lineages.[144] SCF binds with a cell-surface tyrosine kinase receptor called KIT.[145] SCF exists in a soluble circulating form and two distinct transmembrane forms.[144] All forms of SCF are produced by fibroblasts and endothelial cells.[146, 147] SCF enhances the effects of other colony-stimulating factors on hematopoietic cells in culture.[148] It promotes mast cell production by fetal liver cells[149] and cord blood progenitors.[150] SCF also plays a role in the early stages of lymphocyte development[151] and the normal fetal development of gut-associated lymphoid tissue.[152] Absence of SCF or KIT in mice leads to perinatal death from severe macrocytic anemia.[153]

SCF messenger RNA is present in the yolk sac, liver, thymus, and marrow of the fetal mouse, and its expression correlates with the periods of transition from yolk sac to fetal liver to bone marrow hematopoiesis.[151] SCF is thought to be involved in the migration of other cell types such as germ cells and melanocytes.[154]

Interleukin-3

IL-3 is produced by activated T cells and promotes the differentiation of human basophils and hematopoietic progenitor cells.[155–157] IL-3, GM-CSF, and IL-5 produce similar hematopoietic effects by signaling through a common receptor subunit called beta c. IL-3 can maximize the development of erythroid progenitors from fetal mouse liver cells grown in culture with erythropoietin.[158] IL-3 is expressed very early in rat fetal development; it is present in the day 7 yolk sac.[159] It also is produced by the placenta in the mouse.[72] Its function in human fetal development has not been established.

Interleukin-15

IL-15 is a T cell growth factor that resembles IL-2 in biologic activity, but unlike IL-2, it is produced by macrophages.[160] IL-15 is an activator of T cells and NK cells. It promotes immunoglobulin production from B cells. It is not known what role this cytokine plays in the development of the immune system.

Granulocyte Colony-Stimulating Factor

G-CSF is a promoter of neutrophil production and differentiation.[161] G-CSF is present in developing fetal bone as early as 6 weeks postconception[38] and in the fetal liver at least as early as 8 weeks postconception.[19] Monocytes in the fetal liver and bone marrow produce G-CSF in response to IL-1.[86] Mice deficient in G-CSF have decreased hematopoietic progenitors and neutropenia.[162]

Granulocyte-Macrophage Colony-Stimulating Factor

GM-CSF is a pleiotropic cytokine that acts on most hematopoietic cell types.[163, 164] It stimulates proliferation and differentiation of granulocyte and macrophages[164] and promotes phagocytosis, chemotaxis, adhesion, and tumor lysis.[165] GM-CSF is produced by T lymphocytes, macrophages, endothelial cells, trophoblasts, and decidua and the epithelial lining of the bronchi, trachea, and amnion. GM-CSF is present in the yolk sac of the day 7 fetal rat.[159] It is also present in the amniotic fluid, increasing with gestational age. GM-CSF is produced by the fetal lung epithelium and is involved with pulmonary homeostasis.[166]

GM-CSF–deficient mice have normal hematopoiesis but develop alveolar proteinosis caused by the accumulation of surfactant and proteins in the alveolar space.[167, 168] In transgenic mice overexpressing GM-CSF, macrophage proliferation and activation cause widespread abnormalities and death.[169] Mice lacking G-CSF and GM-CSF have more severe neutropenia during the first 2 weeks of life than mice lacking G-CSF alone, suggesting that GM-CSF contributes to neutrophil production and that G-CSF and GM-CSF have redundant effects.[170]

Macrophage Colony-Stimulating Factor

Macrophage colony-stimulating factor (M-CSF) is an essential growth factor for monocytes and macrophages.[171] It is secreted by monocytes, endothelial cells, and fibroblasts[42] and acts on nearby cells. Circulating M-CSF has no recognized physiologic affect.[172] M-CSF is present in the human fetal liver and developing fetal bone as early as 6 weeks postconception.[19]

Mice that are deficient in M-CSF lack osteoclasts and develop osteopetrosis and are secondarily deficient in G-CSF.[173] At birth these mice have a deficiency of monocytes but over time show hematopoietic recovery,[174] demonstrating the ability of the hematopoietic system to use alternative compensatory mechanisms, possibly through cytokines with partially overlapping functions.[170]

Interleukin-7

IL-7 may be an important regulator for the earliest stages of T cell development[175] and is essential for B lymphopoiesis in mice.[176] IL-7 is produced by stromal cells in the bone marrow and the fetal thymic epithelium.[177, 178] Expression of this cytokine by thymic cells in the fetal mouse is markedly increased compared with the adult.[179] IL-7 is thought to be stored within bone marrow stromal cells and is secreted directly to adjacent B cells in a tightly regulated manner.[180]

Studies of the effects of IL-7 on human fetal marrow cells are contradictory. In one study, exogenous IL-7 caused proliferation of fetal B cell precursors, which was potentiated by increased numbers of stromal cells, suggesting it acts in conjunction with another factor produced by the bone marrow stroma.[181] However, another study showed that adding IL-7 or anti-IL-7 receptor antibody to human fetal stem cells grown in bone marrow stromal culture had no influence on B cell development.[182] IL-7 promotes $\gamma\delta$ chain formation and expression of CD8 in fetal mouse thymocytes.[183] IL-7 treatment causes proliferation of immature T cells and expression of the $\gamma\delta$ receptor.[184] It stimulates the proliferation and colony formation of $CD4^+$, $CD8^+$ double-positive, and $CD4^+$ thymocytes from human fetal thymocytes in vitro.[175] IL-7–deficient mice have a defect in early steps of lymphopoiesis, with apoptosis of T cell progenitors. Addition of IL-7 allows the cells to survive. This suggests that IL-7 is required for survival of lymphocyte precursors before TCR rearrangement.[178, 185]

Interleukin-11

IL-11 is a pleiotropic cytokine produced by osteoblasts, alveolar cells, and bronchial epithelial cells, and it acts on hematopoietic, hepatic, stromal epithelial, neural, and osteoclastic cells. It stimulates the growth of myeloid colonies from stem cells in mice. This cytokine is produced by bone marrow stroma and stimulates megakaryopoiesis and production of macrophages. Fetal production of this cytokine is unreported.

CONCLUSIONS

The development of a functional immune system is a highly complex process. The first mechanisms that develop in the human fetus are systems of natural immunity similar to those in less complex animals. By the eighth week after conception, lymphocytes are present, and by the 11th week, cell-mediated immunity begins to develop. During the 11th through 18th weeks, lymph nodes are developing in the intestines and periphery. Functional immunity continues to develop after birth.

Scientists are only beginning to understand the mechanisms that control the development of the immune system and the differences among the immune systems of fetuses, neonates, and adults. New technologies in molecular genetics will allow researchers to dissect the events that control the development of immunity at a molecular level. Such knowledge will promote the development of treatments for congenital immunodeficiencies and further our ability to care for infected premature and term neonates.

References

1. Raghunathan R, Miller M, Wuest C, Faust J: Ontogeny of the immune system: fetal lamb as a model. Pediatr Res 1984;18:451.
2. Zurawski G, de Vries JE: Interleukin 13 elicits a subset of the activities of its close relative interleukin 4. Stem Cells (Dayt) 1994;12:169.
3. Dudley DJ, Wiedmeier S: The ontogeny of the immune response: perinatal perspectives. Semin Perinatol 1991;15:184.
4. Janeway CAG: Approaching the asymptote? Evolution and revolution in immunology. Cold Spring Harbor Symp Quant Biol 1989;54:1.
5. Sharp JG, Crouse DA, Purtilo DT: Ontogeny and regulation of the immune system. Arch Pathol Lab Med 1987;111:1106.
6. Beck G, Habicht GS: The evolution of the immune system: immunity and the invertebrates. Sci Am 1996;275:60.
7. Orkin SH: Molecular genetics of chronic granulomatous disease. Ann Immunol 1989;7:277.
8. Segal AW, Jones OT, Webster D, Allison AC: Absence of a newly described cytochrome *b* from neutrophils of patients with chronic granulomatous disease. Lancet 1978;2:446.
9. Litman G: Sharks and the origin of vertebrate immunity. Sci Am 1996;275:67.
10. Wolpert L: The Triumph of the Embryo. New York: Oxford University Press, 1991.
11. Allison AC, Nawata Y: Cytokines mediating the proliferation and differentiation of B-1 lymphocytes and their role in ontogeny and phylogeny. Ann N Y Acad Sci 1992;651:200.
12. Dieterlen-Lievre F: On the origin of haemopoietic stem cells in the avian embryo: and experimental approach. J Embryol Exp Morphol 1975;33:607.
13. Yoder MC, Hiatt K: Engraftment of embryonic hematopoietic cells in conditioned newborn recipients. Blood 1997;89:2176.
14. Huyhn A, Dommergues M, Izac B, et al: Characterization of hematopoietic progenitors from human yolk sacs and embryos. Blood 1995;86:4474.
15. Tavassoli M: Embryonic and fetal hemopoiesis: an overview. Blood Cells 1991;1:269.
16. Enzan H: Electron microscopic studies of macrophages in early human yolk sacs. Acta Pathol Jpn 1986;36:49.
17. Kelemen E, Calvo W, Fliedner TM: Atlas of Human Hemopoietic Development. New York: Springer-Verlag, 1979.
18. Kelemen EJM: Macrophages are the first differentiated blood cells formed in human embryonic liver. Exp Hematol 1980;8:996.
19. Slayton WB, Juul SE, Calhoun DA, et al: Hematopoiesis in the liver and marrow of human fetuses at 5 to 16 weeks postconception: quantitative assessment of macrophage and neutrophil populations. Pediatr Res 1998;43, 774.
20. Charboard P, Tavian M, Humeau L, Peault B: Early ontogeny of the human marrow from long bones: an immunohistochemical study of hematopoiesis and its micro-environment. Blood 1996;78:4109.
21. Haynes BF, Denning SM, Singer KH, Kurtzberg J: Ontogeny of T cell precursors: a model for the initial stages of human T-cell development. Immunol Today 1989;10:87.
22. Haynes BF, Martin ME, Kay HH, Kurtzberg J: Early events in human T cell ontogeny: phenotypic characterization and immunohistologic localization of T cell precursors in early human fetal tissues. J Exp Med 1988;168:1061.
23. Calhoun DA, Li Y, Braylan RC, Christensen RD: Assessment of the contribution of the spleen to granulocytopoiesis and erythropoiesis of the mid-gestation human fetus. Early Hum Dev 1996;46:217.
24. MacDonald TT, Spencer J: Ontogeny of the gut-associated lymphoid system in man. Acta Paediatr Suppl 1994;395:3.
25. Van Furth R: Cellular biology of pulmonary macrophages. Int Arch Allergy Appl Immunol 1985; 76(Suppl 1):21.
26. Sorokin SP, McNelly NA, Hoyt RF: CFU-rAM, the origin of lung macrophages, and the macrophage lineage. Am J Physiol 1992;263:L299.
27. Naito M, Takahashi T, Nishikawa S: Development, differentiation, and maturation of macrophages in the fetal mouse liver. J Leukoc Biol 1990;48:27.
28. Hinchliffe JR, Johnson DR: The Development of the Vertebrate Limb. Oxford: Clarendon Press, 1980.
29. Hofman F, Danilovs J, Husmann L, Taylor C: Ontogeny of B cell markers in the human fetal liver. J Immunol 1984;133:1197.
30. De Felici M, Heasman J, Wylie CC, McLaren A: Macrophages in the urogenital ridge of the mid-gestation mouse fetus. Cell Differ 1986;18:119.
31. Perry VH, Hume DA, Gordon S: Immunocytochemical localization of macrophages and microglia in the adult and developing mouse brain. Neuroscience 1985;15:313.
32. Hume DA, Perry VH, Gordon S: Immunohistochemical localization of macrophage-specific antigen in developing mouse embryos: phagocytosis of dying neurons and differentiation of microglial cells to form a regular array in the plexiform layers. J Cell Biol 1983;97:253.
33. Hopkinson-Wooley J, Hughes D, Gordon S, Martin P: Macrophage recruitment during limb development and wound healing in the embryonic and foetal mouse. J Cell Sci 1984;107:1159.
34. Lang RA, Bishop JM: Macrophages are required for cell death and tissue remodeling in the developing mouse eye. Cell 1993;74:453.
35. Naito M, Takahashi K, Takahashi H, Kojima M: Ontogenic Development of Kuppfer Cells. Amsterdam: Elsevier Biomedical Press, 1982.
36. Kutteh W, Rainey W, Carr B: Regulation of interleukin-6 production in human fetal Kupffer cells. Scand J Immunol 1991;33:607.
37. Fukuda T: Electron microscopic studies on human hepatic hemopoiesis. Virchows Arch B 1974;16:249.

38. Slayton WB, Li Y, Calhoun DA: The first appearance of neutrophils in the human fetal bone marrow cavity. Early Hum Dev 1998;53:129.
39. Buccheri V, Shetty V, Yoshida N, et al: The role of an anti-myeloperoxidase antibody in the diagnosis and classification of acute leukaemia, a comparison with light and electron microscopy. Br J Haematol 1992;80:62.
40. Christensen RD, Rothstein G: Pre- and postnatal development of granulocytic stem cells in the rat. Pediatr Res 1984;18:599.
41. Christensen RD, Hill HR, Rothstein G: Granulocytic stem cell CFU(c) proliferation in experimental group B streptococcal sepsis. Pediatr Res 1983;17:278.
42. Abbas AK, Lichtman AH, Pober JS (eds): Cellular and Molecular Immunology, 2nd ed. Philadelphia: WB Saunders, 1994.
43. Henkart P, Yue CC: The role of cytoplasmic granules in lymphocyte cytotoxicity. Prog Allergy 1998;40:82.
44. Phillips JH, Hori T, Nagler A, et al: Ontogeny of human natural killer (NK) cells: fetal NK cells mediate cytolytic function and express cytoplasmic CD3 epsilon, delta proteins. J Exp Med 1992;175:1055.
45. Lopez C: Role of natural killer cells in resistance to virus infections. In Lopez C (ed): Immunology and Pathogenesis of Persistent Virus Infections. Washington, DC: American Society of Microbiology, 1988, pp 39–53.
46. Colten HR, Godberger G: Ontogeny of serum complement proteins. Pediatrics 1979;64:775.
47. Ballow M, Fung F, Good RA, et al: Developmental aspects of complement components in the newborn. Clin Exp Immunol 1974;18:257.
48. Lobach DF, Haynes BF: Ontogeny of the human thymus during fetal development. J Clin Immunol 1987;7:81.
49. Allison JP, Lanier LL: Structure, function, and serology of the T-cell antigen receptor complex. Annu Rev Immunol 1987;5:503.
50. Krangel MS, Yssel H, Brocklehurst C, Spits H: A distinct wave of human T cell receptor gamma/delta lymphocytes in the early fetal thymus: evidence for controlled gene rearrangement and cytokine production. J Exp Med 1990;172:847.
51. Freedman MS, D'Souza S, Antel JP: Gamma-delta T-cell-human glial cell interactions. I. In vitro induction of gamma-delta T-cell expansion by human glial cells. J Neuroimmunol 1997;74:135.
52. Adkins B, Mueller C, Okada CY, et al: Early events in T-cell maturation. Annu Rev Immunol 1987;5:325.
53. Haynes B: The role of the thymic microenvironment in promotion of early stages of human T cell maturation. Clin Res 1986;34:422.
54. Germain RH, Marguiles DM: The biochemistry and cell biology of antigen processing and presentation. Annu Rev Immunol 1993;11:403.
55. Kingsley G, Pitzalis C, Waugh AP, Panayi GS: Correlation of immunoregulatory function with cell phenotype in cord blood lymphocytes. Clin Exp Immunol 1988;73:40.
56. Paganelli R, Cherchi M, Scala E, et al: Activated and "memory" phenotype of circulating T lymphocytes in intrauterine life. Cell Immunol 1994;155:486.
57. Bruning T, Daiminger A, Enders G: Diagnostic value of CD45RO expression on circulating T lymphocytes of fetuses and newborn infants with pre-, peri- or early post-natal infections. Clin Exp Immunol 1997; 107:306.
58. Granberg C, Hirvonen T: Cell-mediated lympholysis by fetal and neonatal lymphocytes in sheep and man. Cell Immunol 1980;51:15.
59. Granberg C, Manninen K, Toivanen P: Cell-mediated lympholysis by human neonatal lymphocytes. Clin Immunol Immunopathol 1976;6:256.
60. Bendelac A, Matzinger P, Seder RA, et al: Activation events during thymic selection. J Exp Med 1992;175:731.
61. Wilson CB, Penix L, Melvin A, Lewis DB: Lymphokine regulation and the role of abnormal regulation in immunodeficiency. Clin Immunol Immunopathol 1993;67:S25.
62. Durandy A, De Saint-Basile G, Lisowska-Grospierre B, et al: Undetectable CD40 ligand expression on T cells and low B cell responses to CD40 binding agonists in human newborns. J Immunol 1995;154:1560.
63. Lawton AR, Cooper MD: B-cell ontogeny: immunoglobulin genes and their expression. Pediatrics 1979;64:750.
64. Gathings WE, Lawton AR, Cooper MD: Immunofluorescent studies on the development of pre-B cells, B lymphocytes, and immunoglobulin isotype diversity in humans. Eur J Immunol 1977;7:804.
65. Coffman RL, Seymour BW, Lebman DA, et al: The role of helper T cell products in mouse B cell differentiation and isotype regulation. Immunol Rev 1988;102:5.
66. Waddick KG, Uckun FM: CD5 antigen-positive B lymphocytes in human B cell ontogeny during fetal development and after autologous bone marrow transplantation. Exp Hematol 1993;21:791.
67. Plater-Zyberk C, Lam K, Kennedy TD, et al: Increased representation of a subpopulation of early B cells in the peripheral blood of patients with rheumatoid arthritis. Adv Exp Biol Med 1985;186:957.
68. Casali P, Burastero SE, Nakamura M, et al: Human lymphocytes making rheumatoid factor and antibody to ssDNA belong to Leu-1^{+} B-cell subset. Science 1987;236:77.
69. Gathings W, Kubagawa H, Cooper M: A distinctive pattern of B cell immaturity in perinatal humans. Immunol Rev 1981;57:107.
70. Cooper M: Current concepts: B lymphocytes-normal development and function. N Engl J Med 1987;317:1452.
71. Mellander L, Carlsson B, Hanson LA: Secretory IgA, and IgM antibodies to *E. coli* and poliovirus type 1 antigens occur in amniotic fluid, meconium and saliva from newborns. A neonatal immune response without antigenic exposure: a result of anti-idiotypic induction? Clin Exp Immunol 1985;63:555.
72. Lin H, Mosmann TR, Guilbert L, et al: Synthesis of T helper 2-type cytokines at the maternal-fetal interface. J Immunol 1993;151:4562.
73. Formby B: Immunologic response in pregnancy: its role in endocrine disorders of pregnancy and influence on the course of maternal autoimmune diseases. Endocrinol Metab Clin North Am 1995;24:187.
74. Stallmach T, Hebisch G, Joller-Jemelka HI, et al: Cytokine production and visualized effects in the feto-maternal unit: quantitative and topographic data on cytokines during intrauterine disease. Lab Invest 1995;73:384.
75. Beck G, Habicht GS: Primitive cytokines: harbingers of vertebrate defense. Immunol Today 1991;88:9518.
76. Johnston JA, Bacon CM, Riedy MC, O'Shea JJ: Signaling by IL-2 and related cytokines: JAKs, STATs, and relationship to immunodeficiency. J Leukoc Biol 1996;60:441.
77. Shields DC, Harmon DL, Nunez F, Whitehead AS: The evolution of haematopoietic cytokine/receptor complexes. Cytokine 1995;7:679.

78. Bennett WA, Lagoo-Deenadayalan S, Brackin MN, et al: Cytokine expression by models of human trophoblast as assessed by semiquantitative reverse transcription–polymerase chain reaction technique. Am J Reprod Immunol 1996;36:285.
79. Aboagye-Mathieson G, Toth FD, Zdrvkovic M, Ebbesen P: Human trophoblast interferons: production and possible roles in early pregnancy. Early Pregnancy 1995;1:45.
80. Muller U, Steinhoff U, Reis LFL, et al: Functional role of type I and type II interferons in antiviral defense. Science 1994;264:1918.
81. Kutteh WH, Rainey WE, Beutler B, Carr BR: Tumor necrosis factor-alpha and interleukin 1-beta production of human fetal Kupffer cells. Am J Obstet Gynecol 1991;165:112.
82. Reuben JM, Gonik B, Li S, et al: Induction of cytokines in normal placental cells by the human immunodeficiency virus. Lymphokine Cytokine Res 1991;10:195.
83. Saksela E, Jaattela M: Tumor necrosis factor in the human fetoplacentary unit. Int J Dev Biol 1989;33:173.
84. Romero R, Mazor M, Brandt F, et al: Tumor necrosis factor in preterm and term labor. Am J Obstet Gynecol 1992;27:1576.
85. Pasparakis M, Alexopoulou L, Episkopou V, Kollias G: Immune and inflammatory responses in TNF alpha-deficient mice: a critical requirement for TNF alpha in the formation of primary B cell follicles, follicular dendritic cell networks and germinal centers, and in the maturation of the humoral immune response. J Exp Med 1996;184:1397.
86. Ohls RK, Li Y, Abdel-Mageed A, et al: Neutrophil pool sizes and granulocyte colony-stimulating factor production in human mid-trimester fetuses. Pediatr Res 1995;37:806.
87. Wood GW, Greenwood JH: Murine CD4$^-$CD8$^-$ thymocytes are stimulated by interleukin-2 to proliferate in vitro in chemically defined medium. Thymus 1991;18:15.
88. Romero R, Mazor M, Brandt F, et al: Interleukin-1-alpha and interleukin-1-beta in preterm and term human parturition. Am J Reprod Immunol 1992;27:117.
89. Scott SM, Buenaflor G, Orth D: Immunoreactive human epidermal growth factor concentrations in amniotic fluid, umbilical artery and vein serum, and placenta in full-term and preterm infants. Biol Neonate 1989;56:246.
90. Bry K, Lappalainen U, Waffarn F, et al: Influence of fetal gender on the concentration of interleukin-1 receptor antagonist in amniotic fluid and in newborn urine. Pediatr Res 1994;35:130.
91. Zheng H, Fletcher D, Kozak W, et al: Resistance to fever induction and impaired acute-phase response in interleukin-1 beta-deficient mice. Immunity 1995;3:9.
92. Kishimoto T: The biology of interleukin-6. Blood 1989;74:1.
93. Hirano T, Yasukawa K, Harada H, et al: Complementary DNA for a novel human interleukin (BSF-2) that induces B lymphocytes to produce immunoglobulin. Nature 1986;324:73.
94. Noma T, Mizuta T, Rosen A, et al: Enhancement of the interleukin 2 receptor expression on T cells by multiple B-lymphotropic lymphokines. Immunol Lett 1987;15:249.
95. Castell JV, Gomez-Lechon MJ, Hirano DM, et al: Recombinant human interleukin-6 (IL-6/BSF-2/HSF) regulates the synthesis of acute phase proteins in human hepatocytes. FEBS Lett 1988;234:17.
96. Liechty KW, Koenig JM, Mitchell MD, et al: Production of interleukin-6 by fetal and maternal cells in vivo during intraamniotic infection and in vitro after stimulation with interleukin-1. Pediatr Res 1991;29:1–4.
97. Romani L, Mencacci A, Cenci E, et al: Impaired neutrophil response and CD4$^+$ T helper cell 1 development in interleukin-6–deficient mice infected with *Candida albicans*. J Exp Med 1996;183:1345.
98. Kozak W, Poli V, Soszynski D, et al: Sickness behavior in mice deficient in interleukin-6 during turpentine abscess and influenza pneumonitis. Am J Physiol 1997;272:R621.
99. von Luettichau I, Nelson PJ, Pattison JM, et al: RANTES chemokine expression in diseased and normal human tissues. Cytokine 1996;8:89.
100. Gao JL, Wynn TA, Chang Y, et al: Impaired host defense, hematopoiesis, granulomatous inflammation and type 1–type 2 cytokine balance in mice lacking CC chemokine receptor 1. J Exp Med 1997;185:1959.
101. Shu S, Naylor P, Touraine JL, Hadden JW: IL-1, ICAM-1, LFA-3, and hydrocortisone differentially regulate cytokine secretion by human fetal thymic epithelial cells. Thymus 1996;24:89.
102. Shimoya K, Matsuzaki N, Taniguchi T, et al: Interleukin-8 in cord sera: a sensitive and specific marker for the detection of preterm chorioamnionitis. J Infect Dis 1992;165:957.
103. Zhou P, Goldstein S, Devadas K, et al: Human CD4$^+$ cells transfected with IL-16 cDNA are resistant to HIV-1 infection: inhibition of mRNA expression. Nat Med 1997;3:659.
104. Lim KG, Wan HC, Bozza PT, et al: Human eosinophils elaborate the lymphocyte chemoattractants: IL-16 (lymphocyte chemoattractant factor) and RANTES. J Immunol 1996;156:2566.
105. Maciaszek JW, Parada NA, Cruikshank WW, et al: IL-16 represses HIV-1 promoter activity. J Immunol 1997;158:5.
106. Smith KA: Interleukin 2: inception, impact and implications. Science 1988;240:1169.
107. Nawata Y, Stall AM, Herzenberg LA, et al: Surface immunoglobulin ligands and cytokines differentially affect proliferation and antibody production of human CD5$^+$ and CD5$^-$ B-lymphocytes. Int Immunol 1990;2:603.
108. Moingeon P, Rodewald HR, McConkey D, et al: Generation of natural killer cells from both Fc gamma RII/III$^+$ and Fc gamma RII/III$^-$ murine fetal liver progenitors. Blood 1993;82:1453.
109. Tanaka T, Takeuchi Y, Shiohara T, et al: In utero treatment with monoclonal antibody to IL-2 receptor beta-chain completely abrogates development of Thy-1$^+$ dendritic epidermal cells. Int Immunol 1992;4:487.
110. Noma Y, Sideras T, Naito T, et al: Cloning of cDNA encoding the murine IgG1 induction actor by a novel strategy using SP6 promoter. Nature 1986;319:640.
111. Punnonen J, Aversa GG, Vandekerckhove B, et al: Induction of isotype switching and Ig production by CD5$^+$ and CD10$^+$ human fetal B cells. J Immunol 1992;148:3398.
112. Malahotra I, Ouma J, Wamachi A, et al: In utero exposure to helminth and mycobacterial antigens generates cytokine responses similar to that observed in adults. J Clin Invest 1997;99:1759.
113. Graham CH, Lysiak JJ, McCrae KR, Lala PK: Localization of transforming growth factor-beta at the human fetal-maternal interface: role in trophoblast growth and differentiation. Biol Reprod 1992;46:561.
114. Lin RY, Sullivan KM, Argenta PA, et al: Exogenous

transforming growth factor-beta amplifies its own expression and induces scar formation in a model of human fetal tissue repair. Ann Surg 1995;222:146.
115. Boivin GP, Ormsby I, Jones-Carson J, et al: Germfree and barrier -raised TGF beta 1–deficient mice have similar inflammatory lesions. Transgenic Res 1997;6:197.
116. Letterio JJ, Geiser AG, Kulkarni AB, et al: Autoimmunity associated with TGF-beta1-deficiency in mice is dependent on MHC class II antigen expression. J Exp Med 1996;98:2109.
117. Dalton DK, Pitts-Meek S, Keshav S, et al: Multiple defects of immune cell function in mice with disrupted interferon-gamma genes. Science 1993;259:1739.
118. Huang S, Hendriks W, Althage A, et al: Immune response in mice that lack the interferon-gamma receptor. Science 1993;259:1742.
119. Fu YX, Huang G, Matsumoto M, et al: Independent signals regulate development of primary and secondary follicle structure in spleen and mesenteric lymph nodes. Proc Natl Acad Sci U S A 1997;94:5739.
120. Fu YX, Molina H, Matsumoto M, et al: Lymphotoxin-alpha (LT-alpha) supports development of splenic follicular structure that is required for IgG responses. J Exp Med 1997;185:2111.
121. Kinashi T, Harada N, Severinson E, et al: Cloning of complementary DNA encoding T-cell replacing factor and identity with B-cell growth factor, II. Nature 1986;324:70.
122. Mould AW, Matthaei KI, Foster PS: Relationship between interleukin-5 and eotaxin for the selective accumulation of eosinophils in mice. J Clin Invest 1997;99:1064.
123. Takamoto M, Ovington KS, Behm CA, et al: Eosinophilia, parasite burden and lung damage in Toxocara canis infection in C57BL/6 mice genetically deficient in IL-5. Immunology 1997;90:511.
124. Moore KW, O'Garra A, de Waal Malefyt R, et al: Interleukin-10. Annu Rev Immunol 1993;11:165.
125. Matthes T, Werener FC, Tang H, et al: Cytokine mRNA expression during an in vitro response of human B lymphocytes: kinetics of B cell tumor necrosis factor alpha, interleukin (IL)-6, IL-10, and transforming growth factor beta 1 mRNAs. J Exp Med 1993;178:521.
126. de Waal Malefyt R, Abrams J, Bennet B, et al: Interleukin 10 (IL-10) inhibits cytokine synthesis by human monocytes: an autoregulatory role of IL-10. J Exp Med 1991;174:1209.
127. de Vries JE: Immunosuppressive and anti-inflammatory properties of interleukin 10. Ann Med 1995;27:537.
128. Roth I, Corry DB, Locksley RM, et al: Human placental cytotrophoblasts produce the immunosuppressive cytokine interleukin 10. J Exp Med 1996;184:539.
129. van Hogezand RA, Verspaget HW: New therapies for inflammatory bowel disease: an update on chimeric anti-TNF alpha antibodies and IL-10 therapy. Scan J Gastroenterol Suppl 1997;223:105.
130. Fluckiger AC, Garrone P, Durand I, et al: Interleukin-10 (IL-10) upregulates functional high affinity IL-2 receptors on normal and leukemic B lymphocytes. J Exp Med 1993;178:1473.
131. Rousset F, Garcia E, Defrance T, et al: Interleukin-2 is a potent growth and differentiation factor for activated human B lymphocytes. Proc Natl Acad Sci U S A 1992;89:1890.
132. Germann T, Rude E: Interleukin 12. Int Arch Allergy Immunol 1995;108:103.
133. Becher B, Dodelet V, Fedorowicz V, Antel JP: Soluble tumor necrosis factor receptor inhibits interleukin 12 production by stimulated human adult microglial cells in vitro. J Clin Invest 1996;98:1539.
134. de Vries JE, Zurawski G: Immunoregulatory properties of IL-13: its potential role in atopic disease. Int Arch Allergy Immunol 1995;106:175.
135. Punnonen J, Cocks BG, de Vries JE: IL-4 induces germ-line IgE heavy chain gene transcription in human fetal pre-B cells: evidence for differential expression of functional IL-4 and IL-13 receptors during B cell ontogeny. J Immunol 1995;155:4248.
136. Fossiez F, Djossou O, Chomarat P, et al: T cell interleukin-17 induces stromal cells to produce proinflammatory and hematopoietic cytokines. J Exp Med 1996;183:2593.
137. Kennedy J, Rossi DL, Zurawski SM, et al: Mouse IL-17: a cytokine preferentially expressed by alpha beta $TCR^+ CD4^- CD8^-$ T cells. J Interferon Cytokine Res 1996;40:1050.
138. Taniguchi M, Nagaoka K, Kunikata T, et al: Characterization of anti-human interleukin-18 (IL-18)/interferon-gamma–inducing factor (IGIF) monoclonal antibodies and their application in the measurement of human IL-18 by ELISA. J Immunol Methods 1997;206:107.
139. Ushio S, Namba M, Okura T, et al: Cloning of the cDNA for human IFN-gamma–inducing factor, expression in *Escherichia coli*, and studies on the biologic activities of the protein. J Immunol 1996;156:4274.
140. Stoll S, Muller G, Kurimoto M, et al: Production of IL-18 (IFN-gamma–inducing factor) messenger RNA and functional protein by murine keratinocytes. J Immunol 1997;159:298.
141. Udagawa N, Horwood NJ, Elliott J, et al: Interleukin-18 (interferon-gamma–inducing factor) is produced by osteoblasts and acts via granulocyte/macrophage colony-stimulating factor and not via interferon-gamma to inhibit osteoclast formation. J Exp Med 1997;185:1005.
142. Conti B, Jahng JW, Tinti C, et al: Induction of interferon-gamma inducing factor in the adrenal cortex. J Biol Chem 1997;272:2035.
143. Micallef MJ, Tanimoto T, Kohno K, et al: Interleukin 18 induces the sequential activation of natural killer cells and cytotoxic T lymphocytes to protect syngeneic mice from transplantation with Meth A sarcoma. Cancer Res 1997;57:4557.
144. Broudy VC: Biology of stem cell factor. Blood 1997;90:1345.
145. Chabot B, Stephenson D, Chapman V, et al: The protooncogene c-kit encoding a transmembrane tyrosine kinase receptor maps to the mouse W locus. Nature 1988;335:88.
146. Linenberger ML, Jacobson FW, Bennett LG, et al: Stem cell factor production by human marrow stromal fibroblasts. Exp Hematol 1995;23:1104.
147. Heinrich MC, Dooley DC, Freed AC, et al: Constitutive expression of steel factor gene by human stromal cells. Blood 1993;82:771.
148. Bernstein ID, Andrews RG, Zsebo KM: Recombinant human stem cell factor enhances the formation of colonies by $CD34^+$ cord blood cells in the presence of recombinant human stem cell factor. Blood 1991;77:2316.
149. Irani AA, Nilsson G, Miettinen U, et al: Recombinant human stem cell factor stimulates differentiation of mast cells from dispersed human fetal liver cells. Blood 1992;80:3009.
150. Mitsui H, Furitsu T, Dvorak AM, et al: Development of human mast cells from umbilical cord blood cells

by recombinant human and murine c-kit ligand. Proc Natl Acad Sci U S A 1993;90:735.
151. Palacios R, Nishikawa SI: Developmentally regulated cell surface expression and function of c-kit receptor during lymphocyte ontogeny in the embryo and adult mice. Development 1992;115:1133.
152. Laky K, Lefrancois L, Puddington L: Age dependent lymphoproliferative disorder due to stem cell factor receptor deficiency. J Immunol 1997;158:1417.
153. Besmer P, Manova K, Duttlinger R, et al: The kit-ligand (steel factor) and its receptor c-kit/W: pleiotropic roles in gametogenesis and melanogenesis. Dev Suppl 1993;125:125.
154. Keshet E, Lyman SD, Williams DE, et al: Embryonic RNA expression patterns of the c-kit receptor and its cognate ligand suggest multiple functional roles in mouse development. EMBO J 1991;10:2425.
155. Valent P, Schmidt G, Besemer J, et al: Interleukin-3 is a differentiation factor for human basophils. Blood 1989;73:1763.
156. Saito H, Hatake K, Dvorak AM, et al: Selective differentiation and proliferation of hematopoietic cells induced by recombinant human interleukins. Proc Natl Acad Sci U S A 1988;85:2288.
157. Seldin DC, Caulfield JP, Hein A, et al: Biochemical and phenotypic characterization of human basophilic cells derived from dispersed fetal liver with murine T cell factors. J Immunol 1986;136:2222.
158. Yu H, Bauer B, Lipke GK, et al: Apoptosis and hematopoiesis in murine fetal liver. Blood 1993;81:373.
159. Yamashita A: Role of yolk sac endodermal cells with special reference to the fetal macrophage differentiation. J Leukoc Biol 1996;59:139.
160. Doherty TM, Seder RA, Sher A: Induction and regulation of IL-15 expression in murine macrophages. J Immunol 1996;156:735.
161. Dimetri G, Griffin J: Granulocyte colony-stimulating factor and its receptor. Blood 1991;78:2791.
162. Lieschke G, Grail D, Hodgson G, et al: Mice lacking granulocyte colony-stimulating factor have chronic neutropenia, granulocyte and macrophage progenitor cell deficiency, and impaired neutrophil mobilization. Blood 1994;84:1737.
163. Clark SC, Kamen R: The human hematopoietic colony-stimulating factors. Science 1987;236:1229.
164. Metcalf D: The molecular biology and functions of the granulocyte-macrophage colony-stimulating factors. Blood 1986;67:257.
165. Gasson JC: Molecular physiology of granulocyte-macrophage colony-stimulating factor. Blood 1991; 77:1131.
166. Bry K, Hallman M, Teramo K, et al: Granulocyte-macrophage colony-stimulating factor in amniotic fluid and in airway specimens of newborn infants. Pediatr Res 1997;41:105.
167. Stanley E, Lieschke GJ, Grail D, et al: Granulocyte/macrophage colony-stimulating factor-deficient mice show no major perturbation of hematopoiesis but develop a characteristic pulmonary pathology. Proc Natl Acad Sci U S A 1004;91:5592.
168. Dranoff G, Crawford AD, Sadelain M, et al: Involvement of granulocyte-macrophage colony stimulating factor in pulmonary homeostasis. Science 1994; 264:713.
169. Metcalf D, Moore JG: Divergent disease patterns in granulocyte-macrophage colony-stimulating factor transgenic mice associated with different transgene insertion sites. Proc Natl Acad Sci U S A 1988; 85:7767.
170. Seymour JF, Lieschke GJ, Grail D, et al: Mice lacking both granulocyte colony-stimulating factor (CSF) and granulocyte-macrophage CSF have impaired reproductive capacity, perturbed neonatal granulopoiesis, lung disease, amyloidosis, and reduced long-term survival. Blood 1997;90:3037.
171. Ralph P, Sampson-Johannes A: Macrophage growth and stimulating factor, M-CSF. Prog Clin Biol Res 1990;338:43.
172. Chen BD: In vivo administration of recombinant human interleukin-1 and macrophage colony-stimulating factor (M-CSF) induces a rapid loss of M-CSF receptors in mouse bone marrow cells and peritoneal macrophages: effect of administration route. Blood 1991;77:1923.
173. Wiktor-Jedrzejczak W, Bartocci A, Ferrante AW, et al: Total absence of colony-stimulating factor 1 in the macrophage deficient osteopetrotic (op/op) mouse. Proc Natl Acad Sci U S A 1990;87:4828.
174. Begg SK, Radley JM, Pollard JW, et al: Delayed hematopoietic development in osteopetrotic (op/op) mice. J Exp Med 1993;177:237.
175. Uckun FM, Tuel Ahlgren L, Obuz V, et al: Interleukin 7 receptor engagement stimulates tyrosine phosphorylation, inositol phospholipid turnover, proliferation, and selective differentiation to the CD4 lineage by human thymocytes. Proc Natl Acad Sci U S A 1991;88:6323.
176. von Freeden-Jeffry U, Vieira P, Lucian LA, et al: Lymphopenia in interleukin (IL-7) gene-deleted mice identifies IL-7 as a non-redundant cytokine. J Exp Med 1995;181:1519.
177. Funk PE, Stephan RP, Witte PL: Vascular cell adhesion molecule 1 positive reticular cells express interleukin-7 and stem cell factor in the bone marrow. Blood 1994;83:2661.
178. Oosterwegel MA, Haks MC, Jeffery U, et al: Induction of TCR gene rearrangements in uncommitted stem cells by a subset of IL-7, MHC class-II–expressing thymic stromal cells. Immunity 1997;6:351.
179. Appasamy PM: IL 7-induced T cell receptor-gamma gene expression by pre-T cells in murine fetal liver cultures. J Immunol 1992;149:1649.
180. Stephan RP, Reilly CR, Witte PL: Impaired ability of bone marrow stromal cells to support B-lymphopoiesis with age. Blood 1998;91:75.
181. Moreau I, Duvert V, Banchereau J, Saeland S: Culture of human fetal B-cell precursors on bone marrow stroma maintains highly proliferative CD20dim cells. Blood 1993;81:1170.
182. Prieyl JA, LeBien TW: Interleukin 7 independent development of human B cells. Proc Natl Acad Sci U S A 1996;93:10348.
183. Watanabe Y, Sudo T, Minato N, et al: Interleukin 7 preferentially supports the growth of gamma delta T cell receptor-bearing T cells from fetal thymocytes in vitro. Int Immunol 1991;3:1067.
184. Plum J, De Smedt M, Leclercq G: Exogenous IL-7 promotes the growth of $CD3^-CD4^-CD8^-CD44^+CD25^{+/-}$ precursor cells and blocks the differentiation pathway of TCR-alpha beta cells in fetal thymus organ culture. J Immunol 1993;150:2706.
185. von Freeden-Jeffrey U, Solavason N, Howard M, Murray R: The earliest T lineage-committed cells depend on IL-7 for Bcl-2 expression and normal cell cycle progression. Immunity 1997;7:147.

CHAPTER 3

Fetal Megakaryocytopoiesis

Martha C. Sola, M.D.

Platelets were first described in the early part of the 19th century, but it was not until 1906 that Wright recognized megakaryocytes as their origin.[1] Since then, the study of the mechanisms responsible for platelet production has focused on megakaryocytes. Through the years, however, it became evident that many factors complicated the study of these large and unusual cells. First, they are rare and among the most fragile cells in the bone marrow, composing only 0.03% to 0.1% of the nucleated marrow cells.[2] Second, the development of reproducible assay methods to culture megakaryocyte progenitors was hampered by the sensitivity of these cells to the inhibitory effects of certain cytokines (e.g., transforming growth factor-β [TGF-β]) that are common in the fetal bovine serum used in the assays for other types of hematopoietic progenitors.[3] Third, reliable distinction between megakaryocyte colonies and those of the granulocyte-monocyte lineage requires immunocytochemical staining for specific megakaryocyte antigens, such as GPIIb/IIIa.

Several scientific advances during the past 2 decades contributed greatly to understanding the process of megakaryocytopoiesis: improved culture methods for megakaryocytes,[4, 5] application of flow cytometric techniques to the study of megakaryocytopoiesis,[6, 7] and purification and cloning of thrombopoietin (TPO),[8] the most important physiologic regulator of platelet production.

MEGAKARYOCYTOPOIESIS

In studying developing granulocytes, the concept of *pools* has been widely used. Myeloblasts, promyelocytes, and myelocytes (i.e., cells with the capacity for cell division) are collectively designated the *neutrophil proliferative pool*, and metamyelocytes, band neutrophils, and segmented neutrophils (i.e., cells that have lost the capacity for cell division) are collectively known as the *neutrophil storage pool.*[9]

In a similar manner, the megakaryocyte compartment in the bone marrow has been described as consisting of two pools (Fig. 3–1).[10] One is composed of cells that are morphologically indistinguishable from other blasts but are committed to the megakaryocyte lineage. These *megakaryocyte progenitors* retain a high proliferative capacity and ultimately determine the number of megakaryocytes in the bone marrow. The other pool consists of nondividing cells in terminal stages of megakaryocyte differentiation. These cells, which are directly responsible for the number of platelets produced, are morphologically recognizable as *megakaryocytes* and undergo endoreduplication or endomitosis, a process in which the ploidy of the cell increases without undergoing cellular division. Some researchers add a third pool of cells to this classification, the *transitional cells* or *megakaryocyte precursors*.[11, 12] These cells are difficult to identify morphologically and are characterized by decreased proliferative potential and increased ploidy. They represent the transition between the megakaryocyte progenitors and the megakaryocytes and are viewed by some investigators as early or immature megakaryocytes (i.e., megakaryoblasts).

This chapter reviews the process of platelet production—the progenitors, megakaryocyte maturation, proplatelet formation, and platelet shedding. In each section, any differences between the adult and the fetus or neonate are addressed. The in vitro and in vivo effects of cytokines that participate in the process of megakaryocytopoiesis are described, with a special emphasis on TPO.

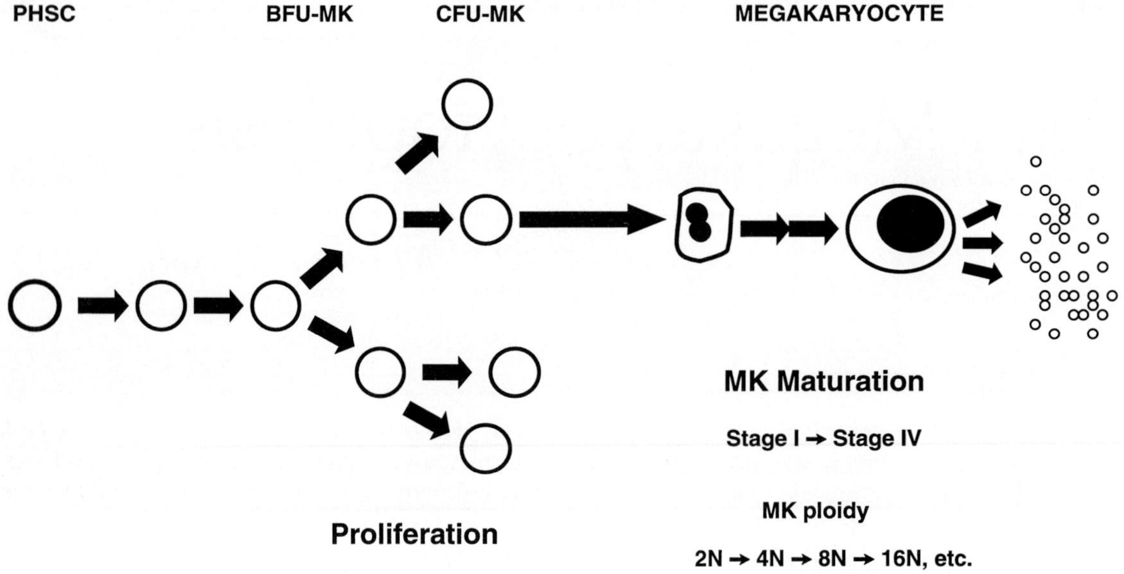

Figure 3–1. Simplified scheme of megakaryocytopoiesis. Megakaryocyte progenitors, such as burst-forming unit–megakaryocyte (BFU-MK) and colony-forming unit–megakaryocyte (CFU-MK), are cells that arise from pluripotent hematopoietic stem cells (PHSC) and have a high proliferative potential, determining the number of megakaryocytes (MK) in the bone marrow. Megakaryocytes are nondividing cells that undergo endoreduplication or endomitosis, a process in which the ploidy of the cell increases without undergoing cellular division.

Progenitors

Characterization

Megakaryocyte progenitors arise from pluripotent hematopoietic stem cells by a process that is still undefined but for which several theories have been proposed. Megakaryocyte progenitors can be identified by two methods: a culture system in which they are identified by their ability to form megakaryocyte colonies and by immunologic staining that allows characterization on the basis of the specific antigens expressed. Using these methods, two different megakaryocyte progenitor cells have been identified: the burst-forming unit–megakaryocyte (BFU-MK), which is the more primitive megakaryocyte progenitor,[13, 14] and the colony-forming unit–megakaryocyte (CFU-MK), which is the more differentiated progenitor.[10, 15] The two progenitor types can be differentiated on the basis of several parameters that disclose the more primitive nature of the BFU-MK (Table 3–1):

1. CFU-MK–derived colonies appear in vitro sooner than BFU-MK–derived colonies.
2. CFU-MK–derived colonies are smaller (3 to 50 cells/colony) and primarily unifocal (Fig. 3–2), whereas BFU-MK–derived colonies are larger (>50 cells/colony) and are composed of multiple foci of development (Fig. 3–3).
3. CFU-MK colony formation is severely reduced by exposure to 5-fluorouracil, but BFU-MK colony formation is unaffected by this

Table 3–1. **Comparison of Primitive Megakaryocyte Progenitors (BFU-MK) and Differentiated Megakaryocyte Progenitors (CFU-MK)**

Characteristic	BFU-MK	CFU-MK
Appearance in culture	Later	Earlier
Cells/colony	>50	3–50
Foci of development	Two or more	One
Immunologic phenotype	$CD34^+HLA\text{-}DR^-$	$CD34^+HLA\text{-}DR^+$
Site of predominance	Peripheral blood and marrow	Bone marrow

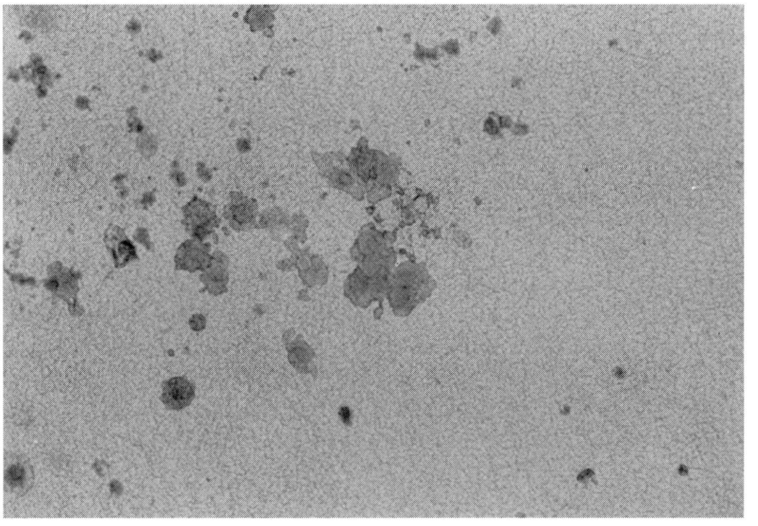

Figure 3–2. Colony-forming unit–megakaryocyte–derived colonies cultured from the peripheral blood of a preterm neonate with thrombocytopenia. Light-density mononuclear cells isolated from the peripheral blood were cultured in a collagen-based, serum-free media with 10 ng/mL of recombinant interleukin-3, 10 ng/mL of recombinant interleukin-6, and 100 ng/mL of recombinant thrombopoietin. After fixation, the colonies were stained with a monoclonal antibody against GPIIb/IIIa (CD41) to allow identification. The colonies are small, composed of only 3 to 20 megakaryocytes.

treatment, suggesting that CFU-MKs tend to be actively cycling and that BFU-MKs are relatively quiescent.

4. When immunologically phenotyped, CFU-MKs express CD34 and HLA-DR ($CD34^+$, $HLA\text{-}DR^+$ cells), whereas BFU-MKs only express CD34 ($CD34^+$, $HLA\text{-}DR^-$ cells).

After both types of megakaryocyte progenitors were identified and characterized, several investigators studied their presence in human bone marrow and peripheral blood. Zauli and colleagues[16] found that the number of CFU-MK in adult bone marrow largely exceeds that of BFU-MK, with a 2.3:1 CFU-MK to BFU-MK ratio. In contrast, the CFU-MK to BFU-MK ratio in the peripheral blood is about 0.5:1. These investigators found a similar number of BFU-MKs in bone marrow and peripheral blood $CD34^+$-enriched samples, but the number of CFU-MKs was significantly lower in peripheral blood than in marrow. It is therefore a *relative absence* of CFU-MKs from the peripheral blood that accounts for the different ratios. The proliferative and immunologic characteristics of these progenitors are similar whether in the marrow or in the blood.

Fetal and Neonatal Progenitors

The study of fetal megakaryocytopoiesis is intrinsically difficult because of the limited

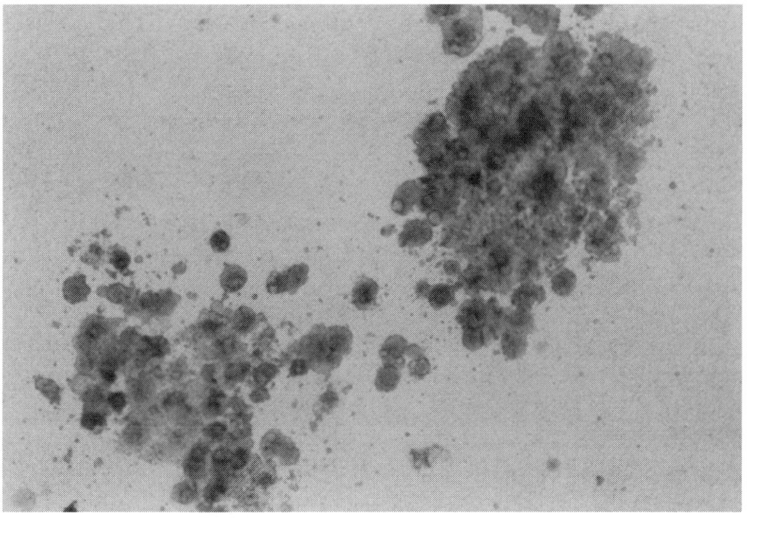

Figure 3–3. Burst-forming unit–megakaryocyte–derived colonies cultured from the peripheral blood of a preterm neonate with thrombocytopenia. The culture conditions were the same described in Figure 3–2, but these larger colonies are each composed of more than 50 cells.

availability of bone marrow specimens from living, healthy fetuses, coupled with the rarity of megakaryocytes in the fetal marrow. For these reasons, most studies have been performed using umbilical cord blood, from which large quantities of megakaryocyte progenitors can be readily obtained. Olson and associates[17] found a significantly higher concentration of CFU-MK in term and preterm cord blood (>30 weeks' gestation) than in adult peripheral blood. They also found that, when stimulated with previously irradiated aplastic canine serum, cord blood CFU-MK–derived colonies contained significantly more cells than adult colonies.

In 1993, Zauli and coworkers[18] studied the characteristics of BFU-MKs and CFU-MKs obtained from human fetal blood and compared them with those from the marrow of adults. They used highly enriched hematopoietic progenitor ($CD34^+$) populations obtained from the blood of fetuses between 18 and 22 weeks of gestation and cultured these in a serum-free fibrin clot assay. As is the case in adult blood, BFU-MKs predominate in fetal blood, with a CFU-MK to BFU-MK ratio of 0.4:1. Whether the ratio in fetal bone marrow mimics the ratio in adult bone marrow is unknown. The same investigators found no differences between fetal and adult megakaryocyte progenitors in their immunologic profiles for the expression of CD34 and HLA-DR. However, they observed significant differences in the morphology and size of fetal BFU-MK–derived colonies. The fetal BFU-MK–derived colonies were significantly larger and were usually composed of only one or two foci of development, but the adult BFU-MK–derived colonies always were multifocal. In contrast to Olson's findings, these investigators did not observe any morphologic or size differences between fetal and adult CFU-MK–derived colonies. However, when the time course of these colonies was studied in culture, fetal CFU-MK–derived and BFU-MK–derived colonies appeared significantly earlier than their counterparts from adults.

Other investigators have reported the existence, in fetal bone marrow, of a megakaryocyte progenitor with an unusually high proliferative potential. Bruno and colleagues[19] described a high proliferative potential cell–MK (HPPC-MK) in fetal bone marrow that gives rise to large, unifocal colonies (>300 cells). This cell, not observed in adult bone marrow cultures, may represent a more primitive megakaryocyte progenitor. Its characteristics strongly resemble a primitive megakaryocyte progenitor found in mouse bone marrow preparations.[20] Nishihira and associates,[21] studying cultures of cord blood (26 to 41 weeks' gestation) with optimal concentrations of recombinant TPO (rTPO), found that all colonies consisted of more than 50 cells and that 50% had more than 500 cells. It is unclear whether these colonies should be classified as BFU-MK–derived or HPPC-MK–derived colonies.

The development of a miniaturized assay system to study megakaryocyte progenitors made it possible to study these cells in the peripheral blood of neonates. Using this technique, Murray and coworkers[22] showed that preterm neonates (24 to 36 weeks) had higher circulating concentrations of all megakaryocyte progenitors than term neonates: BFU-MK, 414 ± 61 versus 151 ± 18 colonies/mL; CFU-MK, 2444 ± 337 versus 869 ± 64 colonies/mL (CFU-MK to BFU-MK ratio of 6:1). These findings are concordant with the gestational age–related decrease in the concentrations of other committed progenitors previously described.[23] However, they differ from Zauli's observations of a predominance of the more primitive progenitors (BFU-MK) in cord blood.[18] Murray and colleagues also reported a predominance of BFU-MK in cord blood obtained by cordocentesis from mid-trimester pregnancies, raising the possibility that the ratio of circulating MK progenitors changes at birth.

Megakaryocytes

Characterization

Unlike their progenitors, the megakaryocytes themselves have lost proliferative abilities and undergo a complex maturational process. Through this process, they evolve from small, mononuclear cells that are indistinguishable from monocytes to very large, polyploid cells that are easily recognized as mature megakaryocytes (Fig. 3–4). Based on different morphologic parameters, including size, ploidy, and presence of granules and demarcation membranes, the process of megakaryocyte maturation has been divided into four stages (Table 3–2): stage I, or

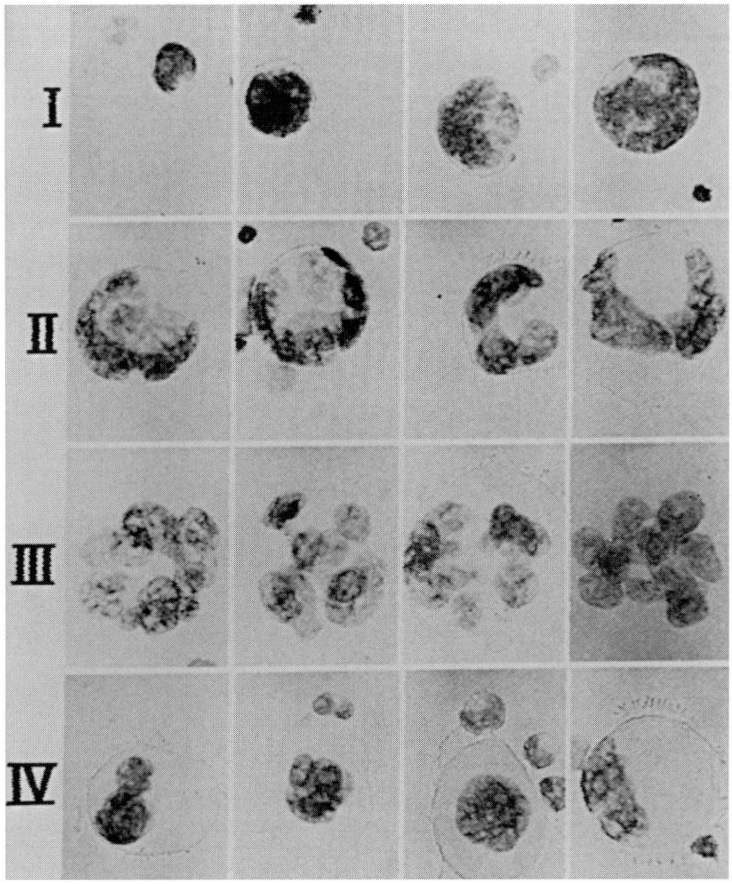

Figure 3–4. Photomicrographs of maturation stages of Feulgen-stained guinea-pig megakaryocytes (original magnification ×760). Each row illustrates representative nuclear configurations of maturation stages I, II, III, and IV, respectively. (From Levine RF, Hazzard KC, Lamberg JD: The significance of megakaryocyte size. Blood 1982;60:1123.)

megakaryoblast; stage II, or promegakaryocyte; stage III, or granular megakaryocyte; and stage IV, or mature megakaryocyte.[24]

Throughout this process, the nucleus and the cytoplasm undergo significant changes. Nuclear differentiation is characterized by endoreduplication or endomitosis, a process in which a cell increases ploidy without undergoing cellular division. This increase in ploidy level correlates with an increase in megakaryocyte size and maturational stage[24] and with increased platelet shedding.[25, 26] The ploidy of megakaryocytes can be measured on stained individual cells in a cytospin[27, 28] or a colony[29] or by flow cytometric analysis of megakaryocytes from bone marrow aspirates.[6, 27, 30] Using the latter technique, the modal ploidy has been found to be 16N in normal adult bone marrow. Quantitative platelet disorders affect the number and ploidy of megakaryocytes; patients with hyporegenerative thrombocytopenia have increased numbers of low-ploidy cells (53% are ≤8N), and patients with thrombocytopenia caused by increased platelet destruction have increased numbers of high-ploidy cells (39% are ≥32N).[30] The cytoplasm also undergoes significant changes through the maturational process, characterized by the proliferation and organization of granules and demarcation membranes.[24]

Morphologic classification of megakaryocytes in different stages of maturation is often difficult. Electron microscopy allows the recognition of the immature megakaryocytes based on the presence of few granules and demarcation membranes in their cytoplasm. However, immunologic staining of surface glycoproteins specific to the megakaryocytes has become the gold standard for identification of these cells and has brought a new perspective to the study of megakaryocytopoiesis.[31, 32]

Several surface proteins are present on megakaryocytes at all stages of development: GPIIb/IIIa (CD41), GPIIIa (CD61), and GPIb (CD42a).[11, 33] GPIIb/IIIa is restricted to the platelet lineage and allows reliable identification of these cells.[12] The analysis of different surface

Table 3–2. **Cytologic Characteristics of Megakaryocyte Maturation Stages**

Stage	Nuclear Morphology	Cytoplasmic Staining (Wright-Giemsa)	Approximate Size Range (μm)	Demarcation Membranes	Granules	Suggested Name
I	Compact (lobed)	Basophilic	6–24	Present by electron microscopy	Few present by electron microscopy	Megakaryoblast
II	Horseshoe	Pink center	14–30	Proliferating to center of cell	Starting to increase	Promegakaryocyte
III	Multilobed	Increasingly more pink than blue	16–56	Extensive but asymmetric	Great numbers	Granular megakaryocyte
IV	Compact but highly lobulated	Eosinophilic	20–50	Evenly distributed	Organized into "platelet fields"	Mature megakaryocyte

Adapted from Williams N, Levine RF: The origin, development and regulation of megakaryocytes. Br J Haematol 1982;52:174.

markers in megakaryocytes and their progenitors at various stages of development has greatly contributed to the understanding of the process of thrombopoiesis. For example, the expression of GPIb is associated with a higher level of megakaryocyte maturation,[11] and the expression of HLA-DR is restricted to the more immature megakaryocytes and to some progenitors (i.e., CFU-MKs). CD34 is found on all megakaryocyte progenitors but not on mature megakaryocytes.

The exact timing of appearance or disappearance of these markers is unclear. Debili and associates[34] determined the stage along megakaryocyte differentiation at which CD34 is turned off. By flow cytometry, they found three populations of small cells: $CD34^+$ $GPIIIa^-$, $CD34^+GPIIIa^+$, and $CD34^-GPIIIa^+$ cells. Morphologically, the two $GPIIIa^+$ populations were immature megakaryocytes, and approximately 45% were capable of undergoing at least one cell division. Twenty-two percent of the $CD34^+GPIIIa^+$ cells were polyploid (>4N). Their findings revealed significant overlap in the expression of these antigens and showed that a population of immature megakaryocytes retains low proliferative capacities. The cells with increasing ploidy and decreasing proliferative potential correspond to the *transitional cells*, *megakaryocyte precursors*, or *promegakaryoblasts* described by other researchers as the intermediate step between the progenitors and the megakaryocytes.[11, 12, 33] One transitional cell may also be the megakaryoblast, the earliest cell of the megakaryocyte lineage.

Fetal and Neonatal Megakaryocytes

Megakaryocytes are first detected in the liver and circulatory system at 8 weeks postconception, and the first platelets appear at 5 weeks.[35, 36] Using different techniques, several investigators have evaluated the size and ploidy of megakaryocytes in the fetus and neonate. Graeve and de Alarcon studied the size and maturational stage of fetal bone marrow megakaryocytes from 20 human fetuses of 12 to 21 weeks' gestation. They found that, at all stages of maturation, the fetal megakaryocytes were smaller than adult megakaryocytes and that there was no significant variation in size over the gestational age range studied.[37] The ploidy distribution of the fetal megakaryocytes also had a shift to the left compared with the adult megakaryocytes, with a higher proportion of immature megakaryocytes. These investigators also examined the few megakaryocytes present in liver and spleen biopsy specimens obtained from the same fetuses and found no differences with those in the bone marrow.

Hegyi and coworkers[38] cultured megakaryocytes from livers obtained from 8- to 20-week fetuses and from cord blood and compared their size, level of maturity, and ploidy with that of cultured adult bone marrow megakaryocytes. In contrast to other reports,[37, 39] they found a progressive shift to higher ploidy classes and an increase in megakaryocyte size during development. Only 2N and 4N megakaryocytes were usually present in 8- to 10-week cultures. Using ultrastructural techniques, they also evaluated the maturity stage of these small liver megakaryocytes and found they had all the cytoplasmic components of a mature cell, with multiple granules and a well-developed demarcation membrane system. This finding supported previous observations by Kelemen, who stated that "megakaryocytes with only one to four nuclei produce the platelets of the fetus."[35] Hegyi and colleagues also cultured adult marrow cells in the presence of 20% supernatant of fetal liver cultures and found no differences in the ploidy distribution.[38] This finding suggested that the low ploidy in the fetal cultures was not caused by the secretion of a fetal endogenous factor that prevented endomitosis. Later studies[40] confirmed a developmentally regulated shift toward larger and more mature megakaryocytes during gestation. Despite this shift, 78% of megakaryocytes in the bone marrow of fetuses of 7 to 8 months' gestation have a ploidy 8N or less, compared with only 33% of the megakaryocytes in adult bone marrow.

Studies on preterm and term cord blood have found significantly larger numbers of circulating megakaryocytes than in adult blood. As in the fetus, however, cord blood megakaryocytes are significantly smaller than the circulating megakaryocytes of adults, and many of them have diameters as small as 13 μm. Levine and associates[41] studied the characteristics of megakaryocytes isolated from term cord blood. They reported that more than one third of the megakaryocytes had unusually decreased nuclear lobulations and were micromegakaryocytes but were otherwise mature cells. The investigators suggested that these small but mature cells, also described by Hegyi in fetal livers,[38] are the result of a left shift in the megakaryocyte ploidy.

In summary, megakaryocytes of the fetus are smaller and have a lower ploidy than megakaryocytes of neonates, although they otherwise exhibit the features of mature megakaryocytes. Megakaryocytes of neonates are smaller than those of adults. Adult-size megakaryocytes appear by 2 years of age, but the evolution of the process of megakaryocytopoiesis in the first year of life is poorly understood because of the lack of normal marrow specimens from children of this age.[12] Because larger megakaryocytes generate more platelets than do smaller megakaryocytes, it is reasonable to assume that megakaryocytes of neonates produce fewer platelets than their adult counterparts. The normal platelet counts found in fetuses and neonates are probably maintained by an increased proliferative rate of the fetal megakaryocyte progenitors.

Platelet Production

The process of platelet production and release is one of the least understood steps of thrombopoiesis. Two main theories have been proposed to explain the formation of platelets from megakaryocytes. Several investigators have postulated that small buds, *proplatelets*, are formed from megakaryocytes and then released as platelets,[42–44] a process that mainly occurs in the bone marrow.[45–47] Other investigators have hypothesized that platelets are released from megakaryocytes mainly in the lungs as a consequence of shear forces, a theory sustained by the fact that circulating megakaryocytes have been documented[48, 49] and that they are more abundant in the lungs than in any other organ except bone marrow.[50]

Levine and coworkers[51] evaluated the number and characteristics of the megakaryocytes in pulmonary arterial blood and in aortic blood obtained from 20 hematologically normal adults during routine cardiac catheterization. They found that 10 times as many intact megakaryocytes entered the lungs as exited and that the exiting megakaryocytes had significantly less cytoplasm than did those going in. Based on measurements of megakaryocyte and platelet volume, platelet count, and cardiac output, they calculated that 133×10^9 platelets were produced daily in the lungs by this method, enough to match the expected daily production rate. Although their findings strongly supported the hypothesis of platelet production in the pulmonary circulation, investigators have been unable to reproduce in vitro the production of platelets or the separation of megakaryocyte nuclei from cytoplasm by high shear forces. In the fetus, circulating megakaryocytes also have been seen in the placental circulation,[52] but it is unclear whether this finding is relevant to the process of platelet production.

CYTOKINES

Thrombopoietin

Characterization

In 1958, Kelemen first used the term *thrombopoietin* to refer to a putative humoral regulator of the circulating concentration of platelets.[53] During the subsequent 36 years, multiple studies were conducted using the serum of thrombocytopenic animals and patients[54, 55] and media from human embryonic kidney cell cultures[56, 57] as the biologic sources that might contain TPO. However, every attempt to isolate and purify TPO from these sources failed, until the discovery of MPL, an "orphan" member of the hematopoietic growth factor receptor superfamily,[58] found to be expressed almost exclusively in $CD34^+$ cells, megakaryocytes, and platelets.[59–61] This discovery started an active search for the MPL ligand, which culminated in 1994, when five independent groups almost simultaneously isolated the protein. Each group used a different approach, and each assigned the purified protein a different name: MPL ligand,[62] TPO,[63] megakaryocyte growth and development factor (MGDF),[64] or megapoietin.[65] Except for species-related differences, however, all groups sequenced the same protein. Thirty-six years after Kelemen's original postulate, TPO had been found.

Using fluorescence in situ hybridization, the gene that encodes TPO was localized to the long arm of human chromosome 3.[66, 67] The gene is composed of five coding exons, similar to the five erythropoietin exons.[68] The protein is composed of 332 amino acids, divided into two domains: an active amino-terminal half (153 amino acids) with marked homology to erythropoietin and a carboxyl-terminal domain with 179 amino acids.[67]

The site of production of TPO has been the subject of significant research. Several investigators have demonstrated that TPO mRNA is expressed primarily in liver and kidney and to a lesser extent in many other tissues.[63, 69, 70] Bone marrow stromal cells also produce TPO and may play a key role in the response to thrombocytopenia.[71–73] However, some evidence suggests that the interaction of the stromal cells with megakaryocytes can inhibit the process of platelet production.[73] Further studies are necessary to better delineate the mechanisms regulating TPO production in normal and pathologic states.

Since TPO was purified and cloned, multiple in vitro and in vivo studies have been conducted to characterize the role of the newly discovered cytokine. For many years, the process of platelet production was considered to be regulated by at least two specific growth factors: a megakaryocyte colony-stimulating factor (MK-CSF), acting primarily on megakaryocyte progenitors, and TPO, acting on the late stages of megakaryocytopoiesis. After rTPO was available, it became evident that TPO acted as an MK-CSF and as a maturational factor.[74, 75] Since then, multiple studies have proven that TPO is a potent stimulator of all stages of megakaryocyte growth and development,[76, 77] although its role in the terminal stages of megakaryocytopoiesis and proplatelet formation is less clearly established.[78–80] In vitro studies suggested that it plays a role in platelet activation, mostly priming the platelets to the aggregatory effects of other agonists,[81] but these effects have not been confirmed in vivo.[82]

MPL and TPO knock-out mice models have been generated.[83, 84] The megakaryocyte and blood platelet concentrations of these mice are only 10% to 15% of normal controls, confirming that TPO is a primary regulator of platelet production and that alternative pathways exist for megakaryocytopoiesis.

Significant attention has been directed to the effects of TPO on other hematologic cell lines. In vitro, TPO alone can significantly stimulate the proliferation and survival of erythroid, myeloid, and multipotential progenitors.[85] Similarly, TPO can enhance erythropoietin-induced erythroid burst formation from CD34$^+$ cells.[86] Both effects probably are mediated by TPO's ability to inhibit apoptosis of primitive progenitor cells.[87, 88]

Multiple in vivo animal studies, mostly involving mice and nonhuman primates, have confirmed the role of TPO as a potent stimulator of platelet production. The full-length rTPO molecule and a recombinant human polypeptide that contains the receptor-binding N-terminal domain of TPO (rhMGDF) have been the subject of multiple studies. When injected into normal animals,[89–93] rTPO or rhMGDF induced significant thrombocytosis, with peak mean platelet counts up to 670% of baseline. When administered to animals exposed to myelosuppressive chemotherapy, rhMGDF ameliorated or completely prevented the associated thrombocytopenia,[89] and it accelerated red blood cell and neutrophil recovery.[94, 95] Studies using myelosuppressed mice and primates have shown a synergistic effect for rTPO and recombinant granulocyte colony-stimulating factor or granulocyte-macrophage colony-stimulating factor (GM-CSF) in the prevention of the thrombocytopenia and neutropenia associated with marrow suppressive chemotherapy.[96–99] The pegylated form of rhMGDF (PEG-rhMGDF) is 5 to 10 times more potent in vivo than the unconjugated polypeptide, as demonstrated in normal nonhuman primates,[92] and has been the formulation chosen for most of the human studies published.

Several phase I and II human trials have demonstrated the efficacy of rTPO and PEG-rhMGDF as a potent stimulator of platelet production in nonthrombocytopenic adults[100, 101] and in patients with chemotherapy-induced thrombocytopenia.[102, 103] Only mild side effects have been reported, including isolated thromboembolic events in treated patients, sometimes when the platelet count was not abnormally elevated. It has been postulated that these cases were related to the predisposition for thrombotic events of patients with malignancies. Although rTPO has not been tested in cases of thrombocytopenia unassociated with the administration of myelosuppressive agents, it is reasonable to speculate that it may be beneficial in treating many diseases and syndromes. In support of this hypothesis, studies using rhesus monkeys infected with the human immunodeficiency virus showed a 10-fold increase in platelet counts after administration of three doses of PEG-rhMGDF.[104]

Thrombopoietin in Neonates

In most cases of neonatal thrombocytopenia the cause is unknown, but studies suggest that the mechanism in many cases of otherwise unexplained thrombocytopenia is reduced platelet production associated with a decreased megakaryocyte mass.[105, 106] However, little is known about the role of TPO in the neonatal population, and no studies have tested rTPO administration in this age group.

In 1996, Nishihira and colleagues[21] investigated the effects of rTPO on megakaryocyte progenitors isolated from nonthrombocytopenic human cord blood at different gestational ages. Their results demonstrated that rTPO alone supports the growth of megakaryocyte colonies and that progenitors of preterm infants tend to be more sensitive to rTPO than progenitors of term neonates. Murray and associates[107] measured plasma TPO levels at birth in healthy term (n = 17) and preterm babies (n = 16) and in preterm babies with early thrombocytopenia (n = 13). They showed that the median TPO levels were similar in term (145 pg/mL) and preterm (132 pg/mL) infants and that thrombocytopenic preterm infants did not have a significant increase in TPO (median of 185 pg/mL). Among their thrombocytopenic neonates, 24% were small for gestational age, and 45% were born to women with pregnancy-induced hypertension. The TPO levels, however, were measured at birth and not at the time of the thrombocytopenia, raising a question about whether these thrombocytopenic neonates would have had higher TPO concentrations at the time of their platelet nadir. As part of the same study, the researchers cultured megakaryocyte progenitors from the blood of term and preterm neonates with different concentrations of rTPO and showed a greater response in preterm infants (Fig. 3–5). Nishihira and Murray performed their studies using megakaryocyte progenitors isolated from cord blood or peripheral blood of the neonates; the responsiveness of neonatal bone marrow progenitors to rTPO has not been tested.

Van de Ven and coworkers[108] investigated the in vivo effects of interleukin (IL)-3 and IL-11 in combination with rTPO on neonatal rat hematopoiesis. They found that rTPO alone, at a dosage of 10 μg/kg/d for 14 days, significantly increased the platelet count and the absolute neutrophil count of newborn Sprague-Dawley rats without affecting the hematocrit or red blood cell count. The platelet counts induced by rTPO alone were significantly higher than those achieved by IL-11 or IL-6 administration, and no additive effect was observed when rTPO was combined sequentially with IL-3 or administered simultaneously with IL-3 or IL-11.

Other Cytokines

Characterization

Before the isolation and cloning of TPO, multiple cytokines underwent scrutiny in an attempt to identify the main physiologic regulators of platelet production. IL-6 was extensively studied in vitro and in vivo. In vitro studies using long-term murine bone marrow cultures and cord blood megakaryocyte progenitors showed an increase in megakaryocyte size and ploidy in response to IL-6,[109, 110] suggesting a primarily maturational effect. Further studies investigating the effects of rIL-6 on cultured human progenitors also demonstrated some proliferative effects (i.e., increased number of megakaryocyte colonies and of cells comprising individual colonies), although these were significantly less than those induced by IL-3 or GM-CSF.[111] In a similar culture system, IL-6, stem cell factor, or their combination in the presence of IL-3 increased the number of polyploid megakaryocytes up to fourfold.[112] These results suggested that IL-6 acts on the early and late stages of megakaryocytopoiesis, but the effects are not as potent as those seen with other cytokines.

Multiple in vivo studies using murine and primate models confirmed the effects of rIL-6 on thrombopoiesis. Normal mice treated with rIL-6 exhibited an increase in the size and ploidy of megakaryocytes. However, no effect was observed on the megakaryocyte frequency

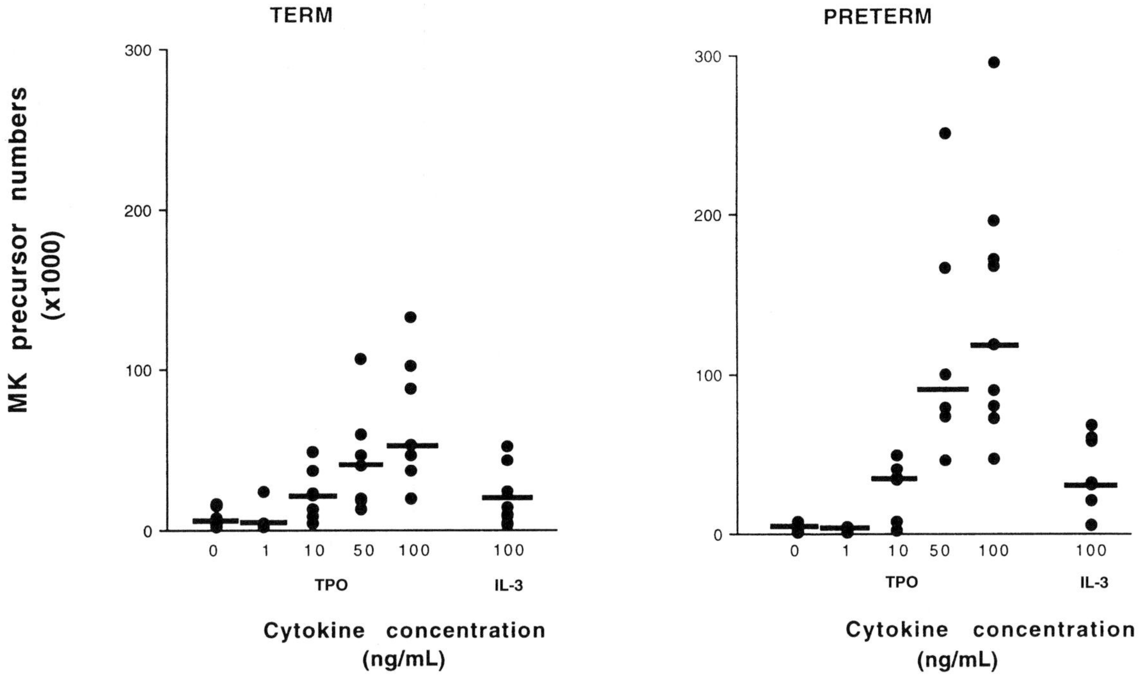

Figure 3–5. Dose-response characteristics of megakaryocyte (MK) progenitors from healthy term and preterm babies and cultured in various concentrations of thrombopoietin (TPO) and interleukin-3 (IL-3). MK progenitors in both groups show significant proliferation over baseline (no TPO) at 50 and 100 ng/mL of TPO (*P* <.01 for both comparisons). MK progenitors in both groups also show proliferation over baseline (no TPO) at 100 ng/mL of IL-3; however, this is significantly less pronounced than with 100 ng/mL of TPO (*P* <.05). (Adapted from Murray NA, Watts TL, Roberts IAG: Endogenous thrombopoietin levels and effect of recombinant human thrombopoietin on megakaryocyte precursors in term and preterm babies. Pediatr Res 1998;43:148; © 1998, The Williams & Wilkins Company, Baltimore.)

or on the mean platelet volume.[113] Similarly, in healthy and irradiated primates, rIL-6 did not increase the number of bone marrow megakaryocytes, but it induced a rightward shift in the megakaryocyte ploidy.[114] Long-term administration of rIL-6 to normal primates induced a twofold to threefold increase in platelet count, but the number of bone marrow megakaryocytes did not increase.[115] The platelet count decreased after 4 weeks of treatment, despite continuing IL-6 administration. This decline was associated with the development of high titers of neutralizing anti-IL-6 antibodies. These observations suggest that IL-6 acts in vivo mainly as a maturational factor but not as a megakaryocyte colony-stimulating factor.

In a phase I-II study, rIL-6 was administered at different doses (0.5 to 20 μg/kg/d) to 20 patients with breast cancer or non-small cell lung cancer.[116] Administration of rIL-6 increased platelet counts and leukocytes, but significant side effects (mainly fever, flulike symptoms, and local erythema) were observed at even the smallest doses. Nausea, anemia, and a reversible increase in the liver enzymes were observed at doses of 2.5 μg/kg/d or higher.

Several investigators studied the effects of rIL-11 on human megakaryocytopoiesis in vitro. In a manner similar to rIL-6, rIL-11 induces a shift in the megakaryocyte ploidy toward higher values.[117] However, rIL-11 alone has little or no effect on CFU-MK–derived or BFU-MK–derived colony formation unless it is combined with rIL-3.[118] In mice, the administration of rIL-11 induces a significant increase in the peripheral platelet count, the number of megakaryocyte progenitors, and the megakaryocyte ploidy.[119] The platelet count increase is significantly enhanced when rIL-11 is administered by continuous subcutaneous infusion compared with subcutaneous injection.[120] In a clinical trial, 12 women with advanced breast cancer were treated with rIL-11 at doses of 10, 25, 50, or 75 μg/kg/d. The two highest doses were associated with increases in bone marrow megakaryocyte frequency and mean ploidy. Two of the three patients treated with the highest dose also showed a 3- to 10-fold increase in the number of committed megakaryocyte progenitors.[121] When administered to patients receiving chemotherapy,[122] treatment with rIL-11 significantly decreased the requirement for platelet transfusions (32%) compared with the placebo-treated group (59%). Most adverse events associated with rIL-11 administration were associated with fluid retention and were only mild to moderate in severity.

Whereas IL-6 and IL-11 have been considered maturational factors with mild proliferative activity, other cytokines have been found to act mainly on the early megakaryocyte progenitors. In vitro, IL-3 and GM-CSF have induced proliferation of megakaryocytic progenitors in a dose-dependent manner.[123] At maximal concentrations, IL-3 alone has a greater ability to promote megakaryocyte colony formation than GM-CSF, but the factors act synergistically when suboptimal concentrations of IL-3 are used.[124]

Kaushansky and coworkers[77] demonstrated that neutralizing the biologic activity of TPO in a culture system eliminated the formation of megakaryocytes in response to the KIT ligand, IL-6, IL-11, or some combination of these factors. However, IL-3 alone or in combination was able to at least partially support the proliferation and initial stages of megakaryocyte differentiation, although the full maturation of the megakaryocytes required TPO. They postulated the existence of two populations of megakaryocyte progenitors: one completely dependent on TPO for proliferation and maturation and one able to proliferate in response to IL-3 but dependent on TPO for full maturation.

Numerous additional growth factors participate in the process of megakaryocytopoiesis, but their roles have been less clearly defined. They include erythropoietin,[125] stem cell factor,[126–129] IL-1,[130] basic fibroblast growth factor,[131] interferon-γ,[132] and platelet-derived growth factor.[133] Some cytokines inhibit thrombopoiesis, including TGF-β[134] and platelet factor 4 (PF4).[135]

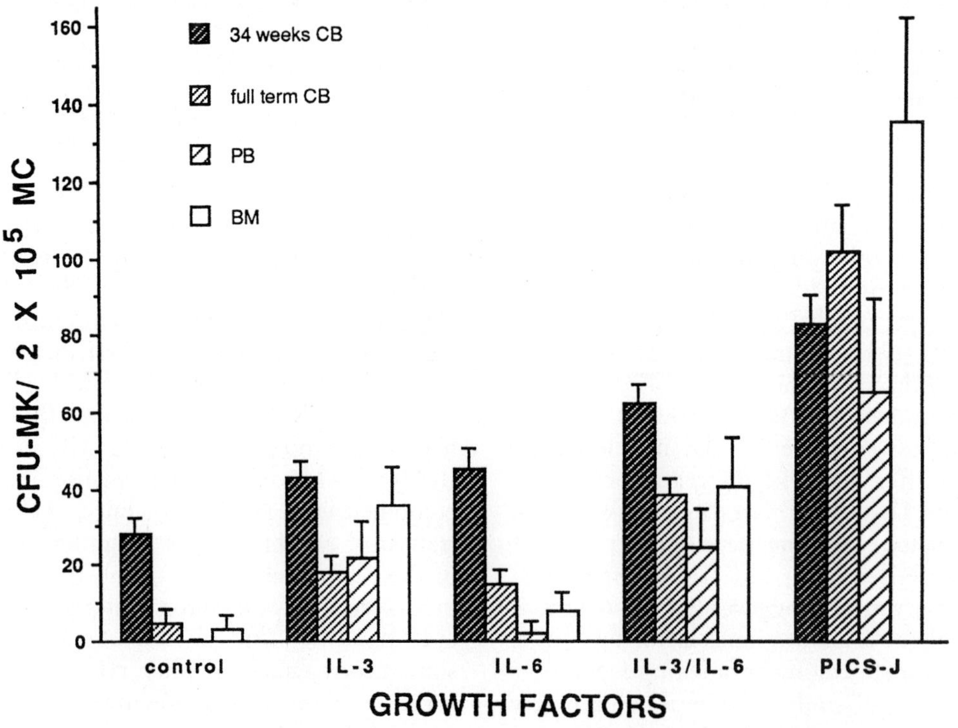

Figure 3–6. Effect of growth factors on megakaryocyte colony-forming units (CFU-MK). MK colonies were grown in plasma clots from 34-week preterm cord blood (n = 5), term cord blood (CB) (n = 8), peripheral blood (PB) (n = 10), or bone marrow (BM) (n = 7) using several growth factors: 5 ng/mL of interleukin-3 (IL-3), 100 units/mL of interleukin-6 (IL-6), and a 10% concentration of postirradiation aplastic canine serum (PICS-J). Results are recorded as the average number of CFU-MK counted ± SD. (From Deutsch VR, Olson TA, Nagler A, et al: The response of cord blood megakaryocyte progenitors to IL-3, IL-6 and aplastic canine serum varies with gestational age. Br J Haematol 1995;89:10.)

Response of Neonatal Progenitors and Megakaryocytes to Cytokines

Deutsch and colleagues investigated the responses of cord blood megakaryocyte progenitors from different gestational ages to IL-3, IL-6, IL-3 plus IL-6, and aplastic canine serum, and compared the results with the responses of progenitors obtained from adult peripheral blood and bone marrow.[136] As shown in Figure 3–6, preterm cord blood (34 weeks' gestation) generated a high number of spontaneous CFU-MK colonies, whereas only insignificant numbers of spontaneous colonies were observed in term cord blood, adult peripheral blood, or adult bone marrow cultures. IL-3 and IL-6 greatly stimulated proliferation of CFU-MKs in preterm cord blood, generating almost equal numbers of CFU-MKs to those of IL-3–stimulated adult bone marrow. This result contrasted with the almost absent proliferative activity of IL-6 in adult blood and bone marrow cultures. IL-3 and IL-6 acted synergistically in preterm and term cord blood cultures. In all sources of progenitor cells, the postirradiation aplastic canine serum was the most potent stimulator of the megakaryocyte progenitors, probably reflecting its high concentrations of TPO.

In summary, these studies demonstrated that cord blood megakaryocyte progenitors are exquisitely sensitive to exogenous cytokines and showed an inverse relationship between the magnitude of the response and gestational age. These findings were in concordance with previous reports[18] of a higher sensitivity of fetal megakaryocyte progenitors (18 to 22 weeks' gestation) to rGM-CSF and to rIL-3 in vitro. As in adults, purified TGF-β1 showed clear dose-dependent inhibition of fetal megakaryocyte progenitors.

Cairo and associates[137] treated newborn rats with 7 days of rIL-6. Although they observed a significant increase in the day 1 platelet and neutrophil counts, rIL-6 failed to induce a sustained increase in the platelet or neutrophil count during the remaining 7 days of administration. They did not observe any significant increase in the hematocrit.

References

1. Wright JH: The origin and nature of the blood plates. Boston Med Surg J 1906;154:643.
2. Levine RF: Isolation and characterization of normal human megakaryocytes. Br J Haematol 1980;45:487.
3. Berthier R, Valiron O, Schweitzer A, et al: Serum-free medium allows the optimal growth of human megakaryocyte progenitors compared with human plasma supplemented cultures: role of TGFβ. Stem Cells 1993;11:120.
4. Hogge D, Fanning SF, Bockhold K, et al: Quantitation and characterization of human megakaryocyte colony-forming cells using a standardized serum-free assay. Br J Haematol 1997;96:790.
5. Mazur EM, Basilico D, Newton JL, et al: Isolation of large numbers of enriched human megakaryocytes from liquid cultures of normal peripheral blood progenitor cells. Blood 1990;76:1771.
6. Tomer A, Harker LA, Burstein SA: Flow cytometric analysis of normal human megakaryocytes. Blood 1988;71:1244.
7. Scharf TA, McMillan R, Ruggeri ZM, et al: Bernard-Soulier syndrome: quantitative characterization of megakaryocytes and platelets by flow cytometric and platelet kinetic measurements. Eur J Haematol 1994;52:193.
8. Lok S, Kaushansky K, Holly RD, et al: Cloning and expression of murine thrombopoietin cDNA and stimulation of platelet production in vivo. Nature 1994;369:565.
9. Sola M, Christensen RD: Use of hematopoietic growth factors in the neonatal intensive care unit. J Intens Care Med 1997;12:187.
10. Mazur EM, Hoffman R: Human megakaryocyte progenitors. In Golde DW (ed): Hematopoiesis. New York: Churchill Livingstone, 1984, p 133.
11. Vinci G, Tabilio A, Deschamps JF, et al: Immunological study of in vitro maturation of human megakaryocytes. Br J Haematol 1984;56:589.
12. Olson TA: Developmental megakaryocytopoiesis. In Polin RA, Fox WW (eds): Fetal and Neonatal Physiology, 2nd ed. Philadelphia: WB Saunders, 1998, p 1787.
13. Long MW, Gragowski LL, Heffner CH, et al: Phorbol diesters stimulate the development of an early murine progenitor cell: the burst-forming unit–megakaryocyte. J Clin Invest 1985;76:431.
14. Briddell RA, Brandt JE, Straneve JE, et al: Characterization of the human burst-forming unit–megakaryocyte. Blood 1989;74:145.
15. Mazur EM, Hoffman R, Bruno E: Regulation of human megakaryocytopoiesis: an in vitro analysis. J Clin Invest 1981;68:733.
16. Zauli G, Vitale L, Brunelli MA, et al: Prevalence of the primitive megakaryocyte progenitors (BFU-meg) in adult human peripheral blood. Exp Hematol 1992;20:850.
17. Olson TA, Levine RF, Mazur EM, et al: Megakaryocytes and megakaryocyte progenitors in human cord blood. Am J Pediatr Hematol Oncol 1992;14:241.
18. Zauli G, Valvassori L, Capitani S: Presence and characteristics of circulating megakaryocyte progenitor cells in human fetal blood. Blood 1993;81:385.
19. Bruno E, Murray LJ, DiGiusto R, et al: Detection of a primitive megakaryocyte progenitor cell in human fetal bone marrow. Exp Hematol 1996;24:552.
20. Jackson H, Williams N, Bertoncello I, et al: Classes of primitive murine megakaryocytic progenitor cells. Exp Hematol 1994;22:954.
21. Nishihira H, Toyoda Y, Miyazaki H, et al: Growth of macroscopic human megakaryocyte colonies from cord blood in culture with recombinant human thrombopoietin (c-mpl ligand) and the effects of gestational

age on frequency of colonies. Br J Haematol 1996;92:23.
22. Murray NA, Roberts IAG: Circulating megakaryocytes and their progenitors (BFU-MK and CFU-MK) in term and pre-term neonates. Br J Haematol 1995;89:41.
23. Clapp DW, Baley JE, Gerson SL: Gestational age-dependent changes in circulating hematopoietic stem-cells in newborn infants. J Lab Clin Med 1989;113:422.
24. Williams N, Levine RF: The origin, development and regulation of megakaryocytes. Br J Haematol 1982;52:173.
25. Levine RF, Hazzard KC, Lamberg JD: The significance of megakaryocyte size. Blood 1982;60:1122.
26. Harker LA: Kinetics of thrombopoiesis. J Clin Invest 1968;47:458.
27. Levine RF, Bunn PA, Hazzard KC, et al: Flow cytometric analysis of megakaryocyte ploidy: comparison with Feulgen microdensitometry and discovery that 8N is the predominant ploidy class in guinea pig and monkey marrow. Blood 1980;56:210.
28. Mazur EM, Lindquist DL, de Alarcon PA, et al: Evaluation of bone marrow megakaryocyte ploidy distributions in persons with normal and abnormal platelet counts. J Lab Clin Med 1988;111:194.
29. Levin J, Levin FC, Penington D, et al: Measurement of ploidy distribution in megakaryocyte colonies obtained from culture: with studies of the effects of thrombocytopenia. Blood 1981;57:287.
30. Tomer A, Friese P, Conklin R, et al: Flow cytometric analysis of megakaryocytes from patients with abnormal platelet counts. Blood 1989;74:594.
31. Levene RB, Lamaziere J-M, Broxmeyer HE, et al: Human megakaryocytes. V. Changes in the phenotypic profile of differentiating megakaryocytes. J Exp Med 1985;161:457.
32. Mazur EM, Hoffman R, Chasis J, et al: Immunofluorescent identification of human megakaryocyte colonies using an antiplatelet glycoprotein antiserum. Blood 1981;57:277.
33. Rabellino EM, Levene RB, Leung LLK: Human megakaryocytes. II. Expression of platelet proteins in early marrow megakaryocytes. J Exp Med 1981;154:88.
34. Debili N, Issaad C, Masse JM, et al: Expression of CD34 and platelet glycoproteins during human megakaryocytic differentiation. Blood 1992;80:3022.
35. Kelemen E, Calvo W, Fliedner TM: Atlas of Human Hemopoietic Development. Berlin: Springer-Verlag, 1979, p 51.
36. Fukuda T: Fetal hemopoiesis. I. Electron microscopic studies on human yolk sac hemopoiesis. Virchows Arch B 1973;14:197.
37. Allen Graeve JL, de Alarcon PA: Megakaryocytopoiesis in the human fetus. Arch Dis Child 1989;64:481.
38. Hegyi E, Nakazawa M, Debili N, et al: Developmental changes in human megakaryocyte ploidy. Exp Hematol 1991;19:87.
39. De Alarcon PA, Graeve JLA: Analysis of megakaryocyte ploidy in fetal bone marrow biopsies using a new adaptation of the Feulgen technique to measure DNA content and estimate megakaryocyte ploidy from biopsy specimens. Pediatr Res 1996;39:166.
40. Ma DC, Sun YH, Chang KZ, et al: Developmental change of megakaryocyte maturation and DNA ploidy in human fetus. Eur J Haematol 1996;57:121.
41. Levine RF, Olson TA, Shoff PK, et al: Mature micromegakaryocytes: an unusual developmental pattern in term infants. Br J Haematol 1996;94:391.
42. Choi ES, Nichol JL, Hokom MM, et al: Platelets generated in vitro from proplatelet-displaying human megakaryocytes are functional. Blood 1995;85:402.
43. Tong M, Seth P, Penington DG: Proplatelets and stress platelets. Blood 1987;69:522.
44. Cramer EM, Norol F, Guichard J, et al: Ultrastructure of platelet formation by human megakaryocytes cultured with the Mpl ligand. Blood 1997;89:2336.
45. Radley JM, Haller CJ: Fate of senescent megakaryocytes in the bone marrow. Br J Haematol 1983;53:277.
46. Tavassoli M, Aoki M: Migration of entire megakaryocytes through the marrow-blood barrier. Br J Haematol 1981;48:25.
47. Harker LA, Finch CA: Thrombokinetics in man. J Clin Invest 1969;48:963.
48. Kaufman RM, Airo R, Pollack S, et al: Circulating megakaryocytes and platelet release in the lung. Blood 1965;26:720.
49. Pedersen NT, Cohn J: Intact megakaryocytes in the venous blood as a marker for thrombopoiesis. Scand J Haematol 1981;27:57.
50. Brill R, Halpern MM: The frequency of megakaryocytes in autopsy sections. Blood 1948;3:286.
51. Levine RF, Eldor A, Shoff PK, et al: Circulating megakaryocytes: delivery of large numbers of intact, mature megakaryocytes to the lungs. Eur J Haematol 1993;51:233.
52. Woods MJ, et al: The placenta: a site of platelet production? Platelets 1992;3:211.
53. Kelemen E, Cserhati I, Tanos B: Demonstration and some properties of human thrombopoietin in thrombocythemic sera. Acta Haematol 1958;20:350.
54. Hill RJ, Levin J, Levin FC: Correlation of in vitro and in vivo biological activities during the partial purification of thrombopoietin. Exp Hematol 1992;20:354.
55. Hill RJ, Warren MK, Levin J, et al: Evidence that interleukin-6 does not play a role in the stimulation of platelet production after induction of acute thrombocytopenia. Blood 1992;80:346.
56. McDonald TP, Jackson CW: Thrombopoietin derived from human embryonic kidney cells stimulates an increase in DNA content of murine megakaryocytes in vivo. Exp Hematol 1990;18:758.
57. McDonald TP, Wendling F, Vainchenker W, et al: Thrombopoietin from human embryonic kidney cells is the same factor as c-mpl-ligand. Blood 1995;85:292.
58. Vigon I, Mornon J-P, Cocault L, et al: Molecular cloning and characterization of MPL, the human homolog of the v-mpl oncogene: Identification of a member of the hematopoietic growth factor receptor superfamily. Proc Natl Acad Sci U S A 1992;89:5640.
59. Methia N, Louache F, Vainchenker W, et al: Oligodeoxynucleotides antisense to the proto-oncogene c-mpl specifically inhibit in vitro megakaryocytopoiesis. Blood 1993;82:1395.
60. Mignotte V, Vigon I, Boucher de Crevecoeur E, et al: Structure and transcription of the human c-mpl gene (MPL). Genomics 1994;20:5.
61. Columbyova l, Loda M, Scadden DT: Thrombopoietin receptor expression in human cancer cell lines and primary tissues. Cancer Res 1995;55:3509.
62. de Sauvage FJ, Hass PE, Spencer SD, et al: Stimulation of megakaryocytopoiesis and thrombopoiesis by the c-Mpl ligand. Nature 1994;369:533.
63. Lok S, Kaushansky K, Holly RD, et al: Cloning and expression of murine thrombopoietin cDNA and stimulation of platelet production in vivo. Nature 1994;369:565.
64. Bartley TD, Bogenberger J, Hunt P, et al: Identification and cloning of a megakaryocyte growth and de-

velopment factor that is a ligand for the cytokine receptor Mpl. Cell 1994;77:1117.
65. Kuter DJ, Beeler DL, Rosenberg RD: The purification of megapoietin: a physiological regulator of megakaryocyte growth and platelet production. Proc Natl Acad Sci U S A 1994;91:11104.
66. Foster DC, Sprecher CA, Grant FJ, et al: Human thrombopoietin: gene structure, cDNA sequence, expression, and chromosomal localization. Proc Natl Acad Sci U S A 1994;91:13023.
67. Gurney AL, Kuang W-J, Xie M-H, et al: Genomic structure, chromosomal localization, and conserved alternative splice forms of thrombopoietin. Blood 1995;85:981.
68. Chang M, McNinch J, Basu R, et al: Cloning and characterization of the human megakaryocyte growth and development factor (MGDF) gene. J Biol Chem 1995;270:511.
69. Stoffel R, Wiestner A, Skoda RC: Thrombopoietin in thrombocytopenic mice: evidence against regulation at the mRNA level and for a direct regulatory role of platelets. Blood 1996;87:567.
70. McCarty JM, Sprugel KH, Fox NE, et al: Murine thrombopoietin mRNA levels are modulated by platelet count. Blood 1995;86:3668.
71. Sungaran R, Markovic B, Chong BH: Localization and regulation of thrombopoietin mRNA expression in human kidney, liver, bone marrow and spleen using in situ hybridization. Blood 1997;89:101.
72. Guerriero A, Worford L, Holland HK, et al: Thrombopoietin is synthesized by bone marrow stromal cells. Blood 1997;90:3444.
73. Nagahisa H, Nagata Y, Ohnuki T, et al: Bone marrow stromal cells produce thrombopoietin and stimulate megakaryocyte growth and maturation but suppress proplatelet formation. Blood 1996;87:1309.
74. Zeigler FC, de Sauvage F, Widmer HR, et al: In vitro megakaryocytopoietic and thrombopoietic activity of c-mpl ligand (TPO) on purified murine hematopoietic stem cells. Blood 1994;84:4045.
75. Debili N, Wendling F, Katz A, et al: The Mpl-ligand or thrombopoietin or megakaryocyte growth and differentiative factor has both direct proliferative and differentiative activities on human megakaryocyte progenitors. Blood 1995;86:2516.
76. Banu N, Wang JF, Deng B, et al: Modulation of megakaryocytopoiesis by thrombopoietin: The c-Mpl ligand. Blood 1995;86:1331.
77. Kaushansky K, Broudy VC, Lin N: Thrombopoietin, the Mpl ligand, is essential for full megakaryocyte development. Proc Natl Acad Sci U S A 1995;92:3234.
78. Toshiharu I, Ishida Y, Kashiwagi R, et al: Recombinant human c-Mpl ligand is not a direct stimulator of proplatelet formation in mature human megakaryocytes. Br J Haematol 1996;94:387.
79. Choi ES, Hokom MM, Chen JL, et al: The role of megakaryocyte growth and development factor in terminal stages of thrombopoiesis. Br J Haematol 1996;95:227.
80. Bunting S, Widmer R, Lipari T, et al: Normal platelets and megakaryocytes are produced in vivo in the absence of thrombopoietin. Blood 1997;90:3423.
81. Chen J, Herceg-Harjacek L, Groopman JE, et al: Regulation of platelet activation in vitro by the c-Mpl ligand, thrombopoietin. Blood 1995;86:4054.
82. O'Malley CJ, Rasko JE, Basser RL, et al: Administration of pegylated recombinant human megakaryocyte growth and development factor to humans stimulates the production of functional platelets that show no evidence of in vivo activation. Blood 1996;88:3288.
83. De Sauvage F, Carver-Moore K, Luoh S, et al: Physiological regulation of early and late stages of megakaryocytopoiesis by thrombopoietin. J Exp Med 1996;183:651.
84. Gurney AL, Carver-Moore K, de Sauvage FJ, et al: Thrombocytopenia in c-mpl–deficient mice. Science 1994;265:1445.
85. Yoshida M, Tsuji K, Ebihara Y, et al: Thrombopoietin alone stimulates the early proliferation and survival of human erythroid, myeloid and multipotential progenitors in serum-free culture. Br J Haematol 1997;98:254.
86. Kobayashi M, Laver JH, Kato T: Recombinant human thrombopoietin (Mpl ligand) enhances proliferation of erythroid progenitors. Blood 1995;86:2494.
87. Ratajczak MZ, Ratajczak J, Marlicz W: Recombinant human thrombopoietin (Tpo) stimulates erythropoiesis by inhibiting erythroid progenitor cell apoptosis. Br J Haematol 1997;98:8.
88. Borge OJ, Ramsfjell V, Cui L, et al: Ability of early acting cytokines to directly promote survival and suppress apoptosis of human primitive $CD34^+CD38^-$ bone marrow cells with multilineage potential at the single-cell level: key role of thrombopoietin. Blood 1997;90:2282.
89. Ulich TR, del Castillo J, Yin S, et al: Megakaryocyte growth and development factor ameliorates carboplatin-induced thrombocytopenia in mice. Blood 1995;86:971.
90. Farese AM, Hunt P, Boone T, et al: Recombinant human megakaryocyte growth and development factor stimulates thrombocytopoiesis in normal nonhuman primates. Blood 1996;86:54.
91. Harker LA, Hunt P, Marzec UM, et al: Regulation of platelet production and function by megakaryocyte growth and development factor in nonhuman primates. Blood 1996;87:1833.
92. Harker LA, Marzec UM, Hunt P, et al: Dose-response effects of pegylated human megakaryocyte growth and development factor on platelet production and function in nonhuman primates. Blood 1996;88:511.
93. Daw NC, Arnold JT, Abushullaih BA, et al: A single intravenous dose of murine megakaryocyte growth and development factor potently stimulates platelet production, challenging the necessity for daily administration. Blood 1998;91:466.
94. Grossmann A, Lenox J, Ren HP, et al: Thrombopoietin accelerates platelet, red blood cell, and neutrophil recovery in myelosuppressed mice. Exp Hematol 1996;24:1238.
95. Neelis KJ, Qingliang L, Thomas GR, et al: Prevention of thrombocytopenia by thrombopoietin in myelosuppressed rhesus monkeys accompanied by prominent erythropoietic stimulation and iron depletion. Blood 1997;90:58.
96. Grossmann A, Lenox J, Deisher TA, et al: Synergistic effects of thrombopoietin and granulocyte colony-stimulating factor on neutrophil recovery in myelosuppressed mice. Blood 1996;88:3363.
97. Harker LA, Marzec UM, Kelly AB, et al: Prevention of thrombocytopenia and neutropenia in a nonhuman primate model of marrow suppressive chemotherapy by combining pegylated recombinant human megakaryocyte growth and development factor and recombinant human granulocyte colony-stimulating factor. Blood 1997;89:155.
98. Neelis KJ, Hartong SCC, Egeland T, et al: The efficacy of single-dose administration of thrombopoietin with coadministration of either granulocyte/macrophage of granulocyte colony-stimulating factor in myelosuppressed rhesus monkeys. Blood 1997;90:2565.

99. Neelis KJ, Dubbelman YD, Qingliang L, et al: Simultaneous administration of Tpo and G-CSF after cytoreductive treatment of rhesus monkeys prevents thrombocytopenia, accelerates platelet and red cell reconstitution, alleviates neutropenia, and promotes the recovery of immature bone marrow cells. Exp Hematol 1997;25:1084.
100. Basser RL, Rasko JEJ, Clarke K, et al: Thrombopoietic effects of pegylated recombinant human megakaryocyte growth and development factor (PEG-rHuMGDF) in patients with advanced cancer. Lancet 1996;348:1279.
101. Vadhan-Raj S, Murray LJ, Bueso-Ramos C, et al: Stimulation of megakaryocyte and platelet production by a single dose of recombinant human thrombopoietin in patients with cancer. Ann Intern Med 1997;126:673.
102. Fanucchi M, Glaspy J, Crawford J, et al: Effects of polyethylene glycol-conjugated recombinant human megakaryocyte growth and development factor on platelet counts after chemotherapy for lung cancer. N Engl J Med 1997;336:404.
103. Basser RL, Rasko JEJ, Clarke K, et al: Randomized, blinded, placebo-controlled phase I trial of pegylated recombinant human megakaryocyte growth and development factor with filgrastim after dose-intensive chemotherapy in patients with advanced cancer. Blood 1997;89:3118.
104. Harker LA, Marzec UM, Novembre F, et al: Treatment of thrombocytopenia in chimpanzees infected with human immunodeficiency virus by pegylated recombinant human megakaryocyte growth and development factor. Blood 1998;91:4427.
105. Murray NA, Roberts IAG: Circulating megakaryocytes and their progenitors in early thrombocytopenia in preterm neonates. Pediatr Res 1996;40:112.
106. Mehta P, Vasa R, Neumann L, et al: Thrombocytopenia in the high-risk infant. J Pediatr 1980;97:791.
107. Murray NA, Watts TL, Roberts IAG: Endogenous thrombopoietin levels and effect of recombinant human thrombopoietin on megakaryocyte precursors in term and preterm babies. Pediatr Res 1998;43:148.
108. van de Ven C, Fernandez GW, Herbst T, et al: Sequential treatment with rmIL-3 or simultaneous treatment with rmIL-3 or rhIL-11 with thrombopoietin (TPO) fails to enhance in vivo neonatal rat thrombocytopoiesis. Exp Hematol 1997;25:1005.
109. Mei RL, Burstein SA: Megakaryocytic maturation in murine long-term bone marrow culture: role of interleukin-6. Blood 1991;78:1438.
110. Imai T, Koike K, Kubo T, et al: Interleukin-6 supports human megakaryocytic proliferation and differentiation in vitro. Blood 1991;78:1969.
111. Bruno E, Hoffman R: Effect of interleukin 6 on in vitro human megakaryocytopoiesis: its interactions with other cytokines. Exp Hematol 1989;17:1038.
112. Debili N, Masse JM, Katz A: Effects of the recombinant hematopoietic growth factors interleukin-3, interleukin-6, stem cell factor, and leukemia inhibitory factor on the megakaryocytic differentiation of $CD34^+$ cells. Blood 1993;82:84.
113. Hill RJ, Warren MK, Stenberg P, et al: Stimulation of megakaryocytopoiesis in mice by human recombinant interleukin-6. Blood 1991;77:42.
114. Zeidler C, Kanz L, Hurkuck F, et al: In vivo effects of interleukin-6 on thrombopoiesis in healthy and irradiated primates. Blood 1992:80:2740.
115. Ryffel B, Car BD, Woerly G, et al: Long-term interleukin-6 administration stimulates sustained thrombopoiesis and acute-phase protein synthesis in a small primate—the marmoset. Blood 1994;83:2093.
116. Van Gameren MM, Willemse PHB, Mulder NH: Effects of recombinant human interleukin-6 in cancer patients: a phase I-II study. Blood 1994;84:1434.
117. Teramura M, Kobayashi S, Hoshino S, et al: Interleukin-11 enhances human megakaryocytopoiesis in vitro. Blood 1992;79:327.
118. Bruno E, Briddell RA, Cooper RJ, et al: Effects of recombinant interleukin 11 on human megakaryocyte progenitor cells. Exp Hematol 1991;19:378.
119. Neben TY, Loebelenz J, Hayes L, et al: Recombinant human interleukin-11 stimulates megakaryocytopoiesis and increases peripheral platelets in normal and splenectomized mice. Blood 1993;81:901.
120. Leonard JP, Neben TY, Kozitza MK, et al: Constant subcutaneous infusion of rhIL-11 in mice: efficient delivery enhances biological activity. Exp Hematol 1996;24:270.
121. Orazi A, Cooper RJ, Tong J, et al: Effects of recombinant human interleukin-11 (Neumega rhIL-11 growth factor) on megakaryocytopoiesis in human bone marrow. Exp Hematol 1996;24:1289.
122. Isaacs C, Robert NJ, Bailey FA, et al: Randomized placebo-controlled study of recombinant human interleukin-11 to prevent chemotherapy-induced thrombocytopenia in patients with breast cancer receiving dose-intensive cyclophosphamide and doxorubicin. J Clin Oncol 1997;15:3368.
123. Teramura M, Katahira J, Hoshino S, et al: Effect of recombinant hemopoietic growth factors on human megakaryocyte colony formation in serum-free cultures. Exp Hematol 1989;17:1011.
124. Lu L, Briddell RA, Graham CD, et al: Effect of recombinant and purified human haematopoietic growth factors on in vitro colony formation by enriched populations of human megakaryocyte progenitor cells. Br J Haematol 1988;70:149.
125. Cardier JE, Erickson-Miller CL, Murphy MJ: Differential effect of erythropoietin and GM-CSF on megakaryocytopoiesis from primitive bone marrow cells in serum-free conditions. Stem Cells 1997;15:286.
126. Grossi A, Vannucchi AM, Bacci P, et al: In vivo administration of stem cell factor enhances both proliferation and maturation of murine megakaryocytes. Haematologica 1995;80:18.
127. Piacibello W, Sanavio F, Bresso P, et al: Stem cell factor improvement of proliferation and maintenance of hemopoietic progenitors in myelodysplastic syndromes. Leukemia 1994;8:250.
128. Imai T, Nakahata T: Stem cell factor promotes proliferation of human primitive megakaryocytic progenitors, but not megakaryocytic maturation. Int J Hematol 1994;59:91.
129. Avraham H, Vannier E, Cowley S, et al: Effects of the stem cell factor, c-kit ligand, on human megakaryocytic cells. Blood 1992;79:365.
130. Briddell RA, Brandt JE, Leemhuis TB, et al: Role of cytokines in sustaining long-term human megakaryocytopoiesis in vitro. Blood 1992;79:332.
131. Avraham H, Banu N, Scadden DT, et al: Modulation of megakaryocytopoiesis by human basic fibroblast growth factor. Blood 1994;83:2126.
132. Muraoka K, Tsuji K, Yoshida M, et al: Thrombopoietin-independent effect of interferon-gamma on the proliferation of human megakaryocyte progenitors. Br J Haematol 1997;98:265.
133. Yang M, Chesterman CN, Chong BH: Recombinant PDGF enhances megakaryocytopoiesis in vitro. Br J Haematol 1995;91:285.
134. Han ZC, Bellucci S, Wan HY, et al: New insights into

the regulation of megakaryocytopoiesis by haematopoietic and fibroblastic growth factors and transforming growth factor beta 1. Br J Haematol 1992;81:1.

135. Gewirtz AM, Zhang J, Ratajczak J, et al: Chemokine regulation of human megakaryocytopoiesis. Blood 1995;86:2559.

136. Deutsch VR, Olson TA, Nagler A, et al: The response of cord blood megakaryocyte progenitors to IL-3, IL-6 and aplastic canine serum varies with gestational age. Br J Haematol 1995;89:8.

137. Cairo MS, Plunkett M, Clark S, et al: In vivo hematological effects of seven days of rhIL-6 in neonatal rats. Am J Pediatr Hematol Oncol 1992;14:44.

CHAPTER 4

Nonhematopoietic Actions of Hematopoietic Growth Factors in the Fetus and Neonate

Sandra E. Juul, M.D., Ph.D.

Hematopoietic growth factors usually are classified as those responsible for the regulation of myeloid and erythroid growth and differentiation, called colony-stimulating factors (CSFs), and those concerned with immunity, called lymphokines. Once sequenced, lymphokines are assigned interleukin (IL) numbers. More than 20 hematopoietic growth factors have been identified and sequenced. Hematopoietic growth factors have extensive functional overlap (redundancy), and each growth factor has a multiplicity of biologic actions (pleiotropy). More than one hematopoietic growth factor controls cells in any cell lineage, and most such factors affect cells in more than one lineage.[1–4] Redundancy and pleiotropy of hematopoietic growth factors have been well established in hematopoiesis and appear also to characterize their nonhematopoietic functions.

Many hematopoietic cytokines were discovered by virtue of their clonogenic, growth-promoting effects on hematopoietic progenitors or because of their specific immune functions. Effects of these factors initially were assumed to be specific to the hematopoietic system, but functional receptors for several of these factors have been demonstrated at nonhematopoietic sites, including the reproductive system and the central nervous system (CNS).[5–8] Complex interactions involving the CNS, the neuroendocrine system, and the immune system are beginning to be delineated.[9, 10] Glia and neurons produce many of the cytokines once thought to be restricted to the hematopoietic system. They also express receptors for these peptides, suggesting the capability of paracrine and autocrine interaction during neurodevelopment and roles in the maintenance of brain homeostasis during adult years.[8, 11–14] Much information has accumulated regarding the specific roles of hematopoietic cytokines in hematopoiesis. One area of active research concerns the roles of these factors in nonhematopoietic systems, and this chapter reviews these functions.

STRUCTURAL CHARACTERISTICS OF HEMATOPOIETIC GROWTH FACTORS AND THEIR RECEPTORS

Erythropoietin (EPO), granulocyte-macrophage colony-stimulating factor (GM-CSF), and granulocyte colony-stimulating factor (G-CSF) belong to a family of hematopoietic growth factors that includes growth hormone, prolactin, and IL-2 through IL-7.[15–17] These cytokines share a predicted tertiary structure containing four antiparallel α helixes with different-sized connecting loops. Hematopoietic growth factors function by binding to specific cell-surface receptors. Specific ligand binding results in allosteric changes in the receptor molecules that, depending on the type of receptor, results in protein kinase activation, as with macrophage colony-stimulating factor (M-CSF),[16–18] or in a cascade of intracellular signaling through the Janus kinase-2 (JAK-2) kinase mechanism, as characterized by EPO.[19, 20]

The receptors for most hematopoietic growth factors (except CSF-1R [formerly FMS] and KIT, which are tyrosine kinase receptors) belong to a receptor superfamily. Family members include specific receptors for GM-CSF, G-CSF, IL-3 through IL-7, growth hormone, prolactin, neurociliary trophic factor, and thrombopoietin. Members of this family share certain features, including four conserved Cys residues, a common binding domain, and absence of a tyrosine kinase domain in the cytoplasmic domain. Most of these cytokine receptors have a characteristic five-residue motif in the extracellular domain (Trp-Ser-X-Trp-Ser [WSXWS], in which X is any amino acid) that is critical for proper folding of the extracellular region and for hormone binding. The growth hormone receptor and prolactin receptor have similar primary structures, but both lack the WSXWS motif. Receptors in this superfamily are characterized by two sets of antiparallel amphipathic β sheets connected through a hinge region of variable size, which together form a pocket for the ligand.[16, 17, 21–28] These cytokine receptors are often assembled as multiple subunit complexes and have been grouped into subfamilies based on the pattern subunit formation.[1, 29] In some cases (e.g., GM-CSF receptor), an accessory protein contributes to the stability of the receptor complex.[24]

ERYTHROPOIETIN

EPO is a major determinant of tissue oxygenation during health and disease and performs this function by regulating production of red blood cells. Abnormalities of EPO or EPO receptor (EPOR) regulation or function result in disease states such as polycythemia vera[30] or anemia of prematurity,[31] and absence of EPO or its receptor leads to fetal death around embryonic day 13 in mouse knock-out models.[32]

Administration of recombinant EPO (rEPO) has gained acceptance in treating many clinical situations, including the anemia of prematurity,[33] chronic renal failure,[34] and certain chronic inflammatory conditions associated with chronic anemia.[35] This treatment is viewed as physiologic, because it supplements low concentrations of circulating EPO in circumstances of associated bone marrow erythroid hypoplasia.[36] Side effects of such therapy include an increased feeling of well-being, neuromuscular enhancement,[37] hypertension,[38–40] neutropenia, and fever with influenza-like symptoms.[41]

In the past, EPO was thought to act specifically and exclusively on hematopoietic cells. However, the effects of EPO are more widespread, and the presence of functional EPOR has been documented in a variety of nonhematopoietic tissues in animal models, in vitro cell culture studies, and in humans.[14, 42–58] Nonerythroid cell types on which EPOR has been shown include liver stromal cells,[54] endothelial cells,[42, 43, 45, 57] mesangial cells,[59] smooth muscle cells,[59] placental tissues,[55, 60] and cells of neuronal origin.[14, 49–51, 56, 58, 61–63] EPO has a mitogenic effect on several of these cell types in vitro.[42, 54, 64] Wald and colleagues[64] reported that addition of rEPO to cardiomyocytes resulted in mitogenic and chemotactic responses, similar to rEPO's action on endothelial cells, and that this response was most likely mediated by Na^+,K^+-ATPase activity. After stimulation with rEPO, influx of calcium and modulation of cAMP levels have been reported for several cell types, including endothelial cells, smooth muscle cells, and PC12 cells.[46, 51, 59, 65–67]

Carlini and coworkers[45, 46] reported that incubation of endothelial cells with rEPO increases endothelin-1 synthesis and release and that this response involves calcium signaling. This dose-dependent effect of rEPO on endothelial cells has been confirmed by other workers[68] and might contribute to the hypertension seen in dialysis patients treated with rEPO.[69]

Another potentially important effect of rEPO on endothelial cells is that of angiogenesis.[47] Brain capillary endothelial cells express a functional membrane-bound EPOR and a soluble EPOR. It was hypothesized by Yamaji and colleagues[57] that, under conditions of hypoxia, EPO might act as a competence factor for these cells and contribute to the growth of new capillary vessels in the brain.

One function proposed for EPO has been as

a general morphogen and inducer of neurogenesis during early development.[70] Yasuda and associates[70] identified widespread distribution of EPO and EPOR in the developing mouse embryo by a combination of reverse transcriptase–polymerase chain reaction (RT-PCR) and immunolocalization. EPORs are also present in many organs of the developing human fetus, including the brain, eye, heart, small bowel, adrenal, liver, and kidney (Fig. 4–1).[71] Human placenta synthesizes EPO.[60] Physiologically relevant circulating concentrations of EPO may be present from early gestation, functioning in concert with other somatic growth factors to influence the growth and development of fetal organs by way of interaction with specific EPORs.

Another possible source of EPO in the neonate is breast milk.[72] Significant concentrations of EPO have been found in human milk, and specific binding of recombinant human EPO (rhEPO) to EPOR in rat gastric mucosal cells has been documented.[53] Human small bowel mucosa expresses the EPOR (see Fig. 4–1*F*), milk-borne EPO can resist proteolytic digestion at physiologic pH, and increased erythropoietic indices have been documented in nursing rat pups following a hemorrhagic insult to the dam.[73] These data support an absorptive role for the EPORs in the small bowel mucosa. An alternative role for enteral EPO might be its local effects on villous enterocytes.

The distribution of EPO and EPORs within the developing human CNS has potential ramifications for neurodevelopment. Serum concentrations of EPO increase markedly and rapidly during hypoxia. Increased EPO concentrations in fetal serum and amniotic fluid have been identified as markers of a distressed fetus in utero.[73–77] In animals, production of EPO within the brain increases during periods of hypoxia.[78] The significance of these findings and their relevance to developing humans was previously unknown. It has been shown, however, by RT-PCR and immunolocalization that EPO and EPOR are present in the developing human brain as early as 5 weeks after conception.[14, 58] EPO is present in the cerebrospinal fluid of normal preterm and term infants, and this EPO concentration decreases with age, although low concentrations persist into adulthood (Fig. 4–2).[79] No correlations between blood and cerebrospinal fluid concentrations of EPO have been found,[80] and no neurodevelopmental differences between infants treated with rEPO and untreated infants have been reported. This is of particular interest, because rEPO is sometimes used in the treatment of anemia of prematurity, and because the function of EPO within the CNS is not yet understood, it is reassuring to know that systemic rEPO treatment probably does not directly affect CNS function.

There is increasing evidence that the EPORs expressed in neural tissues are functional. Early studies showed that addition of rEPO to neural cells resulted in increased monoamine concentrations and increased intracellular calcium concentrations.[49, 51, 61] Circumstantial evidence that EPO and EPOR may serve a role in neurogenesis is provided by the presence of this ligand-receptor pair in the embryonic and fetal murine brain, with evidence of developmental regulation.[70, 81] EPO increases in vivo survival of lesioned rat cholinergic septal neurons produced by fimbria-fornix transections and augments choline acetyltransferase activity in cultured neurons.[49, 56] EPO may also function as a neurotropic factor, influencing neuronal development, differentiation, maintenance, and regeneration.[49, 82]

EPO can be neuroprotective when cultured neurons and neuron precursor cells are exposed to hypoxia,[14] and pretreatment of cultured neurons with physiologic concentrations of rEPO for more than 8 hours can prevent glutamate-induced neuronal death.[63] Ultraviolet radiation–induced apoptosis can also be decreased by pretreatment of NT2 cells with 50 mU/mL of rEPO (Fig. 4–3). EPO is neuroprotective for several different types of neurons in diverse circumstances, suggesting that it may be an important mechanism for neural preservation in adverse conditions.

The temporal and cellular distribution of EPO and EPOR in the developing human CNS has been identified using a combination of RT-PCR and immunohistochemistry.[80] The mRNAs for EPO and EPOR were detected as early as 5 weeks' gestation and persisted through 24 weeks after conception. After documenting the specificity of antibody staining by Western blotting, cellular localization of EPO and EPOR were determined by immunolocalization. In the early cerebral hemisphere of 5 to 6 weeks postconception, EPO and EPOR localized to the periventricular layer of neuro-

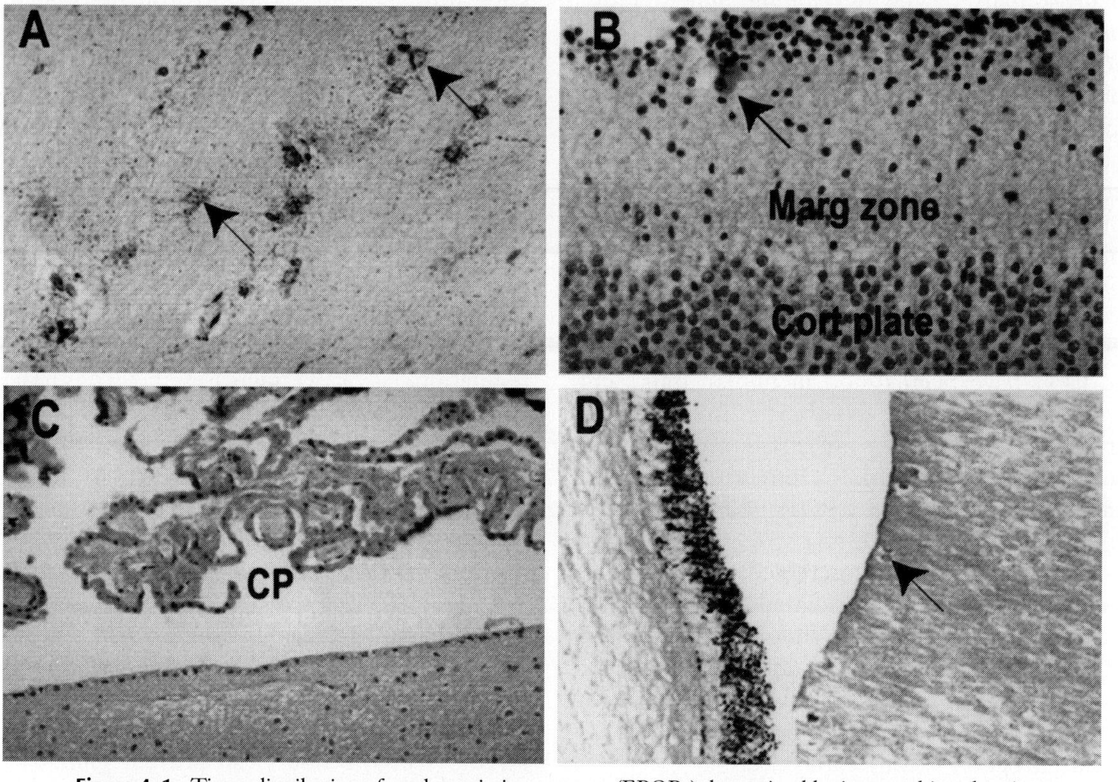

Figure 4–1. Tissue distribution of erythropoietin receptors (EPORs) determined by immunohistochemistry. Tissues from various times during development have been stained with an affinity-purified rabbit polyclonal antibody raised against amino acids 489 to 508 of the carboxyl terminus of the precursor form of human EPOR. Negative controls for these reactions included preincubation with a specific blocking peptide and substitution of preimmune sera for primary antibody. *A* through *C* show specific immunoreactive cell types within the brain. *A*, In this example of astrocyte immunoreactivity within the deep white matter of an adult brain, single astrocytes *(arrows)* are identified (original magnification ×400). *B*, Cajal Retzius neurons *(arrow)* are identified in the subpial granular layer of the developing 20-week brain, as are the underlying marginal zone and cortical plate (original magnification ×400). *C*, Positive staining of choroid plexus (CP) from an adult brain (original magnification ×200). *D*, Immunoreactivity of the neural retina at 8 weeks' gestation (original magnification ×400). An arrow identifies a mitotic cell. Although the strongest immunoreactivity occurs at the mitotic surface, the entire cell layer is moderately reactive.

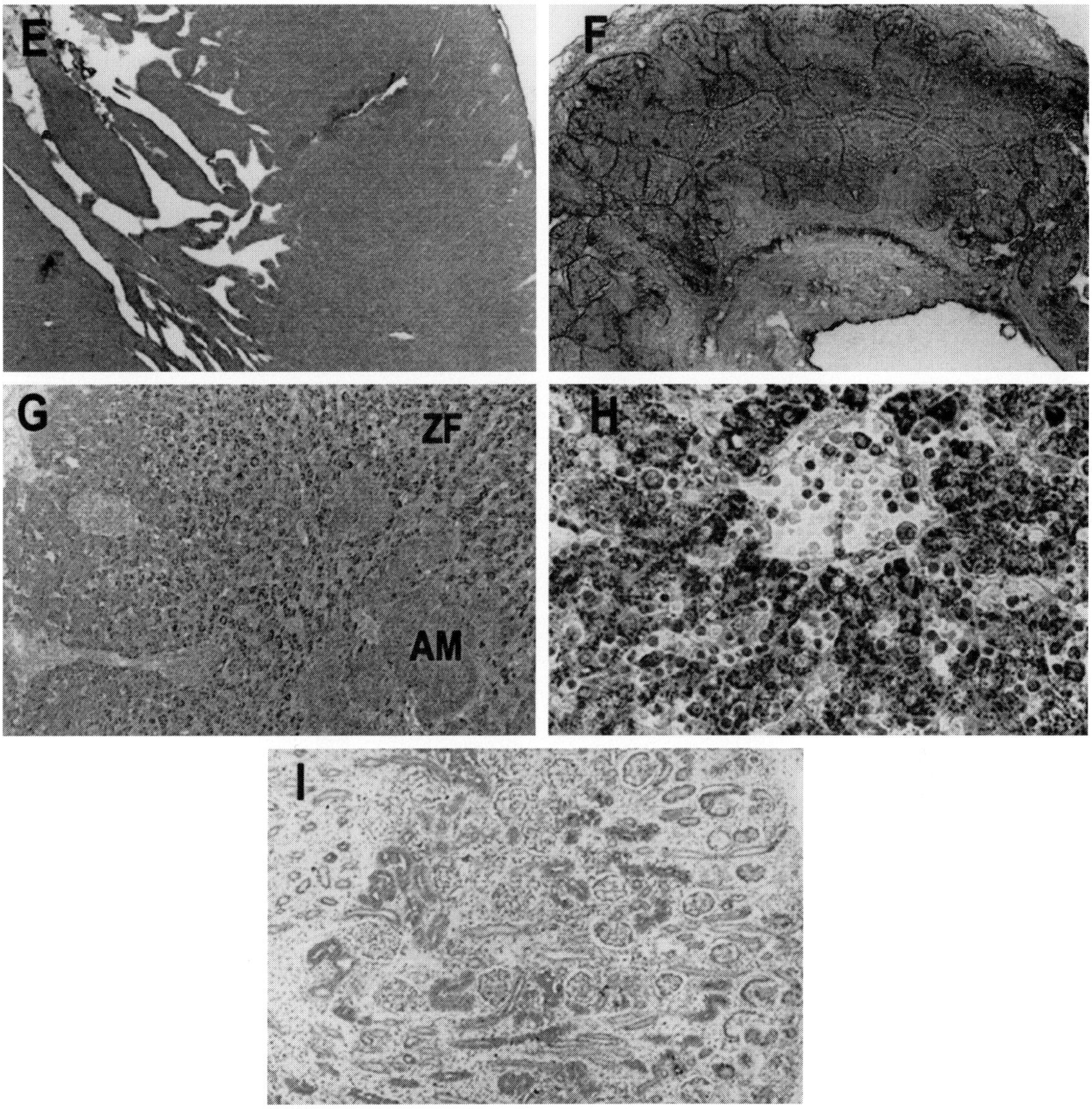

Figure 4–1 *Continued. E,* At 18 weeks after conception, the myocardium is strongly immunoreactive (original magnification ×40). *F,* Portion of the small bowel from an 8-week postconception fetus (original magnification ×100). *G,* Adrenal medulla (AM) and the zona fasciculata (ZF) of the adrenal cortex. Immunoreactivity for EPOR is present in all zones of the adrenal cortex and in the AM. *H,* Liver at 18 weeks of gestation. Notice the strong reactivity of the liver parenchymal cells and the nascent hematopoietic cells. *I,* In a kidney at 22 weeks after conception, immunoreactivity occurs primarily in the proximal tubules.

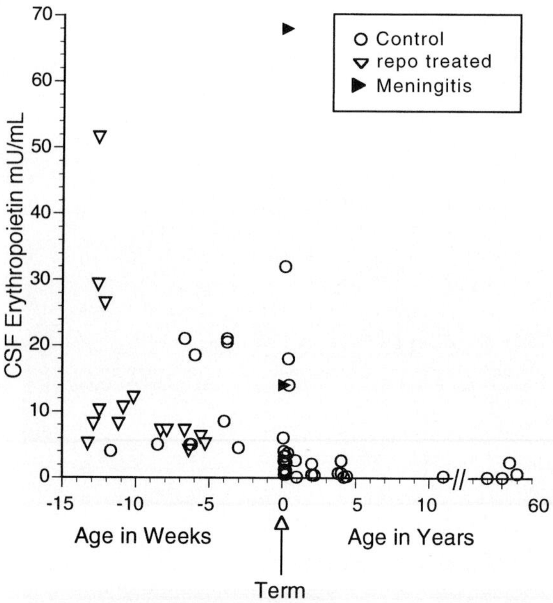

Figure 4–2. Erythropoietin (EPO) concentrations in the cerebrospinal fluid (CSF) of 80 subjects. The concentration of EPO was measured in the spinal fluid of 80 subjects by specific enzyme-linked immunosorbent assay. Control individuals (no rEPO therapy) are identified by open circles, infants receiving treatment with rEPO are denoted by open triangles, and the two patients with meningitis (neither received rEPO) are shown by filled triangles. Erythropoietin concentrations (mU/mL) are reported on the y-axis. Corrected age is plotted in weeks along the x-axis up to term gestation *(arrow)*. After term gestation, age is plotted in years.

epithelial cells (Fig. 4–4*A, B*). As development progressed, a difference in the pattern of expression of these two proteins became apparent. At 10 weeks' postconception, EPO immunoreactivity was present throughout the cortical wall, with the most intense immunoreactivity observed in the ventricular and subventricular zones (see Fig. 4–4*C*). EPOR was localized primarily to the subventricular zone, with little staining evident in the ventricular zone (see Fig. 4–4*D*). The ventricular zone is the germinal zone for nascent neurons, which migrate along radial glial fibers to populate the six layers of the cortex.[83] The subventricular zone contains multipotential progenitor cells that do not express mature neuronal or glial antigens.[84] In vivo, the fate of cells derived from the subventricular zone is restricted to oligodendrocytes and astrocytes.[85] In vitro, these cells have the potential to develop into neurons.

With increased fetal maturity, the diffuse staining of broad zones of developing cortex seen in early gestation are replaced by more specific cellular staining for EPO and EPOR. At 20 weeks' postconception, specific cellular staining for EPO and EPOR is present in the dentate nucleus of the hypothalamus (see Fig. 4–4*E, F*) and in astrocytic cells in the subventricular region. At 32 weeks' gestation, diffuse EPO immunoreactivity is identified in the pyramidal cell layer and in other populations of neurons, although a subpopulation of astrocytes also stains with EPO antibody (see Fig. 4–4*G*). In contrast, EPOR staining is most prominent in cells of astrocytic character and location (see Figs. 4–1A and 4–4 *H*), although a few specific cell types such as Cajal Retzius neurons and cells of the choroid plexus continue to show immunoreactivity for EPO and EPOR (see Fig. 4–1*B, C*). EPOR staining in the brains of teenagers and adults is localized to astrocytes and neurons, suggesting a maturational change in the distribution of the receptor. The presence of the receptor in neurons and astrocytes suggests

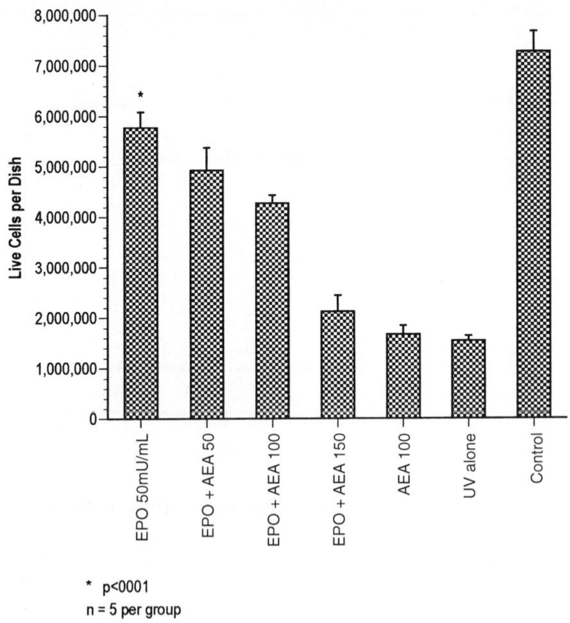

Figure 4–3. Live cell counts after 13 seconds of ultraviolet (UV) radiation exposure. NT2 cells (human neuronal precursor cell line) were preincubated overnight at 37°C under the following conditions: 50 mU/mL of recombinant erythropoietin (rEPO); 50 mU/mL rEPO plus 50 μL/mL anti-EPO neutralizing antibody (AEA); 50 mU/mL rEPO plus 100 μL/mL AEA; 50 mU/mL rEPO plus 150 μL/mL AEA; 150 μL/mL AEA alone; or no additives with or without UV exposure. Cells were then exposed to 13 seconds of UV light, and 24 hours later, the surviving live cells were trypsinized, spun down, and counted by hemocytometer. Live cells per plate are plotted on the y-axis, with the condition plotted on the x-axis.

autocrine and paracrine functions for EPO within the brain.

Predominance of EPOR staining in astrocytes in human fetal brains is at some variance with published studies using murine models, which suggest that EPORs are present primarily on neurons. However, differences in species, in vivo and in vitro techniques, and maturity of the source of cultured cells probably explain these discrepancies. Although synthesis of EPO within the rodent brain is up-regulated during hypoxia, the mechanism by which up-regulation occurs is unknown; neither has the specific cell type in which synthesis is up-regulated been identified, although it is thought to be in astrocytes.[61, 78] EPO synthesis may occur in different cell types under conditions of normal homeostasis or conditions of stress such as hypoxemia.[14] EPO probably has effects on neuronal and glial functions.

Distribution of EPO and its receptor is more widespread in the developing human than was initially postulated. The receptor is widely distributed during early fetal development, leading to the speculation that EPO acts in concert with other growth factors to optimize growth and development during this period. Although further investigation is required to understand EPO's nonhematopoietic roles, it is likely that many of the mechanisms of action that have been worked out for hematopoiesis may be at work in nonhematopoietic systems.

GRANULOCYTE-MACROPHAGE COLONY-STIMULATING FACTOR

GM-CSF is a multipotential hematopoietic growth factor that has overlapping functions with IL-3, although it acts on slightly more mature progenitor cells.[86–88] This 23-kd glycoprotein was initially identified by its ability to promote in vitro proliferation and differentiation of hematopoietic progenitors to neutrophils and macrophages and, to a lesser extent, the generation of eosinophils, erythrocytes, megakaryocytes, and dendritic cells.[89–91] The in vivo function of murine GM-CSF has been studied in the mouse knock-out model. Although GM-CSF is not an essential growth factor for basal hematopoiesis, its absence leads to progressive accumulation of surfactant lipids and proteins in the alveolar space, characteristic of the idiopathic human disorder of pulmonary alveolar proteinosis.[92, 93] This pulmonary abnormality can be reversed by GM-CSF expression targeted to the respiratory epithelium in transgenic mice.[94]

In addition to its effects on lung homeostasis, GM-CSF appears to have specific effects within the CNS. Centrally acting GM-CSF can be produced within the brain by astrocytes, can be stimulated by cytokines such as tumor necrosis factor-α (TNF-α) or IL-6,[95–98] or can cross the blood-brain barrier to act as an important signaling molecule between the CNS and the periphery.[99] GM-CSF also modulates the growth and state of activation of several types of glial cells, including astrocytes, oligodendrocytes, and microglia.[100–102] Much like EPO, GM-CSF augments choline acetyltransferase activity in mouse embryonic primary septal neurons and in the cholinergic hybridoma cell line SN6 in vitro in a dose-dependent manner. GM-CSF can promote survival of septal cholinergic neurons of adult rats after fimbria-fornix transections, suggesting that it may function as a neurotropic factor to influence the differentiation, maintenance, and regeneration of cholinergic neurons.[49, 56] When GM-CSF is used in combination with IL-3 to stimulate cells, neurite extension is increased.[103] GM-CSF therefore may have important neuroimmune and neuroregenerative functions.

GRANULOCYTE COLONY-STIMULATING FACTOR

G-CSF is a hematopoietic growth factor that selectively promotes proliferation, differentiation, and maturation of neutrophils.[104, 105] It also affects the function of mature neutrophils, prolonging their survival and increasing their chemotactic and bacteriocidal activities. Less information is available about the nonhematopoietic effects of G-CSF than about those of EPO and GM-CSF, but its effects within the CNS appear to overlap those of GM-CSF. Addition of rG-CSF to primary septal neurons or to the cholinergic neuronal cell line SN6 improves choline acetyltransferase activity and cell survival after fimbria-fornix transection.[49] Human astrocytes

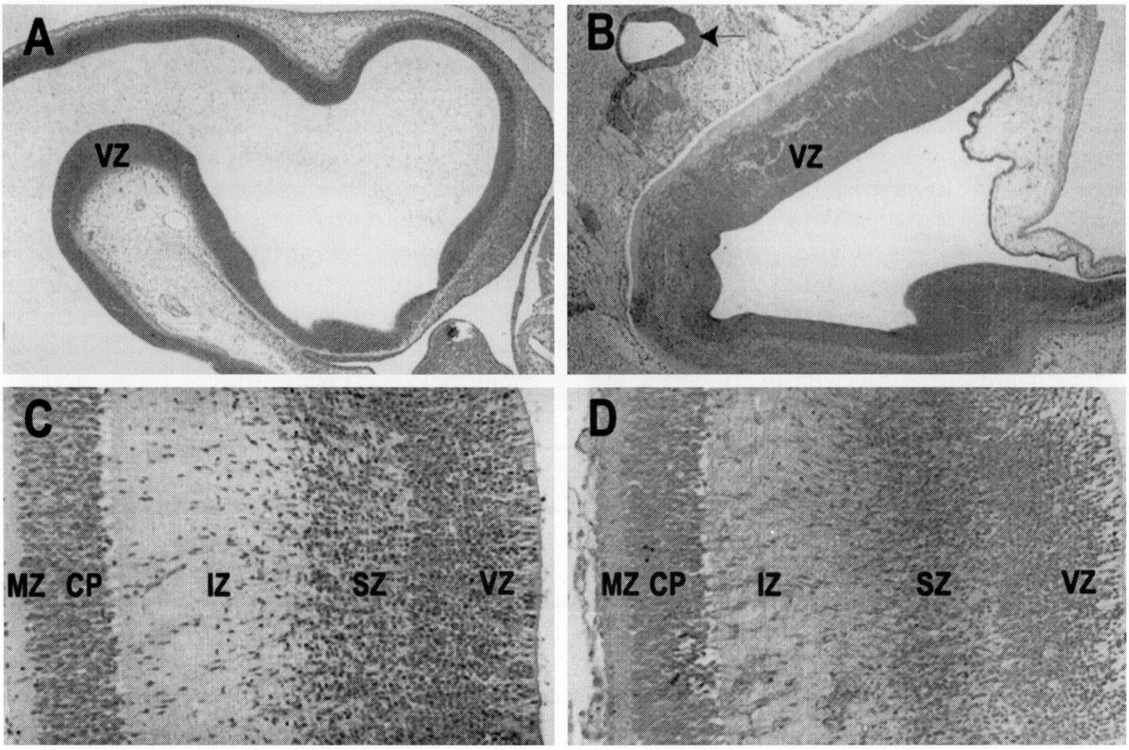

Figure 4–4. Immunohistochemical localization of erythropoietin (EPO) and erythropoietin receptors (EPOR) with neurodevelopment. EPO immunoreactivity is shown in the left panels, and EPOR immunoreactivity in the right panels. *A* and *B*, Diffuse immunostaining of the ventricular zone (V) from fetuses at 5 and 6 weeks' gestation, respectively. The arrow in *B* identifies the otic vesicle. *C* and *D*, Cross sections through the cerebral cortex of a 10-week fetus demonstrate the divergence in EPO and EPOR patterns of immunoreactivity, respectively. The five discrete regions of the cerebral cortex at this stage of development are labeled: ventricular zone (VZ), subventricular zone (SZ), intermediate zone (IZ), cortical plate (CP), and marginal zone (MZ).

in culture do not constitutively produce G-CSF or GM-CSF. However, when stimulated by cytokines such as IL-1β or TNF-α, high levels of specific mRNAs and protein production are found, suggesting a role in the neural-immune axis.[7]

MACROPHAGE COLONY-STIMULATING FACTOR

M-CSF, also known as colony-stimulating factor-1 (CSF-1), was initially identified as a growth factor for mononuclear phagocytes.[106] Developmental and functional studies using mice have demonstrated the importance of this growth factor in placental regulation,[107, 108] male and female fertility,[109, 110] and bone remodeling (i.e., the importance of osteoclasts).[111, 112] The relevance of M-CSF to human pregnancy has been suggested by its presence in human reproductive tissues.[113, 114]

In a study investigating the potential role of hematopoietic cytokines in the development of fetal mouse brain, Chang and coworkers[115] analyzed the production of multiple cytokines, including IL-1α, IL-2 through IL-7, M-CSF, G-CSF, and GM-CSF, by S1-nuclease protection analysis. Only M-CSF transcripts were produced constitutively in normal brain tissue, and these were detected from embryonic day 13 through adulthood, as were transcripts encoding the M-CSF receptor (CSF-1R).[115] Synthesis of M-CSF by astrocytes has been confirmed by other workers,[116–118] and it may be essential for microglial maturation and differentiation.[119, 120] In cell culture experiments, M-CSF treatment of neurons from normal embryonic brain resulted in dose-dependent improved survival and promoted process outgrowth, whereas M-CSF treatment of neurons cultured from the M-CSF

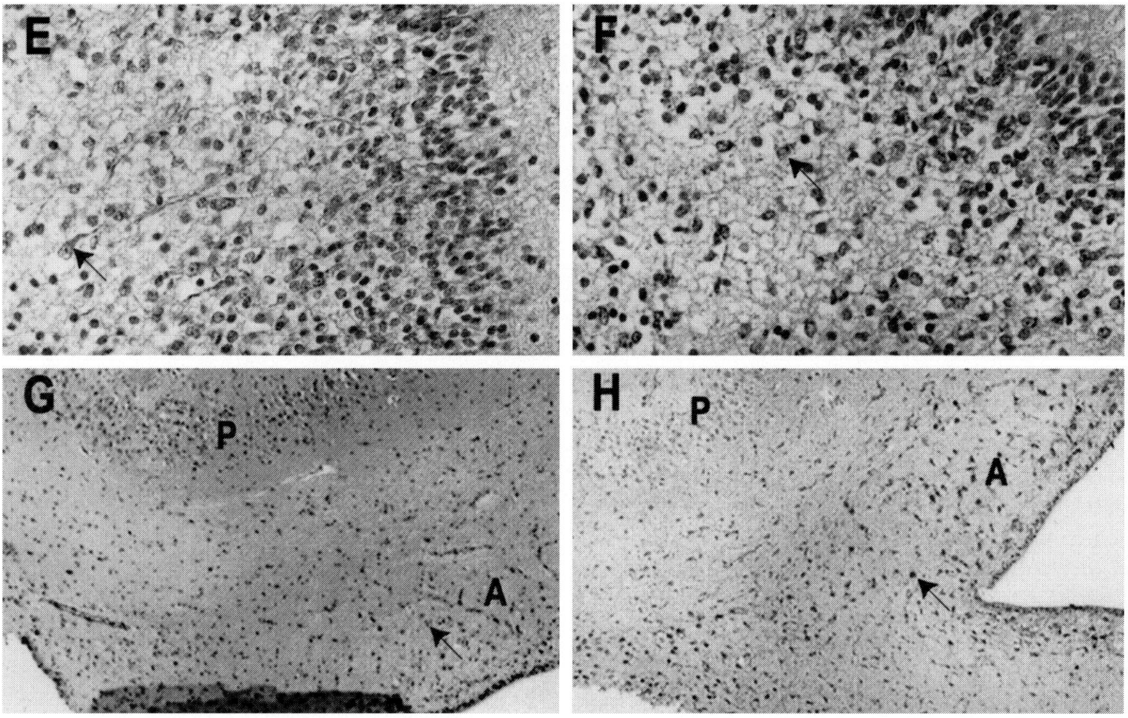

Figure 4–4 *Continued. E* and *F,* Adjacent sections of hippocampus taken from a 20-week fetus. Arrows identify specific cells that are immunoreactive. *G* and *H,* Adjacent sections from a 32-week fetal brain demonstrate the diffuse EPO immunoreactivity of the parietal cell layer (P), with additional immunoreactivity of scattered astrocytes *(arrow)* in the alveus (A). EPOR immunoreactivity is more specific to the astrocytes in the alveus *(arrow).*

null mutation *(op/op)* promoted significantly less process outgrowth.[121]

Preliminary neuropathologic studies on brains of *op/op* mice identified no cytoarchitectural or histopathologic abnormalities, although brain weight was less than that of normal and heterozygous littermates.[115] More in-depth studies of this null mutation mouse have, however, identified significant neurosensory deficits, with abnormal brain stem auditory and visual evoked potentials, aberrant neuronal function within the visual cortex, alterations in the cortical circuitry balancing excitation and inhibition, and increased neuronal vulnerability to injury.[121, 122] These animals have an abnormal microglial response to hypoxia that results in larger infarcts after a standard vascular insult. Exogenous M-CSF improved the survival of neurons in the ischemic lesion of normal and *op/op* animals.[123, 124] This suggests that M-CSF has a role in neurodevelopment and possibly in neuroprotection. It also illustrates that normal structure does not necessarily imply normal function. As the function of hematopoietic cytokines are evaluated in nonhematopoietic systems, this is an important concept to remember.

INTERLEUKIN-1

IL-1α and IL-1β are two distinct gene products recognized by the same cell-surface receptor (IL-1R). These cytokines are classic "alarm peptides" synthesized in response to noxious stimuli such as infection, the increase of which results in a reaction cascade known as the *acute-phase response.*

In addition to its immunogenic activities, IL-1 has many effects within the CNS. These are mediated through the specific IL-1 receptor and have been identified in many specific subpopulations of neurons and in glial cells.[125–130] Brain structures to which IL-1R have been localized include the anterior olfactory nucleus, medial thalamic nucleus, posterior thalamic nucleus, basolateral amygdaloid nucleus, ventromedial hypothalamic nucleus, arcuate nucleus, median eminence, mesencephalic trigeminal nucleus, motor trigeminal nucleus, facial nucleus, and Purkinje cells of the cerebellum.[125, 130, 131] Astrocytes and glial cells are sources of IL-1 within the brain, and systemically administered rIL-1 has significant CNS effects.[132–134]

IL-1α has been implicated as a neurotropic factor in the CNS, a function that appears to be developmentally specific.[135] During normal neurodevelopment, IL-1 is produced by ameboid microglia, and this IL-1 has growth-promoting effects on astroglia.[118, 136, 137] In primary cell cultures of spinal cord dorsal root ganglion from 9-day-old rats, treatment or pretreatment with IL-1α improves neuronal survival, an effect that can be mediated by nerve growth factor.[135, 138] These effects are, however, age dependent; IL-1α treatment of cultures from 1-month-old animals produce neuronal cell death.[135]

IL-1 is up-regulated during periods of stress or injury.[139–141] The effects of rIL-1 given by intravenous, intraperitoneal, or intracerebral injection mimic many of the physiologic responses to pathologic states (e.g., infection) or stressful events. For example, IL-1 appears to be involved in up-regulation of temperature[10, 142, 143] and sleep,[144, 145] and in down-regulation of appetite,[145] symptoms that often accompany systemic illness. IL-1β is a potent activator of the hypothalamic-pituitary-adrenal axis, and many of its effects are mediated by the release of corticotropin-releasing hormone and activation of the sympathetic nervous system.[142, 146, 147] Administration of rIL-1β peripherally or centrally results in corticosteroid release from the adrenals.[146, 148–151] Some studies indicate that the stimulatory effect of IL-1 on the hypothalamus is mediated by the cyclooxygenase metabolites of arachidonic acid and, among others, by prostaglandin $F_{2\alpha}$.[152, 153]

The role of IL-1 in brain damage from stroke or ischemia has been investigated. During middle cerebral artery occlusion in rats, IL-1 expression increases. The volume of the resulting infarct is markedly reduced by administration of IL-1R antagonist (IL-1Ra).[154] Other studies support the role of IL-1 in ischemic brain damage, revealing potent, sustained, neuroprotective effects of recombinant human IL-1Ra in the cortex and striatum and suggesting that IL-1 may influence cortical damage through the release of specific substances or activation of polysynaptic pathways.[155, 156] The brain's response to IL-1 is age related, and this may be one reason for the changing sensitivity of brain to hypoxic-ischemic injury with age.[157]

Large amounts of nitric oxide are produced in the brain in response to pathologic stimuli such as infectious agents, ischemia, and trauma. IL-1β stimulates inducible nitric oxide synthase (iNOS) mRNA expression and iNOS-enzyme activity in brain microvascular endothelial cells,[158] in glia,[134] and in hypothalamic cell cultures.[159] IL-1β also induces calcium-independent NOS activity in cultured cerebellar granule neurons.[160] This may be another mechanism by which IL-1 affects homeostasis.

In addition to the neuroimmune axis, there appears to be an immune-brain-gut interaction such that peripheral or central injection of rIL-1 results in dose-related inhibition of gastric acid output.[161, 162] This effect is mediated through central IL-1 receptors and through prostaglandin- and corticotropin-releasing factor–dependent mechanisms.[163]

INTERLEUKIN-2

IL-2 is a 15.5-kd, single-chain protein that enhances T and B lymphocyte proliferation and differentiation after antigenic stimulation and induces growth and activation of natural killer (NK) cells and thymocytes.[164, 165] IL-2 interacts with a specific membrane-associated receptor (IL-2R) that consists of variable subunits: a low-affinity, glycosylated p55 subunit (IL-2Rα chain), a higher-affinity glycosylated p75 subunit (IL-2Rβ chain), and an intermediate-affinity p95–110 subunit (IL-2Rδ chain).[166]

In addition to its presence on the surface of specific cells of the immune system, the IL-2R has been localized to specific regions of murine forebrain, including the hippocampus, the frontal cortex, and the striatum.[167–169] Recombinant IL-2 has been used as a chemotherapeutic agent to bolster the cytolytic functions of lymphoid cells, but a wide range of toxic effects have occurred, particularly symptoms referable to the CNS.[166] These included somnolence, depression, confusion, convulsions, coma, and psychiatric disorders.[166, 170] Increased concentrations of IL-2 in the spinal fluid of schizophrenic patients have been associated with recurrence of psychotic symptoms.[171]

Because of the range of CNS symptoms that

have been observed with the administration of rIL-2, several studies have investigated the importance of IL-2 in the CNS. In vitro studies have shown that IL-2 has a survival or growth-promoting effect on cortical, striatal, hippocampal, and septal neurons and on oligodendrocytes.[12, 172, 173] IL-2 also has dose-dependent potentiating or inhibitory effects on hippocampal acetylcholine release, effects that appear to be mediated in part by γ-aminobutyric acid.[174] Dopamine release from rat striatal cells and mesencephalic cells can be stimulated by IL-2.[175, 176] In a study comparing the effects of IL-2 on sympathetic and sensory neurons, only sympathetic neurons showed a neurotropic response.[177]

Intraventricular injection of IL-2 in rats results in a marked decrease in neuron discharge frequency in the ventromedial nucleus of hypothalamus and a marked increase in the supraoptic and paraventricular nuclei. Because the supraoptic and paraventricular nuclei secrete antidiuretic hormone, their excitation may contribute to the water retention observed during rIL-2 treatment.[178] Chronic (14-day) exposure of rat brains to intracerebral rIL-2 is associated with increased plasma levels of corticosterone. Immunohistochemical evaluations of these brains showed an accumulation of non-neural, major histocompatibility complex class II–positive cells and T and B lymphocytes within the infused brain hemisphere. Reactive astrogliosis, microglial activation, endothelial up-regulation of adhesion molecules, myelin damage, and neuronal loss were also observed in this model, suggesting that persistently elevated central levels of IL-2 lead to nervous tissue injury.[179]

INTERLEUKIN-3

IL-3, also known as multi-CSF, acts on a wide range of hematopoietic cells to stimulate their proliferation and differentiation.[3] It interacts with its cognate receptor, which in humans is composed of a ligand-specific α subunit and a β subunit that is common to GM-CSF and IL-5.[24]

Null mutations for the β subunit result in animals with lymphocytic infiltration of lung parenchyma, with areas resembling alveolar proteinosis and low basal numbers of circulating eosinophils.[180] Like many of the other hematopoietic cytokines, IL-3 appears to be active in brain tissue. It enhances neurite outgrowth of cholinergic neurons and increases choline acetyltransferase activity,[49, 56, 181] and these effects are mediated by interaction with its cognate receptor. In vivo, rIL-3 infused into the lateral ventricles of rats after unilateral axotomy of the septohippocampal pathways results in significant numbers of acetylcholinesterase-positive neurons remaining in the septal region,[181] suggesting that IL-3 may act on cholinergic neurons, as well as being a neurotropic factor influencing the differentiation, maintenance, and regeneration.

INTERLEUKIN-6

IL-6 was first identified as a product of monocytes, but it has since been shown to be produced by a variety of somatic and CNS cell types, including fibroblasts, endothelial cells, astrocytes, and microglia, and by cells from human astrocytomas.[182] IL-6 mRNA production in brain has been localized to the Purkinje cells and hippocampal neurons,[183] and functional receptors have been demonstrated on PC12 cells, sympathetic neurons, cholinergic neurons, and cultured astrocytes.[184–187] TNF-α is one cytokine involved in the up-regulation of IL-6R expression, and corticosteroids down-regulate receptor expression.[187]

IL-6 does not affect differentiation of cultured embryonic rat septal cholinergic neurons,[188] but it can induce differentiation of PC12 cells, immature adrenal chromaffin-like cells that undergo differentiation to sympathetic neuron–like cells. The mechanism by which IL-6 induces PC12 differentiation is through induction of an active RAS-GTP complex.[189] Studies conflict about whether IL-6 is expressed during normal neurodevelopment, with some studies showing constitutive expression[190] and others refuting this finding.[115, 118] Although the role of IL-6 in neurodevelopment is unclear, there is convincing evidence that it plays a role in the modulation of inflammatory or pathologic events. For example, elevated IL-6 concentrations have been measured biochemically in the brains of Alzheimer's patients, and IL-6 immunoreactivity has been identified at the site of primitive plaques, raising a question about whether IL-6 contributes to brain injury in this disease.[191] Transgenic mice, in which human IL-6 expression has been targeted to neurons, develop reactive astrocytosis and an increase in ramified microglial cells, but they do not show evidence of neuron damage.[192] IL-6 also is associated with intrauterine infection, with elevated amniotic fluid concentrations of IL-6 corresponding with neonatal white matter damage in human infants.[193, 194] IL-6 may affect the susceptibility of certain neurons to damage by altering the intracellular calcium responses to neurotransmittors.[195]

In contrast to the data suggesting that IL-6 is harmful to the CNS, several studies show that IL-6 has significant neurotropic effects on cholinergic neurons. It enhances choline acetyltransferase activity[188] and improves neuronal survival, an effect that is dose dependent, blocked by specific neutralizing antibody, and is independent of nerve growth factor.[188, 196] Preincubation of PC12 cells with IL-6 prevents the apoptotic cell death induced by serum deprivation or the calcium ionophore A23187.[197] Rat astrocytes subjected to an hypoxic-ischemic insult release IL-6 in a time-dependent manner. Conditioned media from these stimulated astrocytes have a neuroprotective effect on differentiated PC12 cells that is blocked by specific neutralizing antibody, suggesting the possibility of a paracrine neurotropic effect during brain ischemia.[198]

Another central effect of IL-6 is to stimulate the human hypothalamic-pituitary-adrenal axis. IL-6 administered intravenously results in marked elevations of plasma corticotropin, cortisol, and plasma arginine vasopressin concentrations. This effect is not mediated by an increase in IL-1 or TNF-α concentrations; concentrations of these cytokines do not increase after dosing with IL-6.[199]

INTERLEUKIN-12

IL-12 is a 75-kd heterodimeric cytokine composed of two chains (p35 and p40). It stimulates activated T cells and synergizes with IL-2 in inducing cytotoxic lymphocyte proliferation.[200] In the CNS, IL-12 secretion is stimulated by microglial cells but not by astrocytes or by lipopolysaccharide (LPS) alone, or by LPS in combination with interferon-δ.[201–204] This upregulation of IL-12 is inhibited by IL-10, prostaglandin E_2, and cAMP-elevating agents. Coculture of microglia with astrocytes or exposure of microglia to astrocyte-conditioned medium modifies the IL-12 response, suggesting a regulatory role for astrocytes in IL-12 production.[201] Increased concentrations of IL-12 activate interferon-δ and TNF-α production, resulting in a substantial increase in type III NOS immunoreactivity in astrocytes. This complex interaction affects regulation of perfusion and may affect maintenance of the blood-brain barrier.[205]

CONCLUSIONS

The functions of hematopoietic cytokines are not limited to the hematopoietic system. A recurring theme in these extrahematopoietic functions is their role in the CNS. Complex interactions occur among the hematopoietic cytokines, the hypothalamic-pituitary axis, and other mediators of inflammation. Each cytokine can have unique effects in the CNS but also may have secondary effects mediated by the stimulation of other cytokines. For example, exposure of neural tissues to IL-1 or TNF-α results in upregulation of IL-6 and IL-8.[7, 206, 207] Other products of inflammation, such as prostaglandins, can also participate in the up- or down-regulation of hematopoietic cytokines.[208] The measured outcome may depend on the balance of cytokines in the local environment.[133, 202, 209–211] Stimulation of this cytokine cascade can result in a regulatory feedback loop, limiting the severity of the response. For example, LPS stimulates IL-1 production with subsequent release of corticotropin-releasing factor, which stimulates corticotropin and corticosteroid production, which inhibits the IL-1 response.

Many of the cytokines discussed are produced within the brain, suggesting autocrine or paracrine CNS function, but they often also function by classic hormonal means: production and release into the bloodstream by cells remote from the site of action. Under certain circumstances, some of these cytokines can cross the blood-brain barrier.[99] Even those that do not cross can exert their effects through the circumventricular organs of the brain, which do not depend on passage from the blood-brain barrier (e.g., area postrema, pineal gland, subfornical organ, median eminence, neurohypophysis). As various recombinant hematopoietic growth factors are brought to clinical trial for neonates, the extrahematopoietic action of these factors must be considered.

References

1. Nicola NA, Metcalf D: Subunit promiscuity among hemopoietic growth factor receptors. Cell 1991;67:1.
2. Nicola NA: Cytokine pleiotropy and redundancy: a view from the receptor. Stem Cells (Dayt) 1994;1:3.
3. Metcalf D: Hematopoietic regulators: redundancy or subtlety? Blood 1993;82:3515.
4. Metcalf D: Implications of the polyfunctionality of hemopoietic regulators. Stem Cells (Dayt) 1994;1:259.
5. Cohen PE, Zhu L, Pollard JW: Absence of colony stimulating factor-1 in osteopetrotic (csfmop/csfmop) mice disrupts estrous cycles and ovulation. Biol Reprod 1997;56:110.
6. Licinio J, Wong ML: Interleukin 1 receptor antagonist gene expression in rat pituitary in the systemic inflammatory response syndrome: pathophysiological implications. Mol Psychiatry 1997;2:99.
7. Aloisi F, Care A, Borsellino G, et al: Production of hemolymphopoietic cytokines (IL-6, IL-8, colony-stimulating factors) by normal human astrocytes in response to IL-1 beta and tumor necrosis factor-alpha. J Immunol 1992;149:2358.
8. Ban E, Haour F, Lenstra R: Brain interleukin 1 gene expression induced by peripheral lipopolysaccharide administration. Cytokine 1992;4:48.
9. Nistico G, De Sarro G: Is interleukin 2 a neuromodulator in the brain? Trends Neurosci 1991;14:146.
10. Miller AJ, Hopkins SJ, Luheshi GN: Sites of action of IL-1 in the development of fever and cytokine responses to tissue inflammation in the rat. Br J Pharmacol 1997;120:1274.
11. Bazan JF: Neuropoietic cytokines in the hematopoietic fold. Neuron 1991;7:197.
12. Awatsuji H, Furukawa Y, Nakajima M, et al: Interleukin-2 as a neurotrophic factor for supporting the survival of neurons cultured from various regions of fetal rat brain. J Neurosci Res 1993;35:305.
13. Balasingam V, Tejada Berges T, Wright E, et al: Reactive astrogliosis in the neonatal mouse brain and its modulation by cytokines. J Neurosci 1994;14:846.
14. Juul SE, Anderson DK, Li Y, Christensen RD: Erythropoietin and erythropoietin receptor in the developing human central nervous system. Pediatr Res 1998;43:40.
15. Bazan JF: Haemopoietic receptors and helical cytokines. Immunol Today 1990;11:350.
16. Nicola NA: Hemopoietic cell growth factors and their receptors. Annu Rev Biochem 1989;58:45.
17. Nicola NA: Structural aspects of cytokine/receptor interactions. Ann N Y Acad Sci 1995;766:253.
18. Nicola NA: Hemopoietic growth factors and their interactions with specific receptors. J Cell Physiol Suppl 1987;5:9.
19. Watowich SS, Hilton DJ, Lodish HF: Activation and inhibition of erythropoietin receptor function: role of receptor dimerization. Mol Cell Biol 1994;14:3535.
20. Miura O, Nakamura N, Quelle FW, et al: Erythropoietin induces association of the JAK2 protein tyrosine kinase with the erythropoietin receptor in vivo. Blood 1994;84:1501.
21. Bazan JF: A novel family of growth factor receptors: a common binding domain in the growth hormone, prolactin, erythropoietin and IL-6 receptors, and the p75 IL-2 receptor beta-chain. Biochem Biophys Res Commun 1989;164:788.
22. Baird PN, D'Andrea RJ, Goodall GJ: Cytokine receptor genes: structure, chromosomal location, and involvement in human disease. Leuk Lymphoma 1995;18:373.
23. Bazan JF: Structural design and molecular evolution of a cytokine receptor superfamily. Proc Natl Acad Sci U S A 1990;87:6934.
24. Brizzi MF, Avanzi GC, Pegoraro L: Hematopoietic growth factor receptors. Int J Cell Cloning 1991;9:274.
25. Cosman D, Lyman SD, Idzerda RL, et al: A new cytokine receptor superfamily. Trends Biochem Sci 1990;15:265.
26. Cosman D: The hematopoietin receptor superfamily. Cytokine 1993;5:95.
27. Gobert S, Porteu F, Pallu S, et al: Tyrosine phosphorylation of the erythropoietin receptor: role for differentiation and mitogenic signal transduction. Blood 1995;86:598.
28. Nicola NA: Receptors for colony-stimulating factors. Br J Haematol 1991;77:133.
29. Watowich SS, Yoshimura A, Longmore GD, et al: Homodimerization and constitutive activation of the erythropoietin receptor. Proc Natl Acad Sci U S A 1992;89:2140.
30. Sokol L, Luhovy M, Guan Y, et al: Primary familial polycythemia: a frameshift mutation in the erythropoietin receptor gene and increased sensitivity of erythroid progenitors to erythropoietin. Blood 1995;86:15.
31. Brown MS, Garcia JF, Phibbs RH, Dallman PR: Decreased response of plasma immunoreactive erythropoietin to "available oxygen" in anemia of prematurity. J Pediatr 1984;105:793.
32. Wu H, Liu X, Jaenisch R, Lodish HF: Generation of committed erythroid BFU-E and CFU-E progenitors does not require erythropoietin or the erythropoietin receptor. Cell 1995;83:59.
33. Shannon KM, Keith JF III, Mentzer WC, et al: Recombinant human erythropoietin stimulates erythropoiesis and reduces erythrocyte transfusions in very low birth weight preterm infants. Pediatrics 1995;95:1.
34. Eschbach JW, Egrie JC, Downing MR, et al: Correction of the anemia of end-stage renal disease with recombinant human erythropoietin: results of a combined phase I and II trial. N Engl J Med 1987;316:73.
35. Porter JC, Leahey A, Polise K, et al: Recombinant human erythropoietin reduces the need for erythrocyte and platelet transfusions in pediatric patients with sarcoma: a randomized, double-blind, placebo-controlled trial. J Pediatr 1996;129:656.
36. Shannon KM: Recombinant erythropoietin in pediatrics: a clinical perspective. Pediatr Ann 1990;19:197.
37. Sobh MA, el Tantawy AE, Said E, et al: Effect of treatment of anaemia with erythropoietin on neuromuscular function in patients on long term haemodialysis. Scand J Urol Nephrol 1992;26:65.
38. Hand MF, Haynes WG, Johnstone HA, et al: Erythropoietin enhances vascular responsiveness to norepinephrine in renal failure. Kidney Int 1995;48:806.
39. Tojo A, Doumoto M, Oka K, et al: Endothelin-mediated effect of erythropoietin on blood pressure and renal hemodynamics in hypertensive rats. Am J Physiol 1996;270:R744.
40. Schmieder RE, Langenfeld MR, Hilgers KF: Endoge-

nous erythropoietin correlates with blood pressure in essential hypertension. Am J Kidney Dis 1997;29:376.
41. Takemasa A, Yorioka N, Yamakido M: Investigations of the influenza-like symptoms associated with recombinant human erythropoietin therapy. J Int Med Res 1997;25:127.
42. Anagnostou A, Lee ES, Kessimian N, et al: Erythropoietin has a mitogenic and positive chemotactic effect on endothelial cells. Proc Natl Acad Sci U S A 1990;87:5978.
43. Anagnostou A, Liu Z, Steiner M, et al: Erythropoietin receptor mRNA expression in human endothelial cells. Proc Natl Acad Sci U S A 1994;91:3974.
44. Buemi M, Allegra A, Lagana A, et al: Is erythropoietin-induced hypertension a phenomenon due to the intracellular Ca^{++} mobilisation? Int Angiol 1994;13:75.
45. Carlini RG, Dusso AS, Obialo CI, et al: Recombinant human erythropoietin (rHuEPO) increases endothelin-1 release by endothelial cells. Kidney Int 1993;43:1010.
46. Carlini RG, Gupta A, Liapis H, Rothstein M: Endothelin-1 release by erythropoietin involves calcium signaling in endothelial cells. J Cardiovasc Pharmacol 1995;26:889.
47. Carlini RG, Reyes AA, Rothstein M: Recombinant human erythropoietinstimulates angiogenesis in vitro. Kidney Int 1995;47:740.
48. Digicaylioglu M, Bichet S, Marti HH, et al: Localization of specific erythropoietin binding sites in defined areas of the mouse brain. Proc Natl Acad Sci U S A 1995;92:3717.
49. Konishi Y, Chui DH, Hirose H, et al: Trophic effect of erythropoietin and other hematopoietic factors on central cholinergic neurons in vitro and in vivo. Brain Res 1993;609:29.
50. Marti HH, Wenger RH, Rivas LA, et al: Erythropoietin gene expression in human, monkey and murine brain. Eur J Neurosci 1996;8:666.
51. Masuda S, Nagao M, Takahata K, et al: Functional erythropoietin receptor of the cells with neural characteristics. Comparison with receptor properties of erythroid cells. J Biol Chem 1993;268:11208.
52. Neusser M, Tepel M, Zidek W: Erythropoietin increases cytosolic free calcium concentration in vascular smooth muscle cells. Cardiovasc Res 1993;27:1233.
53. Okada A, Kinoshita Y, Maekawa T, et al: Erythropoietin stimulates proliferation of rat-cultured gastric mucosal cells. Digestion 1996;57:328.
54. Ohneda O, Yanai N, Obinata M: Erythropoietin as a mitogen for fetal liver stromal cells which support erythropoiesis. Exp Cell Res 1993;208:327.
55. Sawyer ST, Krantz SB, Sawada K: Receptors for erythropoietin in mouse and human erythroid cells and placenta. Blood 1989;74:103.
56. Tabira T, Konishi Y, Gallyas F Jr: Neurotrophic effect of hematopoietic cytokines on cholinergic and other neurons in vitro. Int J Dev Neurosci 1995;13:241.
57. Yamaji R, Okada T, Moriya M, et al: Brain capillary endothelial cells express two forms of erythropoietin receptor mRNA. Eur J Biochem 1996;239:494.
58. Li Y, Juul SE, Morris-Wiman JA, et al: Erythropoietin receptors are expressed in the central nervous system of mid-trimester human fetuses. Pediatr Res 1996;40:376.
59. Morakkabati N, Gollnick F, Meyer R, et al: Erythropoietin induces Ca^{2+} mobilization and contraction in rat mesangial and aortic smooth muscle cultures. Exp Hematol 1996;24:392.
60. Conrad KP, Benyo DF, Westerhausen-Larsen A, Miles TM: Expression of erythropoietin by the human placenta. FASEB J 1996;10:760.
61. Masuda S, Okano M, Yamagishi K, et al: A novel site of erythropoietin production. Oxygen-dependent production in cultured rat astrocytes. J Biol Chem 1994;269:19488.
62. Morishita E, Narita H, Nishida M, et al: Anti-erythropoietin receptor monoclonal antibody: epitope mapping, quantification of the soluble receptor, and detection of the solubilized transmembrane receptor and the receptor-expressing cells. Blood 1996;88:465.
63. Morishita E, Masuda S, Nagao M, et al: Erythropoietin receptor is expressed in rat hippocampal and cerebral cortical neurons, and erythropoietin prevents in vitro glutamate-induced neuronal death. Neuroscience 1997;76:105.
64. Wald MR, Borda ES, Sterin-Borda L: Mitogenic effect of erythropoietin on neonatal rat cardiomyocytes: signal transduction pathways. J Cell Physiol 1996;167:461.
65. Bonanou Tzedaki SA, Sohi MK, Arnstein HR: The role of cAMP and calcium in the stimulation of proliferation of immature erythroblasts by erythropoietin. Exp Cell Res 1987;170:276.
66. Miller BA, Bell LL, Lynch CJ, Cheung JY: Erythropoietin modulation of intracellular calcium: a role for tyrosine phosphorylation. Cell Calcium 1994;16:481.
67. Cheung JY, Zhang XQ, Bokvist K, et al: Modulation of calcium channels in human erythroblasts by erythropoietin. Blood 1997;89:92.
68. Nagai T, AY N, Kohjiro NS, et al: Effects of rHuEpo on cellular proliferation and endothelin-1 production in cultured endothelial cells. Nephrol Dial Transplant 1995;10:1814.
69. Maschio G: Erythropoietin and systemic hypertension. Nephrol Dial Transplant 1995;2:74.
70. Yasuda Y, Nagao M, Okano M, et al: Localization of erythropoietin and erythropoietin-receptor in postimplantation mouse embryos. Dev Growth Differen 1993;35:711.
71. Juul SE, Yachnis AT, Christensen RD: The tissue distribution of Erythropoietin and Erythropoietin receptor in the developing human fetus. in press: Early Hum Dev 1998;52:235.
72. Kling PJ, Sullivan TM, Roberts RA, et al: Human milk as a potential enteral source of erythropoietin. Pediatr Res 1998;43:216.
73. Carmichael RD, LoBue J, Gordon AS: Neonatal erythropoiesis. I. Peripheral blood erythropoietic parameters: data suggest erythropoietin transfer via maternal milk. Endocr Regul 1995;26:83.
74. Teramo KA, Widness JA, Clemons GK, et al: Amniotic fluid erythropoietin correlates with umbilical plasma erythropoietin in normal and abnormal pregnancy. Obstet Gynecol 1987;69:710.
75. Smith JH, Anand KJ, Cotes PM, et al: Antenatal fetal heart rate variation in relation to the respiratory and metabolic status of the compromised human fetus. Br J Obstet Gynaecol 1988;95:980.
76. Voutilainen PE, Widness JA, Clemons GK, et al: Amniotic fluid erythropoietin predicts fetal distress in Rh-immunized pregnancies. Am J Obstet Gynecol 1989;160:429.
77. Mamopoulos M, Bili H, Tsantali C, et al: Erythropoietin umbilical serum levels during labor in women with preeclampsia, diabetes, and preterm labor. Am J Perinatol 1994;11:427.
78. Tan CC, Eckardt K-U, Firth JD, Ratcliffe PJ: Feedback modulation of renal and hepatic erythropoietin mRNA in response to graded anemia and hypoxia. Am J Physiol 1992;263:F474.

79. Juul SE, Harcum J, Li Y, Christensen RD: Erythropoietin is present in the cerebrospinal fluid of neonates. J Pediatr 1997;130:428.
80. Juul SE: Proteoglycans in the developing lung, and, the location and function of erythropoietin in the developing human central nervous system. Ph.D. thesis in developmental biology. University of Chicago, Chicago, 1997.
81. Liu Z-Y, Chin K, Noguchi C: Tissue specific expression of human erythropoietin receptor in transgenic mice. Dev Biol 1994;166:159.
82. Bikfalvi A, Han ZC: Angiogenic factors are hematopoietic growth factors and vice versa. Leukemia 1994;8:523.
83. McConnell SK: Constructing the cerebral cortex: neurogenesis and fate determination. Neuron 1995;15:761.
84. Goldman JE: Lineage, migration, and fate determination of postnatal subventricular zone cells in the mammalian CNS. J Neurooncol 1995;24:61.
85. Levison SW, Goldman JE: Both oligodendrocytes and astrocytes develop from progenitors in the subventricular zone of postnatal rat forebrain. Neuron 1993;10:201.
86. Sieff CA, Emerson SG, Donahue RE, et al: Human recombinant granulocyte-macrophage colony-stimulating factor: a multilineage hematopoietin. Science 1985;230:1171.
87. Clark SC, Kamen R: The human hematopoietic colony stimulating factors. Science 1987;236:1229.
88. Rapoport AP, Abboud CN, DiPersio JF: Granulocyte-macrophage colony-stimulating factor (GM-CSF) and granulocyte colony-stimulating factor (G-CSF): receptor biology, signal transduction, and neutrophil activation. Blood Rev 1992;6:43.
89. Ruef C, Coleman DL: Granulocyte-macrophage colony stimulating factor: Pleiotropic cytokine with potential usefulness. Rev Infect Dis 1990;12:41.
90. Metcalf D: Lineage commitment of hemopoietic progenitor cells in developing blast cell colonies: influence of colony-stimulating factors. Proc Natl Acad Sci U S A 1991;88:11310.
91. Metcalf D, Nicola NA: The clonal proliferation of normal mouse hematopoietic cells: enhancement and suppression by colony-stimulating factor combinations. Blood 1992;79:2861.
92. Dranoff G, Crawford AD, Sadelain M, et al: Involvement of granulocyte-macrophage colony-stimulating factor in pulmonary homeostasis. Science 1994;264:713.
93. Stanley E, Lieschke GJ, Grail D, et al: Granulocyte/macrophage colony-stimulating factor-deficient mice show no major perturbation of hematopoiesis but develop a characteristic pulmonary pathology. Proc Natl Acad Sci U S A 1994;91:5592.
94. Huffman JA, Hull WM, Dranoff G, et al: Pulmonary epithelial cell expression of GM-CSF corrects the alveolar proteinosis in GM-CSF-deficient mice. J Clin Invest 1996;97:649.
95. Lee SC, Liu W, Brosnan CF, Dickerson DW: GM-CSF promotes proliferation of human fetal and adult microglia in pulmonary cultures. Glia 1994;12:309.
96. Malipiero UV, Frei K, Fontana A: Production of hematopoietic colony-stimulating factors by astrocytes. J Immunol 1990;144:3816.
97. Raivich G, Gerhmann J, Kreutzberg GW: Increase of macrophage colony-stimulating factor and granulocyte-macrophage colony-stimulating factor receptors in the regenerating rat facial nucleus. J Neurosci Res 1991;30:682.
98. Tweardy DJ, Glazer EW, Mott PL, Anderson K: Modulation by tumor necrosis factor-alpha of human astroglial cell production of GM-CSF and G-CSF. J Neuroimmunol 1991;32:269.
99. McLay RN, Kimura M, Williams WA, Kastin AJ: Granulocyte-macrophage colony-stimulating factor crosses the blood-brain and blood-spinal cord barriers. Brain 1997;120:2083.
100. Fischer HG, Bielinsky AK, Nitzgen B, et al: Functional dichotomy of mouse microglia developed in vitro: differential effects of macrophage and granulocyte/macrophage colony-stimulating factor on cytokine secretion and antitoxoplasmic activity. J Neuroimmunol 1993;45:193.
101. Baldwin GC, Benveniste EN, Chung GY, et al: Identification and characterization of a high-affinity granulocyte-macrophage colony-stimulating factor receptor on primary rat oligodendrocytes. Blood 1993;82:3279.
102. Guillemin G, Boussin FD, Le Grand R, et al: Granulocyte macrophage colony stimulating factor stimulates in vitro proliferation of astrocytes derived from simian mature brains. Glia 1996;16:71.
103. Kamegai M, Konishi Y, Tabira T: Trophic effect of granulocyte-macrophage colony stimulating factor on central cholinergic neurons in vitro. Brain Res 1990;532:323.
104. Nicola NA: Granulocyte colony-stimulating factor. Immunol Ser 1990;49:77.
105. Lieschke GJ, Grail D, Hodgson G, et al: Mice lacking granulocyte colony-stimulating factor have chronic neutropenia, granulocyte and macrophage progenitor cell deficiency, and impaired neutrophil mobilization. Blood 1994;84:1737.
106. Stanley ER, Guilebert LJ, Tushinski RJ, Bartelmez SH: CSF-1—a mononuclear phagocyte lineage specific haemopoietic growth factor. J Cell Biochem 1983;21:151.
107. Arceci RJ, Shanahan F, Stanley ER, Pollard JW: Temporal expression and location of colony-stimulating factor 1 (CSF-1) and its receptor in the female reproductive tract are consistent with CSF-1–regulated placental development. Proc Natl Acad Sci U S A 1989;86:8818.
108. Pollard JW, Bartocci A, Arceci R, et al: Apparent role of the macrophage growth factor, CSF-1, in placental development. Nature 1987;330:484.
109. Cohen PE, Chisholm O, Arceci RJ, et al: Absence of colony-stimulating factor-1 in osteopetrotic (csfmop/csfmop) mice results in male fertility defects. Biol Reprod 1996;55:310.
110. Pollard JW: Role of colony-stimulating factor-1 in reproduction and development. Mol Reprod Dev 1997;46:54.
111. Wiktor Jedrzejczak W, Urbanowska E, Szperl M: Granulocyte-macrophage colony-stimulating factor corrects macrophage deficiencies, but not osteopetrosis, in the colony-stimulating factor-1-deficient op/op mouse. Endocrinology 1994;134:1932.
112. Wiktor Jedrzejczak W, Urbanowska E, Aukerman SI, et al: Correction by CSF-1 of defects in the osteopetrotic op/op mouse suggests local, developmental, and humoral requirements for this growth factor. Exp Hematol 1991;19:1049.
113. Pampfer S, Tabibzadeh S, Chuan FC, Pollard JW: Expression of colony-stimulating factor-1 (CSF-1) messenger RNA in human endometrial glands during the menstrual cycle: molecular cloning of a novel transcript that predicts a cell surface form of CSF-1. Mol Endocrinol 1991;5:1931.
114. Daiter E, Pampfer S, Yeung YG, et al: Expression of

colony-stimulating factor-1 in the human uterus and placenta. J Clin Endocrinol Metab 1992;74:850.
115. Chang Y, Albright S, Lee F: Cytokines in the central nervous system: expression of macrophage colony stimulating factor and its receptor during development. J Neuroimmunol 1994;52:9.
116. Thery C, Hetier E, Evrard C, Mallat M: Expression of macrophage colony-stimulating factor gene in the mouse brain during development. J Neurosci Res 1990;26:129.
117. Frei K, Nohava K, Malipiero UV, et al: Production of macrophage colony-stimulating factor by astrocytes and brain macrophages. J Neuroimmunol 1992;40:189.
118. Mizuno T, Sawada M, Suzumura A, Marunouchi T: Expression of cytokines during glial differentiation. Brain Res 1994;656:141.
119. Shafit Zagardo B, Sharma N, Berman JW, et al: CSF-1 expression is upregulated in astrocyte cultures by IL-1 and TNF and affects microglial proliferation and morphology in organotypic cultures. Int J Dev Neurosci 1993;11:189.
120. Liu W, Brosnan CF, Dickson DW, Lee SC: Macrophage colony-stimulating factor mediates astrocyte-induced microglial ramification in human fetal central nervous system culture. Am J Pathol 1994;145:48.
121. Dror Michaelson M, Bieri PL, Mehler MF, et al: CSF-1 deficiency in mice results in abnormal brain development. Development 1996;122:2661.
122. Berezovskaya O, Maysinger D, Fedoroff S: The hematopoietic cytokine, colony-stimulating factor 1, is also a growth factor in the CNS: congenital absence of CSF-1 in mice results in abnormal microglial response and increased neuron vulnerability to injury. Int J Dev Neurosci 1995;13:285.
123. Maysinger D, Berezovskaya O, Fedoroff S: The hematopoietic cytokine colony stimulating factor 1 is also a growth factor in the CNS: (II) microencapsulated CSF-1 and LM-10 cells as delivery systems. Exp Neurol 1996;141:47.
124. Fedoroff S, Berezovskaya O, Maysinger D: Role of colony stimulating factor-1 in brain damage caused by ischemia. Neurosci Biobehav Rev 1997;21:187.
125. Ban E, Milon G, Prudhomme N, et al: Receptors for interleukin-1 (alpha and beta) in mouse brain: mapping and neuronal localization in hippocampus. Neuroscience 1991;43:21.
126. Cunningham ET Jr, Wada E, Carter DB, et al: In situ histochemical localization of type I interleukin-1 receptor messenger RNA in the central nervous system, pituitary, and adrenal gland of the mouse. J Neurosci 1992;12:1101.
127. Haour F, Marquette C, Tsiang H, et al: Interleukin-1 receptors in brain and pituitary. Characterization and modulation during infection and stress. Ann N Y Acad Sci 1994;741:324.
128. Parnet P, Amindari S, Wu C, et al: Expression of type I and type II interleukin-1 receptors in mouse brain. Brain Res Mol Brain Res 1994;27:63.
129. Takao T, Tracey DE, Mitchell WM, De Souza EB: Interleukin-1 receptors in mouse brain: characterization and neuronal localization. Endocrinology 1990;127:3070.
130. Yabuuchi K, Minami M, Katsumata S, Satoh M: Localization of type I interleukin-1 receptor mRNA in the rat brain. Brain Res Mol Brain Res 1994;27:27.
131. Cunningham ET Jr, Wada E, Carter DB, et al: Localization of interleukin-1 receptor messenger RNA in murine hippocampus. Endocrinology 1991;128:2666.
132. Yao J, Keri JE, Taffs RE, Colton CA: Characterization of interleukin-1 production by microglia in culture. Brain Res 1992;591:88.
133. Giulian D, Li J, Li X, et al: The impact of microglia-derived cytokines upon gliosis in the CNS. Dev Neurosci 1994;16:128.
134. Romero LI, Tatro JB, Field JA, Reichlin S: Roles of IL-1 and TNF-alpha in endotoxin-induced activation of nitric oxide synthase in cultured rat brain cells. Am J Physiol 1996;270:R326.
135. Brenneman DE, Hill JM, Glazner GW, et al: Interleukin-1 alpha and vasoactive intestinal peptide: enigmatic regulation of neuronal survival. Int J Dev Neurosci 1995;13:187.
136. Giulian D, Li J, Leara B, Keenen C: Phagocytic microglia release cytokines and cytotoxins that regulate the survival of astrocytes and neurons in culture. Neurochem Int 1994;25:227.
137. Giulian D, Vaca K, Johnson B: Secreted peptides as regulators of neuron-glia and glia-glia interactions in the developing nervous system. J Neurosci Res 1988;21:487.
138. Nakao N, Itakura T, Uematsu Y, et al: Pretreatment with interleukin-1 enhances survival of sympathetic ganglionic neuron grafts. Neurol Med Chir (Tokyo) 1994;34:407.
139. Takao T, Hashimoto K, De Souza EB: Interleukin-1 receptors in the brain-endocrine-immune axis. Modulation by stress and infection. Ann N Y Acad Sci 1995;771:372.
140. Takao T, Tojo C, Nishioka T, et al: Corticotropin-releasing factor treatment upregulates interleukin-1 receptors in the mouse pituitary: reversal by dexamethasone. Brain Res 1995;688:219.
141. Takao T, Tojo C, Nishioka T, et al: Stress-induced upregulation of pituitary interleukin-1 receptors is mediated by corticotropin releasing factor. Life Sci 1996;59:L165.
142. Vellucci SV, Parrott RF, da Costa AC, et al: Increased body temperature, cortisol secretion, and hypothalamic expression of c-fos, corticotrophin releasing hormone and interleukin-1 beta mRNAs following central administration of interleukin-1 beta in the sheep. Brain Res Mol Brain Res 1995;29:64.
143. Lin MT: Heatstroke-induced cerebral ischemia and neuronal damage. Involvement of cytokines and monoamines. Ann N Y Acad Sci 1997;813:572.
144. Takahashi S, Fang J, Kapas L, et al: Inhibition of brain interleukin-1 attenuates sleep rebound after sleep deprivation in rabbits. Am J Physiol 1997;273:R677.
145. Plata Salaman CR, Ilyin SE: Interleukin-1beta (IL-1beta)-induced modulation of the hypothalamic IL-1beta system, tumor necrosis factor-alpha, and transforming growth factor-beta 1 mRNAs in obese (fa/fa) and lean (Fa/Fa) Zucker rats: implications to IL-1beta feedback systems and cytokine-cytokine interactions. J Neurosci Res 1997;49:541.
146. Sandi C, Guaza C: Evidence for a role of nitric oxide in the corticotropin-releasing factor release induced by interleukin-1 beta. Eur J Pharmacol 1995;274:17.
147. Smagin GN, Swiergiel AH, Dunn AJ: Peripheral administration of interleukin-1 increases extracellular concentrations of norepinephrine in rat hypothalamus: comparison with plasma corticosterone. Psychoneuroendocrinology 1996;21:83.
148. Day HE, Akil H: Differential pattern of c-fos mRNA in rat brain following central and systemic administration of interleukin-1-beta: implications for mechanism of action. Neuroendocrinology 1996;63:207.
149. van der Meer MJ, Sweep CG, Rijnkels CE, et al: Acute stimulation of the hypothalamic-pituitary-adrenal axis

by IL-1 beta, TNF alpha and IL-6: a dose response study. J Endocrinol Invest 1996;19:175.

150. Zhou D, Shanks N, Riechman SE, et al: Interleukin 6 modulates interleukin-1- and stress-induced activation of the hypothalamic-pituitary-adrenal axis in male rats. Neuroendocrinology 1996;63:227.

151. Schmidt ED, Janszen AW, Wouterlood FG, Tilders FJ: Interleukin-1–induced long-lasting changes in hypothalamic corticotropin-releasing hormone (CRH)–neurons and hyperresponsiveness of the hypothalamus-pituitary-adrenal axis. J Neurosci 1995;15:7417.

152. Bernardini R, Calogero AE, Mauceri G, Chrousos GP: Rat hypothalamic corticotropin-releasing hormone secretion in vitro is stimulated by interleukin-1 in an eicosanoid-dependent manner. Life Sci 1990;47:1601.

153. Katsuura G, Gottschall PE, Dahl RR, Arimura A: Interleukin-1 beta increases prostaglandin E2 in rat astrocyte cultures: modulatory effect of neuropeptides. Endocrinology 1989;124:3125.

154. Yang GY, Zhao YJ, Davidson BL, Betz AL: Overexpression of interleukin-1 receptor antagonist in the mouse brain reduces ischemic brain injury. Brain Res 1997;751:181.

155. Stroemer RP, Rothwell NJ: Cortical protection by localized striatal injection of IL-1ra following cerebral ischemia in the rat. J Cereb Blood Flow Metab 1997;17:597.

156. Loddick SA, Rothwell NJ: Neuroprotective effects of human recombinant interleukin-1 receptor antagonist in focal cerebral ischaemia in the rat. J Cereb Blood Flow Metab 1996;16:932.

157. Murray CA, McGahon B, McBennett S, Lynch MA: Interleukin-1 beta inhibits glutamate release in hippocampus of young, but not aged, rats. Neurobiol Aging 1997;18:343.

158. Bonmann E, Suschek C, Spranger M, Kolb Bachofen V: The dominant role of exogenous or endogenous interleukin-1 beta on expression and activity of inducible nitric oxide synthase in rat microvascular brain endothelial cells. Neurosci Lett 1997;230:109.

159. Brunetti L, Volpe AR, Ragazzoni E, et al: Interleukin-1 beta specifically stimulates nitric oxide production in the hypothalamus. Life Sci 1996;58:L373.

160. Sato I, Kim Y, Himi T, Murota S: Induction of calcium-independent nitric oxide synthase activity in cultured cerebellar granule neurons. Neurosci Lett 1995;184:145.

161. Uehara A, Okumura T, Kitamori S, et al: Gastric antisecretory and antiulcer actions of interleukin-1. Evidence for the presence of an "immune-brain-gut" axis. J Clin Gastroenterol 1992;14:0192.

162. Tache Y, Saperas E: Potent inhibition of gastric acid secretion and ulcer formation by centrally and peripherally administered interleukin-1. Ann N Y Acad Sci 1992;664:353.

163. Suto G, Kiraly A, Tache Y: Interleukin 1 beta inhibits gastric emptying in rats: mediation through prostaglandin and corticotropin-releasing factor. Gastroenterology 1994;106:1568.

164. Smith KA: Interleukin-2: inception, impact, and implications. Science 1988;240:1169.

165. Kintzel PE, Calis KM: Recombinant interleukin-2: a biological response modifier. Drug Rev 1991;10:110.

166. Nistico G: Communications among central nervous system, neuroendocrine and immune systems: interleukin-2. Prog Neurobiol 1993;40:463.

167. Lapchak PA: Immunoautoradiographic localization of interleukin 2-like immunoreactivity and interleukin 2 receptors (Tac antigen-like immunoreactivity) in the rat brain. Neuroscience 1991;44:173.

168. Petitto JM, Huang Z: Molecular cloning of a partial cDNA of the interleukin-2 receptor-beta in normal mouse brain: in situ localization in the hippocampus and expression by neuroblastoma cells. Brain Res 1994;650:140.

169. Petitto JM, Huang Z: Molecular cloning of the coding sequence of an interleukin-2 receptor-alpha subunit cDNA in murine brain. J Neuroimmunol 1995;59:135.

170. Merrill JE: Interleukin-2 effects in the central nervous system. Ann N Y Acad Sci 1990;594:188.

171. McAllister CG, van Kammen DP, Rehn TJ, et al: Increases in CSF levels of interleukin-2 in schizophrenia: effects of recurrence of psychosis and medication status. Am J Psychiatry 1995;152:1291.

172. Sarder M, Saito H, Abe K: Interleukin-2 promotes survival and neurite extension of cultured neurons from fetal rat brain. Brain Res 1993;625:347.

173. Otero GC, Merrill JE: Response of human oligodendrocytes to interleukin-2. Brain Behav Immun 1997;11:24.

174. Seto D, Kar S, Quirion R: Evidence for direct and indirect mechanisms in the potent modulatory action of interleukin-2 on the release of acetylcholine in rat hippocampal slices. Br J Pharmacol 1997;120:1151.

175. Lapchak PA: A role for interleukin-2 in the regulation of striatal dopaminergic function. Neuroreport 1992;3:165.

176. Alonso R, Chaudieu I, Diorio J, et al: Interleukin-2 modulates evoked release of [3H]dopamine in rat cultured mesencephalic cells. J Neurochem 1993;61:1284.

177. Haugen PK, Letourneau PC: Interleukin-2 enhances chick and rat sympathetic, but not sensory, neurite outgrowth. J Neurosci Res 1990;25:443.

178. Bindoni M, Perciavalle V, Berretta S, et al: Interleukin 2 modifies the bioelectric activity of some neurosecretory nuclei in the rat hypothalamus. Brain Res 1988;462:10.

179. Hanisch UK, Neuhaus J, Rowe W, et al: Neurotoxic consequences of central long-term administration of interleukin-2 in rats. Neuroscience 1997;79:799.

180. Nishinakamura R, Nakayama N, Hirabayashi Y, et al: Mice deficient for the IL-3/GM-CSF/IL-5 beta c receptor exhibit lung pathology and impaired immune response, while beta IL3 receptor-deficient mice are normal. Immunity 1995;2:211.

181. Kamegai M, Niijima K, Kunishita T, et al: Interleukin 3 as a trophic factor for central cholinergic neurons in vitro and in vivo. Neuron 1990;4:429.

182. Ringheim GE, Burgher KL, Heroux JA: Interleukin-6 mRNA expression by cortical neurons in culture: evidence for neuronal sources of interleukin-6 production in the brain. J Neuroimmunol 1995;63:113.

183. Gadient RA, Otten U: Identification of interleukin-6 (IL-6)-expressing neurons in the cerebellum and hippocampus of normal adult rats. Neurosci Lett 1994;182:243.

184. Sato T, Nakamura S, Taga T, et al: Induction of neuronal differentiation in PC12 cells by B cell stimulatory factor 2/interleukin 6. Mol Cell Biol 1988;8:3546.

185. Hama T, Kushima Y, Miyamoto M, et al: Interleukin-6 improves the survival of mesencephalic catecholaminergic and septal cholinergic neurons from post natal two-week-old rats in cultures. Neuroscience 1991;40:445.

186. Frei K, Malipiero UV, Leist TP, et al: On the cellular source and function of interleukin-6 produced in the central nervous system in viral disease. Eur J Immunol 1989;19:689.

187. Marz P, Gadient RA, Otten U: Expression of interleukin-6 receptor (IL-6R) and gp130 mRNA in PC12 cells and sympathetic neurons: modulation by tumor necrosis factor alpha (TNF-alpha). Brain Res 1996;706:71.
188. Hama T, Miyamoto M, Tsukui H, et al: Interleukin-6 as a neurotrophic factor for promoting the survival of cultured basal forebrain cholinergic neurons from postnatal rats. Neurosci Lett 1989;104:340.
189. Nakafuku M, Satoh T, Kaziro Y: Differentiation factors, including nerve growth factor, fibroblast growth factor, and interleukin-6, induce an accumulation of an active Ras.GTP complex in rat pheochromocytoma PC12 cells. J Biol Chem 1992;267:19448.
190. Burns TM, Clough JA, Klein RM, et al: Developmental regulation of cytokine expression in the mouse brain. Growth Factors 1993;9:253.
191. Hull M, Strauss S, Berger M, et al: The participation of interleukin-6, a stress-inducible cytokine, in the pathogenesis of Alzheimer's disease. Behav Brain Res 1996;78:37.
192. Fattori E, Lazzaro D, Musiani P, et al: IL-6 expression in neurons of transgenic mice causes reactive astrocytosis and increase in ramified microglial cells but no neuronal damage. Eur J Neurosci 1995;7:2441.
193. Yoon BH, Jun JK, Romero R, et al: Amniotic fluid inflammatory cytokines (interleukin-6, interleukin-1 beta, and tumor necrosis factor-alpha), neonatal brain white matter lesions, and cerebral palsy. Am J Obstet Gynecol 1997;177:19.
194. Dammann O, Leviton A: Maternal intrauterine infection, cytokines, and brain damage in the preterm newborn. Pediatr Res 1997;42:1.
195. Qiu Z, Parsons KL, Gruol DL: Interleukin-6 selectively enhances the intracellular calcium response to NMDA in developing CNS neurons. J Neurosci 1995;15:6688.
196. Kushima Y, Hatanaka H: Interleukin-6 and leukemia inhibitory factor promote the survival of acetylcholinesterase-positive neurons in culture from embryonic rat spinal cord. Neurosci Lett 1992;143:110.
197. Umegaki H, Yamada K, Naito M, et al: Protective effect of interleukin-6 against the death of PC12 cells caused by serum deprivation or by the addition of a calcium ionophore. Biochem Pharmacol 1996;52:911.
198. Maeda Y, Matsumoto M, Hori O, et al: Hypoxia/reoxygenation–mediated induction of astrocyte interleukin 6: a paracrine mechanism potentially enhancing neuron survival. J Exp Med 1994;180:2297.
199. Mastorakos G, Weber JS, Magiakou MA, et al: Hypothalamic-pituitary-adrenal axis activation and stimulation of systemic vasopressin secretion by recombinant interleukin-6 in humans: potential implications for the syndrome of inappropriate vasopressin secretion. J Clin Endocrinol Metab 1994;79:934.
200. Stern AS, Podlaski FJ, Hulmes JD, et al: Purification to homogeneity and partial characterization of cytotoxic lymphocyte maturation factor from human B-lymphoblastoid cells. Proc Natl Acad Sci U S A 1990;88:6808.
201. Aloisi F, Penna G, Cerase J, et al: IL-12 production by central nervous system microglia is inhibited by astrocytes. J Immunol 1997;159:1604.
202. Lodge PA, Sriram S: Regulation of microglial activation by TGF-beta, IL-10, and CSF-1. J Leukoc Biol 1996;60:502.
203. Park JH, Shin SH: Induction of IL-12 gene expression in the brain in septic shock. Biochem Biophys Res Commun 1996;224:391.
204. Stalder AK, Pagenstecher A, Yu NC, et al: Lipopolysaccharide-induced IL-12 expression in the central nervous system and cultured astrocytes and microglia. J Immunol 1997;159:1344.
205. Barna M, Komatsu T, Reiss CS: Activation of type III nitric oxide synthase in astrocytes following a neurotropic viral infection. Virology 1996;223:331.
206. De Simoni MG, De Luigi A, Gemma L, et al: Modulation of systemic interleukin-6 induction by central interleukin-1. Am J Physiol 1993;265:R739.
207. Romero LI, Kakucska I, Lechan RM, Reichlin S: Interleukin-6 (IL-6) is secreted from the brain after intracerebroventricular injection of IL-1 beta in rats. Am J Physiol 1996;270:R518.
208. Fiebich BL, Hull M, Lieb K, et al: Prostaglandin E_2 induces interleukin-6 synthesis in human astrocytoma cells. J Neurochem 1997;68:704.
209. Frei K, Lins H, Fontana A: Production and function of IL-10 in the central nervous system. Schweiz Arch Neurol Psychiatry 1994;145:30.
210. Bell MJ, Kochanek PM, Doughty LA, et al: Interleukin-6 and interleukin-10 in cerebrospinal fluid after severe traumatic brain injury in children. J Neurotrauma 1997;14:451.
211. Benveniste EN, Tang LP, Law RM: Differential regulation of astrocyte TNF-alpha expression by the cytokines TGF-beta, IL-6 and IL-10. Int J Dev Neurosci 1995;13:341.

CHAPTER 5

Bone Marrow Failure Syndromes in the Neonate and Infant

D. Wade Clapp, M.D.

Bone marrow failure is characterized by decreased production of mature red blood cells, white blood cells, and platelets, generating a progressive peripheral blood pancytopenia and hypoplastic marrow. Bone marrow failure in the neonate is rare, but genetic disorders, which account for 25% to 30% of aplastic anemia cases in childhood,[1, 2] often have physical stigmata that are present at delivery and that allow early diagnosis and prospective management of the consequent bone marrow aplasia.

This chapter reviews the pathophysiology and features of bone marrow failure syndromes that manifest in the newborn period and in early infancy. Particular attention is given to physical and laboratory stigmata in the newborn period.

PANCYTOPENIA

The causes of pancytopenia in the neonate and infant are listed in Table 5–1. These disorders and syndromes are discussed in the following section.

Table 5–1. **Pancytopenia in the Neonate and Infant**

Fanconi's anemia
Shwachman-Diamond syndrome
Pearson's syndrome
Reticular dysgenesis
Seckel's syndrome

Fanconi's Anemia

Fanconi's anemia (FA) is a complex autosomal recessive genetic disorder characterized by a diverse range of organ system abnormalities. FA is the most common genetic cause of aplastic anemia.[2–6] FA is found in all races and has been reported to have a carrier frequency of approximately 1 carrier per 300 persons,[2, 7, 8] although some investigators suggest that the heterogeneity of the disease results in underreporting and that the frequency of the gene in the general population may be significantly higher.[9] Manifestation of hematologic symptoms during the newborn period is rare. Approximately 4% of FA patients were diagnosed in the first year of life, and approximately one half of these had hematologic stigmata at the time of diagnosis.[9, 10] Before the 1980s, the genetic diagnosis was most frequently obtained when the patients acquired aplastic anemia or leukemia.[9]

Physical Examination

Patients with FA who are diagnosed at birth have a much higher incidence of multisystem involvement than patients who are diagnosed later in life. Many FA patients have completely normal features. However, physical stigmata provide an important opportunity to identify approximately 50% to 60%[9, 10] of patients with FA. Because most patients who are diagnosed in infancy are not aplastic, recognition of these physical stigmata provides an opportunity to obtain definitive diagnosis by chromosome breakage analysis. The most common physical findings observed in patients with FA are listed in Table 5–2.

Forty-six percent of patients with FA are small for gestational age at birth, and 50% have small stature detected in the first year of life.[9] Common limb anomalies include absent or hypoplastic thumbs and radii and abnormalities of the fingers, which may be enlarged or hypoplastic (Fig. 5–1). Gonadal abnormalities are common in males and females, although they are more easily diagnosed in males. These abnormalities include undescended testes, hypospadias, absent testis, abnormal urethra, micropenis, and atresia or aplasia of the vagina, uterus, or ovary. Approximately 25% of FA patients have cranial abnormalities, which include microcephaly, microphthalmia, and scaphocephaly. The gastrointestinal, renal, cardiac, and musculoskeletal systems are variably affected.

Patients with FA are sometimes misdiagnosed as having the more common VATER syndrome (vertebral or vascular, anal, tracheoesophageal, renal, and radial)[11] or the TAR syndrome (thrombocytopenia with absent radii). Discrimination of FA and TAR can be accomplished by chromosome breakage analysis. The normality of the thumbs is critical in discriminating TAR from FA. If the radii are affected, the thumbs of patients with TAR are always normal, whereas the thumbs of patients with FA are always abnormal.[2] Selected classic features observed in patients with FA are shown in Figure 5–1.

Table 5–2. **Common Physical Abnormalities Associated with Fanconi's Anemia**

Short stature
Radial and thumb abnormalities
Microcephaly
Café au lait spots
Genitourinary abnormalities
Microphthalmia

Laboratory Diagnosis

The major diagnostic laboratory test for FA is chromosome breakage analysis of lymphocytes. Patients with FA have an increased chromosome breakage rate compared with normal individuals after stimulation with phytohemagglutinin (PHA), and this rate is greatly increased when cells are cultured in the presence of diepoxybutane[11, 12] or mitomycin C.[12–15] Evaluation of PHA-stimulated lymphocytes in the presence of a clastogenic agent is essential, because some patients do not have increased numbers of spontaneous breaks. Normal individuals have approximately 0 to 0.06 chromosome breaks per cell, whereas patients with FA have 6 to 8.96 breaks per cell after stimulation with diepoxybutane.[2, 14–16] Although rare, some patients with FA are not hypersensitive to diepoxybutane or mitomycin C.

Culture of lymphocytes in mitomycin C or diepoxybutane distinguish FA from two other chromosome instability syndromes: ataxia telangiectasia and Bloom's syndrome.[17] These two syndromes, like FA, may have an increased incidence of spontaneous chromosome breaks but not an increased rate of chromosome breakage in response to mitomycin C. Prenatal diagnosis can be accomplished by chromosome breakage analysis using chorionic villus sampling or amniocentesis.[12, 15, 16] The cultured cells from these specimens, analogous to many other primary FA cells in these patients, grow slowly.

Laboratory evaluation of patients in whom FA is suspected should include a complete blood cell count including platelets, hemoglobin F (Hb F), and red cell size analysis. Diagnostic evaluation of peripheral blood lymphocytes using diepoxybutane is required, because this test can confirm or exclude nearly all patients affected with the disease. Because only a minority of FA patients present with anemia or pancytopenia as newborns, identification of patients with FA before the onset of bone marrow failure allows expectant management and provides the opportunity to identify other affected siblings and to institute genetic counseling.

Genetics and Complementation Analysis

Somatic cell fusion studies of lymphoblasts have resulted in the identification of at least

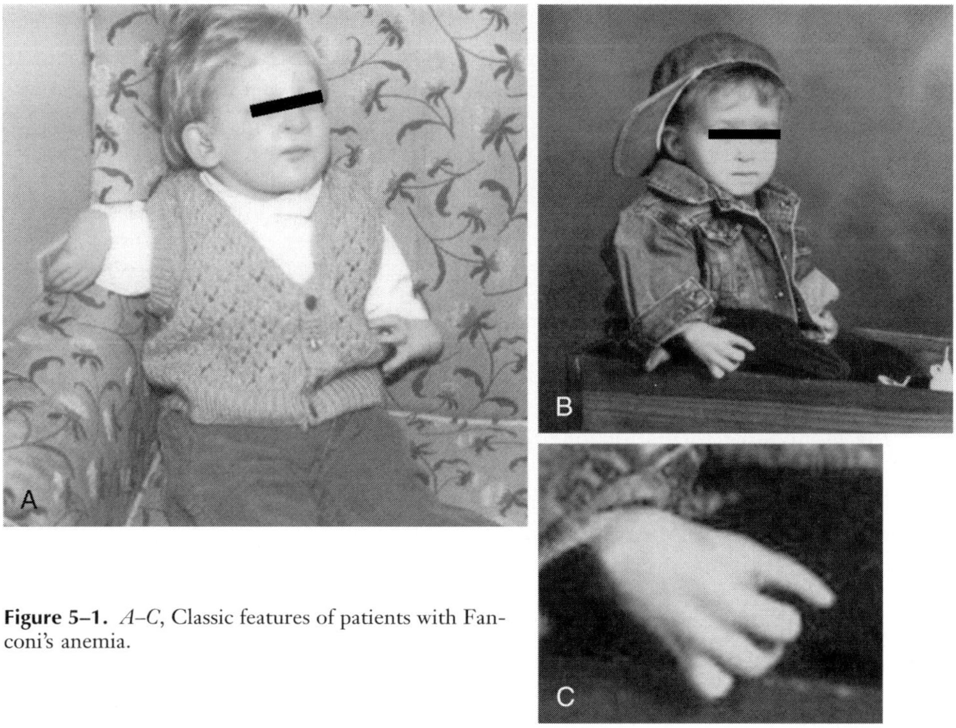

Figure 5–1. *A–C*, Classic features of patients with Fanconi's anemia.

eight FA complementation types and, theoretically, eight genes as well.[18–23] Unlike many other important families of genes, no structural homologues of the FA genes have been identified in yeast or other phylogenetically lower organisms. This lack of identifiable homologues has in part increased the challenge of determining the function of these genes in cellular homeostasis.

The cDNAs of two Fanconi complementation groups have been isolated: FA complementation type C[21] [FACC] and FA complementation type A [FACA].[22, 23] The cDNA of FACC contains 558 amino acids, has 14 exons,[24] and is located principally within the cytoplasm.[24, 25] This was somewhat of a surprise, because a characteristic of FA is a propensity of cells to acquire double-stranded DNA breaks and progressive chromosomal instability. However, it may be that the FA genes encode a cellular pathway that includes a cytoplasmic sensor and genes involved in DNA repair. One group of investigators demonstrated that the *FACA* gene is localized to the nucleus[26] and associates with the *FACC* gene, suggesting that this family of genes may contain its own unique pathway. The predicted protein of this gene is 163 kd, and unlike the product of the *FACC* gene, it appears to contain a partial leucine zipper sequence and nuclear localization sequences.[27] The structure and function of FACA is being evaluated in several laboratories.

Hematopoietic Defects

Whether loss of the FA gene results in an alteration in the stem cell compartment or in more mature multipotent progenitors remains unclear. There is a single case report of a symptomatic FA patient who spontaneously had a complete clinical remission, suggesting that a recombinational event resulted in normal cellular restoration of a stem progenitor cell and that the proliferation advantage of this cell resulted in repopulation of the marrow.[27] If this case report can be generalized to other FA patients, it suggests that even a paucity of normal functioning stem cells should be able to outgrow the uncorrected, mutant cells. This type of clinical situation is ideal for genetic therapy of autologous cells.

Although there may be some question about the role of FA in the stem cell compartment, the hematopoietic defect in FA is evident at the level of the multipotent (e.g., colony-forming unit–granulocyte, erythrocyte, macrophage, megakaryocyte [CFU-GEMM]) progenitor and at the level of the lineage-restricted progenitors (e.g., colony-forming unit–granulocyte-macrophage [CFU-GM], burst-forming unit–erythroid [BFU-E]).[28–33] Even clinically unaffected patients with FA usually have reduced numbers of assayable progenitors cultured from their bone marrow. Restoration of the *FACC* gene *in trans* using recombinant retroviruses has resulted in enhancement but not complete correction of the clonogenic formation of progenitors in FA patients.[34, 35]

No overt immunodeficient component has been recognized in this disease. Murine models containing a disruption of the murine homologue of FACC by homologous recombination are great assets for evaluating the role of FACC in the cell.[36–38]

Shwachman-Diamond Syndrome

Shwachman-Diamond (SD) syndrome is a rare, autosomal recessive, panethnic disorder that most frequently manifests with steatorrhea, abdominal distention, and failure to thrive in the newborn period or early infancy. The pregnancy and birth history of these patients usually is normal, although approximately 10% are small for gestational age. In addition to the exocrine pancreatic insufficiency, patients uniformly develop neutropenia, although thrombocytopenia or anemia sometimes accompany or precede the neutropenia. Nearly 25% of these patients acquire aplastic anemia.[2, 39] On physical examination, patients typically have malnutrition, including a protuberant abdomen; ichthyotic rashes; and decreased height and weight. Patients are predisposed to skin infections and pneumonia as a result of the neutropenia.

Laboratory Findings

The neutropenia in SD may be intermittent or chronic and may be associated with anemia (nearly one third of patients) or thrombocytopenia. Pancytopenia is observed in patients over a wide range of ages from as young as 1 year of age (mean age, 9 years).[2] Culture of bone marrow cells for growth of erythroid and granulocyte-macrophage progenitors results in a decreased absolute number of progenitors in both lineages.[2] Immunoglobulin levels are frequently normal in these patients. Pancreatic insufficiency is determined by evidence of alterations in trypsin, lipase, and amylase.

Outcome

The malabsorption of patients with SD responds to supplementation with pancreatic enzymes. Anemia and thrombocytopenia in patients with SD have been treated symptomatically with transfusions of red blood cells or platelets as needed. Infections are generally responsive to treatment with antibiotics. Approximately 5% of patients with SD acquire leukemic transformations. The leukemia and pancytopenia are important causes of mortality in patients with SD. Data are limited for the administration of recombinant cytokines to ameliorate the neutropenia or anemia in this disease.[40, 41]

Pearson's Syndrome

Pearson's syndrome (PS) is a rare clinical disorder characterized by anemia, metabolic acidosis, and exocrine pancreatic dysfunction.[42, 43] Physical anomalies are uncommon in this disorder, although some patients are small for gestational age. The initial overwhelming problem encountered by most patients with this disorder is a severe metabolic acidosis that is associated with a high morbidity and mortality. Renal and liver insufficiency are common sequelae of this condition. Not all patients have the severe metabolic disease, and some patients have only the refractory sideroblastic anemia that frequently presents within the first month of life. Neutropenia and thrombocytopenia are generally not of clinical significance.

PS results from a deletion of mitochondrial DNA.[42–44] The enzymes involved in these mutations are pivotal in oxidative phosphorylation metabolism and include nicotinamide adenine dinucleotide and cytochrome oxidase. The inheritance pattern of this disease, analogous to other mitochondrial DNA–related diseases, is maternal.[42, 43]

Laboratory Findings

Anemia is diagnosed in the first 6 months in approximately three fourths of patients. Most patients have macrocytic red blood cells, and the bone marrow has distinctive vacuolated myeloid and erythroid precursors. Many aspirates have decreased numbers of erythroblasts and many sideroblasts. The diagnosis usually is made by the histologic features of the vacuolated marrow precursors, evidence of refractory anemia with ringed sideroblasts, and detection of deletions in mitochondrial DNA.[2] There is heterogeneity in the degree of involvement of individual organs and hematopoietic stem or progenitor cells. Some patients are susceptible to clonal hematopoiesis.

Outcome

PS should be considered in newborns with unexplained hydrops fetalis and with unexplained metabolic acidosis, hepatorenal disease, and anemia. The mortality from this disease is principally related to the profound metabolic acidosis and the hepatorenal failure. Anemia is common during infancy, and patients sometimes have reduced numbers of leukocytes and platelets as well. The hematologic manifestations tend to be less severe after 2 to 4 years of age in patients who survive the early metabolic acidosis. Therapy is directed at ameliorating the loss of function of the mitochondrial enzymes. Recombinant cytokines have been used in individual cases.[44]

Reticular Dysgenesis

Reticular dysgenesis manifests in neonates and infants as recurrent and unremitting infections. Patients have lymphopenia, lack cellular and humoral immunity, and have markedly reduced granulocyte counts. There is a marked absence of tonsillar tissue, lymph nodes, thymic development, and splenic follicles.[2, 45]

The inheritance of this disorder remains unclear because of the rarity of the disease, although there is a very high male predominance. Most patients die of infection in the first 6 months of life. Bone marrow transplantation has been used to rescue some patients.[46, 47] One patient who underwent bone marrow transplantation without myeloablation became chimeric with the donor lymphocytes only, analogous to patients with severe combined immunodeficiency. This suggests that pathogenesis occurs at the level of the lymphoid stem or progenitor cell. However, a second patient became chimeric with myeloid and lymphoid elements, indicating that the hematopoietic compartment affected involves a more primitive multipotential stem or progenitor cell.

Seckel's Syndrome

Seckel's syndrome is a rare, autosomal recessive condition. Patients present in the newborn period with microcephaly and dwarfism. An affected infant typically has a receding forehead and chin, antimongoloid palpebral fissures, a high arched palate, hirsutism, and a relatively large nose and eyes. Patients may have severe mental retardation. They are likely to develop aplastic anemia, acute myelogenous leukemia, or malignancies.[48–50] Endogenous chromosome breakage is observed in some patients.[51] However, unlike FA, chromosome breakage does not appear to increase in response to mitomycin C stimulation.

SINGLE-LINEAGE FAILURE

Bone marrow failure can consist of depression of a single variety of hematologic cell (Table 5–3). These disorders are discussed in the following section.

Table 5–3. **Marrow Failure Syndromes of Neonates Consisting of Depression of a Single Variety of Hematologic Cell**

Erythrocytes
Congenital parvovirus infection
Congenital hypoplastic anemia
Neutrophils
Osteopetrosis
Kostmann's syndrome
Platelets
Thrombocytopenia with absent radii

Parvovirus Infection

The B19 parvovirus is most commonly known as the etiologic agent of fifth disease. Fifth disease is a common, transient childhood illness characterized by several days of fever in an otherwise nontoxic-appearing child. An exanthem is associated temporally with abatement of the fever. In normal children and adults, the disease is benign, although it is known to result in erythroid-specific, transient aplastic crises in children.[52] In the fetus, however, B19 is an important cause of spontaneous abortions and nonimmune hydrops fetalis.[53–55] Based on epidemiologic data, almost 10% of fetuses whose mothers acquire a primary parvovirus infection acquire hydrops fetalis.

The crux of the pathogenesis of B19 seems to lie in the tropism of the cellular receptor of the virus for a glycolipid present on erythroid cells and some megakaryocytes.[56] Parvovirus specifically targets lineage-restricted erythroid progenitors (BFU-E) and particularly the colony-forming units–erythrocyte [CFU-E]. The high cellular tropism of B19 for these particular progenitors has resulted in some investigators considering the use of this virus for genetic therapy applications.[57, 58] When the virus infects the erythroid progenitors, it prevents further replication and differentiation.

The diagnosis is established by obtaining IgM antibody or evaluation of serial samples of IgG for parvovirus in the blood of mothers with affected anemic fetuses. Treatment is symptomatic and consists of administration of intrauterine infusions of red blood cells or by an intrauterine partial-exchange transfusion.

Patients who are immunodeficient for a variety of reasons are predisposed to chronic parvovirus infection.[59, 60] This group includes patients who have congenital immunodeficiencies, those being treated with chemotherapy, and patients infected with human immunodeficiency 1 virus (HIV-1). Chronic parvovirus infections, unlike the acute infections in normal patients, are associated with a sustained pure red blood cell aplasia. If perinatal transmission of HIV-1 to infants increases in the next decade, with human immunodeficiency virus in infants, it is possible that chronic parvovirus could be of increasing epidemiologic significance in infants.

Congenital Hypoplastic Anemia

Congenital hypoplastic anemia (CHA) has alternatively been called Diamond-Blackfan syndrome, erythrogenesis imperfecta, and chronic regenerative anemia. Symptoms associated with a progressive anemia appear in the first few months of life. Approximately three fourths of patients present by 4 months of age. There is no clear genetic pattern of inheritance, although affected siblings have been described. Because only a small group of cases of CHA are familial, there are no clear-cut genetic markers for this disease, and prenatal testing is not available.[2]

A variety of abnormal symptoms have been observed in the pregnancy history, including previous stillbirths, preeclampsia, and placental hemorrhage, although it is unclear whether this frequency is above that of the general population.[2, 61–63] CHA patients do seem to have a higher incidence of being small for gestational age. At birth, these patients frequently have constitutional abnormalities, including triphalangeal thumbs, flattening of the thenar eminence, and other dysmorphic head and facial features. Patients with CHA also have a predisposition to renal and skeletal anomalies, especially of the upper limb.[2, 64, 65]

Laboratory Analysis

The complete blood cell count of these patients is remarkable for the anemia and the erythrocyte macrocytosis. The mean cell volume (MCV) of the erythroid cells is often greater than 100 fL. Patients have elevated levels of Hb F and elevated expression of the i antigen. These latter two features of the erythroid cells provide important clues in differentiating patients with congenital hypoplastic anemia from patients with transient erythropenia of childhood, in which the Hb F and i antigen levels are low. Peripheral blood reticulocyte counts are consistently low. The myeloid cells and platelets are normal in patients with CHA, and lymphocytes are normal or somewhat increased. Bone marrow aspirates obtained from these patients have normal myeloid cells and megakaryocytes and have normal bone marrow cellularity. Cells of the erythroid series are decreased in number in most instances, and even when normal, they usually show evidence of maturation arrest.

Pathogenesis

The pathogenesis of this disease remains unclear. Reduced numbers of erythroid progenitors (BFU-E and CFU-E) are assayable from bone marrow cells cultured from patients with CHA.[66, 67] Patients have elevated erythropoietin levels, which probably represents a compensatory response to the anemia.[68] Lymphocyte-conditioned media or serum from patients with CHA inhibit the formation of erythroid progenitors from normal patients in some instances, suggesting that an immunologic inhibition of erythroid growth is involved directly or indirectly in the pathogenesis of the disease. However, inhibition of normal progenitor growth by lymphocytes from CHA patients is not observed uniformly, and culture of erythroid progenitors from CHA marrow in the presence of normal lymphocytes does not restore normal erythroid progenitor growth.[69–72]

Osteopetrosis

The presentation of osteopetrosis in the neonate characteristically includes hepatosplenomegaly, a progressive anemia, craniomegaly, and bone sclerosis. Deafness, blindness, and other cranial nerve palsies are also common. All result from the central pathogenic defect in which osteoclasts fail to normally resorb and remodel bone. The hepatosplenomegaly is a consequence of compensatory extramedullary hematopoiesis in response to constriction of the bone marrow cavity. Similarly, the deafness, blindness, and other cranial nerve abnormalities result from cranial compression.

The pathogenesis of osteopetrosis appears to occur in utero, because a family history of spontaneous abortions and stillbirths is common. The infantile form of osteopetrosis is transmitted as an autosomal recessive trait, although an adult variant that is much less severe is transmitted in an autosomal dominant fashion.[73, 74] Ultrasound methods can be used for prenatal diagnosis. They can evaluate bone density, intrauterine fractures, and macrocephaly.[75, 76]

Patients have no intrinsic abnormality in blood cell formation, although they do have hematologic abnormalities as a result of the compression of the marrow space. Progressive macrocytic anemia with reticulocytosis develops along with elevated myeloid counts. Patients eventually develop thrombocytopenia and have increased hemolysis as a result of splenomegaly. Bone marrow biopsies and aspirates are difficult to obtain because of hypocellularity, fibrosis, and a narrowed marrow cavity.[2]

The median survival of patients with the infantile form of osteopetrosis treated with conventional therapy, including blood cell transfusions, antibiotics for infections, and platelets for hemorrhage, is approximately 4 years. The most common causes of death are related to complications from the overgrowth of bone, resulting in hemorrhage, infection, and impaired host defense. Because osteoclasts are tissue macrophages, bone marrow transplantation is a possibility for treatment of this otherwise lethal disease.[77] In one large series of patients, early bone marrow transplantation restored bone marrow hematopoiesis, stabilized skeletal symptoms, and improved the radiographic appearance.

Kostmann's Syndrome

Kostmann described a group of infants who had chronic neutropenia, pyogenic infections, and early deaths.[78–80] The pregnancy history and neonatal history were generally normal. However, more than 50% of patients become symptomatic in the first month of life, and nearly all patients are symptomatic by 1 year of age.

This disease is transmitted as an autosomal recessive trait. It is panethnic, although the initial descriptions were principally of northern Europeans.[81] The white blood cell counts of these patients usually are profoundly deficient because of a very low absolute number of neutrophils in the peripheral blood. When bone marrow is cultured from these patients, the number of granulocyte macrophage progenitors is in many instances normal or even increased. However, cytologic examination of the differentiated cells produced in these colonies shows a paucity of neutrophils and instead a propensity of monocytes and eosinophils. Other blood cell indices such as hemoglobin and platelets are normal, suggesting a maturation arrest in the granulocyte lineage.

Patients with Kostmann's syndrome have increasingly been treated with recombinant granulocyte–colony stimulating factor (G-CSF).[40, 82] More than 90% of patients respond to this therapy. This is not trivial in a disease for which death from sepsis previously occurred at a mean of slightly more than 2 years. However, the use of recombinant G-CSF is not without risks, because there are increasing reports of patients with Kostmann's syndrome who develop a myeloid leukemia after treatment with recombinant G-CSF.[83–85] Whether there is a direct correlation between chronic G-CSF administration and the development of myeloid leukemia in Kostmann's syndrome patients is unclear. These patients may instead have an underlying bone marrow defect that predisposes them to leukemia, and treatment with G-CSF prolongs survival of patients who are already predisposed to the disease.

Thrombocytopenia with Absent Radii Syndrome

TAR syndrome is easily recognized in neonates by the bilateral absence of radii, normal thumbs, and thrombocytopenia.[2, 65, 86, 87] The status of the thumbs is important in differentiating patients with TAR from patients with FA. Patients with FA with involved radii have no thumbs, whereas patients with TAR always have normal thumbs. Petechiae and bloody stools are common in these patients in infancy. Despite thrombocytopenia in infancy, qualitative platelet function is normal.

The platelet counts normalize after the first year of life. Patients with TAR do not have subsequent hematologic sequelae.

Neurofibromatosis Type 1

Neurofibromatosis type 1 (NF1) is a common, autosomal dominant genetic disorder with variable penetrance. Mutations of the *NF1* gene cause an autosomal dominant disorder with an incidence of 1 case per 4000 persons.[88] The most common physical sign in the newborn period is café au lait lesions. Affected individuals are predisposed to develop benign and malignant neoplasms that primarily arise in cells derived from the embryonic neural crest.[88–96]

Infants and young children with NF1 are at a markedly increased risk (200- to 500-fold) of developing malignant myeloid disorders and comprise as many as 30% of de novo cases of preleukemia in the pediatric age group.[89, 97–100] Juvenile chronic myelogenous leukemia (JCML), also called juvenile myelomonocytic leukemia, is a myeloproliferative syndrome characterized by leukocytosis, thrombocytopenia, and hepatosplenomegaly with infiltrates of myeloid cells. It is the most common leukemia seen in children with NF1.[97, 98, 101–104] Genetic and biochemical data from studies of human leukemias have shown that *NF1* functions as a tumor suppressor gene in hematopoietic cells by negatively regulating the signaling of RAS, a GTPase-activating protein.[96, 97, 103, 105–107]

A hallmark of low-density blood and bone marrow cells from children with JCML is an abnormal pattern of in vitro progenitor growth that is characterized by the appearance of factor-independent myeloid colonies in methylcellulose cultures.[89, 98] A second consistent finding is that JCML cells form higher numbers of colonies derived from lineage-restricted colony-forming unit–granulocyte-macrophage (CFU-GM) progenitors in the presence of low concentrations of granulocyte-macrophage colony-stimulating factor (GM-CSF), although no mutations have been detected in the GM-CSF receptors of these patients.[99, 105] Hypersensitive growth has not been observed in cultures in which interleukin-3 or G-CSF was added, and these results led to the hypothesis that a specific defect within the GM-CSF signal transduction pathway plays a central role in the pathogenesis of JCML.[89, 98]

Two murine models have hematopoietic phenotypes that are remarkably similar to those of patients with JCML.[108–111] The *NF1*-deficient mouse dies in utero from apparent hydrops fetalis, but the fetal liver cells are hypersensitive to GM-CSF, analogous to patients with JCML, and irradiated mice reconstituted with fetal liver cells develop myeloproliferative disease and activation of the RAS pathway in primary progenitor cells. These mice provide a model for investigating the role of neurofibromin in regulating RAS signaling in hematopoietic cells and the pathogenesis of JCML.

Bloom's Syndrome

Bloom's syndrome is a rare genetic disorder characterized by genomic instability. Infants affected with this disorder usually are small for gestational age and have feeding difficulties. As they mature, they develop the classic triad of small features, microcephaly, and hypersensitivity to the sun.[2, 65] Some children also have hypogonadism, café au lait spots, microsomia, and various distal limb abnormalities such as syndactyly, supernumerary digits, or absence of toes. Somatic cells from patients with Bloom's syndrome acquire excessive numbers of mutations throughout the genome in cultured but otherwise unstressed cells and in fresh, unmanipulated cells.[112]

Children with this disease are highly predisposed to the acquisition of malignancies.[113] The affected gene of Bloom's syndrome has been identified[114] and found to have homology to RecQ helicases, a subfamily of DNA and RNA helicases thought to have a role in DNA repair.

References

1. Fanconi G: Familiare infantile perniziosaartige Anamie (pernizioses Blutbild und Konstitution). Jahrbuch Kinder 1927;117:257.
2. Alter B, Young N: The bone marrow failure syndromes. In Nathan D, Oski F (eds): Hematology of Infancy and Childhood, 5th ed. Philadelphia: WB Saunders, 1998, p 27.
3. Fanconi G: Familial constitutional panmyelocytopathy, Fanconi's anemia. Semin Hematol 1967;4:233.
4. Alter B: Annotation: Fanconi's anaemia and its variability. Br J Haematol 1993;85:9.
5. Auerbach A, Schroeder T: First announcement of the Fanconi Anemia International Registry. Blood 1982;60:1054.
6. Glanz A, Fraser F: Spectrum of anomalies in Fanconi anaemia. J Med Genet 1982;19:412.
7. Schroeder T, Tilgen D, Kruger D, et al: Formal genetics of Fanconi's anemia. Hum Genet 1976;32:257.
8. Swift M: Fanconi anaemia: cellular abnormalities and clinical predisposition to malignant disease. In 37 CFS: Congenital Disorders of Erythropoiesis. Amsterdam: Elsevier North-Holland, 1976, p 115.
9. Auerbach A: Fanconi anemia. Dermatol Clin 1995;13:41.
10. Giampietro P, Adler-Brecher B, Verlander P, et al: The need for more accurate and timely diagnosis in Fanconi anemia: a report for the International Fanconi Anemia Registry. Pediatrics 1993;91:1116.
11. Wang H, Hunter A, Clifford B, et al: VACTERL with hydrocephalus: spontaneous chromosome breakage and rearrangement in a family showing apparent sex-linked recessive inheritance. Am J Med Genet 1993;47:114.
12. Auerbach A, Zhang M, Ghosh R, et al: Clastogen-induced chromosomal breakage as a marker for first trimester prenatal diagnosis of Fanconi anemia. Hum Genet 1986;73:86.
13. Auerbach A, Adler B, Chaganti R: Prenatal and postnatal diagnosis and carrier detection of Fanconi anemia by a cytogenetic method. Pediatrics 1981;67:128.
14. Auerbach A, Rogatko A, Schroeder-Kurth T: International Fanconi anemia registry: relation of clinical symptoms to diepoxybutane sensitivity. Blood 1989;73:391.
15. Auerbach A, Sagi M, Adler B: Fanconi anemia: prenatal diagnosis in 30 fetuses at risk. Pediatrics 1985;76:794.
16. Auerbach A, Ghosh R, Pollio P, et al: Diepoxybutane (DEB) test for prenatal and postnatal diagnosis of Fanconi anemia. In Schroeder-Kurth T, Auerbach A, Obe G (eds): Fanconi Anemia: Clinical, Cytogenetic, and Experimental Aspects. Heidelberg: Springer-Verlag, 1989, p 71.
17. Meyn M: Chromosome instability syndromes: lessons for carcinogenesis. Curr Top Microbiol Immunol 1997;221:71.
18. Joenje H, Oostra A, Wijker M, et al: Evidence for at least eight Fanconi anemia genes. Am J Hum Genet 1997;61:940.
19. Strathdee C, Duncan A, Buchwald M: Evidence for at least four Fanconi anemia genes, including FACC on chromosome 9. Nat Genet 1992;1:196.
20. Pronk J, Gibson R, Savoia A, et al: Localization of the Fanconi anemia complementation group A gene to chromosome 16q24.3. Nat Genet 1995;22:338.
21. Strathdee C, Gavish H, Shannon W, et al: Cloning of cDNAs for Fanconi's anaemia by functional complementation. Nature 1992;356:763.
22. LoTenFoe J, Rooimans M, Bosnoyan-Collins L, et al: Expression cloning of a cDNA for the major Fanconi anaemia gene, FAA. Nat Genet 1996;14:320.
23. Consortium FABC: Positional cloning of the Fanconi anaemia group A gene. Nat Genet 1996;14:324.
24. Gibson R, Buchwald M, Roberts R, et al: Characterization of the exon structure of the Fanconi anaemia group C gene by vectorette PCR. Hum Mol Genet 1993;2:35.
25. Youssoufian H: Localization of Fanconi anemia C protein to the cytoplasm of mammalian cells. Proc Natl Acad Sci USA 1994;91:7975.
26. Kupfer GM, Naf D, Suliman A, et al: The Fanconi anemia proteins, FAA and FAC, interact to form a nuclear complex. Nat Genet 1997;17:487.
27. D'Andrea A, Grompe M: Molecular biology of Fanconi anemia: implications for diagnosis and therapy. Blood 1997;90:1725.
28. Daneshbod-Skibba G, Martin J, Shahidi N: Myeloid and erythroid colony growth in non-anaemic patients with Fanconi's anaemia. Br J Haematol 1980;44:33.
29. Lui V, Ragab A, Findley H, et al: Bone marrow cultures in children with Fanconi anemia and the TAR syndrome. J Pediatr 1977;91:952.
30. Saunders E, Freedman M: Constitutional aplastic anemia: defective haematopoietic stem cell growth in vitro. Br J Haematol 1978;40:277.
31. Chu J: Granulopoiesis in Fanconi's aplastic anemia. Proc Soc Exp Biol Med 1979;161:609.
32. Prindull G, Jentsch E, Hansmann I: Fanconi's anemia developing erythroleukemia. Scand J Haematol 1979;23:59.
33. Auerbach A, Weiner M, Warburton D, et al: Acute myeloid leukemia as the first hematologic manifestation of Fanconi anemia. Am J Hematol 1982;12:289.
34. Walsh C, Grompe M, Vanin E, et al: A functionally

active retrovirus vector for gene therapy in Fanconi anemia group C. Blood 1994;84:453.
35. Freie B, Dutt P, Clapp D: Correction of Fanconi anemia type C phenotypic abnormalities using a clinically suitable retroviral vector infection protocol. Cell Transplant 1996;5:385.
36. Chen M, Tomkins D, Auerbach W, et al: Inactivation of Fac in mice produces inducible chromosomal instability and reduced fertility reminiscent of Fanconi anaemia. Nat Genet 1996;12:1.
37. Haneline L: Multiple inhibitory cytokines induce deregulated progenitor growth and apoptosis in hematopoietic cells from Fac −/− mice. Blood 1998;91:4092.
38. Whitney M, Royle G, Low M, et al: Germ cell defects and hematopoietic hypersensitivity to γ-interferon in mice with a targeted disruption of the Fanconi anemia C gene. Blood 1996;88:49.
39. Ozsoylu S, Argun G: Tryptic activity of the duodenal juice in aplastic anemia. J Pediatr 1967;70:60.
40. Dale D, Bonilla M, Davis M, et al: A randomized controlled phase III trial of recombinant human granulocyte colony-stimulating factor (filgrastim) for treatment of severe chronic neutropenia. Blood 1993;81:2496.
41. Paley C, Murphy S: Treatment of neutropenia in Schwachman-Diamond syndrome (SDS) with recombinant human granulocyte stimulating factor (rh-G-CSF). Blood 1991;74:324a.
42. Rotig A, Cormier V, Blanchi S, et al: Pearson's marrow-pancreas syndrome: a multisystem disorder in infancy. J Clin Invest 1990;86:1601.
43. Pearson H, Jobel J, Kocoshis S, et al: A new syndrome of refractory sideroblastic anemia with vacuolization of marrow precursors and exocrine pancreatic dysfunction. J Pediatr 1979;95:976.
44. Blaw M, Mize C: Juvenile Pearson syndrome. J Child Neurol 1993;5:186.
45. De Vaal O, Seynhaeve V: Reticular dysgenesia. Lancet 1959;2:1123.
46. Levinsky R, Tiedeman K: Successful bone marrow transplantation for reticular dysgenesis. Lancet 1983;1:671.
47. Roper M, Parmley R, Crist W, et al: Severe congenital leukopenia (reticular dysgenesis). Am J Dis Child 1985;139:832.
48. Majewski F, Goecke T: Studies of microcephalic primordial dwarfism, I: Approach to the delineation of the Seckel syndrome. Am J Med Genet 1982;12:7.
49. Seemanova E, Passarge E, Beneskova D, et al: Familial microcephaly with normal intelligence and risk for lymphoreticular malignancies: a new autosomal recessive disorder. Am J Med Genet 1985;20:639.
50. Hayani A, Suarez C, Molnar Z, et al: Acute myeloid leukemia in a patient with Seckel syndrome. J Med Genet 1994;31:148.
51. Butler M, Hall B: Do some patients with Seckel's syndrome have hematologic problems and/or chromosomal breakage? Am J Med Genet 1987;27:645.
52. Wodzinski M, Lilleyman J: Transient erythroblastopenia of childhood due to human parvovirus B19 infection. Br J Haematol 1989;73:127.
53. Andersen H, Drew J, Beischer N, et al: Nonimmune hydrops fetalis: changing contribution to perinatal mortality. Br J Obstet Gynecol 1983;90:636.
54. Hall S, Cohen B: Prospective of human parvovirus (B19) in pregnancy. BMJ 1990;300:1166.
55. Kinney J, Anderson L: Risk of adverse outcomes of pregnancy after human parvovirus infection. J Infect Dis 1988;157:663.
56. Srivastava A, Bruno E: Parvovirus B19-induced perturbation of human megakaryopoiesis in vitro. Blood 1990;76:1997.
57. Broxmeyer HE, Cooper S, Etienne JM, et al: Cord blood transplantation and the potential for gene therapy–gene transduction using a recombinant adeno-associated viral vector. Ann N Y Acad Sci 1995;770:105.
58. Ponnazhagan S, Mukerjee P, Wang X, et al: Adeno-associated virus 2–mediated transduction of primary human bone marrow-derived CD34$^+$ hematopoietic progenitor cells: donor variation and correlation of gene expression with cellular differentiation. J Virol 1997;71:8262.
59. Clark D, Dessypris E, Krantz S: Studies on pure red blood cell aplasia. XI. Results of immunosuppressive treatment of 37 patients. Blood 1984;63:277.
60. Kurtzmann G, Ozawa K: Chronic bone marrow failure due to persistent parvovirus infection. N Engl J Med 1987;317:287.
61. Bertolani M, Baroncini A: Malattia de Blackfan-Diamond con genitali ambigui. Pediatr Med Chir 1993;15:589.
62. Madanat F, Arnaout M: Red cell aplasia resembling Diamond-Blackfan anemia in seven children in a family. Am J Pediatr Hematol Oncol 1994;16:260.
63. Yetgin S, Balci S: Aase-Smith syndrome: report of a new case with unusual features. Turk J Pediatr 1994;36:239.
64. Cathie I: Erythrogenesis imperfecta. Arch Dis Child 1950;25:313.
65. Jones K: Smith's Recognizable Patterns of Human Malformation, 5th ed. Philadelphia: WB Saunders, 1997.
66. McGuckin C, Ball S, Gordon-Smith E: Diamond-Blackfan anaemia: three patterns of in vitro response to haemopoietic growth factors. Br J Haematol 1995;89:457.
67. Casadevall N, Croisille L: Age-related alterations in erythroid and granulopoietic progenitors in Diamond-Blackfan anaemia. Br J Haematol 1994;87:369.
68. Hammond D, Shore N, Movassaghi N: Production, utilization and excretion of erythropoietin. I. Chronic anemias. II. Aplastic crisis. III. Erythropoietic effects of normal plasma. Ann N Y Acad Sci 1968;149:516.
69. Steinberg M, Coleman M, Pennebaker J: Diamond-Blackfan syndrome: evidence for T-cell mediated suppression of erythroid development and a serum blocking factor associated with remission. Br J Haematol 1979;41:57.
70. Hoffman R, Zanjani E: Diamond-Blackfan syndrome: lymphocyte-mediated suppression of erythropoiesis. Science 1976;193:899.
71. Nathan D, Clarke B: Erythroid precursors in congenital hypoplastic (Diamond-Blackfan) anemia. J Clin Invest 1978;61:489.
72. Nathan D, Hillman D: Normal erythropoietic helper T cells in congenital hypoplastic (Diamond-Blackfan) anemia. N Engl J Med 1978;298:1049.
73. Shapiro F: Osteopetrosis: current clinical considerations. Orthop Rel Res 1993;294:34.
74. Gerritsen E, Vossen J: Autosomal recessive osteopetrosis: variability of findings at diagnosis and during the natural course. Pediatrics 1994;93:247.
75. Khazen N, Faverly D: Lethal osteopetrosis with multiple fractures in utero. Am J Med Genet 1986;23:811.
76. Golbus M, Koerper M, Hall B: Failure to diagnose osteopetrosis in utero. Lancet 1976;2:1246.
77. Gerritsen E, Vossen J: Bone marrow transplantation for autosomal recessive osteopetrosis: a report from the working part on inborn errors of the European

Bone Marrow Transplantation Group. J Pediatr 1994;125:896.
78. Kostmann R: Infantile genetic agranulocytosis: a review with presentation of ten new cases. Acta Paediatr Scand 1975;64:362.
79. Kostmann R: Infantile genetic granulocytosis: a new recessive lethal disease in man. Acta Paediatr Scand 1956;64:362.
80. Kostmann R: Infantile genetic agranulocytosis: a new recessive lethal disease in man. Acta Paediatr Scand 1956;45:1.
81. Iselius L, Gustavson K: Spatial distribution of the gene for infantile genetic agranulocytosis. Hum Hered 1984;34:358.
82. Donadieu J, Boutard P: A phase II study of recombinant human granulocyte colony-stimulating factor (rHuG-CSF, Lenograstim) in the treatment of agranulocytosis in children. Nouv Rev Fr Hematol 1994;36:441.
83. Rosen R, Kang S-J: Congenital agranulocytosis terminating in acute myelomonocytic leukemia. J Pediatr 1979;94:406.
84. Weinblatt M, Scimeca P: Transformation of congenital neutropenia into monosomy 7 and acute nonlymphoblastic leukemia in a child treated with granulocyte colony-stimulating factor. J Pediatr 1995;126:263.
85. Imashuku S, Hibi S: Myelodysplasia and acute myeloid leukaemia in cases of aplastic anaemia and congenital neutropenia G-CSF administration. Br J Haematol 1995;89:188.
86. Hall J, Levin J: Thrombocytopenia with absent radius (TAR). Medicine (Baltimore) 1969;48:411.
87. Hall J: Thrombocytopenia and absent radius (TAR) syndrome. J Med Genet 1987;24:79.
88. Skuse G, Kosciolek B, Rowley P: Molecular genetic analysis of tumors in von Recklinghausen neurofibromatosis: loss of heterozygosity for chromosome 17. Genes Chromosomes Cancer 1989;1:36.
89. Emanuel P, Bates L, Castleberry R, et al: Selective hypersensitivity to granulocyte-macrophage colony-stimulating factor by juvenile chronic myeloid leukemia hematopoietic progenitors. Blood 1991;77:925.
90. Xu G, O'Connell P, Viskochil D, et al: The neurofibromatosis type 1 gene encodes a protein related to GAP. Cell 1990;62:599.
91. Hudson SM: Neurofibromatosis: historical perspective, classification and diagnostic criteria. In Hudson SM, Hughes RAC (eds): The Neurofibromatoses: A Pathogenetic and Clinical Overview. London: Chapman & Hall Medical, 1994, p 1.
92. Li Y, Bollag G, Clark R, et al: Somatic mutations in the neurofibromatosis 1 gene in human tumors. Cell 1992;69:275.
93. Matsui I, Tanimura M, Kobayaski N, et al: Neurofibromatosis type 1 and childhood cancer. Cancer 1993;72:2746.
94. Wiestler O, Radner H: Pathology of Neurofibromatosis, 1 and 2: The Neurofibromatoses. London: Chapman & Hall Medical, 1994, p 135.
95. Shannon K, Watterson J, Johnson P, et al: Monosomy 7 myeloproliferative disease in children with neurofibromatosis, type 1: epidemiology and molecular analysis. Blood 1992;79:1311.
96. Shannon K, O'Connell P, Martin G, et al: Loss of the Normal NF1 allele from the bone marrow of children with type 1 neurofibromatosis and malignant myeloid disorders. N Engl J Med 1994;330:597.
97. Boguski M, McCormick F: Proteins regulating Ras and its relatives. Nature 1993;366:643.
98. Emanuel P, Bates L, Zhu S, et al: The role of monocyte-derived hemopoietic growth factors in the regulation of myeloproliferation in juvenile chronic myelogenous leukemia. Exp Hematol 1991;19:1017.
99. Side L, Emanuel P, Taylor B, et al: Mutations of the NF1 gene in children with juvenile myelomonocytic leukemia without clinical evidence of neurofibromatosis, type 1. Blood 1998;92:267.
100. Bagby G, Dinarello C, Neerhout R, et al: Interleukin 1-dependent paracrine granulopoiesis in chronic granulocytic leukemia of the juvenile. J Clin Invest 1988;82:1430.
101. Kitamura T, Sato N, Arai K, et al: Expression cloning of the human IL-3 receptor cDNA reveals a shared β subunit for the human IL-3 and GM-CSF receptors. Cell 1991;66:1165.
102. Bradley T, Hodgson G: Detection of primitive macrophage progenitor cells in mouse bone marrow. Blood 1979;54:1446.
103. Copeland N, Gilbert D, Cho B, et al: Mast cell growth factor maps near the steel locus on mouse chromosome 10 and is deleted in a number of steel alleles. Cell 1990;63:175.
104. Paulson R, Vesely S, Siminovitch K, et al: Signalling by the W/Kit receptor tyrosine kinase is negatively regulated in vivo by the protein tyrosine phosphatase Shp 1. Nat Genet 1996;13:309.
105. Brodeur G: The *NF1* gene in myelopoiesis and childhood myelodysplastic syndromes. N Engl J Med 1994;330:637.
106. Neubauer A, Shannon K, Liu E: Mutations of the ras proto-oncogenes in childhood monosomy 7. Blood 1991;77:594.
107. Yamamoto F, Kasai H, Togashi Y, et al: Elevated level of 8-hydroxydeoxyguanosine in DNA of liver, kidneys, and brain of Long-Evans cinnamon rats. Jpn J Cancer Res 1993;84:508.
108. Zhang Y, Vik T, Ryder J, et al: NF1 regulates hematopoietic progenitor cell growth and Ras signaling in response to multiple cytokines. J Exp Med 1998;187:1893.
109. Jacks T, Shih TS, Schmitt EM, et al: Tumour predisposition in mice heterozygous for a targeted mutation in *NF1*. Nat Genet 1994;7:353.
110. Largaespada D, Brannan C, Jenkins N, et al: NF1 deficiency causes Ras-mediated granulocyte/macrophage colony stimulating factor hypersensitivity and chronic myeloid leukaemia. Nat Genet 1996;12:137.
111. Pan G, Ni J, Wei Y-F, et al: An antagonist decoy receptor and a death domain-containing receptor for TRAIL. Science 1997;277:815.
112. Weksberg R, Smith C: Bloom syndrome: a single complementation group defines patients of diverse ethnic origin. Am J Hum Genet 1988;42:816.
113. German J: Bloom syndrome: a mendelian prototype of somatic mutational disease. Medicine (Baltimore) 1993;72:393.
114. Ellis N, Groden J, Ye T, et al: The Bloom's syndrome gene product is homologous to RecQ helicases. Cell 1995;83:655.

CHAPTER 6

Hematologic Aspects of the Maternal-Fetal Relationship

Darlene A. Calhoun, D.O.

Hematologic relationships between the mother and fetus are complex and intricate. Although the two circulations are fundamentally separate, small numbers of blood cells and occasionally large numbers of such cells move from one circuit to the other. Certain infectious agents and drugs within the mother's circulation routinely gain access into the fetal circulation and cause characteristic hematologic changes in the fetus and neonate. Moreover, various maternal illnesses can affect the hematologic status of the fetus and neonate. This chapter reviews these maternal-fetal issues for neonatologists who deal with problems rooted in these relationships.

MOVEMENT OF BLOOD CELLS BETWEEN MATERNAL AND FETAL CIRCULATIONS

Since the 18th century, it has been realized that the circulation of the human fetus is separated from that of its mother by intervening placental tissue.[1, 2] A representative third trimester placenta is shown in Figure 6–1. Fetal villi can be seen protruding into the intervillous space, which contains maternal blood. Fetal trophoblasts, composed of syncytiotrophoblasts and cytotrophoblasts, line the surface of the villi and are separated from maternal blood by an intervening epithelial layer. The syncytiotrophoblast is a continuous, uninterrupted, multinucleated layer without separating cell borders.[3] The trophoblastic basement membrane separates the trophoblast from the stromal core of the villi. Fetal vessels can be seen within the larger villi and are connected to the fetal circulatory system through the chorionic plate and umbilical cord.[3] Fetal vessels that are adjacent to the trophoblastic layer can lie very close to the maternal circulation.

Despite this apparent barrier to the movement of cells, fetal red blood cells, white blood cells, and platelets are commonly found in the maternal circulation.[4–8] Some have estimated that fetomaternal transfusions occur in about 50% of all pregnancies.[8–11] This movement of cells permits genetic diagnoses to be made using fetal cells contained within maternal blood.[4, 12–15]

In addition to the common movement of relatively small numbers of blood cells between the maternal and fetal circulations, the movement of substantial volumes of blood occurs occasionally. This gives rise to fetal anemia or fetal polycythemia, depending on the net directionality of the transfer, and sometimes results in intrauterine demise.[16, 17] The transplacental passage of red blood cells has been observed as early as the fourth to eighth week of gestation, and chronic conditions resulting from the long-term passage of cellular elements can occur.[11] If the development of anemia is chronic, the fetus can adapt hemodynamically. However, acute hemorrhage can result in the infant being pale and manifesting clinical signs consistent with shock.[8, 18–20]

The passage of leukocytes and platelets from the fetal into the maternal circulation can result in the stimulation of antibody production against antigens located on fetal cells.[21, 22] Neutropenia and thrombocytopenia in the neonate can be caused by transplacental passage of IgG antibodies that are specific for antigens on fetal neutrophils and platelets.

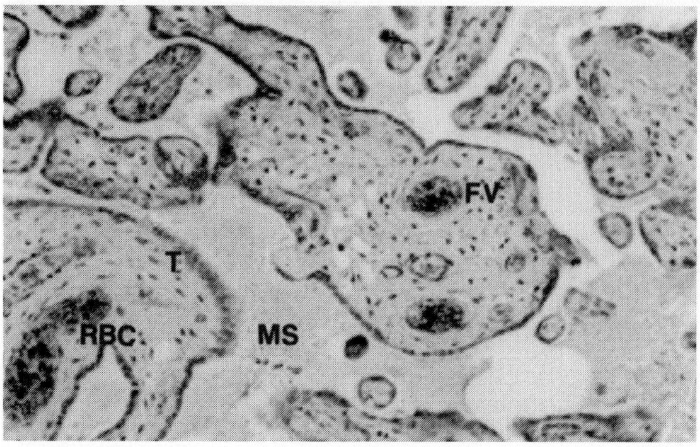

Figure 6–1. Representative villi from a third-trimester placenta. (FV, fetal vessels; MS, maternal space; RBC, red blood cells; T, fetal trophoblasts.)

HEMATOLOGIC MANIFESTATIONS OF TRANSPLACENTALLY ACQUIRED INFECTIONS

Maternal infections acquired during pregnancy are unique in that, although the mother may show minimal or no symptoms related to the infection, the consequences for the fetus can be devastating and include significant hematologic alterations.

TORCH Infections

Classically, this group of infections produced neonatal diseases that were clinically indistinguishable and included *Toxoplasma gondii*, "other" (e.g., *Treponema pallidum*), rubella virus, cytomegalovirus, and herpes simplex virus. Table 6–1 contains some diagnostic features of these infections and compares them with features of erythroblastosis fetalis. Other agents that can cause similar illnesses include human parvovirus, human immunodeficiency virus (HIV), varicella-zoster virus, coxsackie viruses, echoviruses, *Mycobacterium tuberculosis*, and *Plasmodium* sp.

Toxoplasmosis

Epidemiology and General Characteristics

Congenital toxoplasmosis results from the transplacental passage of the intracellular protozoan *T. gondii*, so named because it was first isolated from a North African rodent called the gondi.[23, 24] The domestic cat is the definitive host, and fetal infection can result after a primary infection in a nonimmune mother. The first cases of toxoplasmosis in infants were reported by Wolf and colleagues, who described an encephalomyelitis of infancy.[25] The frequency of congenital infection in the United States is estimated to be 1 in 1000 to 10,000 live births.[26]

In pregnant women with untreated primary toxoplasmosis during the first, second, and third trimesters, the proportion of infected fetuses is 25%, 54%, and 65%, respectively.[26] Infections acquired just before or soon after conception are less likely to result in congenital infection than infections that occur later.[27] However, the most severe neonatal disease usually occurs with first and second trimester infections. Maternal treatment with spiramycin can reduce the incidence of fetal infection by more than 50% and can reduce the severity of fetal disease.[28–30] Mothers with chronic toxoplasmosis do not transmit the disease to subsequent fetuses.

The classic triad of toxoplasmosis—chorioretinitis, hydrocephalus, and intracranial calcifications—is found in the form of the disease that is primarily neurologic.[31] The generalized form of congenital toxoplasmosis is characterized by fever, hepatosplenomegaly, jaundice, skin manifestations, pneumonitis, and diarrhea.[32, 33]

Hematologic Manifestations

Approximately two thirds of infants with congenital toxoplasmosis have inapparent dis-

Table 6–1. **Features of Congenital TORCH Infections Compared with Erythroblastosis Fetalis**

Finding	Congenital Syphilis	Toxoplasmosis (Generalized)	Cytomegalic Inclusion Disease	Rubella Syndrome	Erythroblastosis Fetalis
Jaundice	+ + +	+ + +	+ + +	+	+ + +
Anemia	+ + + +	+ + +	+ +	+ +	+ + +
Thrombocytopenia	+ +	+	+ + +	+ + +	+
Hepatomegaly	+ + + +	+ + +	+ + + +	+ +	+ +
Splenomegaly	+ + + +	+ + + +	+ + + +	+ +	+ + +
Purpura	+ +	+	+ + +	+ + +	+
Rash	+	+	0	+	0
Chorioretinitis	+	+ + +	+	+	0
Intracranial calcifications	0	+	+ + +	?	0
Generalized edema	+ +	+	+	?	+
Other findings	Mucocutaneous lesions, periostitis, snuffles, positive serology	Convulsions, microcephaly, hydrocephaly, lymphadenopathy	Pneumonia, cytomegalic inclusion cells in the urine	Cataract, glaucoma, heart defects, deafness, microcephaly, hydrocephaly, bone lesions, rubella virus recoverable	Positive Coombs' test, evidence of blood group incompatibility between mother and child

0, not described; +, present in approximately 1–25% of cases; + +, present in approximately 26–50% of cases; + + +, present in approximately 51–75% of cases; + + + +, present in approximately 76–100% of cases.

ease at birth. Symptomatic congenital toxoplasmosis can mimic Rh (D) erythroblastosis fetalis in that the infant is pale and hydropic at birth with marked hepatosplenomegaly.[34, 35] Anemia occurs in up to 77% of patients with the generalized form of toxoplasmosis and in as many as 50% of those with the neurologic form.[31, 36] The anemia is often accompanied by reticulocytosis, normoblastemia, and hyperbilirubinemia, suggesting a hemolytic state.

Thrombocytopenia occurs in approximately 10% of affected patients. In a case reported by Beckett and Flynn, platelets were rare on the blood film, with fewer than one or two per 25 oil-immersion fields.[35] However, when bone marrow examinations were performed, adequate numbers of megakaryocytes were observed,[36] suggesting that increased peripheral destruction of platelets was the cause of the thrombocytopenia.

Neutropenia and neutrophilia have been observed in patients with congenital toxoplasmosis, and eosinophilia occurs in 18% to 25%.[31, 36] In a neonate delivered at 33 weeks' gestation with congenital toxoplasmosis, a total white blood cell count of 35,000 cells/mm^3 was reported, and the peripheral blood smear contained 2% segmented and 15% nonsegmented neutrophils, 15% metamyelocytes, 8% myelocytes, 8% blasts, 29% small and 13% large lymphocytes, and 10% eosinophils.[35] Decreased CD4$^+$ lymphocyte counts and diminished CD4 to CD8 ratios are common.[37, 38] The severe organ damage seen in congenital toxoplasmosis may be the result of deficiencies in cell-mediated immune responses to the protozoan.

Syphilis

Epidemiology and General Characteristics

The first major work on syphilis was written by Francisco Lopez de Villaloba in 1498.[39] Congenital syphilis is acquired by the transplacental passage of the spirochete *T. pallidum.* Most infants with congenital syphilis are asymptomatic at birth, but during the third to eighth weeks of life, they can manifest clinical signs, including fever, irritability, snuffles, mucocutaneous lesions, pseudoparalysis with osteochondritis and periostitis, jaundice, and lymphadenopathy. The classic triad of snuffles, palmar and plantar bullae, and splenomegaly may be observed.[40] Hepatosplenomegaly occurs in as many as 50% to 90% of affected infants[40, 41] and is the result of extramedullary hematopoiesis and subacute hepatic and splenic inflammation. Infants with fulminant syphilitic hepatitis can mimic those with metabolic or other infectious causes of acute liver failure by presenting with hypoglycemia, lactic acidosis, encephalopathy, disseminated intravascular coagulation, and shock.[42, 43]

Hematologic Manifestations

Among infants with congenital syphilis, hematologic abnormalities are common.[44] Congenital syphilis is often misdiagnosed as erythroblastosis fetalis or confused with congenital toxoplasmosis, cytomegalic inclusion disease, or congenital leukemia.[45]

Anemia occurs in the 64% of infants younger than 4 weeks and 89% of those older than 4 weeks of age.[46] It appears to be the result of an intense hemolytic process.[47, 48] Occasionally, the anemia may be the result of marrow hypoplasia or aplasia,[48, 49] replacement of bone marrow by syphilitic granulation tissue, or an arrest in maturation of the erythroid cell line.[41] Hydrops fetalis due to severe anemia has been described.[50] The anemic patient characteristically has a negative Coombs' test result and has polychromasia and erythroblastemia with up to 500 nucleated red blood cells per 100 leukocytes.[41]

Thrombocytopenia occurs in as many as 46% of affected neonates.[51] Platelet counts of less than 100,000/mm^3 were reported by Freiman and Super for 13 of 46 infants,[51] and Whitaker and colleagues reported counts as low as 17,000/mm^3 in infants with this disease.[48] Bone marrow examinations of patients in the latter series revealed adequate numbers of megakaryocytes, suggesting decreased platelet survival as the cause of thrombocytopenia.[48]

No characteristic white blood cell count is uniformly seen in infants with congenital syphilis. Leukopenia and leukocytosis have been described, and the differential count can reveal absolute lymphocytosis[52] or an increase in the myeloid series.[53] In a series of patients described by Whitaker and colleagues, white blood cell counts as high as 34,700 cells/mm^3 were observed.[48] Hochsinger described a "constant irritation of the bone marrow, characterized by an outpouring of characteristic leukocytes," including eosinophils.[54]

Jaundice occurs in approximately one third of infants as a result of hepatitis or hemolysis[41] and can be present on the first day of life. Peak bilirubin concentrations of 40 mg/dL have been described with elevations in conjugated and unconjugated bilirubin fractions.

Rubella

Epidemiology and General Characteristics

Rubella was first recognized as a clinical entity by German researchers in the mid-18th century, and they called it "Rötheln."[55] In 1941, Gregg, an Australian ophthalmologist, associated intrauterine acquisition of infection with the production of cataracts and heart disease.[56] After the rubella epidemic of 1964 and 1965, the consequences of fetal rubella infection were acknowledged. Although more than one half of all neonates with congenital rubella are asymptomatic at birth, most manifest one or more symptoms of the disease later. When infection occurs during the first 12 weeks of pregnancy, these consequences can include low birth weight, cataracts, glaucoma, retinitis, deafness, congenital heart disease, and brain lesions associated with microcephaly, meningoencephalitis, or hydrocephalus. Thrombocytopenia, hepatosplenomegaly, neonatal hepatitis, intrahepatic biliary atresia, jaundice, bone lesions, dermal erythropoiesis, and a hemolytic syndrome can occur.

Hematologic Manifestations

The most common hematologic manifestation of the congenital rubella syndrome is thrombocytopenia. The incidence varies from 40% to 80%, and platelet counts are frequently below 50,000/mm^3, with values as low as 3000/mm^3.[57, 58] Although the thrombocytopenia usually is transient, resolving within the first 2 weeks of life, some cases have lasted 2 months.[59] Bone marrow aspirates reveal decreased megakaryocytes and an increased number of phagocytic reticulum cells.[60]

The leukocyte count is variable, and leukopenia[60] and leukocytosis[45] have been reported. Anemia may be related to reduced red blood cell survival.[60] This hemolytic anemia with morphologic abnormalities of the red blood cells can persist for several months, and it can progress to a transient hypoplastic anemia.[61] Altered blood group expression can occur.[62, 63]

Hepatomegaly and splenomegaly occur in 33% to 75% of affected patients. Jaundice occurs in 25%, and an elevated direct bilirubin component can result from hepatic obstruction. The jaundice can persist into the second month of life, and biopsies generally reveal evidence of giant cell hepatitis.[64]

Cytomegalovirus

Epidemiology and General Characteristics

The name of this disease is taken from the Greek words *kytos*, for a hollow container, and *megalos*, meaning large.[65] In 1904, Jesionek and Kiolemenoglov first reported intracytoplasmic inclusion bodies in an infant,[66] and in 1956, the etiologic agent was discovered.[67, 68] In the neonate, disease is acquired transplacentally, usually from an asymptomatic mother, and placental infection can occur exclusive of fetal involvement.[69] Unlike rubella and toxoplasmosis, in utero transmission of cytomegalovirus can occur as a consequence of primary or recurrent infection.[70]

Cytomegalovirus is the most common congenital infection in humans in the United States and is the most common cause of viral infection–induced mental retardation and sensorineural hearing loss.[71–74] Ninety percent of infants show no evidence of disease during the neonatal period.[65, 74] Clinical manifestations include a small-for-gestational-age infant with hepatosplenomegaly, jaundice, purpura and ecchymoses, microcephaly, intracranial calcifications, pneumonia, and chorioretinitis. Although hepatomegaly and splenomegaly are probably the most common physical abnormalities, liver function test results are usually only slightly abnormal.

Hematologic Manifestations

The hematologic manifestations of infants in whom the disease manifested in the first week of life are shown in Table 6–2. Enlargement of the liver and spleen was almost universally present. Jaundice occurred in nearly 75% of patients, with elevations in conjugated and unconjugated bilirubin fractions.[72] The presence of anemia was somewhat variable (as many as 43%) and, if not present in the first few days of life, developed during the following weeks. Thrombocytopenia was observed in about 80% and platelet counts of 6000 to 20,000/mm^3 were reported.[72, 75] Bone marrow examination of these patients revealed a virtual absence of megakaryocytes. An atypical lymphocytosis was seen in some.

Herpes Simplex Virus

Epidemiology and General Characteristics

Infections by the herpes simplex viruses have been recognized since the ancient Greek civilization. *Herpes* means to creep or crawl.[76] Between 1500 and 2000 cases of neonatal herpes simplex virus infection occur each year in the United States, and of these, 4% are congenital, 86% are acquired natally, and 10% are acquired postnatally.[73, 77] Neonatal infections with herpes simplex virus are associated with a mortality rate of 70% if untreated.[78]

The clinical manifestations of infection acquired in utero depend on the time at which the infection occurs in the fetus and are a direct reflection of the site and extent of viral replication.[79] Primary herpes simplex virus infections during the first half of gestation are associated with a significant frequency of spontaneous abortions and stillbirths.[73] These infections can result in microcephaly (60%), microphthalmia (25%), intracranial calcifications (15%), chorioretinitis (45% to 60%), and cutaneous vesicular lesions at the time of birth.[80–84]

Infections acquired during delivery can manifest in a variety of ways. Infants may exhibit lethargy, respiratory distress, fever or hypothermia, seizures, episodes of cyanosis, keratitis, conjunctivitis, and jaundice. Approximately 50% of affected infants have a characteristic papulovesicular rash. Signs typically manifest by the third day of life.

Table 6–2. **Hematologic Findings in Neonates with Confirmed Cytomegalovirus Infection**

Finding	Cases/Total Patients
Hepatomegaly	29/29
Splenomegaly	28/29
Anemia	3/7
Jaundice	21/29
Thrombocytopenia or purpura	20/29

Hematologic Manifestations

Bleeding caused by disseminated intravascular coagulation is the most common hematologic abnormality observed in infants with generalized herpes simplex virus infections, and it has been observed in 40% to 50% of cases. Bleeding is associated with thrombocytopenia and variable deficiencies of fibrinogen and factors V and VIII,[85, 86] and it appears to be a consequence of viral infection–induced disseminated intravascular coagulation and liver failure from hepatitis. A hemolytic anemia resulting from the mechanical fragmentation of erythrocytes has been observed in infants with disseminated herpesvirus infection.[87]

Parvovirus

Epidemiology and General Characteristics

Human parvovirus (B19), also called fifth disease or erythema infectiosum, was discovered in 1975 by Cossart and colleagues.[88] In the United States, approximately 50% of adult women are immune to parvovirus, and maternal risks associated with parvovirus infection are minimal in these women.[89] Clinical manifestations of the disease in women include malaise, arthralgias, and an erythematous, lace-like rash on the face and extremities. The condition is self-limited, and immunity to parvovirus should be lifelong.

Although maternal disease is generally mild, the fetus is at risk for serious complications.

Between 5% and 10% of infants delivered to women who contract the illness during pregnancy are affected.[89] The association of B19 infection with stillbirths was described by Brown and associates in 1984,[90] and additional reports of fetal death associated with maternal parvovirus B19 infection followed.[91–93] The risk to the fetus is greatest when maternal infection occurs in the first 12 weeks of gestation and decreases rapidly after 20 weeks. The fetus appears to be at risk for approximately 4 to 8 weeks after maternal infection.

The consequences of fetal infection with parvovirus B19 range from inapparent infection to life-threatening hydrops fetalis. Two mechanisms appear to be responsible for the hydrops: a direct effect of the virus on the myocardium and destruction of red blood cell precursors in the bone marrow leading to anemia and high output heart failure.

The reasons for the marked differences in fetal response to maternal B19 infection are poorly understood. In an animal model of B19 infection using an erythrotropic simian parvovirus, the timing of infection related to the maternal transfer of IgG antibodies was evaluated.[94] Persistent infection, severe anemia, and hydrops fetalis developed when maternal inoculation and viremia occurred before the transplacental passage of antibodies. When inoculation and viremia developed after the establishment of antibody transfer, pregnancies resulted in live, healthy infants. These findings suggest that infection established before the receipt of maternally derived IgG antibodies is important in the pathophysiology of hydrops fetalis related to B19 infection in the fetus.[94]

Hematologic Manifestations

Fetal infection with parvovirus can result in neonatal hydrops fetalis because of the affinity of B19 for erythroid progenitors. Pathologic findings suggest that the suppression of erythroid progenitors produces bone marrow aplasia, resulting in a chronic fetal anemia and leading to congestive heart failure and development of hydrops.[91] Histologic examination of fetal tissues reveals that erythroid precursor cells in the liver sinusoids are greatly increased.[93]

Unfortunately, no assessment of fetal risk can be made on the basis of current information. Treatment of affected fetuses by intrauterine transfusions has been recommended. If the fetus can be transfused, red blood cell precursors ultimately recover, and normal hematopoiesis is restored.

Human Immunodeficiency Virus

Epidemiology and General Characteristics

The first descriptions of acquired immunodeficiency syndrome (AIDS) in children were published in 1982.[95, 96] Vertical transmission of type 1 HIV (HIV-1) from the mother to the infant accounts for most new cases of pediatric AIDS in the United States.[97] Vertical transmission can occur in utero, intrapartum, or postpartum. Although it is commonly thought that vertical transmission of HIV-1 transmission in the United States occurs chiefly through intrauterine, transplacental spread of the virus, a growing body of evidence indicates that intrapartum transmission may be a major mode of fetal infection.

Maternal factors enhancing the rate at which HIV is transmitted to the fetus include advanced disease, low $CD4^+$ lymphocyte percentage, low absolute $CD4^+$ counts, higher plasma virus titers, P24 antigenemia, coexisting infections, viral strain differences, premature delivery, and obstetric factors such as prolonged rupture of maternal membranes or chorioamnionitis. The precise contribution of each factor is unclear.[98] Preterm infants are about fourfold more likely to become HIV-1 infected than those born at term.[99]

Hematologic Manifestations

Congenitally infected infants are usually asymptomatic during the neonatal period, although hepatomegaly and splenomegaly have been observed in approximately 5% of cases. Infected neonates often have normal blood counts, unlike adult patients who are often lymphopenic. Infants whose mothers have received zidovudine during pregnancy have lower hemoglobin levels than those whose HIV-positive mothers were not given zidovudine.[100] These same infants developed a mild normocytic normochromic anemia with a nadir at 4 weeks of age, earlier than the normal physiologic anemia of newborns. The anemia resolved without intervention except for the use of supplemental iron therapy in two infants.[101] Neutrophil counts of these infants were within normal limits for age.[101] The effects of maternal zidovudine therapy on the fetus and neonate are discussed in more detail later in this chapter.

Autoimmune thrombocytopenic purpura is a common complication of HIV infection.[102] HIV infection complicates up to 2.2% of pregnancies at inner-city hospitals and up to 39% of pregnancies in intravenous drug abusers.[103] An HIV-positive pregnant woman can have thrombocytopenia, and her fetus is then at risk for thrombocytopenia. Glantz and colleagues described a single case in which thrombocytopenia occurred in a neonate delivered of an HIV-positive women with associated autoimmune thrombocytopenia.[104] The diagnosis of thrombocytopenia in the fetuses of these women poses difficulties because of the inherent risk of fetal inoculation during the sampling.

Coxsackie B Virus

Epidemiology and General Characteristics

Kibrick and coworkers first reported that coxsackie B virus infections could result in disease in the neonate.[105] The disease spectrum can range from relatively benign to fulminant[106] and can be acquired by vertical transmission of the virus from a colonized mother.[107, 108] Neonates can be asymptomatic initially, with the development of fever, anorexia, and vomiting after an incubation period of 1 to 5 days. In many infants with myocardial involvement, it is temporary, and recovery occurs over the course of several weeks. In other cases, acute hepatitis, disseminated intravascular coagulation, respiratory distress, renal failure, refractory hypotension, and death ensue.[106] Most cases with severe myocarditis and meningoencephalitis have been the result of infection with types B2 to B5, and coxsackie B1 is a rare cause of disease in the neonate.[106]

Hematologic Manifestations

Purpura and hemorrhage occur in about 13% of neonatal cases. Hemorrhage appears to be related to a depletion of coagulation factors and platelets caused by disseminated intravascular coagulation[109] or hepatic injury with a resultant inability to synthesize certain clotting factors. Jaundice, mild anemia, and hepatic and splenic enlargement have been observed.[106, 110]

Echovirus

Epidemiology and General Characteristics

Neonatal infections related to echovirus occur as a result of perinatal transmission and are most commonly caused by echovirus 9. A febrile, viral-like illness before or during delivery in the mother is often reported. In one series, a striking seasonal occurrence of the viral infection was noticed during late summer or early fall.[111] Echovirus infections acquired from the mother tend to be more serious than those acquired nosocomially. Infants can present with various clinical manifestations, including central nervous system disease and overwhelming systemic infection.[111]

Hematologic Manifestations

Infants with infection can manifest severe hepatic dysfunction and coagulopathy and disseminated intravascular coagulation.[111] Some infants have overwhelming hepatic necrosis.

Tuberculosis

Epidemiology and General Characteristics

Tuberculosis remains one of the leading infectious diseases in the world.[112] In the United States, escalating rates of homelessness and HIV infection have provided a background for its resurgence.[113] Fetal and neonatal tuberculosis can be acquired transplacentally as a result of intra-amniotic infection, aspiration and ingestion of infected amniotic fluid, or postnatally through droplet spread.[114] Placental infection with *M. tuberculosis* can allow direct access of the organisms to the fetal circulation.

Congenital tuberculosis occurs most commonly in infants born to women with primary infection and is the result of *M. tuberculosis* bacillemia. Miliary tuberculosis untreated in the last part of pregnancy places the infant at greatest risk of developing congenital tuberculosis. Diagnosis of neonatal infection is often delayed, because clinical manifestations such as poor feeding and jaundice can mimic neonatal bacterial sepsis.[115] In some infants, bloody diarrhea and abdominal distention have mimicked the typical presentation of necrotizing enterocolitis.[116] A delay in diagnosis and initiation of appropriate treatment can result in neonatal mortality that approaches 30%.[114]

Hematologic Manifestations

Hepatosplenomegaly, jaundice, and disseminated intravascular coagulation as a result of liver failure have been described.[115, 117, 118]

Malaria

Epidemiology and General Characteristics

Even in endemic areas, congenital malaria is a relatively uncommon disease. However, in areas where the disease is endemic, transplacentally acquired infections in neonates can be as high as 9%, with a prevalence of 4% to 30%.[119] Severe fetal infections can result in stillbirths.[120] Because the prevalence of maternal disease is 0% to 23%,[119] maternal parasitemia occurs frequently, but transmission to the fetus usually is prevented by the placenta. Infections in humans have involved all four species of *Plasmodium*. Maternal chloroquine prophylaxis, although safe during pregnancy, does not appear to be effective in preventing fetal infection.[121] The emergence of chloroquine resistance may explain in part the increased prevalence of congenital malaria.[122] This is especially true when the etiologic agent is *P. falciparum*.

Infected neonates are usually asymptomatic at birth but develop manifestations of the disease between 3 and 12 weeks of age. These manifestations cannot be readily distinguished from those of neonatal sepsis.[123] Fever (88%) is followed by pallor and anemia (38%), with loss of appetite and development of listlessness, diarrhea, and jaundice (25%).[124]

Hematologic Manifestations

Nearly 50% of infants have isolated hepatomegaly. In the 31% of neonates with hepatosplenomegaly,[124] progressive hemolytic anemia is common, and the most severely affected infants can resemble those with erythroblastosis fetalis. The anemia is accompanied by reticulocytosis, and serum bilirubin concentrations are increased, with conjugated and unconjugated forms occurring. Neutrophil and platelet counts are variable. The diagnosis of infection can be confirmed by demonstration of the characteristic parasite on a thin or thick blood smear.

NEONATAL HEMATOLOGIC ABNORMALITIES CAUSED BY MATERNAL ANTIBODIES

Thrombocytopenia

Neonatal Alloimmune Thrombocytopenia

Neonatal alloimmune thrombocytopenia (NAIT), also called neonatal isoimmune thrombocytopenia, was first described in the 1950s.[125] This uncommon (1 in 2000 live births) but serious disorder is characterized by a marked thrombocytopenia in the fetus and neonate.[21] Maternal antibodies directed against fetal platelet antigens lead to increased platelet destruction. Intracranial hemorrhage, which can occur in utero as early as 18 weeks of gestation,[126–128] is the most devastating complication of NAIT, affecting 20% of all proven cases and up to 50% of cases occurring antenatally.[21, 129] Approximately 50% of NAIT cases occur during the first pregnancy,[129] and almost 100% of subsequent pregnancies are affected equally or more severely.[21]

Antenatal management directed at preventing intracranial hemorrhage has become a matter of great importance. Prenatal therapeutic strategies directed at increasing the fetal platelet count have included administration of intravenous γ-globulin to the mother[129, 130] and administration of platelet transfusions to the fetus.[126, 131] The antigen system most often involved in NAIT is HPA-1 (e.g., P1[A1]),[132, 133] with other antigen systems involved less frequently.[134–136]

Neonatal Autoimmune Thrombocytopenia

Neonatal thrombocytopenia can be the result of maternal idiopathic thrombocytopenic purpura (ITP), maternal systemic lupus erythematosus, or as a consequence of drugs taken by the mother, including quinine, quinidine, sulfonamides, and digitoxin.[137, 138] The disease closely resembles the alloimmune type, except that the IgG antibody is directed against antigens of maternal origin rather than antigens of paternal (fetal) origin. The risk of neonatal intracranial hemorrhage is only 1% to 2%, a rate markedly reduced compared with the occurrence in alloimmune thrombocytopenia.[130]

Maternal platelet counts are usually reduced, and maternal platelets are often large. In some mothers, increased bone marrow activity can compensate for the accelerated destruction of antibody-sensitized platelets, and the mothers can have normal platelet counts. However, their infants are still at risk for acquired thrombocytopenia as a result of the transplacental passage of IgG-mediated antibodies. Unfortunately, the maternal platelet count and levels of platelet-bound IgG and serum platelet antibody do not predict with certainty which infants will be thrombocytopenic.[139–141]

Neutropenia

Alloimmune Neonatal Neutropenia

Alloimmune neonatal neutropenia is the neutrophil counterpart of hemolytic disease of the newborn. The incidence of the disease is in the range of 1 case per 500 to 2000 neonates.[22, 142] This form of neutropenia occurs when a mother becomes sensitized to a foreign antigen of paternal origin on the neutrophils of her fetus. Specific IgG antibody directed against this antigen is then formed. The antigens most commonly involved are NA1, NA2, NB1, and NC1.[7, 142] The transplacental passage of antibody into the fetal circulation results in neutropenia, which is a self-limited condition in the neonate. The duration of neutropenia usually is a few weeks or months. The severity of the neutropenia is influenced by the titer and subclass of the maternal IgG neutrophil antibody, the phagocytic activity of the infant's reticuloendothelial system, and the capacity of the infant's marrow to compensate for the shortened survival of antibody-sensitized neutrophils.

Alloimmune neutropenia is not a benign disorder, because affected infants with severe neutropenia are at risk for serious bacterial infections such as cellulitis, omphalitis, pneumonia, and meningitis.[7, 143, 144] Numerous treatments, including corticosteroids,[145] intravenous administration of immune globulin,[142, 146, 147] exchange transfusion,[148] and leukocyte transfusions,[149] have been attempted in neonates with alloimmune neonatal neutropenia and serious bacterial infection, but none has been consistently effective in increasing the absolute neutrophil count. Administration of the hematopoietic growth factor recombinant human granulocyte colony-stimulating factor (rhG-CSF) to neonates with this condition has shown promise in producing a rapid and prolonged decrease in the neutropenia induced by NA1 and NA2 antigens.[143]

Autoimmune Neonatal Neutropenia

A transient neutropenia in the neonatal period may reflect transfer of IgG anti-neutrophil antibodies from the mother to the fetus. These cases differ from neonatal alloimmune neutropenia in that, although the antibodies are of maternal origin, the mother can be neutropenic or have a history of an autoimmune disorder such as systemic lupus erythematosus. If the neonate warrants a therapeutic intervention for the neutropenia, high-dose intravenous immunoglobulin can produce a transient increase in the absolute neutrophil count.[150, 151]

Hemolytic Anemia

Erythroblastosis Fetalis

Erythroblastosis fetalis, also called Rh hemolytic disease or hemolytic disease of the newborn, was originally included with clinical syndromes known as icterus gravis neonatorum, congenital anemia of the newborn, and hydrops fetalis.[152] In 1941, Levine and Katzin described the role of Rh antibody in classic erythroblastosis fetalis.[153] The pathophysiology of alloimmune hemolysis caused by Rh incompatibility includes the following features:

1. An Rh-negative mother
2. An Rh-positive fetus
3. Leakage of fetal red blood cells into the maternal circulation
4. Maternal sensitization to the D antigen on the fetal red blood cells
5. Production and transplacental passage of those maternal antibodies to the fetus
6. Attachment of the maternal antibodies to the fetal red blood cell with resultant hemolysis

Rh hemolytic disease occurs in only 1% of first pregnancies involving an Rh-positive fetus, and the likelihood increases with each subsequent pregnancy involving Rh-positive fetuses. The disease spectrum in the fetus and neonate can range from a mild hemolytic anemia to stillbirth with hydrops.

The degree of hemolysis depends on the amount of antibody absorbed. Anemia, hepatosplenomegaly, and hyperbilirubinemia are common. Maternal titers of anti-D antibodies do not accurately predict the severity of fetal hemolysis.

Thrombocytopenia is a well-recognized complication of severe Rh erythroblastosis fetalis.[154, 155] In some instances, the thrombocytopenia precedes exchange transfusions, but in others, it appears to be the direct consequence of transfusions using platelet-poor blood.[156] In a study done by Koenig and Christensen, only patients with severe and moderate disease had thrombocytopenia. The duration of the thrombocytopenia was 216 ± 38 hours (mean ± SD) in the severely affected group and 85 ± 79 hours in moderately affected patients.[156]

Neutropenia was not described as a feature of Rh hemolytic disease[155, 154] until the report of patients by Koenig and Christensen.[156] They described neutropenia lasting 83 ± 33 hours (mean ± SD) in severely affected patients but only 11 ± 7 hours in patients with mild disease. A more detailed description of erythroblastosis fetalis can be found Chapter 10.

Hemolytic Disease of the Neonate Caused by ABO Incompatibility

In 1944, Halbrecht first recognized ABO incompatibility as a cause of hemolytic disease of the neonate.[157] This disease differs from hemolytic disease caused by Rh incompatibility in that it is much milder and can occur in firstborn infants. Jaundice is the primary manifestation, but the anemia is generally mild. The lesser severity of the anemia is attributed to two factors: A and B substances are present on many epithelial surfaces in the body and aid in antibody absorption, and fewer A and B reactive sites are present on erythrocytes, resulting in less absorption of anti-A and anti-B per cell.[158]

The disease results from the transplacental passage of maternal anti-A and anti-B antibodies and their attachment to fetal erythrocytes. The disease is confined to A or B infants of mothers who are group O, because the antibodies found in group O mothers are of the IgG class, whereas those of mothers who are group A or B, who also produce anti-B and anti-A, respectively, are predominantly of the IgM class. When the first born is severely affected, subsequent offspring are usually affected to a similar degree.[159]

The primary manifestation of ABO hemolytic disease is jaundice. It usually appears within the first 24 hours of life and, if untreated, can be severe enough to cause kernicterus and death. Only 10% to 20% of ABO-incompatible infants develop jaundice.

Anemia is usually mild or absent, and pallor is uncommon, although Miller and Petrie reported the case of a stillborn infant at 40 weeks' gestation related to hydrops fetalis caused by ABO incompatibility.[160] The hemoglobin concentration is usually normal but rarely can be as low as 8 mg/dL.[161] Polychromasia, reticulocytosis (up to 30%), and increased numbers of nucleated red blood cells can be seen. An exag-

Table 6–3. **Comparison of Rh and ABO Incompatibility**

Characteristic	Rh	ABO
Blood group set-up		
Mother	Negative	O
Infant	Positive	A or B
Type of antibody	IgG	IgG
Clinical aspects		
Occurrence in first born	5%	40–50%
Predictable severity in subsequent pregnancies	Usually	No
Stillbirth and/or hydrops	Frequent	Rare
Severe anemia	Frequent	Rare
Degree of jaundice	+ + +	+
Hepatosplenomegaly	+ + +	+
Laboratory findings		
Direct Coombs' test (infant)	Positive	Positive or negative
Maternal antibodies	Always present	Not clear-cut
Spherocytes	0	Positive

+, present in approximately 1–25% of cases; + + +, present in approximately 51–75% of cases; 0, not described.

gerated physiologic anemia, as seen in Rh hemolytic disease, is uncommon.[162] Spherocytes (up to 40%) can be seen in neonates with clinically significant ABO hemolytic disease.[163]

Hepatosplenomegaly can occur but less often than occurs with Rh incompatibility. In 1971, Boineau and Hallock reported two infants with severe disease associated with marked hepatosplenomegaly.[161] Bilirubin concentrations parallel the degree of erythrocyte sensitization, and cord blood concentrations correlate with the degree of subsequent hyperbilirubinemia. Nearly 50% of infants with cord blood bilirubin concentrations of 4 mg/dL or greater developed sufficient hyperbilirubinemia to require the institution of phototherapy.[164] As in Rh hemolytic disease, hyperbilirubinemia involves mainly the indirect fraction. Occasionally, when the jaundice is severe, elevation of the direct fraction can develop.

Table 6–3 lists characteristics of Rh and ABO incompatibility. Clinical aspects, laboratory findings, treatments, and response to intravenous immunoglobulin G (IVIG) are compared.

Autoimmune Hemolytic Anemia

Maternal autoimmune hemolytic anemia related to maternal disease can develop during pregnancy. It is characterized as being Coombs' positive, and the passive transfer of IgG antibodies can result in anemia in the fetus.[165–168] Other maternal immune diseases that produce such antibodies include systemic lupus erythematosus and rheumatoid arthritis.

Disease in the neonate usually is a self-limited process, with antibody titers falling during the first months of life. In some infants, the anemia may be severe enough to require treatment, including administration of packed red blood cells or exchange transfusion. The hyperbilirubinemia usually is mild. Maternal antibody may not be specific for antigens on red blood cells, and immune neutropenia, thrombocytopenia, or both can occur.[169, 170] The diagnosis is suggested by the presence of hemolysis that is Coombs' positive, lack of a set up for Rh or ABO incompatibility, and a mother who is also Coombs' positive. Prenatal administration of glucocorticoids to the mother has been used to treat this form of anemia.[167, 168]

EFFECTS OF MATERNAL DISEASES ON THE FETUS AND NEONATE

Conditions Existing Before Pregnancy

Systemic Lupus Erythematosus

The first reported cases of lupus erythematosus cells in the blood of infants born to mothers with systemic disease were made by Bridge and Foley.[171] Since that time, others have described infants affected by the transplacental passage of antibodies.[172–174] Neonatal lupus erythematosus is a rare syndrome characterized by fetal and neonatal congenital heart block, cutaneous lesions, and hematologic abnormalities. It is commonly associated with autoantibodies to antigens such as SS-A/Ro, SS-B/La, and U_1RNP(nRNP).[175, 176] The incidence of neonatal disease is estimated to be 1 case per 20,000 live births.[177]

The hematologic manifestations of neonatal systemic lupus erythematosus are self-limited, usually disappearing coincidentally with the disappearance of the maternal antibodies.[177, 178] Hemolytic anemia,[179] thrombocytopenia,[179–182] and neutropenia[169, 181] occur in 10% to 20% of patients.[175–177] Anemia can result in congestive heart failure. Platelet counts as low as 30,000/mm^3 have been reported,[180] and although the pathogenesis of the thrombocytopenia is unknown, anti–SS-A/Ro antibodies are involved in some instances.[176] Disseminated intravascular coagulation has also been reported.[179] Hepatosplenomegaly and pericarditis are less common manifestations of neonatal lupus and are transient.[183]

Leukemia and Malignancies

In 1866, Friedreich reported the first case of a cancer metastasizing to the fetus.[184] Cancer complicates pregnancy more frequently than appendicitis, thyrotoxicosis, nephrolithiasis, and deep venous thrombosis.[185] The incidence of cancer during pregnancy is approximately 1 case per 1000 to 1500 pregnancies.[186, 187]

Although malignancy in the mother does not usually spread to the fetus, cases of malignancy in the fetus have been reported.[187–190] The malignancies most likely to involve the products of conception include malignant melanoma (33%), hematopoietic malignancies (leukemia and lymphoma) and breast carcinoma (30%), and various types of sarcomas and carcinomas (37%).[187] Eighty-three percent of fetal malignancies were associated with malignant melanomas or hematopoietic malignancies of the mother.[187] Although metastatic involvement of the products of conception is rare, fetal involvement is even less likely and accounted for only 27% of the total cases. In all cases in which the placenta and infant were examined, fetal involvement never occurred without placental involvement.[187]

Monocytic, myelocytic, lymphocytic, and lymphoblastic leukemias have been reported in pregnant women.[191] In the nearly 400 cases of maternal leukemia associated with pregnancy, none of the neonates had leukemia. However, leukemia developed later in two infants whose mothers had the disease. One mother developed the disease on the eighth postpartum day,[192] and the other mother was diagnosed with lymphoblastic leukemia near the time of delivery. The first infant, although initially hematologically normal, developed acute lymphocytic leukemia at 9 months of age. The second infant developed lymphoblastic leukemia at 5 months of age.

Cardiac Disease

The risk of heart disease in the fetuses of women with congenital heart disease is 15% to 50%.[193] Maternal congenital heart diseases with poor fetal outcomes include cyanotic heart disease with high maternal hematocrits, conditions with pulmonary hypertension, cardiomyopathies, and arrhythmias with frequent episodes of symptomatic hypotension.[193] In general, these infants are small for gestational age.

In 1956, Bromberg and coworkers reported that infants of mothers experiencing chronic hypoxia had higher fetal hemoglobin concentrations.[194] Four women with heart failure, two women with severe asthma and cyanosis, and six women who were profoundly anemic were included in this group. In 1962, Kravkova reported that fetuses from mothers with severe heart disease had higher hemoglobin and white cells counts compared with other neonates whose mothers did not have heart disease.[195] Bone marrows of these infants showed increased erythropoietic activity.

Hyperthyroidism

Thyroid disease in the mother can be associated with disease in the neonate. Thyrotoxicosis in the neonate is believed to be a consequence of the transplacental passage of long-acting thyroid stimulator from mother to infant.

Infants can manifest plethora, congestive

heart failure, hepatosplenomegaly, hyperbilirubinemia, and thrombocytopenia.[196] Some of these infants exhibit the hyperviscosity syndrome.[197] Thrombocytopenia has been observed in adults with hyperthyroidism.[198, 199]

Pernicious Anemia

Nearly 60% of patients with pernicious anemia have antibody to intrinsic factor. This IgG antibody can be transferred from the mother to the fetus, and two instances of the transplacental passage of antibody have been described.[200] Neither infant developed anemia.

Diabetes Mellitus

Before the availability of insulin, it was unusual for women with diabetes to conceive and survive and even less likely for the fetus to survive. Effects of maternal diabetes on the fetus include fetal death; macrosomia and resultant birth trauma; cardiac, gastrointestinal, and skeletal anomalies; respiratory distress syndrome; hypoglycemia; hypocalcemia; hypomagnesemia; perinatal asphyxia; and intrauterine growth retardation.[201]

Infants of diabetic mothers can have a variety of hematologic abnormalities, such as increased red cell mass, the hyperviscosity syndrome, hyperbilirubinemia, hyperaggregable platelets, and an increased incidence of thrombosis. In 1969, Warner and Cornblath reported that the venous hematocrit was higher than 64% in 42% of infants of diabetic mothers.[202] When infants of mothers with gestational diabetes were studied, 30% had hematocrits greater than 64%. Although the red blood cell mass in these neonates is normal, the plasma volume is decreased.[203] Widness and associates described increased plasma erythropoietin concentrations in infants of diabetic mothers.[204] Chronically low tissue oxygen levels increase erythropoietin production and erythrocyte mass, leading to neonatal polycythemia and hyperbilirubinemia.[205] Hyperbilirubinemia occurs primarily in those who are large for gestational age,[206–208] and increased heme catabolism probably is responsible for the jaundice.[208]

Infants of diabetic mothers have an increased incidence of thrombosis.[209] It can be as high as 15%, compared with less than 1% for infants of nondiabetic mothers. In an evaluation of plasma coagulation factors, no abnormalities were found that could explain this tendency.[210]

A slight decrease in platelet count has been reported and may be the result of the associated polycythemia or secondary to preeclampsia that frequently occurs in mothers with diabetes.[211] Increased platelet aggregability has been documented by Stuart and Elrad.[212] This hyperaggregability disappeared by the fourth to fifth day of life.

Conditions Occurring During Pregnancy

Pregnancy-Induced Hypertension

The effect of pregnancy-induced hypertension, including preeclampsia or HELLP syndrome (i.e., hemolysis, elevated liver enzymes, and low platelets), on the developing fetus varies with the type and severity of the disorder and according to the gestational age at which it becomes a problem.[213] Mild chronic hypertension slightly increases the risk of intrauterine growth retardation and placental abruption.[213] More severe degrees of chronic hypertension, especially if preeclampsia is superimposed, can have profound effects on the fetus, including death.

The association of maternal hypertension with neonatal neutropenia was first reported by Manroe.[214] This form of neutropenia may occur in as many as 49% of infants delivered of mothers with pregnancy-induced hypertension,[215, 216] and the duration can be 1 hour to 30 days. The prevalence of the condition is greater among infants who were growth retarded, delivered prematurely, or whose mothers had severe hypertension or hypertension and the HELLP syndrome. The mechanism for this form of neonatal neutropenia is reduced neutrophil production. The condition is associated with increased risk for nosocomial infection.[215, 217] G-CSF promotes a rapid increase in circulating neutrophils in these patients,[217–221] and appears to lower their risk of infection, although further study is needed.[219]

Some infants have an associated thrombocytopenia.[215] Most are born to mothers with severe hypertension or with hypertension and HELLP syndrome. In one study, the mean duration of their thrombocytopenia was 48 hours, and the suggested mechanism was decreased platelet production.[222] Term infants of hypertensive mothers were no more likely to be thrombocytopenic than controls; however, premature infants, especially those with intrauterine growth restriction, had a much higher risk of thrombocytopenia.[141] Hyperbilirubinemia has occurred in about one half of infants delivered of women with the HELLP syndrome.[223]

Intra-Amniotic Infection

Infection plays a key role in the pathogenesis of preterm labor and delivery.[224] Microbial invasion of the amniotic cavity can occur as a result of one of four pathways: ascending from the vagina and cervix, hematogenous dissemination through the placenta, retrograde seeding from the peritoneal cavity, and introduction at the time of invasive procedures.[224]

Levels of several cytokines are significantly increased during intra-amniotic infection.[224–233] One of these, G-CSF, is a primary regulator of neutrophil proliferation, differentiation, function, and survival. During intra-amniotic infection, amniotic fluid concentrations of G-CSF obtained from preterm pregnancies with culture-proven intra-amniotic infection are 10 to 100 times higher than concentrations from preterm pregnancies without evidence of infection.[234] Infants delivered of mothers with increased serum, amniotic fluid, and cord blood concentrations of G-CSF have markedly increased serum and urine concentrations of G-CSF compared with gestational age–matched controls. It is unclear whether the G-CSF is of maternal, placental, or fetal origin or a combination of these sources.

Some infants who experience leukemoid reactions in the immediate neonatal period are delivered of mothers with intra-amniotic infection.[235] In one study, 71% of infants in whom leukemoid reactions were present within the first 4 days of life were born to women with evidence of intra-amniotic infection. Although none of these infants had positive blood cultures, hematologic effects resulting from maternal infection could not be excluded. Serum G-CSF concentrations were markedly increased in some of the infants, and for others, it was speculated that the peak concentration of G-CSF preceded the peripheral neutrophilia.

The effect of maternal intra-amniotic infection on the concentration of G-CSF in human milk has been evaluated.[236–238] In mothers with intra-amniotic infection, G-CSF in human milk is 10-fold higher than the concentration in milk of women without infection.[238] It is unknown whether the G-CSF in human milk is functional or could survive the environment of the neonatal intestinal tract. It is also unknown whether G-CSF acts locally within the neonatal gastrointestinal system or is absorbed and acts systemically. The potential hematopoietic and nonhematopoietic roles of G-CSF in human milk are an active area of investigation.

EFFECTS OF MATERNAL DRUG ADMINISTRATION ON THE FETUS AND NEONATE

Placental Transfer of Drugs

Betamethasone

The prophylactic induction of fetal lung maturation through maternal steroid administration has gained increasing clinical acceptance since the original report in 1972 by Liggins and Howie.[239] Administration of antenatal steroids results in fetal blood concentrations that approximate those of the mother.[240]

Glucocorticoids increase leukocyte count by enhancing the release of neutrophils from the bone marrow and by decreasing neutrophil clearance from the circulation.[241] Leukemoid reactions have been described in infants of mothers who have received antenatal steroids.[242–244] Our own evaluation of the mechanism producing leukemoid reactions in neonates did not find an association between this condition and the maternal administration of steroids.[235] When bone marrow aspirations of infants with leukemoid reactions were examined, my colleagues and I did not find the mechanism for leukocytosis seen with steroid administration (i.e., accelerated release of neutrophils from the bone marrow into the blood and diminished egress of neutrophils from the blood into the tissues). All of our infants who experienced a leukemoid reaction after maternal steroid administration had benign courses, and the time to resolution of the leukemoid reaction was less than 1 week. In older children and adults, steroids can produce lymphopenia. When umbilical cord blood was evaluated for the number of CD34+ cells and lymphocytes, no decrease was observed in that obtained from infants who received antenatal steroids.[245]

Granulocyte Colony-Stimulating Factor

A lineage-specific hematopoietic growth factor, G-CSF effects neutrophil function and production. A potential method for diminishing the severity and sequelae of early-onset infection was investigated by Medlock and associates[246] and Novales and colleagues[247] using a pregnant rat model. They observed that rhG-CSF administered to pregnant dams crossed the placenta and increased neutrophil production in utero. Although the concentration of G-CSF transferred to the fetus was low, it was sufficient to stimulate fetal neutrophil production and to improve the outcome of pups experimentally infected with group B streptococci.

Neonates with overwhelming sepsis and neutropenia have been treated with rhG-CSF,[218–220] and two clinical trials evaluating the administration of rhG-CSF to women about to deliver extremely preterm neonates have been completed.[248, 249] The phase I study determined whether rhG-CSF would cross to the fetal circulation and have a biologic effect on the fetus. Twenty-two women about to deliver at less than 30 weeks' gestation were treated with a one-time dose of rh G-CSF (25 μg/kg) or were not treated. Twelve neonates were delivered to the 11 women given rhG-CSF. Ten infants were delivered within 30 hours of the rhG-CSF administration, one was delivered at 54 hours, and one was delivered at 108 hours. In the former group, maternal G-CSF concentrations and blood neutrophil levels were higher than those of control subjects. However, no difference was seen in cord blood neutrophil concentrations. In the latter group, although maternal serum and cord blood G-CSF concentrations were no different than those of control subjects, cord blood neutrophil levels were higher than those of control subjects and remained elevated for 1 week. Administration of rhG-CSF to pregnant women with an imminent preterm delivery can result in transplacental passage of a measurable quantity of G-CSF, and this amount can have a biologic effect on the fetus if given at least 30 hours before delivery.

A second clinical trial was performed to determine whether maternal treatment with rhG-CSF would improve neonatal outcome without adverse maternal affects.[249] A randomized, double-blind, placebo-controlled trial with the administration of a single intravenous dose (25 μg/kg) of rhG-CSF or placebo was given to a total of 20 women in preterm labor (<30 weeks' gestation). Ten of the women delivered within 3 weeks of dosing, and maternal G-CSF concentrations and absolute neutrophil counts at the time of delivery were not different in the G-CSF and the placebo recipients. There was no correlation between maternal and cord blood serum G-CSF concentrations. Although absolute neutrophil counts during the first week of life did not differ in the rhG-CSF treatment and placebo infants, bone marrow neutrophil proliferative pools were higher than in the control group. No difference was observed between the groups in scores for neonatal acute physiology, and there were no maternal problems related to the administration of rhG-CSF. Although these pilot trials suggest that the antenatal administration of rhG-CSF may be less reliable in human subjects than it was in the animal experiments, further studies evaluating intrapartum cytokine therapy are necessary.

Immunoglobulin G

IgG is freely transported across the placenta,[250–252] but transfer is slow and equilibration may take as long as three weeks.[253] Maternal administration of IVIG as an antenatal treatment for the fetuses of women with ITP has been evaluated,[254, 255] but the effects of antenatally administered IVIG on fetal platelet counts have been variable.[141] In one series, IVIG was given for steroid-refractory pregnancies complicated by ITP.[256] Thirty-six percent of the neonates had thrombocytopenia with counts less than 100×10^9/L, and 18% had severe thrombocytopenia with counts less than 50×10^9/L. Fetal thrombocytopenia was not associated with the maternal response to IVIG but was associated with the concentration of IgG of the neonates at birth.

A combined retrospective analysis confirmed that the lack of effect of maternally administered IVIG on fetal platelet counts might be attributed to an insufficient therapeutic level of transferred IgG. In pregnancies at risk for NAIT, improved fetal platelet counts were observed in 70% of the cases, and no intraventricular hemorrhage occurred.[257] There are no recommendations regarding maternal interventions for the purpose of raising the fetal platelet count.[141]

Folic Acid and Vitamin B_{12}

Folate is transported across the placenta against a concentration gradient. Fetal blood contains high concentrations of a folate-binding protein[258] that appears to facilitate extraction of the vitamin by the fetus from the mother. As a result, even neonates delivered of mothers with marginal folate status are not usually deficient.[259] The initially elevated levels of serum folate decline rapidly during the first several weeks of life.[260]

Vitamin B_{12} is also effectively captured by the fetus. This process results in cord blood concentrations that are usually two to three times higher than maternal values, despite the fact that fetal liver contains only one-third the concentration of vitamin B_{12} found in adult liver.[261]

Neither folic acid nor B_{12} deficiency in the mother results in anemia in the immediate newborn period. Prolonged breast-feeding by mothers who have vitamin B_{12} deficiency because of a poor diet or untreated pernicious anemia can produce megaloblastic anemia in the infant.[262, 263]

Zidovudine

Zidovudine (ZDV, AZT) is a synthetic thymidine analogue widely used in the treatment of AIDS. ZDV freely crosses from the maternal circulation into the fetal circulation and inhibits fetal erythropoiesis, as judged by the lower hemoglobin concentrations and hematocrits of neonates whose mothers were treated with ZDV compared with those of infants whose mothers were treated with placebo.[100, 101, 264, 265]

The initial ZDV trials led to widespread acceptance of its use during pregnancy in cases complicated by maternal HIV infection.[100] The transmission of disease to the fetus is markedly altered by the intrapartum administration of ZDV, with transmission rates of 26% for the placebo group and 8% for ZDV-treated women.[100]

Infants treated with ZDV have toxic reactions similar to those of adults but have higher rates of anemia (62.5%) and neutropenia (28%).[266] A heightened sensitivity of the fetus and neonate to the myelotoxic effects of ZDV is suggested by the observation that neonates whose HIV-positive mothers received ZDV during pregnancy were born with lower hemoglobin concentrations than those whose HIV-positive mothers were not given ZDV.[100]

Little is known about the hematologic impact of this therapy on the fetus and neonate. An in vitro study evaluating the effect of ZDV on fetal progenitor cells revealed that mature erythroid progenitors (fetal and neonatal) were the most sensitive progenitors to the adverse effects of ZDV on clonal maturation and that multipotent progenitors were the most resistant cells.[264]

References

1. Sibley C, Boyd R: Mechanisms of transfer across the human placenta. In Polin R, Fox W (eds): Fetal and Neonatal Physiology, 2nd ed. Philadelphia: WB Saunders, 1993, pp 62–74.
2. Baer K: Untersuchungen ueber die GefaBverbindung zwischen Mutter und Frucht in den Saeugethieren. Leipzig: L Voss, 1828.
3. Benirschke K, Kaufmann P: Placental Types. Pathology of the Human Placenta. New York: Springer-Verlag, 1995, pp 1–13.
4. Bianchi D, Klinger K, Vadnais T, et al: Development of a model system to compare cell separation methods for the isolation of fetal cells from maternal blood. Prenat Diagn 1996;16:289.
5. Cohen F, Zuelzer W: The transplacental passage of maternal erythrocytes into the fetus. Am J Obstet Gynecol 1965;93:566.
6. Pearson H, Shulman N, Marder V, et al: Isoimmune neonatal thrombocytopenic purpura: clinical and therapeutic considerations. Blood 1964;23:154.
7. Lalezari P, Radel E: Neutrophil-specific antigens: immunology and clinical significance. Semin Hematol 1974;11:281.
8. Cohen F, Zuelzer W, Gustafson D, et al: Mechanism of isoimmunization. I. The transplacental passage of fetal erythrocytes in heterospecific pregnancies. Blood 1964;26:621.

9. Jones P, McNay A, Walker W: Association between foeto-maternal bleeding and hypertension in pregnancy. BMJ 1969;2:738.
10. McLarey D, Fish S: Fetal erythrocytes in the maternal circulation. Am J Obstet Gynecol 1966;95:824.
11. Zipursky A, Pollock J, Neelands P, et al: The transplacental passage of foetal red blood cells and the pathogenesis of Rh immunisation during pregnancy. Lancet 1963;2:489.
12. Price J, Wlias S, Wachtel S, et al: Prenatal diagnosis with fetal cells isolated from maternal blood by multiparameter flow cytometry. Am J Obstet Gynecol 1991;165:1731.
13. Bianchi D, Mahr A, Zickwolf G, et al: Detection of fetal cells with 47,XY, +21 karyotype in maternal peripheral blood. Hum Genet 1992;90:368.
14. Elias S, Price J, Dockter M, et al: First trimester prenatal diagnosis of trisomy 21 in fetal cells from maternal blood. Lancet 1992;340:1033.
15. Zheng Y, DeMaria M, Zhen D, et al: Flow sorting of fetal erythroblasts using intracytoplasmic anti-fetal haemoglobin: preliminary observations on maternal samples. Prenat Diagn 1995;15:897.
16. Sims D, Barron S, Wadehra V, et al: Massive chronic feto-maternal bleeding associated with placental chorioangiomas. Acta Paediatr Scand 1976;65:271.
17. Blackburn G: Massive fetomaternal hemorrhage due to choriocarcinoma of the uterus. J Pediatr 1954;89:680.
18. Weisert O, Marstrander J: Severe anemia in a newborn caused by protected feto-maternal "transfusion." Acta Paediatr 1960;49:426.
19. Raye J, Gutberlet R, Stahlman M: Symptomatic posthemorrhagic anemia in the newborn. Pediatr Clin North Am 1970;17:401.
20. Shahar E, Birenbaum E, Inbar D, et al: Hypovolemic shock due to extensive fetomaternal hemorrhage. Isr J Med Sci 1981;17:441.
21. Johnson J, Ryan G, al Musa A, et al: Prenatal diagnosis and management of neonatal alloimmune thrombocytopenia. Semin Perinatol 1997;21:45.
22. Levine D, Madyastha P: Isoimmune neonatal neutropenia. Am J Perinatol 1986;3:231.
23. Nicolle C, Manceaux L: Sur une infection a corps de Leishman (ou organismes voisins) du gondi. Compt Rend Acad Sci 1908;147:763.
24. Splendore A: Un nuovo protozoa parassita dei conigli. Incontrato nelle lesioni anatomiche d'una malattia che ricorda in molti punti il Kala-azar dell'uomo. Rev Soc Sci 1908;3:109.
25. Wolf A, Cowen D, Paige B: Human toxoplasmosis: Occurrence in infants as an encephalomyelitis: verification by transmission to animals. Science 1939;89:226.
26. Freij B, Sever J: Toxoplasmosis. Pediatr Rev 1991;12:227.
27. Feldman H: Toxoplasmosis. Pediatrics 1958;22:424.
28. Hohlfeld P, Daffos F, Thulliez P, et al: Fetal toxoplasmosis: outcome of pregnancy and infant follow-up after in utero treatment. J Pediatr 1989;115:765.
29. Ghidini A, Sirtori M, Spelta A, Vergani P: Results of a preventative program for congenital toxoplasmosis. J Reprod Med 1991;36:270.
30. Desmonts G, Couvreur J: Congenital toxoplasmosis: a prospective study of 78 pregnancies. N Engl J Med 1974;290:1110.
31. Eichenwald H: Congenital toxoplasmosis: a study of 150 cases. J Dis Child 1957;94:411.
32. Remington J, Desmonts G: Toxoplasmosis. In Remington J, Klein J (eds): Infectious Diseases of the Fetus and Newborn Infant. Philadelphia: WB Saunders, 1990, pp 89–195.
33. Couvreur J, Desmonts G, Tournier G, et al: A homogeneous series of 20 cases of congenital toxoplasmosis in 0 to 11 month old infants detected prospectively. Ann Pediatr 1984;31:815.
34. Callahan W, Russell W, Smith M: A clinicopathologic study with presentation of five cases and review of the literature. Medicine (Baltimore) 1946;25:343.
35. Beckett R, Flynn F: Toxoplasmosis: report of two new cases, with a classification and with a demonstration of the organisms in the human placenta. N Engl J Med 1953;249:345.
36. Arnaud J, Griscelli C, Couvreur J, Desmonts G: Hematological and immunological abnormalities in congenital toxoplasmosis. Nouv Rev Fr Hematol 1975;15:496.
37. Rajantie J, Siimes M, Taskinen E, et al: White blood cells in infants with congenital toxoplasmosis: transient appearance of cALL antigen on reactive marrow lymphocytes. Scand J Infect Dis 1992;24:227.
38. Hohlfeld P, Forestier F, Marian S, et al: Toxoplasma gondii infection during pregnancy: T lymphocyte subpopulations in mothers and fetuses. Pediatr Infect Dis J 1990;9:878.
39. Goodman H: Notable contributions to the knowledge of syphilis. New York: Froben Press, 1943.
40. Schulz K, Murphy F, Patamasucon P, Meheus A: Congenital syphilis. In Holmes K, Mardh P, Sparling P, et al (eds): Sexually Transmitted Diseases, 2nd ed. New York: McGraw-Hill, 1990, p 821.
41. Sanchez P: Congenital syphilis. Adv Pediatr Infect Dis 1992;7:161.
42. Wright M, Tecklenburg F: Critical illness in congenital syphilis after the newborn period. Clin Pediatr (Phila) 1992;31:247.
43. Noseda G, Roy C, Phan P, et al: Acute hepatic failure in an infant with congenital syphilis. Arch Fr Pediatr 1990;47:445.
44. Berry M, Dajani A: Resurgence of congenital syphilis. Infect Dis Clin North Am 1992;6:19.
45. Oski F, Naiman J: The hematologic aspects of the maternal-fetal relationship. In Oski F, Naiman J (eds): Hematologic Problems in the Newborn, 3rd ed. Philadelphia: WB Saunders, 1982, p 38.
46. Hira S, Bhat G, Patel J, et al: Early congenital syphilis: clinicoradiologic features in 202 patients. Sex Transm Dis 1985;12:177.
47. Risel H: Blutbefunde bei angeborener syphilis. Arch Kinderh 1924;72:136.
48. Whitaker J, Sartain P, Shaheedy M: Hematological aspects of congenital syphilis. J Pediatr 1965;66:629.
49. Baar H, Baar S, Rogers K, Stransky E: Disorders of Blood and Blood-forming Organs in Childhood. New York: Hafner Publishing, 1963, p 469.
50. Barron S, Pass R: Infectious causes of hydrops fetalis. Semin Perinatol 1995;19:493.
51. Freiman I, Super M: Thrombocytopenia and congenital syphilis in South African Bantu infants. Arch Dis Child 1966;41:87.
52. Nitschke E: Blutbenfunde bei angeborener Syphilis. Arch Kinderh 1924;72:136.
53. Baar H, Baar S, Rogers K, Stransky E: Disorders of the Blood and Blood-forming Organs in Childhood. New York: Hafner Publishing, 1963, p 473.
54. Hochsinger C: Syphilis. In Pflaundler M, Schlossman A (eds): The Diseases of Children. Philadelphia: JB Lippincott, 1909, pp 522, 538–539.
55. Wesselhoff C: Rubella (German measles). N Engl J Med 1947;236:943.

56. Gregg N: Congenital cataracts following German measles in the mother. Trans Ophthal Soc 1941;3:35.
57. Rudolph A, Yow M, Phillips C, et al: Transplacental rubella infection in newly born infants. JAMA 1965;191:843.
58. Banatalva J, Horstmann D, Payne M, et al: Rubella syndrome and thrombocytopenic purpura in newborn infants: clinical and virologic observations. N Engl J Med 1965;273:474.
59. Rausen A, London R, Mizrahi A, et al: Generalized bone changes and thrombocytopenic purpura in association with intrauterine rubella. Pediatrics 1965; 36:264.
60. Zinkham W, Medearis D: Blood and bone marrow picture in congenital rubella. J Pediatr 1965;67:A461.
61. Lafer C, Morrison A: Thrombocytopenic purpura progressing to transient hypoplastic anemia in a newborn with rubella syndrome. Pediatrics 1966;38:499.
62. Sherman L, Silberstein L, Berkman E: Altered blood group expression in a patient with congenital rubella infection. Transfusion 1994;24:267.
63. Zinkham W, Medearis DJ, Osborn J: Blood and bone marrow findings in congenital rubella. J Pediatr 1967;71:512.
64. Plotkin S, Oski F, Hartnett E, et al: Some recently recognized manifestations of the rubella syndrome. J Pediatr 1965;67:182.
65. Mustafa M: Cytomegalovirus infection and disease in the immunocompromised host. Pediatr Infect Dis J 1994;13:249.
66. Jesionek A, Kiolemenoglov G: Uber einen befund von protozonartigen Gibilden in den Organ eines hereditarleutischen Fotus. Munch Med Wochenschr 1904;51:1905.
67. Smith M: Propagation of a cytopathogenic virus from salivary gland virus disease of infants in tissue cultures. Am J Pathol 1956;32:641.
68. Weller T, Macauley J, Craig J, et al: Isolation of intranuclear inclusion producing agents from infants with illness resembling cytomegalic inclusion disease. Proc Soc Exp Biol Med 1957;92:4.
69. Hayes K, Gibas H: Placental cytomegalovirus infection without fetal involvement following primary infection in pregnancy. J Pediatr 1971;79:401.
70. Stagno S, Pass R, Dworsky M, et al: Congenital cytomegalovirus infection: the relative importance of primary and recurrent maternal infection. N Engl J Med 1982;306:945.
71. Elek S, Stern H: Development of vaccine against mental retardation caused by cytomegalovirus. Lancet 1974;1:1.
72. Boppana S, Pass R, Britt W, et al: Symptomatic congenital cytomegalovirus infection: neonatal morbidity and mortality. Pediatr Infect Dis J 1992;11:93.
73. Calhoun D, Christensen R: Commonly asked questions regarding infections in neonates. Pediatr Ann 1995;24:583.
74. Alford C, Stagno S, Pass R, Britt W: Congenital and perinatal cytomegalovirus infections. Rev Infect Dis 1990;12:S745.
75. Fowler K, Stagno S, Pass R, et al: The outcome of congenital cytomegalovirus infection in relation to maternal antibody status. N Engl J Med 1992;326:663.
76. Schopfer K, Lauber E, Krech U: Congenital cytomegalovirus infection in newborn infants of mothers infected before pregnancy. Arch Dis Child 1978;53:536.
77. Hanshaw J: Congenital cytomegalovirus infection. Pediatr Ann 1994;23:124.
78. Prober C, Corey L, Brown Z, et al: The management of pregnancies complicated by genital infections with herpes simplex virus. Clin Infect Dis 1992;15:1031.
79. Stagno S, Reynolds D, Huang E, et al: Congenital cytomegalovirus infection: occurrence in an immune population. N Engl J Med 1977;296:1254.
80. South M, Tompkins W, Morris C, et al: Congenital manifestations of the central nervous system associated with genital type (type 2) herpesvirus. J Pediatr 1969;75:13.
81. Montgomery J, Flanders R, Yow M: Congenital herpesvirus infection with possibly related anomalies. Am J Dis Child 1973;125:364.
82. Whitley R: Herpes simplex virus infections of the central nervous system: a review. Am J Med 1988;85:61.
83. Hutto C, Arvin A, Jacobs R, et al: Intrauterine herpes simplex virus infections. J Pediatr 1987;110:97.
84. Parish W: Intrauterine herpes simplex virus infection: hydranencephaly and a nonvesicular rash in an infant. Int J Dermatol 1989;28:397.
85. Lascari A, Wallace P: Disseminated intravascular coagulation in the newborn. Clin Pediatr 1971;10:11.
86. Miller D, Rickels F, Lichtman M, et al: A new variant of hereditary stomatocytosis. Blood 1970;36:839.
87. Nahmias A, Alford C, Korones S: Infection of the newborn with herpesvirus hominis. Adv Pediatr 1970;17:185.
88. Cossart Y, Field A, Cant B, Widdows D: Parvovirus-like particles in human sera. Lancet 1975;1:72.
89. Baley J, Goldfarb J: The immune system. In Fanaroff A, Martin R (eds): Neonatal-Perinatal Medicine Diseases of the Fetus and Neonate, 5th ed. Philadelphia: Mosby–Year Book, 1992, p 678.
90. Brown T, Anand A, Ritchie L, et al: Intrauterine parvovirus infection associated with hydrops fetalis (Letter). Lancet 1984;2:1033.
91. Kinney J, Anderson L, Farrar J, et al: Risk of adverse outcomes of pregnancy following human parvovirus B19 infection. J Infect Dis 1988;157:663.
92. Woernle C, Anderson L, Tattersall P, Davison J: Human parvovirus B19 infection during pregnancy. J Infect Dis 1987;156:17.
93. Anand A, Gray E, Brown T, et al: Human parvovirus infection in pregnancy and hydrops fetalis. N Engl J Med 1987;316:183.
94. O'Sullivan M, Turner A, Gardin J, et al: Experimental induction of hydrops fetalis with simian parvovirus (Abstract). J Soc Gynecol Invest 1998;5:63A.
95. Cowan M, Hellman D, Chudwin D, et al: Maternal transmission of acquired immune deficiency syndrome. Pediatrics 1984;73:382.
96. Unexplained immunodeficiency and opportunistic infections in infants. MMWR Morb Mortal Wkly Rep 1984;31:665.
97. Luzuriage K, Sullivan J: Pathogenesis of vertical HIV-1 infection: implications for intervention and management. Pediatr Ann 1994;23:159.
98. Alexio L, Goodenow M, Sleasman J: Zidovudine administered to women infected with human immunodeficiency virus type 1 and to their neonates reduces pediatric infection independent of an effect on levels of maternal virus. J Pediatr 1997;130:906.
99. European Collaborative Study: Risk factors for mother-to-child transmission of HIV-1. Lancet 1992;339:1007.
100. Connor E, Sperling R, Gelber R, et al: Reduction of maternal-infant transmission of human immunodeficiency virus type 1 with zidovudine treatment: Pediatric AIDS Clinical Trials Group protocol 076 study group. N Engl J Med 1994;331:1173.
101. O'Sullivan M, Boyer P, Scott G, et al: The pharmacokinetics and safety of zidovudine in the third trimester

of pregnancy for women infected with human immunodeficiency virus and their infants: phase I acquired immunodeficiency syndrome clinical trials group study (protocol 082). Am J Obstet Gynecol 1993;168:1510.
102. Ratner L: Human immunodeficiency virus-associated autoimmune thrombocytopenic purpura: a review. Am J Med 1989;86:194.
103. Donagan S, Steger K, Recla L, et al: Seroprevalence of human immunodeficiency virus in parturients at Boston City Hospital: implications for public health and obstetric practice. Am J Obstet Gynecol 1992;167:622.
104. Glantz J, Roberts D: Pregnancy complicated by thrombocytopenia secondary to human immunodeficiency virus infection. Obstet Gynecol 1994;83:825.
105. Kibrick S, Benirschke K: Severe generalized disease (encephalohepatomyocarditis) occurring in the newborn period and due to coxsackie virus group B. Pediatrics 1958;27:857.
106. Chou L, Chang C, Wu L: Neonatal coxsackievirus B1 infection associated with severe hepatitis: report of three cases. Acta Paediatr Sin 1995;36:296.
107. Strong B, Young S: Intrauterine coxsackie virus, group B type 1, infection: viral cultivation from amniotic fluid. Am J Perinatol 1995;12:78.
108. Isacsohn M, Eidelman A, Kaplan M, et al: Neonatal coxsackie group B infections: experience of a single department of neonatology. Isr J Med Sci 1994;30:371.
109. Desmond M: Coxsackie septicemia in newborn with intravascular coagulation. J Pediatr 1968;73:283.
110. Baker D, Phillips C: Maternal and neonatal infection with coxsackie virus. Obstet Gynecol 1980;55:125.
111. Pruekprasert P, Stout C, Patamasucon P: Neonatal enterovirus infection. J Assoc Acad Minor Phys 1995;6:134.
112. Starke J: Tuberculosis: an old disease but a new threat to the mother, fetus, and neonate. Clin Perinatol 1997;24:107.
113. Henderson C: Management of tuberculosis in pregnancy. J Assoc Acad Minor Phys 1995;6:38.
114. Machin G, Honore L, Fanning E, Molesky M: Perinatally acquired neonatal tuberculosis: report of two cases. Pediatr Pathol 1992;12:707.
115. Foo A, Tann K, Chay O: Congenital tuberculosis. Tuber Lung Dis 1993;74:59.
116. Wang J, Chen W, Soong W, et al: Congenital tuberculosis: a case report. Chung Hua I Hsueh Tsa Chih (Taipei) 1990;45:266.
117. Pai P, Parikh P: Congenital miliary tuberculosis. Clin Pediatr 1976;15:376.
118. Morens D, Baublis J, Heidelberger K: Congenital tuberculosis and associated hypoadrenocorticism. South Med J 1979;72:160.
119. Fischer P: Congenital malaria: an African survey. Clin Pediatr (Phila) 1997;36:411.
120. Hennequin C, Bouree P: Malaria of the pregnant woman and newborn. Bull Soc Pathol Exot 1991;84:465.
121. Subramanian D, Moise K, White AJ: Imported malaria in pregnancy: report of four cases and review of management. Clin Infect Dis 1992;15:408.
122. Larkin G, Thuma P: Congenital malaria in an endemic area. Am J Trop Med Hyg 1991;45:587.
123. Akindele J, Sowunmi A, Abohweyere A: Congenital malaria in a hyperendemic area: a preliminary study. Ann Trop Paediatr 1993;13:273.
124. Ibhanesebhor S, Okolo A: Malaria parasitaemia in neonates with predisposing risk factors for neonatal sepsis: report of six cases. Ann Trop Paediatr 1992;12:297.
125. Harrington W, Sprague C, Minnich V, et al: Immunologic mechanisms in idiopathic and neonatal thrombocytopenic purpura. Ann Intern Med 1953;38:433.
126. Udom-Rice I, Bussel J: Fetal and neonatal thrombocytopenia. Blood Rev 1995;9:57.
127. Burrows R, Caco C, Kelton J: Neonatal alloimmune thrombocytopenia: spontaneous in utero intracranial hemorrhage. Am J Hematol 1988;28:98.
128. Herman J, Jumbelic M, Ancona R, Kickler T: In utero cerebral hemorrhage in alloimmune thrombocytopenia. Am J Pediatr Hematol Oncol 1986;8:312.
129. Dickinson J, Marshall L, Phillips J, Barr A: Antenatal diagnosis and management of fetomaternal alloimmune thrombocytopenia. Am J Perinatol 1995;12:333.
130. Bussel J: Neonatal uses of intravenous immunoglobulin. Am J Pediatr Hematol Oncol 1990;12:505.
131. Bussel J, Kaplan C, McFarland J, et al: Recommendations for the evaluation and treatment of neonatal autoimmune and alloimmune thrombocytopenia. Thromb Haemost 1991;65:631.
132. von dem Borne A, van Leeuwen E, von Riesz L, et al: Neonatal alloimmune thrombocytopenia: detection and characterization of the responsible antibodies by the platelet immunofluorescence test. Blood 1981; 57:649.
133. Mueller-Eckhardt C, Kiefel V, Grubert A, et al: 348 Cases of suspected neonatal alloimmune thrombocytopenia. Lancet 1989;1:363.
134. Kroll H, Kiefel V, Santoso S, Mueller-Eckhardt C: Sr(a), a private platelet antigen on glycoprotein IIIa associated with neonatal alloimmune thrombocytopenia. Blood 1990;76:2296.
135. Kaplan C, Morel-Kopp M, Kroll H, et al: HPA-5b (Br(a)) neonatal alloimmune thrombocytopenia: clinical and immunological analysis of 39 cases. Br J Hematol 1990;78:425.
136. Friedman J, Aster R: Neonatal alloimmune thrombocytopenic purpura and congenital porencephaly in two siblings associated with a "new" maternal antiplatelet antibody. Blood 1985;65:1412.
137. Mauer A, De Vaux L, Lahey M: Neonatal and maternal thrombocytopenic purpura due to quinine. Pediatrics 1957;19:84.
138. Merenstein G, O'Loughlin E, Plunket D: Effects of maternal thiazides on platelet counts of newborn infants. J Pediatr 1970;76:766.
139. Kelton J, Inwood M, Barr R, et al: The prenatal prediction of thrombocytopenia in infants of mothers with clinically diagnosed immune thrombocytopenia. Am J Obstet Gynecol 1982;144:449.
140. Clines D, Dusak B, Tomaski A, et al: Immune thrombocytopenic purpura and pregnancy. N Engl J Med 1982;306:826.
141. Burrows R, Kelton J: Perinatal thrombocytopenia. Clin Perinatol 1995;22:779.
142. Minchinton R, McGrath K: Alloimmune neonatal neutropenia—a neglected diagnosis? Med J Aust 1987;147:139.
143. Gilmore M, Stroncek D, Korones D: Treatment of alloimmune neonatal neutropenia with granulocyte colony-stimulating factor. J Pediatr 1994;125:948.
144. Lalezari P: Alloimmune neonatal neutropenia. In Engelfriet C, van Logham J, von dem Borne A (eds): Immunohaematology. Amsterdam: Elsevier, 1984, pp 179–186.
145. Lalezari P, Nussbaum M, Gelman S, Spaet T: Neonatal neutropenia due to maternal isoimmunization. Blood 1960;15:236.
146. Bux J, Jung K, Kauth T, Mueller-Eckhardt C: Serological and clinical aspects of granulocyte antibodies leading to alloimmune neonatal neutropenia. Transfus Med 1992;2:143.

147. Hanada T, Shin R, Hosoi M, et al: Intravenous gamma-globulin in treatment of isoimmune neonatal neutropenia. Eur J Pediatr 1988;148:218.
148. Rios E, Heresi G, Arevalo M: Familial alloimmune neutropenia of NA2 specificity. Am J Pediatr Hematol Oncol 1991;13:296.
149. Carton J, Tchernia G, Celton J, et al: Alloimmune neonatal neutropenia. Am J Pediatr Hematol Oncol 1991;13:21.
150. Bussell J, Lalezari P, Fikrig S: Intravenous treatment with gamma-globulin of autoimmune neutropenia of infancy. J Pediatr 1988;112:298.
151. Leeuwen E, Roord J, Gast G, Plas-Van Dalen C: Neonatal neutropenia due to maternal autoantibodies against neutrophils. BMJ 1983;287:94.
152. Diamond L, Blackfan K, Baty J: Erythroblastosis fetalis and its association with universal edema of fetus, icterus gravis neonatorum, and anemia of the newborn. J Pediatr 1932;1:269.
153. Levine P, Katzin E, et al: Isoimmunization in pregnancy, its possible bearing on the etiology of erythroblastosis fetalis. JAMA 1941;116:825.
154. Zipursky A: Isoimmune hemolytic disease. In Nathan DC, Oski F (eds): Hematology of Infancy and Childhood. Philadelphia: WB Saunders, 1987, p 73.
155. Oski F, Naiman J: Disorders of platelets. In Oski F, Naiman J (eds): Hematologic Problems in the Newborn. Philadelphia: WB Saunders, 1982, pp 175–222.
156. Koenig J, Christensen R: Neutropenia and thrombocytopenia in infants with Rh hemolytic disease. J Perinatol 1989;9:126.
157. Halbrecht I: Role of hemagglutinins anti-A and anti-B in pathogenesis of jaundice of the newborn (icterus neonatorum precox). Am J Dis Child 1944;64:248.
158. Voak D, Williams M: An explanation of the failure of the direct antiglobulin test to detect erythrocyte sensitization in ABO hemolytic disease of the newborn and observations on pinocytosis of IgG anti-A antibodies by infant (cord) red cells. Br J Haematol 1971;20:9.
159. Mollison P, Frame M, Ross M: Differences between Rh (D) negative subjects in response to Rh (D) antigen. Br J Haematol 1970;19:257.
160. Miller D, Petrie S: Fatal erythroblastosis fetalis secondary to ABO incompatibility. Obstet Gynecol 1963;22:773.
161. Boineau F, Hallock J: Two examples of severe fetal disease due to ABO incompatibility. Clin Pediatr 1971;10:180.
162. Kanto W, Marino B, Godwin A, et al: ABO hemolytic disease: a comparative study of clinical severity and delayed anemia. Pediatrics 1978;62:365.
163. Zipursky A, Chintu C, Brown E, et al: The quantitation of spherocytes in ABO hemolytic disease. J Pediatr 1979;94:965.
164. Peevy K, Wiseman H: ABO hemolytic disease of the newborn: evaluation of management and identification of racial and antigenic factors. Pediatrics 1978;61:475.
165. Baumann R, Rubin H: Autoimmune hemolytic anemia during pregnancy with hemolytic disease in the newborn. Blood 1973;41:293.
166. Chaplin H, Cohen R, Bloomberg G, et al: Pregnancy and idiopathic autoimmune hemolytic anemia: a prospective study during 6 months gestation and 3 months post-partum. Br J Haematol 1973;24:219.
167. Benraad C, Scheerder H, Overbeeke M: Autoimmune haemolytic anaemia during pregnancy. Eur J Gynecol Reprod Biol 1994;55:209.
168. Tsai Y, Chang J, Chang J, et al: Idiopathic autoimmune hemolytic anemia during pregnancy. J Formos Med Assoc 1994;93:328.
169. Seip M: Systemic lupus erythematosus in pregnancy with hemolytic anemia, leucopenia and thrombocytopenia in the mother and her newborn infant. Arch Dis Child 1960;35:365.
170. Zuelzer W, Mastrangelo R, Stulberg C, et al: Autoimmune hemolytic anemia: natural history and viral immunologic interactions in childhood. Am J Med 1970;49:80.
171. Bridge R, Foley F: Placental transmission of the lupus erythematosus factor. Am J Med Sci 1965;227:1.
172. Jackson R: Discoid lupus in a newborn infant of a mother with lupus erythematosus. Pediatrics 1964;33:425.
173. Cruveiller J, Harpey J, Veron P, et al: Lupus erythemateux systemique. Arch Fr Pediatr 1970;27:195.
174. Beck J, Rowell N: Transplacental passage of antinuclear antibody. Lancet 1963;1:134.
175. Provost T, Watson R, Gammon W, et al: The neonatal lupus syndrome associated with U(1)RNP (nRNP) antibodies. N Engl J Med 1987;316:1135.
176. Provost T, Watson R, Gaither K, Harley J: The neonatal lupus erythematosus syndrome. J Rheumatol 1987;14:199.
177. Lee L: Neonatal lupus erythematosus. J Invest Dermatol 1993;100:9.
178. Watson R, Lane A, Barnett N, et al: Neonatal lupus erythematosus: a clinical, serological and immunogenetic study with review of the literature. Medicine (Baltimore) 1984;63:362.
179. Winkler R, Nora A, Nora J: Familial congenital complete heart block and maternal systemic lupus erythematosus. Circulation 1977;56:1103.
180. Nathan D, Snapper I: Simultaneous placental transfer of factors responsible for LE cell formation and thrombocytopenia. Am J Med 1958;25:647.
181. Vonderheid E, Koblenzer P, Ming P, et al: Neonatal lupus erythematosus. Arch Dermatol 1976;112:698.
182. Qamar T, Lockshin M, Druzin M, et al: Antibody to cardiolipin and to Ro/La (SS-A/SS-B) antigens in maternal cord serum pairs. Arthritis Rheum 1986;29:S96.
183. Nolan R, Shulman S, Victorica B: Congenital complete heart block associated with maternal mixed connective tissue disease. J Rheumatol 1979;95:420.
184. Friedreich N: Beitrage zur pathologic des krebses. Virchows Arch Pathol Anat 1866;36:30.
185. Shivvers S, Miller D: Preinvasive and invasive breast and cervical cancer prior to or during pregnancy. Clin Perinatol 1997;24:369.
186. Brossard J, Abish S, Bernstein M, et al: Maternal malignancy involving the products of conception: a report of malignant melanoma and medulloblastoma. Am J Pediatr Hematol Oncol 1994;16:380.
187. Read E Jr, Platzer P: Placental metastasis from maternal carcinoma of the lung. Obstet Gynecol 1981;58:387.
188. Brodsky I, Baren M, Kahn S, et al: Metastatic malignant melanoma from mother to fetus. Cancer 1965;18:1048.
189. Holland E: A case of transplacental metastases of malignant melanoma from mother to fetus. J Obstet Gynaecol Br Emp 1949;56:529.
190. Kasdon S: Pregnancy and Hodgkin's disease. Am J Obstet Gynecol 1949;57:282.
191. McLain C: Leukemia in pregnancy. Clin Obstet Gynecol 1974;17:185.
192. Cramblett H, Friedman J, Najjar S: Leukemia in an infant born of a mother with leukemia. N Engl J Med 1958;259:727.
193. McFaul P, Dornan J, Lamki H, et al: Pregnancy com-

plicated by maternal heart disease: a review of 519 women. Br J Obstet Gynaecol 1988;95:861.
194. Bromberg Y, Abrahamov A, Salzberger M: The effect of maternal anoxemia on the foetal haemoglobin of the newborn. J Obstet Gynaecol Br Emp 1956;63:875.
195. Kravkova E: Morphological picture of the blood of the human foetus in pregnancy complicated by heart disease. Akush Ginekol (Mosk) 1962;5:49.
196. Elsas L, Whittemore R, Burrow G: Maternal and neonatal Graves' disease. JAMA 1967;200:250.
197. Bussman Y, Tellman M, Pagliara A: Neonatal thyrotoxicosis associated with the hyperviscosity syndrome. J Pediatr 1977;90:266.
198. Woodruff P: Behavior of blood platelets in thyrotoxicosis. Med J Aust 1040;2:190.
199. Lamberg B, Kwikangas V: Thrombocytopenia and decreased life span of thrombocytes in hyperthyroidism. Ann Clin Res 1971;3:98.
200. Bar-Shany S, Herbert V: Transplacentally acquired antibody to intrinsic factor with vitamin B_{12} deficiency. Blood 1967;30:777.
201. Gabbe S: Congenital anomalies among infants of diabetic mothers. Obstet Gynecol Surv 1977;32:125.
202. Warner R, Cornblath M: Infants of gestational diabetic mothers. Am J Dis Child 1969;117:678.
203. Klebe J, Ingomar C, Norgaard-Pedersen B: Blood volumes in premature infants of diabetic and nondiabetic mothers correlated with the time of clamping of the umbilical cord. Acta Paediatr Scand 1971;61:549.
204. Widness J, Susa J, Garcia J, et al: Increased erythropoiesis and elevated erythropoietin in infants born to diabetic mothers and in hyperinsulinemic rhesus fetuses. J Clin Invest 1981;67:637.
205. Shannon K, Davis J, Kitzmiller J, et al: Erythropoiesis in infants of diabetic mothers. Pediatr Res 1986;30:161.
206. Taylor P, Wolfson J, Bright N: Hyperbilirubinemia in infants of diabetic mothers. Biol Neonate 1963;5:289.
207. Olsen B, Osler M, Pedersen J: Neonatal jaundice in infants of diabetic mothers. Dan Med Bull 1963;10:18.
208. Peevy K, Landaw S, Gross S: Hyperbilirubinemia in infants of diabetic mothers. Pediatrics 1980;66:417.
209. Oppenheimer E, Esterly J: Thrombosis in the newborn: comparison between infants of diabetic and nondiabetic mothers. J Pediatr 1965;67:549.
210. Hathaway W, Mahasan-dana C, Makowski E: Cord blood coagulation studies of high risk pregnant women. Am J Obstet Gynecol 1975;121:51.
211. Kleckner H, Giles H, Corrigan J: The association of maternal and neonatal thrombocytopenia in high risk pregnancies. Am J Obstet Gynecol 1977;128:235.
212. Stuart M, Elrad H: Increased synthesis of platelet malonyaldi-aldehyde and platelet hyperfunction in infants of mothers with diabetes mellitus. J Lab Clin Med 1979;94:12.
213. Wellen I: The infant mortality in specific hypertensive disease of pregnancy and in essential hypertension. Am J Obstet Gynecol 1953;66:36.
214. Manroe B, Weinberg A, Rosenfeld C: The neonatal blood count in health and disease. I. Reference values for neutrophilic cells. J Pediatr 1979;95:89.
215. Koenig J, Christensen R: Incidence, neutrophil kinetics, and natural history of neonatal neutropenia associated with maternal hypertension. N Engl J Med 1989;321:557.
216. Brazy J, Grimm J, Little V: Neonatal manifestations of severe maternal hypertension occurring before the thirty-sixth week of pregnancy. J Pediatr 1982; 100:265.
217. Doran M, Makhlouf R, Katz V, et al: Increased incidence of sepsis at birth in neutropenic infants of mothers with preeclampsia. J Pediatr 1994;125:452.
218. Kocherlakota P, La Gamma E: Preliminary report: rhG-CSF may reduce the incidence of neonatal sepsis in prolonged pre-eclampsia-associated neutropenia. Pediatrics 1998;102:1107.
219. Kocherlakota P, La Gamma E: Human granulocyte colony-stimulating factor may improve outcome attributable to neonatal sepsis complicated by neutropenia. Pediatrics 1997;100:e6.
220. Makhlouf R, Doron M, Bose C, et al: Administration of granulocyte colony-stimulating factor to neutropenic low birth weight infants of mothers with preeclampsia. J Pediatr 1995;126:454.
221. La Gamma E, Alpan O, Kocherlakota P: Effect of granulocyte colony-stimulating factor on preeclampsia-associated neonatal neutropenia. J Pediatr 1995;126:457.
222. Koenig J, Christensen R: The mechanism responsible for diminished neutrophil production in neonates delivered of women with pregnancy-induced hypertension. Am J Obstet Gynecol 1989;165:467.
223. Eeltink C, van Lingen R, Aarnoudse J, et al: Maternal haemolysis, elevated liver enzymes and low platelets syndrome: specific problems in the newborn. Eur J Pediatr 1993;152:160.
224. Gomez R, Ghezzi F, Romero R, et al: Premature labor and intra-amniotic infection. Clin Perinatol 1995;22:281.
225. Romero R, Parvizi S, Oyarzun E, et al: Amniotic fluid interleukin-1 in spontaneous labor at term. J Reprod Med 1990;35:235.
226. Romero R, Avila C, Santhanam U, Sehgal P: Amniotic fluid interleukin-6 in preterm labor. J Clin Invest 1990;85:1392.
227. Romero R, Ceska M, Avila C, et al: Neutrophil attractant/activating peptide-1/interleukin-8 in term and preterm parturition. Am J Obstet Gynecol 1991;165:813.
228. Romero R, Mazor M, Sepulveda W, et al: Tumor necrosis factor in term and preterm labor. Am J Obstet Gynecol 1992;166:1576.
229. Saito S, Kato Y, Ishihara Y, Ichijo M: Amniotic fluid granulocyte colony-stimulating factor in preterm and term labor. Clin Chim Acta 1992;208:105.
230. Saito S, Kasahara T, Yumiko K, et al: Elevation of amniotic fluid interleukin-6 (IL-6), IL-8 and granulocyte colony-stimulating factor (G-CSF) in term and preterm parturition. Cytokine 1993;5:81.
231. Shorter S, Vince G, Starkey P: Production of granulocyte colony-stimulating factor at the materno-foetal interface in human pregnancy. Immunology 1992;75:468.
232. Stallmach T, Hebisch G, Joller-Jemelka H, et al: Cytokine production and visualized effects in the fetomaternal unit: quantitative and topographic data on cytokines during intrauterine disease. Lab Invest 1995;73:384.
233. Weimann E, Reisbach G, Reinsberg J, Lentze M: IL-6 and G-CSF levels in amniotic fluid during the second trimester in normal and abnormal pregnancies. Arch Gynecol Obstet 1995;256:125.
234. Calhoun D, Polliotti B, Christensen R: The concentration of granulocyte colony-stimulating factor (G-CSF) in amniotic fluid (Abstract). J Soc Gynecol Investig 1998;5:176A.
235. Calhoun D, Kirk J, Christensen R: Incidence, significance, and kinetic mechanism responsible for leukemoid reactions in patients in the neonatal intensive

care unit: a prospective evaluation. J Pediatr 1996;129:403.
236. Gilmore W, McKelvey-Martin V, Rutherford S, et al: Human milk contains granulocyte colony stimulating factor. Eur J Clin Nutr 1994;48:222.
237. Wallace J, Ferguson S, Loane P, et al: Cytokines in human breast milk. Br J Biomed Sci 1997;54:85.
238. Calhoun D, Christensen R: Granulocyte colony-stimulating factor (G-CSF) concentrations in human milk (Abstract). Pediatr Res 1998;43:A1502.
239. Liggins G, Howie R: A controlled trial of antepartum glucocorticoid treatment for prevention of the respiratory distress syndrome in premature infants. Pediatrics 1972;50:515.
240. Anderson A, Gessner G, Jeremy J, et al: Placental transfer and metabolism of beta-methasone in human pregnancy. Obstet Gynecol 1977;49:471.
241. Bishop C, Athens J, Cartwright G, et al: Leukokinetic studies. XIV. Blood neutrophil kinetics in chronic, steady-state neutropenia. J Clin Invest 1971;50:1678.
242. Barak M, Cohen A, Herschkowitz S: Total leukocyte and neutrophil count changes associated with antenatal betamethasone administration in premature infants. Acta Paediatr 1992;81:760.
243. Anday E, Harris M: Lekemoid reaction associated with antenatal dexamethasone administration. J Pediatr 1982;101:614.
244. Otero L, Conlon C, Reynolds P, et al: Neonatal leukocytosis associated with prenatal administration of dexamethasone. Pediatrics 1981;68:778.
245. Farid M, Lorenz J, Huard T: The effect of antenatal steroids (ANS) on cord blood stem cells (CD34) in premature infants (Abstract). Pediatr Res 1998; 43:A1387.
246. Medlock E, Kaplan D, Cecchini M, et al: Granulocyte colony-stimulating factor crosses the placenta and stimulates fetal rat granulopoiesis. Blood 1993;81:916.
247. Novales J, Salva A, Modanlou H, et al: Maternal administration of granulocyte colony-stimulating factor improves neonatal rat survival after a lethal group B streptococcal infection. Blood 1993;81:923.
248. Calhoun D, Cesar R, Christensen R: Transplacental passage of recombinant human granulocyte colony-stimulating factor in women with an imminent preterm delivery. Am J Obstet Gynecol 1996;174:1306.
249. Calhoun D, Christensen R: A randomized, double-blind, placebo-controlled pilot trial of recombinant granulocyte colony-stimulating factor administration in women prior to preterm delivery. Am J Obstet Gynecol 1998;179:766.
250. Leach L, Eaton B, Firth J, Contractor S: Immunocytochemical and labelled tracer approaches to uptake and intracellular routing of immunoglobulin-G (IgG) in human placenta. Cell Tissue Res 1991:444.
251. Leach L, Eaton B, Firth J, Contractor S: Uptake and intracellular routing of peroxidase-conjugated immunoglobulin-G by the perfused human placenta. Cell Tissue Res 1990;261:383.
252. Leach J, Sedmak D, Osborne J, et al: Isolation from human placenta of the IgG transporter, FcRn, and localization to the syncytiotrophoblast. J Immunol 1996;157:3317.
253. Mollison PL: Blood transfusion in clinical medicine. 7th ed. Oxford: Blackwell, 1983.
254. McMillan R: Chronic idiopathic thrombocytopenic purpura. N Engl J Med 1981;304:1135.
255. Newland A, Boots M, Patterson K: Intravenous IgG for autoimmune thrombocytopenia in pregnancy. N Engl J Med 1984;310:261.
256. Bessho T, Ida A, Minagawa K, Koyama K: Effects of maternally administered immunoglobulin on platelet counts of neonates born to mothers with autoimmune thrombocytopenia: re-evaluation. Clin Exp Obstet Gynecol 1997;24:53.
257. Kornfeld I, Wilson R, Ballem P, et al: Antenatal invasive and noninvasive management of alloimmune thrombocytopenia. Fetal Diagn Ther 1996;11:210.
258. Kamen B, Caston J: Purification of folate binding protein in normal umbilical cord serum. Proc Natl Acad Sci U S A 1975;72:4261.
259. Pritchard J, Scott D, Whalley P, et al: Infants of mothers with megaloblastic anemia due to folate deficiency. JAMA 1970;211:1982.
260. Shojania A, Gross S: Folic acid deficiency and prematurity. J Pediatr 1964;64:323.
261. Rapazzo M, Solmi H, Hall C: The content of vitamin B12 in adult and foetal tissue: a comparative study. Br J Haematol 1970;18:425.
262. Higgenbottom M, Sweetman L, Nyhan W: A syndrome of methylmalonic aciduria, homocystinuria, megaloblastic anemia, and neurologic abnormalities in a vitamin B_{12} deficient breastfed infant of a strict vegetarian. N Engl J Med 1978;299:317.
263. Lampkin B, Shore N, Chadwick D: Megaloblastic anemia of infancy secondary to maternal pernicious anemia. N Engl J Med 1966;274:1168.
264. Shah M, Li Y, Christensen R: Effects of perinatal zidovudine on hematopoiesis: a comparison of effects on progenitors from human fetuses versus mothers. AIDS 1996;10:1239.
265. Liebes L, Mendoza S, Wilson D, Dancis J: Transfer of zidovudine (AZT) by human placenta. J Infect Dis 1990;161:203.
266. Boucher R, Modlin J, Weller S, et al: Phase 1 evaluation of zidovudine administered to infants exposed at birth to the human immunodeficiency virus. J Pediatr 1993;122:137.

SECTION 2

A Practical Guide to Solving Hematologic Problems of Neonates

CHAPTER 7

Expected Hematologic Values for Term and Preterm Neonates

Robert D. Christensen, M.D.

Defining normal hematologic values for neonates is more problematic than for most other groups of patients. The ranges of values obtained from term infants generally do not apply to preterm infants, and ranges of values obtained for low-birth-weight preterm infants can be very different from ranges obtained for extremely-low-birth-weight micropremes of 24 to 26 weeks' gestation. For example, a venous hematocrit of 38% is within the expected range for a 2-hour-old infant born at 24 weeks' gestation, but this hematocrit is abnormal, constituting an anemic value, for a term infant.

Another problem encountered in defining normal hematologic values for neonates is that normal values for unstable, sick infants may not always be optimal values. For instance, a neonate delivered at 24 weeks' gestation, now 4 weeks old, is expected to have a venous hematocrit of 22% to 28%. However, if such a patient acquires a nosocomial infection, becomes hypoxemic and tachycardic, and is placed on a ventilator, a hematocrit of 22%, although normal, is not optimal for patient care. A higher hematocrit could facilitate better tissue oxygenation and diminish the heart rate. A list of normal values for hematologic parameters of neonates is therefore not always sufficiently informative for the purposes of clinical neonatology.

Making the determination about whether a specific hematologic value for a neonate is normal or abnormal often requires cognizance of the gestational age of the subject, age of the subject (i.e., hours after delivery), specific illness, level of support needed, and the method used for blood sampling (e.g., venous, arterial, capillary). Sometimes knowledge of other factors is pertinent, such as whether "stripping" of the umbilical cord was attempted after delivery; whether a capillary sample was obtained from a warmed or an unwarmed, mottled extremity; and whether serial complete blood count (CBC) samples were drawn from the same or different anatomic sites.

This chapter describes the expected hematologic values for preterm and term infants. It also provides the practical information needed to avoid pitfalls in interpreting these values. Expected values are discussed for circulating erythrocytes, leukocytes, platelets, and bone marrow differential cell counts.

ERYTHROCYTES

Site of Sampling

Erythrocyte values—particularly the hematocrit, hemoglobin concentration, and erythrocyte concentration—obtained from newborn infants vary, somewhat predictably, according to the vascular source from which the sample is obtained (Table 7–1).[1–8] In general, erythrocyte values are higher (i.e., more concentrated) when samples are obtained by lancing capillary beds than when they are drawn directly from an artery or a vein or obtained from an indwelling arterial or venous catheter.

Table 7–1. **The Effect of Site of Blood Sampling on Hematocrits or Hemoglobin Concentrations of Neonates**

Study	Year	Anatomic Sites of Comparison	Observed Average Difference
Vahlquist[1]	1941	Capillary vs. femoral vein	Capillary 10% higher
Oettinger & Mills[2]	1949	Great toe vs. internal jugular	Capillary 21% higher
Mollision[3]	1951	Capillary vs. venous	Capillary 5% higher
Oh & Lind[4]	1966	Heel vs. scalp or femoral vein	Capillary 15% higher*
Moe[5]	1967	Patients with erythroblastosis fetalis: heel vs. umbilical cord	Capillary 25% higher
Linderkamp[6]	1977	Capillary vs. umbilical cord	Capillary 10–21% higher
Rivera & Rudolph[7]	1982	Heel vs. antecubital vein	Capillary 12% higher (up to 20%)
Thurlbeck & McIntosh[8]†	1987	Heel vs. UAC	Capillary 15% higher

UAC, umbilical artery catheter.
*The capillary hematocrit was only 5% higher when the heel was warmed.
†Preterm infants, 24 to 32 weeks' gestation, with respiratory distress.

The specific anatomic site of the vein, artery, or capillary bed sampled appears not to affect the results. For instance, values obtained from a femoral vein appear to be equivalent to those obtained from a scalp vein,[5] and values from an umbilical artery appear to be equivalent to those obtained from a radial artery. Values obtained from a capillary bed, such as from a heel, toe, or finger, are also similar to one another if perfusion of those sites is similar.[5]

As a general rule, capillary blood obtained from a neonate's poorly perfused extremity is a poor source on which to base clinical decisions. The erythrocyte values (i.e., hematocrit, hemoglobin concentration, and erythrocyte count) obtained from such a source are about 15% (range of 5% to 25%) above those of simultaneously obtained venous or arterial blood. Capillary values obtained from a poorly perfused extremity can erroneously indicate the diagnosis of polycythemia and can erroneously exclude anemia. The amount to which the capillary hematocrit is elevated above the venous or arterial hematocrit cannot be accurately predicted in individual cases, but in general, it appears to vary with perfusion of the extremity.

When a CBC is obtained from a sick neonate with poor cutaneous perfusion, the neonatologist interpreting the value should realize that a capillary hematocrit is less informative and less reproducible than a venous or an arterial hematocrit. Oh and Lind[4] and Lindercamp and colleagues[6] found that infants of the shortest gestation generally have the largest difference in capillary and venous hematocrits (Table 7–2). Studies by Oh and Lind[4] and by Moe[5] indicate that warming the extremity before lancing the capillary bed can result in a better correlation between capillary and venous hematocrits. However, when a neonatologist feels it important to detect changes in serial hematocrit samples, it should likewise be important to keep a uniform site of sampling (i.e., all venous or all arterial). When comparing serial hematocrits of an ill neonate, it is at least useful to have the sample site clearly documented on the laboratory result.

Effect of Gestational Age on Erythrocyte Values

The marked improvements in survival of extremely low-birth-weight infants during the past decade have resulted in a new population of neonatal intensive care unit patients. Because

Table 7–2. **Effect of Gestational Age on Capillary and Venous Hematocrit Differences**

Gestational Age (wk)	Number of Patients	Capillary Hematocrit (% of Venous Hematocrit)
26–30	22	120*
31–32	18	112
33–35	13	117
36–41	39	112

*$P < .05$ compared with term
From Oh W, Lind J: Venous and capillary hematocrit in newborn infants and placental transfusion. Acta Paediatr Scand 1966;55:38.

of the shift to smaller infants of younger gestational age, studies were needed to establish the expected values for hemoglobin, hematocrit, and other elements of the CBC. In an early study, Oh and Lind[4] observed that the difference in hematocrit, with capillary values higher than venous values, was even more marked in extremely-low-birth-weight infants (see Table 7–2).

In another early study, Walker and Turnbull observed that fetuses in the first and early second trimester had much lower cord blood hemoglobin concentrations than those in the third trimester (Fig. 7–1).[9] Zaizov and Matoth reported the effect of gestational age on red blood cell values obtained for 135 neonates during their first day of life.[10] Forestier and colleagues reported similar data by ultrasound-guided intrauterine techniques using blood obtained from 409 fetuses.[11] McIntosh and associates reported counts of 101 preterm infants who had appropriate weights for gestational age and 42 who were small for gestational age.[12] A summary of the values are given in Table 7–3. It is not clear why the fetuses studied by Forestier and coworkers in utero (first three lines of Table 7–3) had substantially lower hematocrits and hemoglobin concentrations than those for the umbilical cord blood samples of Zaizov and Matoh that were obtained at delivery (last eight lines of Table 7–3). Perhaps the fetal values were somewhat diluted by drawing a very small blood sample into a fixed amount of anticoagulant. Alternatively, these differences are real but unexplained.

Time of Blood Sampling Relative to Delivery

During the first few hours after delivery, increases in the neonate's hematocrit, hemoglobin, and erythrocyte count are normal. The usual explanation for this effect is hemoconcentration of erythrocytes received at delivery from a placental transfusion. The magnitude of increase in erythrocyte values over the first hours of life varies in part in proportion to the volume of the placental transfusion received. However, placental blood transfusion is probably only a partial explanation for the increase in erythrocyte values observed over the first hours of life. Gairdner and coworkers attempted to prevent cord transfusion by clamping the cord as soon

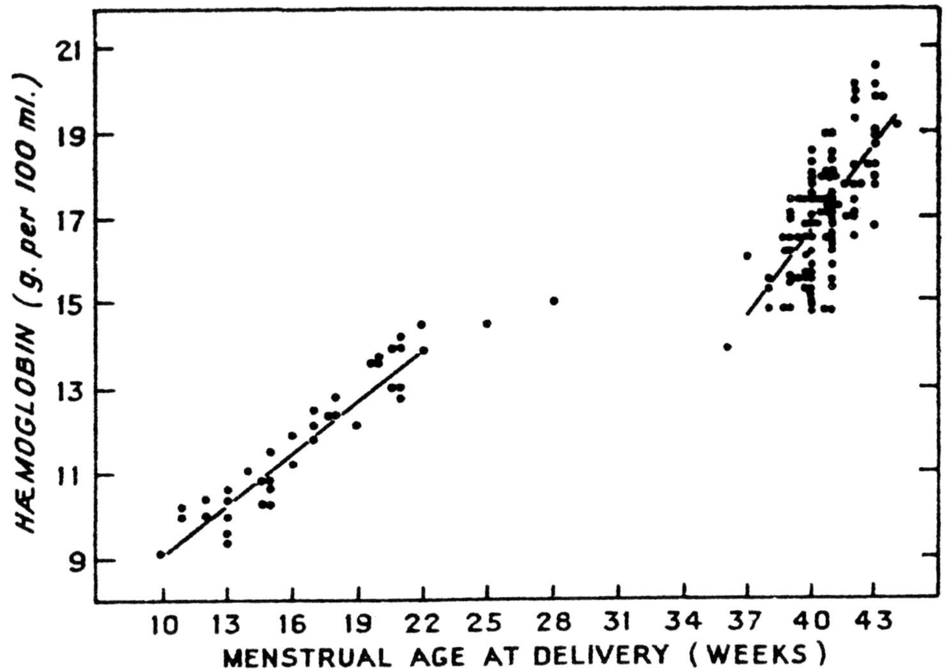

Figure 7–1. Umbilical cord blood hemoglobin concentration as a function of gestational age. (From Walker JL, Turnbull EPN: Haemoglobin and red cells in the human foetus and their relation to the oxygen content of the blood in the vessels of the umbilical cord. Lancet 1953;2:312. © by The Lancet Ltd., 1953.)

Table 7–3. **The Effect of Gestational Age of Fetuses In Utero and Newborn Infants on Their Hematocrit, Hemoglobin, Mean Corpuscular Volume, and Reticulocytes**

Gestational Age (wk)	Hematocrit (%)†	Hemoglobin (g/dL)	MCV (fL)	Reticulocytes (%)
18–20*	36 ± 3	11.5 ± 0.8	134 ± 9	NR
21–22*	38 ± 3	12.3 ± 0.9	130 ± 6	NR
22–23*	38 ± 1	12.4 ± 0.2	125 ± 1	NR
24–25	63 ± 4	19.4 ± 1.5	135 ± 0	6.0 ± 0.5
26–27	62 ± 8	19.0 ± 2.5	132 ± 14	9.6 ± 3.2
28–29	60 ± 7	19.3 ± 1.8	131 ± 14	7.5 ± 2.5
30–31	60 ± 8	19.1 ± 2.2	127 ± 13	5.8 ± 2.0
32–33	60 ± 8	18.5 ± 2.0	123 ± 16	5.0 ± 1.9
34–35	61 ± 7	19.6 ± 2.1	122 ± 10	3.9 ± 1.6
36–37	64 ± 7	19.2 ± 1.7	121 ± 12	4.2 ± 1.8
Term	61 ± 7	19.3 ± 2.2	119 ± 9	3.2 ± 1.4

NR, not reported; MCV, mean corpuscular volume.
*Fetuses in utero.
†Values reported as the mean ± SD.
Data from Zaizov R, Matoth Y: Red cell values on the first postnatal day during the last 16 weeks of gestation. Am J Hematol 1976;1:275; Forestier F, Daffos F, Galacteros F, et al: Hematological values of 163 normal fetuses between 18 and 30 weeks of gestation. Pediatr Res 1986;20:342; and McIntosh N, Kempson C, Tyler RM: Blood counts in extremely low birth weight infants. Arch Dis Child 1988;63:74.

as possible but still observed an increase in hemoglobin concentration (from 16.6 to 19.1 g/dL) over the 8 hours after delivery.[13] When a neonate fails to have the expected increase in hematocrit, hemoglobin concentration, and erythrocyte count over the first hours of life, the neonatologist may consider the possibility that hemorrhage or hemolysis has occurred.

About 100 mL of blood usually can be withdrawn from the placental vessels at term by using the technique of catheterizing the vessels and washing out the blood.[14] Direct venipuncture of the placental end of the umbilical vein after cord clamping generally yields somewhat less blood (50 to 60 mL). The blood within the umbilical cord and placenta is about one third of the entire circulating blood volume of the fetus.

Normally, after a term fetus is delivered, the umbilical arteries constrict in response to the increasing Po_2, retarding the flow of blood from the neonate into the placenta. The umbilical vein, however, fails to significantly constrict, permitting blood to flow in a direction partly controlled by gravity—from the placenta to the neonate or vice versa. In the time between delivery and clamping of the umbilical cord, the direction of the umbilical venous blood flow usually is from the placenta to the infant. If, however, the neonate is held in a position significantly above the placenta, blood can flow through the umbilical vein from the neonate to the placenta.[15, 16]

Hemoglobin Concentration

The concentration of hemoglobin in the blood can be quantified by manual or automated techniques. The standard assay for hemoglobin determination, approved by the World Health Organization, is simple but highly reproducible.[17] It involves the conversion of the several forms of hemoglobin in the blood, including oxyhemoglobin, carboxyhemoglobin, and the minor quantities of other hemoglobin species present, to a single compound, hemoglobincyanide, which is then determined spectrophotometrically. The hemoglobin concentration and the hematocrit are for the most part different measurements of the same biologic variable. However, because the hemoglobin concentration is a direct measurement but the hematocrit usually is a calculated value, as explained later, the hemoglobin concentration has sometimes been a slightly preferred method.

Many studies have reported a normal range of hemoglobin values from the umbilical cord blood of healthy term infants (Table 7–4). The summation of these reports indicates an overall average hemoglobin concentration at term of 16.8 g/dL, with a range of 13.7 to 20.1 g/dL. Values less than 13.7 g/dL could be considered anemic and more than 20.1 g/dL could be considered polycythemic.

The umbilical cord blood hemoglobin concentrations (see Table 7–4) were obtained almost exclusively from neonates delivered in the third trimester. At 16 weeks of gestation, 1 dL of fetal blood has about 10 g of hemoglobin, and this concentration reaches about 15 g/dL at 32 to 34 weeks. Burman and Morris reported that the expected (normal) hemoglobin value in female fetuses could be determined by this formula: 7 + the gestational age in months.[26] A girl delivered at 7 months' gestation would be expected to have a hemoglobin concentration of 7 plus 7, or 14 g/dL. They reported that this relationship did not hold true for male fetuses, who reached a value of about 16 g/dL by 32 weeks and then remained constant through term. Postmature infants do not have higher hemoglobin concentrations than those delivered at term, unless chronic hypoxemia has occurred.

Hematocrit

In 1929, Dr. Wintrobe described a clinical laboratory test that he called the *volume of packed red blood cells* (VPRC).[27] The test was performed by centrifuging blood in a specifically designed glass tube called a *hematocrit*. Originally, hematocrit was the name of the tube used in the measurement, not the measurement itself. Usage subsequently changed, and the term hematocrit now typically indicates the measurement, and the term VPRC is rarely used.

The hematocrit measurement is the proportion of the blood sample occupied by erythrocytes. The units are given as a percentage or as a fraction (liters of red blood cells/liter of blood). Because neonates and young children do not have a liter of blood in their entire circulation, children's hospital laboratories usually express the hematocrit as a percentage.

Originally, the result of the hematocrit test was read directly from the tube after a standardized centrifugation as the proportion of the height of the total column of blood occupied by the column of red cells. Although an extremely simple concept, this test constituted a significant advance in clinical medicine. It was highly successful and became widely used, probably because the results were very reproducible and useful in patient care and because the test could be performed without complicated or expensive instrumentation. Subsequent modifications of the hematocrit test to permit using small blood samples led to its applicability to neonates. Ten years after it was described for testing adults, Waugh and colleagues reported that the hematocrit of normal infants, averaging 51.3%, was higher than that of normal adults.[28]

Most hospital laboratories no longer use centrifugation methods for hematocrit determinations; instead, aperture-impedance instruments calculate the hematocrit. This is done by electronically measuring the mean red blood cell volume and multiplying this number by the erythrocyte concentration, also measured electronically. The mean volume of the erythrocytes multiplied by their number per microliter yields the volume of red blood cells per microliter, or the hematocrit. Other types of cell counters calculate the hematocrit using laser optics, correlating the magnitude of a light pulse generated by passing a red blood cell through a laser with the cell's volume.

Many neonatologist have noticed that, when manual and electronic methods for hematocrit

Table 7–4. **Hemoglobin Concentration in Umbilical Cord Blood**

Study	Year	Mean Hemoglobin (g/dL)	Range	Number of Observations
Mugrage and Andresen[18]	1936	17.1	13–20	40
Guest et al.[19]	1938	17.9	13–22	34
Waugh et al.[20]	1939	15.4	11.9–18.7	52
DeMarsh et al.[21]	1941	15.8	12.5–19.5	33
Dochain et al.[22]	1952	17.9	14.4–21.6	40
Walker and Turnbull[9]	1953	16.5	14.0–20.5	145
Marks et al.[23]	1955	16.9	12.3–22.0	221
Guest and Brown[24]	1957	17.1	13.0–25.0	59
Rooth and Sjostedt[25]	1957	16.7	11.2–26.6	414
Burman and Morris[26]	1974	16.2	2.3 SD	140

determination are used on an individual patient, a consistent difference occurs between the two, a difference usually not seen in testing older children and adults. Neonates tend to have a slightly higher spun hematocrit than automated hematocrit. The reason for this involves the phenomenon of trapped plasma in the spun hematocrit determinations. When blood is centrifuged in a hematocrit tube, a small amount of plasma is always "trapped" between the erythrocytes, slightly elevating the measured hematocrit value. The amount of trapped plasma is insignificant in most cases, usually in the range of 1% to 3% of the plasma volume, as determined by radioiodinated serum albumin labeling experiments.[29] However, in samples with a very high hematocrit and in samples with a very large erythrocyte concentration, more plasma becomes trapped when the cells are centrifuged. Because neonates have considerably higher hematocrits and larger erythrocytes than adults, this additional plasma trapping tends to make the spun hematocrit a higher value than the automated, calculated value (which is not subject to the plasma trapping pitfall). When the neonatologist feels that it is clinically important to closely follow a hematocrit value, this difference between spun and automated values should be recognized and a consistent methodology used.

The hematocrit, just like the hemoglobin concentration and the erythrocyte count, normally increases during the first hours of life and then slowly declines. By the end of the first week of life, it is close to the original cord blood value (Table 7–5).

Erythrocyte Count

The erythrocyte count, or the number of erythrocytes in a volume of blood, usually is determined electronically by a particle counter. Many children's hospital clinical laboratories choose to express the erythrocyte count as cells per 1 μL of blood, but most adult clinical hematology services express the count in units of cells per 1 L of blood. Whether it is expressed as cells per microliter (usually $\times\ 10^6$) or cells per liter (usually $\times\ 10^{12}$), it is equivalent, but because small children do not have a liter of blood in their entire circulating blood volume, it is somewhat peculiar to select the latter option.

Erythrocyte Indices

In addition to devising the hematocrit, Dr. Wintrobe introduced the concept of *erythrocyte indices* and described methods for their calculation.[27] Virtually every CBC includes a report of these indices. The original manual methods for making the measurements with which the erythrocyte indices were calculated have been replaced almost entirely by automated instruments, which provide measurements that are much more precise and reproducible. Although often overlooked, these indices can provide the neonatologist with valuable information not otherwise available.

The *mean corpuscular volume* (MCV) is a measure of the average size of the circulating erythrocytes. It is expressed in femtoliters (fL, 10^{-15} L). Most modern automated cell counters, using laser optics or aperture-impedance, measure the MCV of erythrocytes directly. As originally described, however, the MCV was calculated after measuring the hematocrit and the erythrocyte count by this formula:

$$\text{MCV (fL)} = \frac{\text{Hematocrit (L/L)} \times 1000}{\text{Erythrocyte count } (\times 10^{12}/\text{L})}$$

Table 7–5. **Mean Erythrocyte Values Over the First 2 Weeks of Life in Healthy Term Infants**

Test	Cord Blood	Day 1	Day 3	Day 7	Day 14
Hemoglobin (g/dL)	16.8	18.4	17.8	17.0	16.8
Hematocrit (%)	53	58	55	54	52
Red blood cells (10^6/μL)	5.2	5.8	5.6	5.2	5.1
MCV (fL)	108	108	99	98	96
MCH (pg)	34	35	33	33	32
MCHC (g/dL)	31.7	32.5	33.0	33.0	33.0
Reticulocytes (/μL)	300,000	300,000	50,000	0	0
Nucleated RBC (/μL)	500	200	0	0	0

MCV, mean corpuscular volume; MCH, mean corpuscular hemoglobin; MCHC, mean corpuscular hemoglobin concentration; RBC, red blood cells.

The *mean corpuscular hemoglobin* (MCH) is a measure of the amount of hemoglobin in an average circulating erythrocyte. It is expressed in picograms of hemoglobin (pg, 10^{-12} g) and is given by this formula:

$$\text{MCH (pg)} = \frac{\text{Hemoglobin (g/L)}}{\text{Erythrocyte count } (\times 10^{12}/\text{L})}$$

The *mean corpuscular hemoglobin concentration* (MCHC) is a measure of the concentration of hemoglobin in an average circulating erythrocyte, and is expressed in units of grams of hemoglobin per deciliter of packed red blood cells (g/dL):

$$\text{MCHC (g/dL)} = \frac{\text{Hemoglobin (g/dL)}}{\text{Hematocrit (L/L)}}$$

Healthy neonates have a much higher MCV than do healthy adults. The MCV falls, however, over the first weeks of life. The MCV of a term infant (108 ± 8 fL at birth) should have fallen by 3 to 4 months of life to the level of a normal adult (88 ± 8 fL). Thereafter, the MCV continues to decline, reaching nadir levels during the fourth to sixth months and then slowly increasing to adult values after the first year. The MCV of preterm infants is larger than that of term infants, and in general, the more preterm the infant, the larger the MCV. The lower limit of normal for an MCV in a term neonate during the first days of life is about 100 fL. When a newborn infant has an MCV of less than 94 fL, α-thalassemia trait or iron deficiency should be considered.

Like the MCV, the MCH is higher in healthy neonates (33 to 41 pg) than in healthy adults (27 to 31 pg) and is higher still in preterm infants. The MCHC of preterm and term neonates, however, is in the same range in adults; although the neonate's erythrocytes are larger and contain more hemoglobin on the basis of the increased size, the hemoglobin within the erythrocyte is neither more nor less concentrated than it is in the erythrocytes of adults. Erythrocyte indices of Central African neonates do not differ from those of neonates from other parts of the world, although the hematocrits of these neonates are somewhat lower.[30]

The MCHC can be a sensitive and specific screen for hereditary spherocytosis. Michaels and associates compared automated MCHC measurements from 112 children with hereditary spherocytosis who had not undergone splenectomy with 112 matched healthy children.[31] She observed that the MCHC of the group with hereditary spherocytosis was 35.9 g/dL, significantly higher than the controls (34.3 g/dL, $P < .001$). These patients also had significantly higher erythrocyte distribution widths (19.3 versus 12.6, $P < .001$). Because the children in that report were all older than 2 years, it is not clear what MCHC and red blood cell distribution width (RDW) values might identify newborn infants who have hereditary spherocytosis.

In addition to the erythrocyte indices, the RDW and the hemoglobin distribution width (HDW) are commonly reported on automated CBCs. The RDW is a measure of the homogeneity of red blood cell size, and the HDW is a measure of the homogeneity of red blood cell hemoglobin. The RDW is expressed as a percentage, meaning the percent of erythrocytes that fall outside (smaller or larger) the standard gated population of erythrocytes. An elevated RDW value reflects an abnormal divergence of erythrocyte size. The RDW begins to increase in cases of iron deficiency before any other change in erythrocyte indices or concentrations. The HDW is expressed in grams per deciliter (g/dL) and provides an index of divergence of hemoglobin concentration within erythrocytes. The RDW provides a numeric assessment of anisocytosis, and the HDW provides a numeric assessment of anisochromasia.

Reticulocyte Count

Because erythroid precursor cells clonally mature within the bone marrow, their nucleus becomes pyknotic and is extruded (usually at the orthochromatic normoblast stage), and the cells are thereafter released into the circulating blood. Cytoplasmic organelles, such as ribosomes, mitochondria, and the Golgi complex, generally persist for some time after the erythrocytes have been released into the blood. Supravital stains such as new methylene blue and brilliant cresyl blue stain the nucleic acid within these organelles. New methylene blue is a distinct chemical stain; regular methylene blue stains reticulocytes poorly.

Erythrocytes that have been recently released from the bone marrow into the blood and still contain organelles have a reticulum of blue stain and are called *reticulocytes*.[32] Normally, erythrocytes that have been in the circulation for 24 hours or less stain as reticulocytes. Thereafter, they lose the organelles and fail to stain as reticulocytes. The quantity of reticulum (i.e., nucleic acid) within an erythrocyte diminishes as the cell matures. In the youngest reticulocytes, the reticulum is densely packed, and in the oldest reticulocytes, only a few scattered threads are found. Reticulocytes are on average about 20% larger than mature erythrocytes.[33] Scanning electron microscopy has shown that reticulocytes are not generally bilaterally indented disks like mature erythrocytes, but rather are irregularly shaped and polylobulated.

A neonatologist usually orders a reticulocyte count to assess the level of erythrocyte production, because high reticulocyte counts signify increased erythropoiesis and counts of 0 signify a low level of effective erythropoiesis. Reticulocytes can be reported in at least three different ways, which may sometimes be confusing: as a percentage, as an absolute number, or as a corrected value.

A reticulocyte percentage is the percentage of erythrocytes that stain as reticulocytes. An obvious limitation of this method is that it fails to account for differences in the absolute number of erythrocytes. For example, each of two neonates may have a reticulocyte count of 5%. The neonatologist may be tempted to conclude that the two patients have similar degrees of erythrocyte production. However, the first patient is anemic, with an erythrocyte count of 2 $\times$ $10^6/\mu L$, and the other is not anemic, with an erythrocyte count of 4 $\times$ $10^6/\mu L$. The anemic infant actually has only one-half the number of reticulocytes in the circulation (5% of 2 $\times$ 10^6, or 100,000 reticulocytes/μL of blood) as does the normal infant (5% of 4 $\times$ 10^6, or 200,000 reticulocytes/μL of blood). Failure to recognize this pitfall can give the neonatologist the false impression that the anemic patient is mounting an appropriate increase in erythrocyte production.

Reporting the reticulocyte count as an *absolute number* appears to be gaining popularity in neonatal intensive care units. In reporting the results of clinical trials of recombinant erythropoietin administration to preterm neonates this method was more common than was the reporting a percentage, because it gives a clearer comparison of effective erythropoiesis between groups, despite differences in hematocrit.

A third method of reporting reticulocytes is by using one or two corrections. Generally, one correction is made for hematocrit. The reticulocyte percentage is adjusted to a standard hematocrit, usually 45% (0.45 L/L). The correction is applied as follows:

$$\text{Corrected reticulocyte count} = \text{Patient's reticulocyte count (\%)} \times \frac{\text{Patient's hematocrit (L/L)}}{0.45\ \text{(L/L)}}$$

This correction usually is appropriate for neonatal patients and provides a better framework for assessing the level of effective erythropoiesis, because it normalizes all values to a standard hematocrit.

Another type of correction is sometimes made for *shift reticulocytes*. This correction accounts for the observation that, whereas reticulocytes generally survive in the circulation for only about 1 day, during increased erythropoiesis, even younger reticulocytes can be released from the marrow to the blood (i.e., shifted). These shift reticulocytes, prematurely released from the marrow into the blood, survive longer than 1 day in the blood before loosing their organelles, giving the false impression that the reticulocyte count is high. When reticulocytes survive in the circulation for 2 days, rather than 1 day, the correction for shift reticulocytes is made by reducing the percentage reported in half. To apply this correction, the degree of shift is assumed to be related to the intensity of stimulation of the marrow by erythropoietin. The examiner assumes that the maturation time of the reticulocyte in the circulation is 1 day when the hematocrit is normal, 1.5 days when the hematocrit is reduced moderately, and 2.0 days when the hematocrit is reduced markedly. With a hematocrit of 20%, the physician assumes a marked erythropoietic effort, causing a shift in premature reticulocytes that survive 2 days in the circulation:

$$\text{Corrected reticulocyte count} = \frac{\text{Patient's reticulocyte count (\%)}}{2.0}$$

The shift reticulocyte count correction is rarely used by neonatologists. The correction for shift reticulocytes is only appropriate when the anemia is the result of hemorrhage or hemolysis, because it assumes that erythrocyte production has increased in response to the anemia. If the anemia is the result of hypoproduction of erythrocytes, the reticulocyte count correction for shift reticulocytes would not be valid. Because relative hypoproduction of erythrocytes is thought to be a common component of anemia in preterm infants, the use of this correction would be misleading.

On the first day of life, normal term infants have reticulocyte values of 4% to 7%[34] and absolute reticulocyte counts of 200,000 to 400,000/μL. Infants delivered prematurely have somewhat higher reticulocyte counts than those born at term. Values of 6% to 10% and absolute counts of 400,000 to 550,000/μL are common in low-birth-weight infants.[35] In healthy neonates, reticulocyte levels fall markedly over the first few days of life.[36] By the fourth day of life, the reticulocytes may be 0% to 1%, with an absolute count of 0 to 50,000/μL.

Erythrocyte Morphology

Using erythrocytes suspended in wet preparations that contain 0.2% glutaraldehyde, Zipursky enumerated the various morphologic forms of erythrocytes in term and preterm infants and in adults.[37] He observed considerable heterogeneity among erythrocytes of infants, particularly preterm infants (Fig. 7–2). Whereas

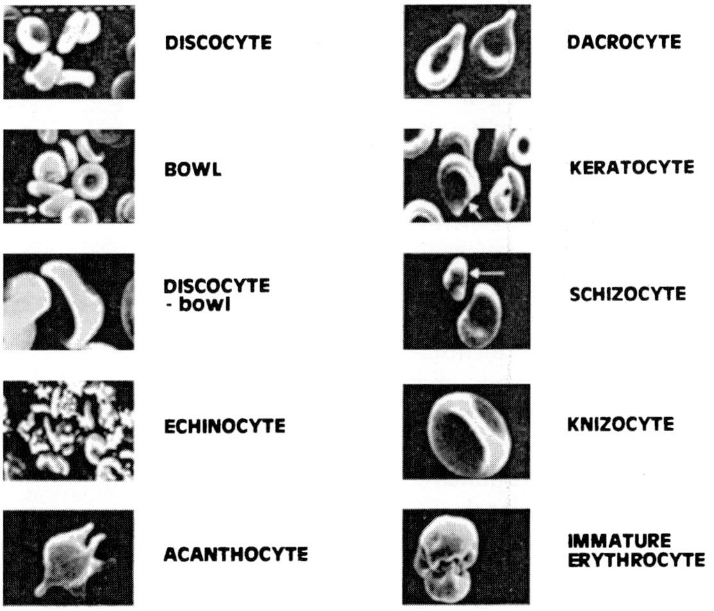

Figure 7–2. A variety of morphologic abnormalities of the erythrocyte are observed in premature infants, term infants, and normal adults. (From Zipursky A: Erythrocyte morphology in newborn infants: a new look. Pediatr Res 1977;11:843.)

THE ERYTHROCYTE DIFFERENTIAL COUNT
(Median and 5% to 95% range)

Cell Type	Premature Infant	Term Infant	Normal Adult
Discocyte	39.5 (18-57)	43 (18-62)	78 (42-94)
Bowl	29.0 (13-53)	40 (14-58)	18 (4-50)
Discocyte-Bowl	3.0 (0-10)	2 (0-5)	2 (0-4)
Spherocyte	0.0 (0-3)	0 (0-1)	0 (0-0)
Echinocyte	5.5 (1-23)	1 (0-4)	0 (0-3)
Acanthocyte	0.0 (0-2)	1 (0-2)	0 (0-1)
Dacrocyte	1.0 (0-5)	1 (0-3)	0 (0-1)
Keratocyte	3.0 (0-7)	2 (0-5)	0 (0-1)
Schizocyte	2.0 (0-5)	0 (0-2)	0 (0-1)
Knizocyte	3.0 (0-11)	3 (0-8)	1 (0-5)
Immature erythrocyte	1.0 (0-6)	0 (0-2)	0 (0-0)

78% of erythrocytes from adults were discocytes, only about 40% of the erythrocytes of neonates had this characteristic shape. Morphologic abnormalities of the erythrocytes of neonates have also been reported using other methods. For instance, interference-contrast microscopy shows pits or craters on the surface of about 2.6% of erythrocytes of healthy adults. In contrast, about 25% of the erythrocytes of term infants and about one half of the erythrocytes of preterm infants have pits.[38] It is believed that these pits are cytoplasmic vacuoles and represent hypofunction of the spleen or reticuloendothelial system, but their significance is not clear.

LEUKOCYTES

Many of the neonatologists who obtained their clinical training in the 1960s and 1970s received the instruction that a CBC was not helpful in evaluating neonates for sepsis. The 1972 edition of *Holt's Pediatrics* stated that "the blood count is of relatively little help in the diagnosis of sepsis neonatorum."[39] This was a prevalent teaching of the time, and when the first cases of group B streptococcal infection were reported, no mention was made of the blood leukocyte counts or the differential cells counts of these infants. It therefore was not clear whether any or all of these patients had neutropenia, neutrophilia, or a leukocyte left shift. The notion that the CBC was not a useful test to perform on neonatal patients was based on the extreme variability of neutrophil counts in neonates and the apparent lack of correlation between the blood neutrophil findings and the presence of infection.

The attitudes of neonatologists about the utility of CBCs began to change after publications of Xanthou,[40] Zipursky and colleagues,[41] Akenzua and associates,[42] and Manroe and coworkers.[43] These reports showed differences in blood neutrophil concentrations in groups of infected compared with noninfected neonates, and they pointed out that neutropenia, accompanied by a high ratio of immature neutrophils (bands and metamyelocytes) to total neutrophils (segmented neutrophils and band neutrophils and metamyelocytes) was particularly common in neonates with sepsis.

Site of Sampling

My colleagues and I observed that leukocyte concentrations and neutrophil concentrations were lower when blood was drawn from an umbilical artery catheter or other arterial line than when simultaneously drawn by venipuncture or capillary stick.[44] The arterial values were about 75% of the venous or capillary values. We also observed that, after moderate exercise in the form of chest physical therapy, the leukocyte counts increased to about 115% of the baseline value, but this was not accompanied by a change in the differential count. This relation of blood leukocyte count to site of sampling was also observed in preterm infants (24 to 32 weeks' gestation) who had respiratory distress syndrome by Thurlbeck and McIntosh.[8] They obtained CBCs through umbilical artery catheters, venipuncture, and heel sticks and found that arterial neutrophil concentrations averaged $3.5 \pm 1.5 \times 10^3/\mu L$, compared with capillary values of $5.5 \pm 3 \times 10^3/\mu L$ ($P < .01$).

Lower leukocyte and neutrophil concentration in arterial blood than venous or capillary blood was observed in experimental animals.[45] The explanation appears to be related to the differences in blood flow of arterial compared with capillary or venous blood. The pulsatile flow of arterial blood appears to "push" the larger cells toward the periphery of the vessel, whereas the leukocytes and erythrocytes are more uniformly mixed in capillary and venous circulation.[45]

Leukocyte Counts in Term Infants

In 1979, Manroe and associates from the University of Texas Southwestern Medical Center in Dallas published normal reference ranges for blood neutrophil concentrations in neonates and for the proportion of circulating neutrophils that were immature (nonsegmented) [Figs. 7–3 and 7–4]. They reported values for neonates of 26 to 44 weeks' gestation and with birth weights of 660 to 5000 g.[43] The data were obtained from 1974 to 1976, when the survival of very-low-birth-weight (VLBW) infants was 42% (compared with 79% a decade later). The number of VLBW infants represented in the Manroe study was limited. This study's publica-

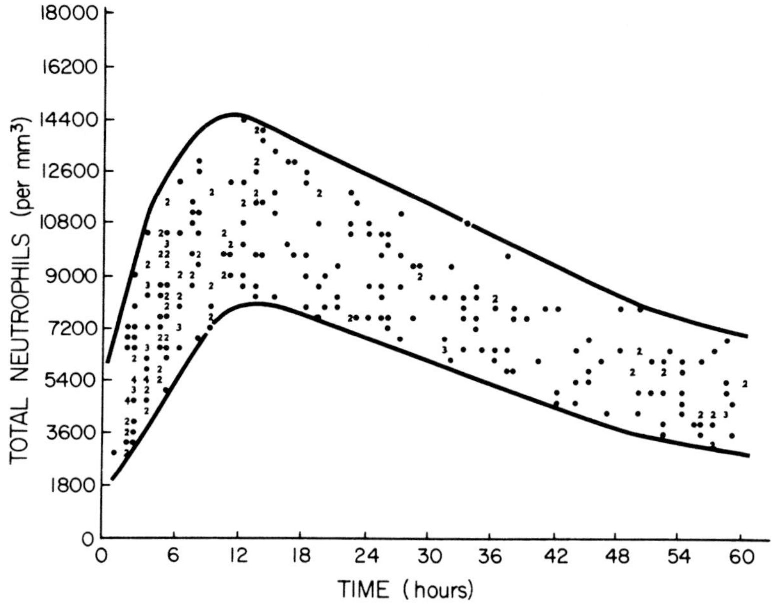

Figure 7–3. The absolute blood neutrophil concentration of normal infants during the first 60 hours after birth. Dots represent single values, and numerals represent the number of values at that same point. (From Manroe BL, Weinberg AG, Rosenfeld CR, et al: The neonatal blood count in health and disease. I. Reference values for neutrophilic cells. J Pediatr 1979;95:89.)

tion constituted a landmark; for the first time, neonatologists could determine with some confidence whether their patient had a blood neutrophil count that was low, normal, or high.

Leukocyte Counts in Preterm Infants

Several studies suggested that the normal values reported by Manroe might not be applicable to VLBW infants. One of the first of these was a report by Coulombel and coworkers of 132 neonates with CBCs obtained during their first 12 hours of life.[46] Blood was sometimes obtained from capillary samples and other times from umbilical venous or arterial catheters. All 132 infants had a clinical reason for obtaining a CBC, although this report excluded those with culture-positive evidence of bacterial infection. The researchers observed an inverse relationship between gestational age and blood neutrophil concentration.

In 1982, Lloyd and Oto reported serial leu-

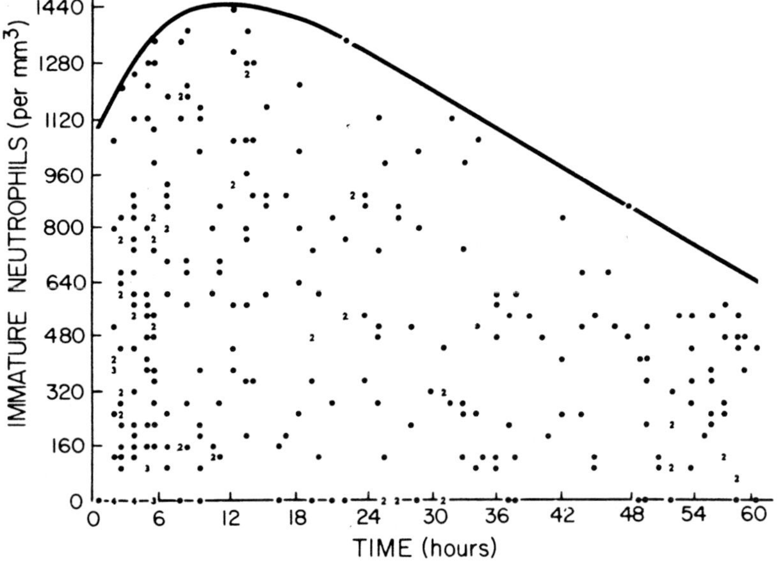

Figure 7–4. The range of absolute concentrations of immature (nonsegmented) neutrophils in the blood of normal infants during the first 60 hours after birth. Dots represent single values, and numerals represent the number of values at that same point. (From Manroe BL, Weinberg AG, Rosenfeld CR, et al: The neonatal blood count in health and disease. I. Reference values for neutrophilic cells. J Pediatr 1979;95:89.)

kocyte counts from 24 preterm infants, all less than 33 weeks' gestation.[47] They observed that the group's blood neutrophil concentrations were lower than those reported by Manroe (predominantly term infants). In 1994, Mouzinho and colleagues reported the results of 1799 blood leukocyte and differential counts obtained from 193 VLBW infants.[48] After excluding counts from neonates with perinatal and/or neonatal complications, values from normal VLBW neonates were displayed and compared with the Manroe reference ranges (Fig. 7–5). Infants of younger gestations had reference ranges for blood neutrophils that differed significantly from those of larger, older neonates. The VLBW infants had the same upper limit boundary for absolute neutrophil count of the larger, older infants, but their lower limit boundary was significantly less than the boundary of the older infants. As shown in Figure 7–5, the lower boundary for normal was set at about 1100/uL.

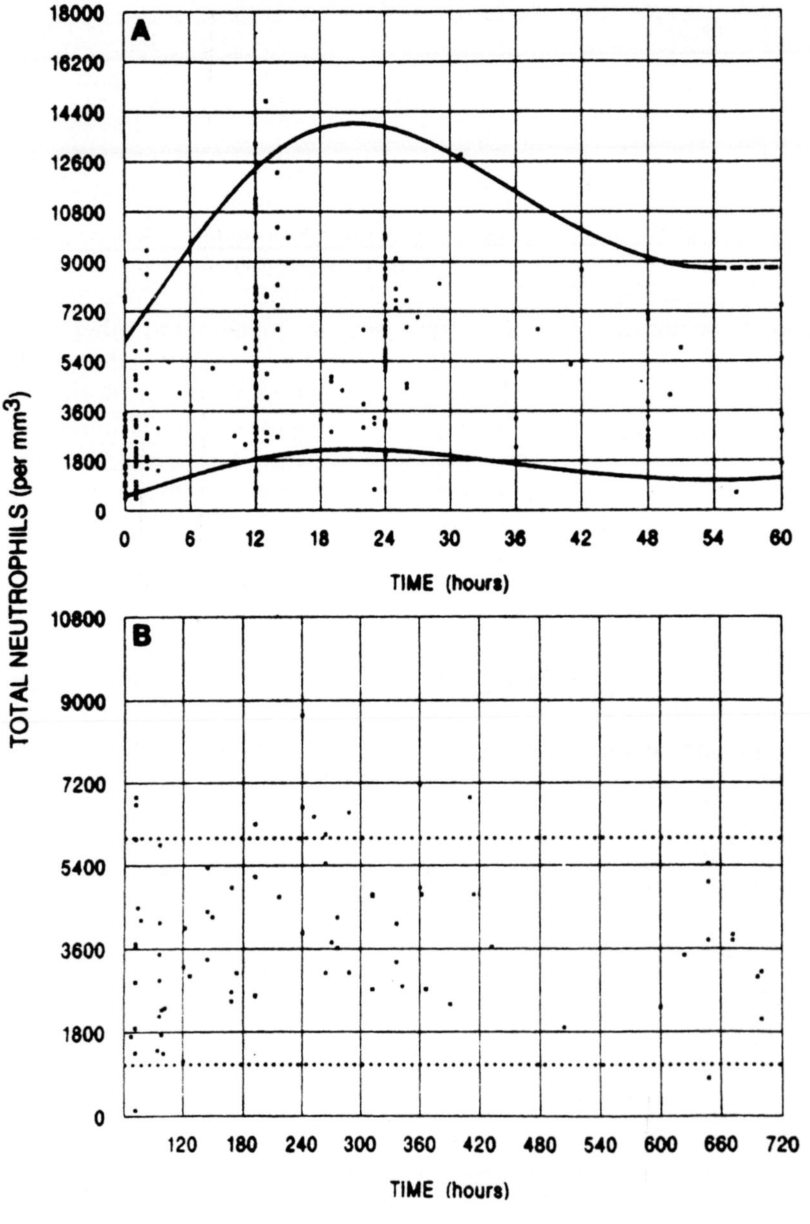

Figure 7–5. The absolute blood neutrophil concentration of very-low-birth-weight infants. Dots represent single values. (From Mouzinho A, Rosenfeld CR, Sanchez PJ, Risser R: Revised reference ranges for circulating neutrophils in very-low-birth-weight neonates. Pediatrics 1994;94:76. Copyright American Academy of Pediatrics 1994.)

Eosinophils

Eosinophilia is not a rare finding in the neonatal intensive care unit. In growing preterm infants, a nonspecific low-grade eosinophilia is so common as to warrant the label of *eosinophilia of prematurity.* Despite its frequent occurrence, the cause and the significance of this condition are uncertain.

Blood eosinophils can increase from their normally very low concentrations to very high concentrations without a concomitant increase in the concentration of other leukocytes. This attests to a unique controlling mechanism. Interleukin-5 (IL-5) probably plays a role as a regulator of eosinophil production. Evidence for this includes the reports of Lee and associates[49] and Dent and coworkers,[50] who produced transgenic mice that constitutively overexpressed IL-5. These animals had a profound eosinophilia, generally equaling 60% of circulating leukocytes. However, mice with a targeted gene disruption of IL-5 and consequently no IL-5 production (i.e., IL-5 knock-out mice) have a reduced number of blood and marrow eosinophils but have no other apparent hematologic defects.[51]

Further evidence that IL-5 regulates eosinophil production comes from studies of Rennick and colleagues[52] and Sher and associates,[53] who used specific neutralizing antibody directed against IL-5 and observed that such inhibits the eosinophilia otherwise seen in parasitized mice. More evidence that IL-5 stimulates eosinophil production comes from the work of Lu and colleagues,[54] who determined that recombinant murine IL-5 had the greatest effect of any factor tested on colony generation of eosinophilic progenitors.

Evidence that IL-5 is a regulator of eosinophil production in humans was provided by Brugnoni and associates, who reported a patient with hypereosinophilia caused by a population of T cells that secreted large amounts of IL-5.[55] Glucocorticoid administration to atopic patients, which can result in an abrupt drop in blood eosinophil concentrations, suppresses the expression of IL-5.[56] Interferon-α, which has beneficial effects in many eosinophil-mediated disorders, also inhibits IL-5 gene expression.[57] In a manner reminiscent of the actions of granulocyte colony-stimulating factor on neutrophils, IL-5 stimulates eosinophil function and eosinophil production. Walsh and coworkers observed that IL-5 enhances the adhesion of human eosinophils by a mechanism dependent on CD11/18 family of adhesions glycoproteins.[58] IL-5 does not enhance adhesion of neutrophils, however. Taken together, this information indicates that IL-5 is a significant physiologic regulator of eosinophil production and function.

Defining the normal range of eosinophils in the blood of neonates has been attempted in relatively few studies. Medoff and Barbero[59] reported that during the first 12 hours of life, absolute blood eosinophil concentrations range from 20 to 850/μL. On the basis of this report, eosinophilia on the first day of life would be defined as an absolute blood eosinophil count of more than 850/μL. Xanthou reported that, by the fifth day of life, eosinophil concentrations had a much greater range than on the first day, with values of 100 to 2500/μL.[60] By day 5, eosinophilia would be diagnosed if the count was more than 2500/μL. It is not clear whether these numbers should be used to define eosinophilia in preterm infants.

According to the reports of Medoff and Xanthou, absolute eosinophil counts of less than 20/μL on the first day of life and less than 100/μL after the first 5 days should define eosinopenia. However, the diagnosis of eosinopenia in the neonatal intensive care unit is made rarely, because so many apparently normal infants have no eosinophils identified on individual differential cell counts. In contrast to this statement, Burell suggested that a complete lack of eosinophils in neonates should be considered an abnormality.[61] He found that a complete absence of eosinophils was common in infants who fared poorly and subsequently died. He reported that on the day of death there was generally a complete absence of blood eosinophils. Bass reported that blood eosinophil concentrations declined rapidly in the presence of bacterial infection.[62]

By defining eosinophilia as blood concentration of more than 700/μL (a definition of eosinophilia sometimes used in adult medicine), Gibson and coworkers[63] found that about 75% of preterm infants develop eosinophilia. They also observed that this eosinophilia of prematurity generally occurs during a period in which an anabolic state is established. This anabolic state and the accompanying eosinophilia usually are seen in the second or third week of life, and the eosinophilia persists for many days and sometimes for weeks. Portuguez-Molavasi reported that at least one episode of eosinophilia (defined as an absolute eosinophil count of more than 1000/μL) occurred in 35% of all infants admitted to an intensive care nursery.[64] Craver reported that eosinophils can be seen in the cerebrospinal fluid weeks after intraventricular hemorrhage,[65] but the significance of this finding is not clear, and this finding did not correlate with blood eosinophil counts.

Although several reports suggest that the eosinophilia of prematurity is benign, the work of Patel and colleagues suggests otherwise.[66] In a retrospective evaluation of 261 admissions to their intensive care unit, eosinophilia (>1000 eosinophils/μL) was found in 33 patients. When age-matched pairs of patients with or without eosinophilia were compared, the development of sepsis was much higher in those who had eosinophilia. All of the 10 neonates born at 26 weeks' gestation or younger who developed eosinophilia also developed at least one nosocomial infection. Twenty of 23 infants born at more than 26 weeks' gestation who developed eosinophilia also had sepsis, compared with only 4 of 23 matched infants who did not have eosinophilia. Whether eosinophilia preceded, was concomitant with, or came after the infections is not clear, but these researchers warn of the correlation between eosinophilia and sepsis, particularly with gram-negative organisms.

What is the pathophysiology and what is the clinical significance of the eosinophilia of prematurity? Odelram and associates[67] addressed this question using the observation that high blood concentrations of eosinophils are often seen in atopic diseases. They attempted to correlate eosinophil counts in neonates with the subsequent development of atopy, determined at the age of 18 months, but little or no correlation was found. Yamamoto and coworkers[68] observed that blood eosinophils counts might be somewhat elevated in neonates who develop chronic lung disease and suggested that eosinophils might become activated in certain patients with hyaline membrane disease and that these cells could subsequently appear in the airways. This postulation accounts for the timing of the eosinophilia of prematurity and the development of chronic lung disease, but not all infants with the eosinophilia of prematurity develop chronic lung disease, and not all neonates with chronic lung disease have eosinophilia. Others have postulated that medications or constituents of hyperalimentation solutions are responsible for the eosinophilia. These issues remain unresolved.

Similarly, it is not clear whether IL-5 production or IL-5 serum concentrations are increased in neonates with eosinophilia. If Xanthou's[60] definition of eosinophilia (>2500/μL) is used instead of the usual definition used for older children or adults (1000/μL), the observer finds relatively few neonates with eosinophilia.

PLATELETS

Site of Sampling

Foley and colleagues observed that platelet counts obtained from the umbilical vein at the time of delivery are higher than counts simultaneously obtained from the umbilical artery.[69] However, Pedersen and associates reported that the umbilical vein contains a lower concentration of megakaryocytes (47/mL) than the umbilical artery (66/mL) and that circulating megakaryocytes are considerably higher in both vessels than in peripheral blood of adults (5/mL).[70] Thurlbeck and McIntosh[8] reported no difference in platelet counts drawn from umbilical arterial lines, venipunctures, or heel stick. Unlike the case for neutrophils and erythrocytes, it does not appear that any significant differences exist in platelet concentrations of blood obtained from capillary, venous, or arterial blood of neonates. It therefore is common practice to obtain platelet counts from the most convenient sampling site, without concern of a potential sampling-site difference.

Lower and Upper Limits of Normal

Healthy term and preterm infants have platelet counts in the same range (150,000 to 450,000/μL), which is also the same range found in older children and adults. Perhaps preterm infants have slightly lower platelet counts than term infants, although the overlap is considerable. For instance, Arad and coworkers[71] observed that 119 term neonates had platelet counts of 323,336 ± 106,918/μL (mean ± SD) and that 36 neonates with birth weights of less than 2 kg had counts of 283,805 ± 114,130/μL ($P < .05$). A slightly lower range of platelet counts in preterm infants was also found by Hathaway and Bonnar,[72] who concluded that a platelet count of less than 150,000/μL at any gestational age should be taken as an indication of thrombocytopenia.

A slight but statistically significant elevation in the platelet count occurs over the first weeks of life. Tan and colleagues[73] obtained daily CBCs on 105 healthy full-term neonates during their first week of life and observed an increasing platelet count. Arad and associates[71] and Sasanakul and coworkers[74] also observed a slight but significant increase in platelet count over the first weeks of life. In contrast, infants who develop hyaline membrane disease generally have declining platelet counts over the first days of life. Kohelet and colleagues[75] observed that infants with hyaline membrane disease had a platelet count nadir on day 4. They also observed that the infants with hyaline membrane disease who required the highest FIO_2 had the greatest fall in platelet count. Although the kinetic mechanism responsible was not evaluated, the fact that a fall began soon after birth suggests that accelerated platelet destruction or platelet sequestration was responsible (perhaps in pulmonary capillary beds).

Mean Platelet Volume and Platelet Distribution Width

The mean platelet volume is a measure of the average size of circulating platelets. It is analogous to the MCV used to assess erythrocyte size. The platelet distribution width (PDW), like the erythrocyte distribution width, is a measure of the distribution of various sized platelets in the circulation. Patrick and associates[76] quantified the MPV and PDW from 143 healthy newborn infants (78 term and 65 preterm). The platelet counts and MPVs were significantly higher in term infants than in preterm infants, but the PDW was significantly lower in term than in preterm infants. Arad and coworkers[71] studied 119 neonates with birth weights greater than 2 kg and 36 with lower birth weights. Like Patrick, they reported slightly higher platelet counts in the larger infants, but unlike Patrick, they observed no difference in MPV between the larger infants (MPV = 8.67 ± 1.03 fL) and smaller infants (MPV = 8.89 ± 1.10 fL).

Serial MPV measurements were obtained on 18 neonatal intensive care unit patients who developed nosocomial sepsis with coagulase-negative staphylococci.[77] The MPVs of these infants increased whether or not thrombocytopenia occurred during the infection, suggesting that an increase in platelet production accompanied the infection. Patrick and Lazarchick[76] also observed that high MPVs occur during bacterial infections in neonates. In a sample of 156 infants, they found a high specificity (95%) for an MPV of greater than 10.8 fL in detecting bacteriemia. They recommended that changes in MPV and PDW would be helpful in the diagnosis of nosocomial infections in neonates.

Reticulated Platelets

Newly synthesized platelets generally have a higher content of ribonucleic acid than platelets that have been circulating for several days. These newly produced platelets can be recognized by flow cytometric analysis after RNA staining with thiazole orange. Such platelets have been called *reticulated platelets* to reflect their similarity to reticulocytes.[78] Between 3% and 5% of the circulating platelets of healthy term neonates and LBW infants are recognized as reticulated platelets (Table 7–6). Peterec and colleagues[78] reported that infants of less than 30 weeks' gestation had reticulated platelet percentages about twice those of term infants, although with a very large variation (8.8% ± 5.1%). Joseph and associates[79] observed that adults (n = 18) had a slightly but significantly higher percentage of reticulated platelets than did healthy term neonates (n = 42). They observed no difference in reticulated platelet count between infants depending on mode of delivery.

BONE MARROW

Aspiration of cells from a neonate's bone marrow occasionally provides important information not otherwise available to the neonatol-

Table 7–6. **Normal Platelet Values for Term and Preterm Neonates**

Neonate	Platelets (per μL)*	MPV (fL)	Reticulated Plt (Percent)	Circulating Platelet Progenitors: BFU-MK	CFU-MK	Megakaryocytes
				(per 10^3 circulating mononuclear cells)		
Term infant	310,000 ± 68,000	8.7 ± 1.0	4.0 ± 2.4	663 ± 174	3267 ± 530	37 ± 8
LBW infant	290,000 ± 70,000	8.9 ± 1.1	4.6 ± 1.7		NR	
VLBW infant	275,000 ± 60,000	NR	8.8 ± 5.1		NR	

MPV, mean platelet volume; fL, femtoliter (10^{-15}L); Ptl, platelets; BFU-MK, burst-forming unit–megakaryocyte; CFU-MK, colony-forming unit–megakaryocyte; LBW, low birth weight (<2500 g); VLBW, very low birth weight (<1500 g); NR, not reported.

*All values are reported as the mean ± SD.

Adapted from Hathaway and Bonnar,[72] Arad et al,[71] Murray and Roberts,[80, 81] and Peterec et al.[78]

ogist. In cases of a persistent cytopenia, a neonatologist might want information relating to the state of production of the cells in question. As an example, a persistent thrombocytopenia could be the kinetic result of decreased platelet production or of increased platelet destruction or use. A bone marrow examination can sometimes help differentiate these conditions. In cases of decreased platelet production, the marrow contains few megakaryocytes, but in cases of increased platelet use, the proportion of megakaryocytes should be increased.

Unfortunately, bone marrow aspirates of neonates are often very diluted with peripheral blood, which can lead to misinterpretations about the state of production. This limitation can be minimized by taking care to withdraw the smallest possible marrow sample, thereby not overdiluting the specimen with peripheral blood. The limitation can be further minimized or eliminated by using a needle-biopsy technique.

Marrow is accessible from essentially any bone in the neonate. We have found that the flat part of the proximal tibia is a simple and reliable site from which to obtain a marrow sample, because this site is easy to stabilize, the landmarks are obvious, and the amount of tissue between the skin and the bone is small. Figure 7–6 illustrates the method we use for marrow

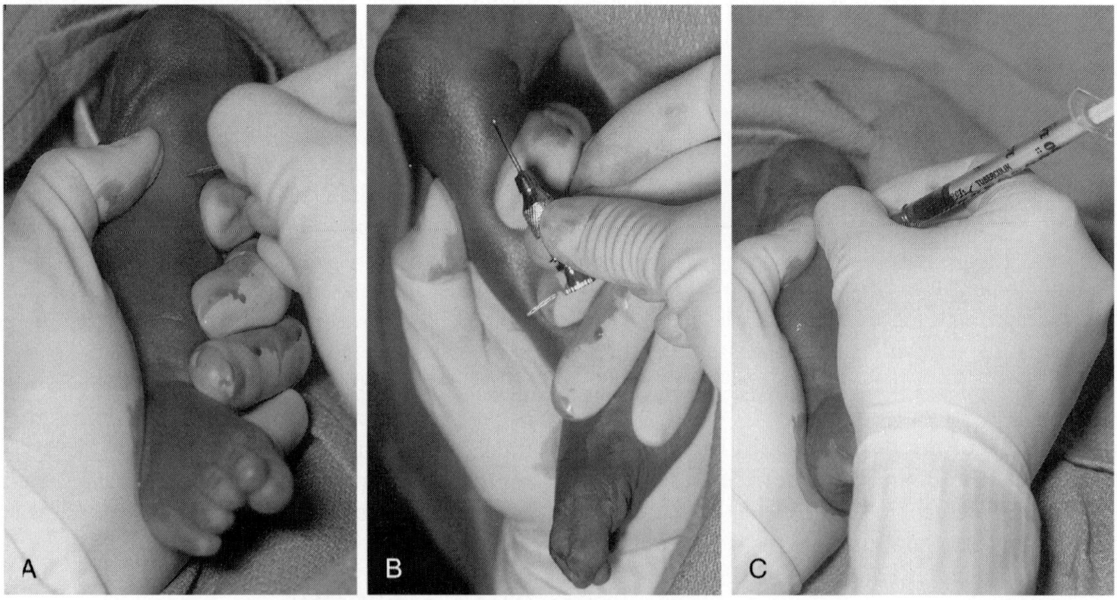

Figure 7–6. A technique for tibial bone marrow aspiration in a newborn infant. *A*, The right-handed operator holds the tibia firmly in a gloved left hand, while the right hand is used to prepare and sterilely drape the area and then to inject the 1% solution of lidocaine, which is used as a local anesthetic. *B*, A 19-gauge, ½-inch Osgood marrow needle fitted with a trocar is twisted carefully through the anesthetized periosteum, with the mid-tibia clearly between the left thumb and forefinger. *C*, The needle is correctly positioned when it is solidly in place and when, on aspiration, marrow cells enter the aspirating syringe.

aspiration of a preterm or term neonate. The (right-handed) operator holds the tibia firmly in a gloved left hand, while the right hand is used to prepare and sterilely drape the area and then to inject 1% lidocaine as a local anesthetic. My colleagues and I typically inject 0.1 mL of lidocaine (without epinephrine) subcutaneously, holding the needle in place for several seconds, after which we advance the needle and inject another 0.1 mL directly into the periosteum. A few minutes later, the operator holds the 19-gauge, ½-inch needle (Osgood marrow needle fitted with a trocar) in the right hand and twists it carefully through the anesthetized periosteum, with the mid-tibia clearly marked directly between the left thumb and forefinger. The needle is directed toward the middle of the tibial shaft to enter the middle of the marrow cavity. The needle is correctly positioned when it is solidly in place and when, on aspiration, marrow enters the aspirating syringe.

If only a microscopic analysis of the bone marrow cells is to be accomplished, only a few drops of marrow should be aspirated. If flow cytometry, a karyotype analysis, or a hematopoietic progenitor cell culture is needed, more cells are needed, and up to 0.25 mL of marrow can sometimes be aspirated. Volumes exceeding this amount, particularly in very small preterm infants, essentially always draw significant amounts of peripheral blood through the marrow and result in a dilute specimen, which may be difficult to interpret.

Little information is available on bone marrow biopsies in neonates. Although the issue of cellularity is much more accurately assessed with a biopsy specimen than with an aspirate, neonatologists have been reluctant to perform this somewhat more invasive procedure, particularly on very small and ill neonates. We have found success in obtaining marrow needle biopsies, even in the smallest preterm infants in our neonatal intensive care unit, by using a modification of the aspiration method.

After the operator feels the Osgood needle penetrating the cortex of the tibia, the stylet (trocar) is withdrawn. The hollow needle is then advanced into the marrow space an additional 3 to 5 mm. Advancing the needle without a stylet cores a small segment of marrow into the needle. A syringe is then attached to the needle hub, and minimal suction is applied for about 1

Table 7–7. **Differential Cell Counts of Nucleated Cells Aspirated from the Bone Marrow of Normal Infants at Term and from Healthy Adult Men**

Cell Types	Term Neonates (% [mean ± SD])	Healthy Adults (% [mean %, 95% CL])
Nucleated erythroid		
Proerythroblast	0.02 ± 0.06	0.6; 0.1–1.1
Basophilic erythroblast	0.24 ± 0.25	1.4; 0.4–2.4
Polychromatic erythroblast	13.06 ± 6.78	21.6; 13.1–30.1
Orthochromatic erythroblast	0.69 ± 0.73	2.0; 0.3–3.7
Neutrophils		
Neutrophil "proliferative pool"		
Promyelocytes	0.79 ± 0.91	3.3; 1.9–4.7
Myelocytes	3.95 ± 2.93	12.7; 8.5–16.9
Neutrophil "storage pool"		
Metamyelocytes	19.37 ± 4.84	15.9; 7.1–24.7
Band neutrophils	28.89 ± 7.56	12.4; 9.4–15.4
Segmented neutrophils	7.37 ± 4.64	7.4; 3.8–11.0
Myeloid:erythroid ratio	4.3:1	2.3:1; 1.1:1–3.5:1
Eosinophils	2.70 ± 1.27	3.1; 1.1–5.2
Basophils	0.12 ± 0.20	0.1
Macrophages-monocytes	0.88 ± 0.85	0.3; 0.0–0.6
Lymphocytes	14.42 ± 5.54	16.2; 8.6–23.8
Megakaryocytes	0.06 ± 0.15	0.1
Plasma cells	0.00 ± 0.02	1.3; 0.0–3.5
Undifferentiated blasts	0.31 ± 0.31	0.9; 0.1–1.7
Unknown or damaged	6.01 ± 3.02	

Data for term neonates from Rosse C, Kraemer MJ, Dillon TL, et al: Bone marrow cell populations of normal infants: the predominance of lymphocytes. J Lab Clin Med 1977;89:1228, and from Shapiro LM, Bassen FA: Sternal marrow changes during first week of life. Am J Med Sci 1941;202:341.

second. This process helps secure the small-core marrow biopsy specimen within the needle. The syringe and the attached needle are then withdrawn, and the core of marrow is pushed out of the needle by reintroducing the stylet. The core can be placed into fixative and subsequently sectioned and stained, or it can be smeared on coverglasses.

Anticipated results of bone marrow differential counts are shown in Table 7–7. Studies in 1941 and 1952 used marrow aspirates obtained from normal neonates, but this practice is no longer permitted. The normal values for marrow nucleated cell concentrations in neonates are available, but normal values for laboratory tests that were devised since 1952 (e.g., concentrations of hematopoietic progenitor cells) are not available. In modern practice, bone marrow aspirates are only performed on neonates if a clinical reason exists to do so or the patient is enrolled in a study that requires a bone marrow study. These subjects therefore are not strictly normal subjects, and the results should not be considered normal values.

References

1. Vahlquist B: Das Serumeisen. Eine padiatrischklinische und experimentelle studie. Acta Paediatrica 1941;28:1.
2. Oettinger L Jr, Mills WB: Simultaneous capillary and venous hemoglobin determinations in the newborn infant. J Pediatr 1949;35:362.
3. Mollision PL: Blood Transfusion in Clinical Medicine, 3rd ed. Oxford: Blackwell, 1951.
4. Oh W, Lind J: Venous and capillary hematocrit in newborn infants and placental transfusion. Acta Paediatr Scand 1966;55:38.
5. Moe PJ: Umbilical cord blood and capillary blood in the evaluation of anemia in erythroblastosis fetalis. Acta Paediatr Scand 1967;56:391.
6. Linderkamp O, Versmold HT, Strohhacker I, et al: Capillary-venous hematocrit differences in newborn infants. I. Relationship to blood volume, peripheral blood flow, and acid-base parameters. Eur J Pediatr 1977;127:9.
7. Rivera LM, Rudolph N: Postnatal persistence of capillary-venous differences in hematocrit and hemoglobin values in low-birth-weight and term infants. Pediatrics 1982;70:956.
8. Thurlbeck SM, McIntosh N: Preterm blood counts vary with sampling site. Arch Dis Child 1987;62:74.
9. Walker JL, Turnbull EPN: Haemoglobin and red cells in the human foetus and their relation to the oxygen content of the blood in the vessels of the umbilical cord. Lancet 1953;2:312.
10. Zaizov R, Matoth Y: Red cell values on the first postnatal day during the last 16 weeks of gestation. Am J Hematol 1976;1:275.
11. Forestier F, Daffos F, Galacteros F, et al: Hematological values of 163 normal fetuses between 18 and 30 weeks of gestation. Pediatr Res 1986;20:342.
12. McIntosh N, Kempson C, Tyler RM: Blood counts in extremely low birth weight infants. Arch Dis Child 1988;63:74.
13. Gairdner D, Marks J, Bosco JD: Blood formation in infancy: the normal bone marrow. Arch Dis Child 1952;27:124.
14. Turner CW, Luzins J, Hutcheson C: A modified harvest technique for cord blood hematopoietic stem cells. Bone Marrow Transplant 1992;10:89.
15. Yao AC, Lind J: Placental transfusion. Am J Dis Child 1974;127:128.
16. Yao AC, Lind J: Blood flow in the umbilical vessels during the third stage of labor. Biol Neonate 1974;25:186.
17. International Committee for Standardization in Haematology: Recommendations for reference method for haemoglobinometry in human blood. J Clin Pathol 1978;31:139.
18. Mugrage ER, Andresen MI: Values for red blood cells of average infants and children. Am J Dis Child 1936;51:775.
19. Guest GM, Brown EW, Wing M: Erythrocytes and hemoglobin of the blood in infancy and in childhood. Am J Dis Child 1938;56:529.
20. Waugh TR, Merchant FT, Maugham GB: Blood studies on the newborn. Am J Med Sci 1939;198:646.
21. DeMarsh QB, Alt HL, Windle WF: The effect of depriving the infant of its placental blood. JAMA 1941;116:2568.
22. Dochain J, Lemage L, Lambrechts A: Principales donnees hematologiques chez le nouveaune normal. Arch Fr Pediatr 1952;9:274.
23. Marks J Gairdner D, Roscoe JD: Blood formation in infancy. III. Cord blood. Arch Dis Child 1955;30:117.
24. Guest GM, Brown EW: Erythrocytes and hemoglobin of the blood in infancy and childhood. Am J Dis Child 1957;93:486.
25. Rooth G, Sjostedt S: Haemoglobin in cord blood in normal and prolonged pregnancy. Arch Dis Child 1957;32:91.
26. Burman D, Morris AF: Cord haemoglobin in low birthweight infants. Arch Dis Child 1974;49:382.
27. Wintrobe MM: A simple and accurate hematocrit. J Lab Clin Med 1929;15:287.
28. Waugh TF, Merchant FT, Maugham GB: Blood studies on newborn; determination of hemoglobin, volume of packed red cells, reticulocytes and fragility of erythrocytes over 9 day period. Am J Med Sci 1939;198:646.
29. Kjeldsberg CR: Principles of hematologic examination. In Lee GR, Bithell TC, Foerster J, et al (eds): Wintrobe's Clinical Hematology, 9th ed. Philadelphia: Lea & Febiger, 1993, p 8.
30. Scott-Emuakpor AB, Okolo AA, Omene JA, Ukpe SI: Normal hematological values of the African neonate. Blut 1985;51:11.
31. Michaels LA, Cohen AR, Zhao H, et al: Screening for hereditary spherocytosis by use of automated erythrocyte indexes. J Pediatr 1997;130:97;57.
32. Dessypris EN: Erythropoiesis. In Lee GR, Bithell TC, Foerster J, et al (eds): Wintrobe's Clinical Hematology, 9th ed. Philadelphia: Lea & Febiger, 1993, pp 138–141.
33. Killmann SA: On the size of normal human reticulocytes. Acta Med Scand 1964;176:529.
34. Seip M: The reticulocyte level and the erythrocyte production judged from reticulocyte studies in newborn infants during the first week of life. Acta Paediatr 1955;44:355.
35. Wegelius R: On changes in peripheral blood picture of

newborn infant immediately after birth. Acta Paediatr 1948;35:1.
36. Humbert JR, Abelson H, Hathaway WE, et al: Polycythemia in small for gestational age infants. J Pediatr 1969;75:812.
37. Zipursky A: Erythrocyte morphology in newborn infants: a new look. Pediatr Res 1977;11:843.
38. Pearson HA, McIntosh S, Rooks Y, et al: Interference phase microscopic enumeration of pitted RBC and splenic hypofunction in sickle cell anemia. Pediatr Res 1978;12:471.
39. Barnett HL Einhorn AH: Pediatrics, 15th ed. New York: Appleton-Century-Crofts, 1972, p 597.
40. Xanthou M: Leukocyte blood picture in healthy full term and premature babies during the neonatal period. Arch Dis Child 1970;45:242.
41. Zipursky A, Palko J, Milner R, et al: The hematology of bacterial infections in premature infants. Pediatrics 1976;57:829.
42. Akenzua GI, Hui YT, Milner R, et al: Neutrophil and band counts in the diagnosis of neonatal infection. Pediatrics 1974;54:38.
43. Manroe BL, Weinberg AG, Rosenfeld CR, et al: The neonatal blood count in health and disease. I. Reference values for neutrophilic cells. J Pediatr 1979;95:89.
44. Christensen RD, Rothstein G: Pitfalls in the interpretation of leukocytes counts of newborn infants. Am J Clin Pathol 1979;72:608.
45. Chervenick PA, Boggs DR, Marsh JC, et al: Quantitative studies of blood and bone marrow neutrophils in normal mice. Am J Physiol 1968;215:353.
46. Coulombel L, Dehan M, Tehernia G, et al: The number of polymorphonuclear leukocytes in relation to gestational age in the newborn. Acta Paediatr Scand 1979;68:709.
47. Lloyd BW, Oto A: Normal values for mature and immature neutrophils in very preterm babies. Arch Dis Child 1982;57:233.
48. Mouzinho A, Rosenfeld CR, Sanchez PJ, Risser R: Revised reference ranges for circulating neutrophils in very-low-birth-weight neonates. Pediatrics 1994;94:76.
49. Lee NA, McGarry MP: Larson KA, et al: Expression of IL-5 in the thymocytes/T cells leads to the development of a massive eosinophilia, extramedullary eosinophilopoiesis, and unique histopathologies. J Immunol 1997;158:1332.
50. Dent LA, Strath M, Mellor AL, Sanderson CJ: Eosinophilia in transgenic mice expressing interleukin 5. J Exp Med 1990;172:1425.
51. Hara T, Miyajima A: Function and signal transduction mediated by the interleukin 3 receptor system in hematopoiesis. Stem Cells 1996;14:605.
52. Rennick DM, Thompson-Snipes L, Coffman RL, et al: In vivo administration of antibody to interleukin-5 inhibits increased generation of eosinophils and their progenitors in bone marrow of parasitized mice. Blood 1990;76:312.
53. Sher A, Coffman RL, Hieny S, et al: Interleukin-5 is required for the blood and tissue eosinophilia but not granuloma formation induced by infection with *Schistosoma mansoni*. Proc Natl Acad Sci U S A 1990;87:61.
54. Lu L, Lin ZN, Shen RN, et al: Influence of interleukins 3, 5, and 6 on the growth of eosinophil progenitors in highly enriched human bone marrow in the absence of serum. Exp Hematol 1990;18:1180.
55. Brugnoni D, Airo R, Rossi G, et al: A case of hypereosinophilic syndrome is associated with the expansion of a CD3-CD4+ T-cell population able to secrete large amounts of interleukin-5. Blood 1996;87:1416.
56. Okayama H, Fushimi T, Shimura S, et al: Glucocorticoids suppress production and gene expression of interleukin-5 by peripheral blood mononuclear cells in atopic patients and normal subjects. J Allergy Clin Immunol 1994;93:1006.
57. Krishnaswamy G, Smith JK, Srikanth S, et al: Lymphoblastoid interferon-alpha inhibits T cell proliferation and expression of eosinophil-activating cytokines. J Interferon Cytokine Res 1996;16:819.
58. Walsh GM, Hartnell A, Wardlaw AJ: IL-5 enhances the *in vitro* adhesion of human eosinophils, but not neutrophils, in a leukocyte integrin (CD11/18)-dependent manner. Immunology 1994;71:258.
59. Medoff HS, Barbero GJ: Total blood eosinophil counts in the newborn period. Pediatrics 1950;6:737.
60. Xanthou M: Leucocyte blood picture in ill newborn babies. Arch Dis Child 1972;47:741.
61. Burell JM: A comparative study of the circulating eosinophil levels in babies. Arch Dis Child 1952;27:337.
62. Bass DA: Behavior of eosinophil leukocytes in acute inflammation. II Eosinophil dynamics during acute inflammation. J Clin Invest 1975;56:870.
63. Gibson JG Jr, Vaucher Y, Corrigan JJ: Eosinophilia in premature infants: relationship to weight gain. J Pediatr 1979;95:99.
64. Portuguez-Molavasi A, Cote-Boileau T, Aranda JV: Eosinophilia in the newborn, possible role in adverse drug reactions. Pediatr Res 1980;14:537.
65. Craver RD: The cytology of cerebrospinal fluid associated with neonatal intraventricular hemorrhage. Pediatr Pathol Lab Med 1996;16:713.
66. Patel L, Garvey B, Arnon S, Roberts IA: Eosinophilia in newborn infants. Acta Paediatr 1994;83:797.
67. Odelram H, Bjorksten B, Leander E, Kjellman NI: Predictors of atopy in newborn babies. Allergy 1995;50:585.
68. Yamamoto C, Kojima T, Hattori K, et al: Eosinophilia in premature infants: correlation with chronic lung disease. Acta Paediatr 1996;85:1232.
69. Foley ME, Clayton JK, McNicol GP: Haemostatic mechanisms in maternal, umbilical vein and umbilical artery blood at the time of delivery. Br J Obstet Gynaecol 1977;84:81.
70. Pedersen NT, Petersen S: Megakaryocytes in the foetal circulation and in cubital venous blood in the mother before and after delivery. Scand J Haematol 1980;25:5.
71. Arad ID, Alpan G, Sznajderman SD, Eldor A: The mean platelet volume in the neonatal period. Am J Perinatol 1986;3:1.
72. Hathaway WE, Bonnar J: Perinatal Coagulation. New York, Grune and Stratton, 1978.
73. Tan KL, Yip YY, Low SH: Haematological status of full-term healthy infants in the first week of life. Ann Acad Med Singapore 1985;14:572.
74. Sasanakul W, Singalavanija S, Hathirat P, et al: Hemogram in normal newborn babies with special reference to platelet count. Southeast Asian J Trop Med Public Health 1993;1(Suppl 1):237.
75. Kohelet D, Perlman M, Hanna G, Ballin A: Reduced platelet counts in neonatal respiratory distress syndrome. Biol Neonate 1990;57:334.
76. Patrick CH, Lazarchick J: The effect of bacteremia on automated platelet measurements in neonates. Am J Clin Pathol 1990;93:391.
77. O'Connor TA, Ringer KM, Gaddis ML: Mean platelet volume during coagulase-negative staphylococcal sepsis in neonates. Am J Clin Pathol 1993;99:69.
78. Peterec SM, Brennan SA, Tinder HM, et al: Reticulated platelet values in normal and thrombocytopenic neonates. J Pediatr 1996;129:269.

79. Joseph MA, Adams D, Maragos J, Saving KL: Flow cytometry of neonatal platelet RNA. J Pediatr Hematol Oncol 1966;18:277.
80. Murray NA, Roberts IA: Circulating megakaryocytes and their progenitors (BFU-MK and CFU-MK) in term and preterm neonates. Br J Haematol 1995;89:41.
81. Murray NA, Roberts IA: Circulating megakaryocytes and their progenitors in early thrombocytopenia in preterm neonates. Pediatr Res 1996;40:112.
82. Rosse C, Kraemer MJ, Dillon TL, et al: Bone marrow cell populations of normal infants: the predominance of lymphocytes. J Lab Clin Med 1977;89:1228.
83. Shapiro LM, Bassen FA: Sternal marrow changes during first week of life. Am J Med Sci 1941;202:341.

CHAPTER 8

Evaluation and Treatment of Anemia in the Neonate

Robin K. Ohls, M.D.

The newborn period marks a time when red blood cell (RBC) values can vary remarkably. Determining whether an infant is anemic becomes a challenge. Anemia can occur at various times in the neonatal period. This chapter reviews the natural adaptation to extrauterine life with respect to erythropoiesis and discusses anemias that fall into one of three general categories: hemorrhage, hemolysis, and inadequate erythrocyte production.

ERYTHROPOIETIC ADAPTATION TO EXTRAUTERINE LIFE

Erythropoiesis in utero is controlled by erythroid growth factors produced solely by the fetus. Erythropoietin (EPO) is the primary regulator of erythropoiesis in adults and appears to be the controlling factor for fetal erythropoiesis. EPO does not cross the placenta in humans, monkeys, or sheep,[1–3] and stimulation of maternal EPO production does not result in stimulation of fetal red cell production.[4] Moreover, suppression of maternal erythropoiesis by hypertransfusion does not suppress fetal erythropoiesis.[5]

The exact mechanism regulating the expression of EPO is unknown, but it is thought to be controlled by an oxygen-sensing mechanism in the liver and kidney.[6] Hypoxia and anemia stimulate erythropoiesis by stimulating mRNA transcription and EPO protein production.[7] Promoter and enhancer elements within the EPO gene are responsive to hypoxia. The liver has a decreased sensitivity to hypoxia compared with the kidney, producing one-tenth the EPO in response to stimuli.[8, 9] The liver also appears to require more prolonged hypoxia to achieve an EPO response.[10, 11] Other hormones or factors that enhance EPO production or its effects include testosterone, estrogen, thyroid hormone, prostaglandins, vitamin E, and lipoproteins.[12–19] It is not known what factors regulate the switch of EPO production from the liver to the kidney nor whether the human fetal kidney produces EPO. It appears that renal production of EPO is unnecessary for normal fetal erythropoiesis, as evidenced by the normal serum EPO concentrations and normal hematocrits of anephric fetuses.[20, 21]

EPO concentrations have been measured in cord blood during the third trimester, and they gradually increase until birth.[22–24] EPO measurements made on cord blood from infants of laboring and nonlaboring mothers[25] and from infants undergoing labor stress[26–28] may reflect hypoxic stress during labor and delivery. An increase in nucleated red blood cells is often associated with chronic in utero hypoxic stress, but acute stress (less than 24 hours) may be associated with elevated EPO concentrations alone. Serum EPO concentrations at birth normally range 5 to 100 mU/mL. For comparison, serum EPO concentrations in anemic, nonuremic adults range 300 to 400 mU/mL.[29]

Physiologic Anemia in Neonates

In term infants, improved oxygenation after birth results in decreased erythrocyte production, reflecting a natural adaptation to the extrauterine environment. The hemoglobin concentration decreases over the first 2 to 3 months of life, remains stable over the next several weeks,

Table 8–1. **Expected Hemoglobin Values (g/dL) in Low Birth Weight Infants**

Birth Weight (g)	Age (wk) 2	4	6	8	10
800–1000	16.0 (14.8–17.2)	10.0 (6.8–13.2)	8.7 (7.0–10.2)	8.0 (7.1–9.8)	8.0 (6.9–10.2)
1001–1200	16.4 (14.1–18.7)	12.8 (7.8–15.3)	10.5 (7.2–12.3)	9.1 (7.8–10.4)	8.5 (7.0–10.0)
1201–1400	16.2 (13.6–18.8)	13.4 (8.8–16.2)	10.9 (8.5–13.3)	9.9 (8.0–11.8)	9.8 (8.4–11.3)
1401–1500	15.6 (13.4–17.8)	11.7 (9.7–13.7)	10.5 (9.1–11.9)	9.8 (8.4–12.0)	9.9 (8.4–11.4)
1501–2000	15.6 (13.5–17.7)	11.0 (9.6–14.0)	9.6 (8.8–11.5)	9.8 (8.4–12.1)	10.1 (8.6–11.8)

From Stockman JA, Oski FA: Red blood cell values in low birth weight infants during the first seven weeks of life. Am J Dis Child 1980;134:945.

and then slowly rises in the fourth to sixth month of life.[30] The decrease in hemoglobin concentration has been called a *physiologic nadir* rather than true anemia.

In preterm infants, adaptive mechanisms to the extrauterine environment may be incomplete. Preterm infants generally have a drop in hemoglobin to lower values than those seen in term infants, and the nadir varies with the degree of prematurity. Hemoglobin concentrations between 7 and 8 g/dL occur commonly in preterm infants who have not undergone significant phlebotomy losses.[31, 32] Declines in hemoglobin concentration based on birth weight and gestational age can be seen in Table 8–1.

In preterm infants, decreasing central venous oxygen tensions correlate with increasing EPO concentrations.[33] A low central venous oxygen tension appears to be a sensitive indicator of anemia and represents one of the many variables that determine oxygen supply and demand. These variables also include hemoglobin concentration, red cell oxygen affinity, intravascular volume, oxygen consumption, heart rate, cardiac stroke volume, and arterial oxygenation. The hemoglobin concentration is only one of many important variables determining oxygen delivery in term and preterm infants.[34]

Pathologic Anemia in Neonates

Anemia is defined as an inability of the circulating erythrocytes to meet the oxygen demands of the tissues. In this sense, many of the conditions affecting newborn erythropoiesis represent early alterations from "normal" values, not true anemia. This issue becomes paramount in determining treatment strategies, which often involve erythrocyte transfusions. The importance of discovering the cause of an infant's altered hematocrit lies in potentially preventing a future anemic state when immediate action (usually a transfusion) is required. It is critical to gather information beyond the hemoglobin or hematocrit to define a pathologic state. For example, an infant with an hematocrit of 29% would not be considered anemic if 46 days old, born at 28 weeks' gestation, on room air with a heart rate of 130 per minute, and had an absolute reticulocyte count of 380,000 cells/μL while receiving recombinant EPO therapy. However, a term infant with the same hematocrit would be anemic if 2 hours old, with a heart rate of 190 per minute, an oxygen requirement, and a history of placental abruption around the time of delivery.

Anemia can occur at any time in life and is the result of one or more of three main causes: hemorrhage (internal or external to the body), increased destruction of red cells (hemolysis), or inadequate production of red cells. Severe anemia presenting in the first hours of life probably represents acute hemorrhage or significant hemolysis due to isoimmunization. Anemia presenting after the first day or two of life may be caused by new or continued hemorrhage, immune-mediated hemolysis, or nonimmune hemolysis. The task for the neonatologist is to decipher the evidence to prevent a further drop in red cell volume (if possible) and to treat the anemia appropriately.

HEMORRHAGE

Hemorrhage is a common cause of anemia in neonates. Blood loss can occur before birth, during delivery, or after delivery, and it can be associated with obstetric accidents and maternal hemorrhage or can be caused by internal hemorrhage or recurrent phlebotomy losses after birth. Maternal factors that increase the incidence of hemorrhage include third-trimester bleeding with placenta previa, placental abruption, vasa previa, emergency cesarean section, twin gestation, amniocentesis, and percutaneous umbilical blood sampling (PUBS).

The clinical manifestations of hemorrhage at birth depend on the extent and duration of blood loss. When acute massive blood loss has occurred, the infant is extremely pale and requires immediate volume expansion and transfusion. The hemoglobin may be normal initially or may be low and usually falls further within 6 to 8 hours after birth. Internal hemorrhage should be suspected when a 24- to 48-hour-old neonate has evidence of hypovolemic shock without signs of external blood loss.

As many as one fourth of patients admitted to newborn intensive care units have a 20% to 30% decrease in their red cell volume because of hemorrhage.[35] Blood loss can equal 50% or more of the total blood volume after a severe hemorrhage. Hemorrhagic anemia in the newborn period can be divided into three general categories: prenatal hemorrhage from the fetus into the maternal circulation or into a twin; hemorrhage due to obstetric accidents of the placenta or cord around the time of delivery; and hemorrhage due to trauma, disseminated intravascular coagulation (DIC) and sepsis, or phlebotomy loss (Table 8–2). Severe hemorrhage produces pallor and shock and must be recognized immediately to prevent significant organ damage or death.

Perinatal Practices and Blood Volume

The placenta and umbilical cord contain 75 to 125 mL of blood at term, or approximately one fourth to one third of the fetal blood volume.[36] Umbilical arteries constrict shortly after birth, but the umbilical vein remains dilated, and blood flows in the direction of gravity. Infants held below the level of the placenta can receive one half of the placental blood volume (30 to 50 mL) in 1 minute. Conversely, infants held above the placenta can lose 20 to 30 mL of blood back into the placenta per minute.[37] The blood volume of infants with early cord clamping averages 72 mL/kg, and the volume of infants with delayed cord clamping averages 93 mL/kg.

Linderkamp and colleagues compared postnatal alterations in blood viscosity, hematocrit,

Table 8–2. **Causes of Hemorrhage in the Perinatal Period**

Before delivery

- Chronic and/or acute twin-to-twin transfusion syndrome
- Chronic and/or acute fetal-maternal hemorrhage
- Hemorrhage after percutaneous umbilical blood sampling
- Traumatic amniocentesis
- Maternal trauma
- Trauma after external cephalic version

During delivery

- Placental abruption
- Placenta previa
- Vasa previa
- Trauma or incision of placenta during cesarean section
- Ruptured normal or abnormal (varices, aneurysms) umbilical cord
- Cord or placental hematoma
- Velamentous insertion of the cord
- Nuchal cord

During or after delivery

- Subgaleal hemorrhage
- Cephalohematoma
- Intraventricular or intrahemorrhage (prematurity, trauma, isoimmune thrombocytopenia)
- Hemorrhage associated with disseminated intravascular coagulation or sepsis
- Organ trauma (liver, spleen, adrenal, renal)
- Pulmonary hemorrhage
- Iatrogenic blood loss (phlebotomy, central line accidents, arterial line accidents)

plasma viscosity, red cell aggregation, and red cell deformability in the first 5 days of postnatal life in term neonates with early (less than 10 seconds) and late (3 minutes) cord clamping.[38] The residual placental blood volume decreased from 52 ± 8 mL/kg of neonatal body weight after early cord clamping to 15 ± 4 mL/kg after later cord clamping. The neonatal blood volume was 50% higher in the late cord-clamped infants than in the early cord-clamped infants.

Preterm infants have slightly larger blood volumes (89 to 105 mL/kg) because of an increased plasma volume. At 30 weeks' gestation, one half of the approximately 120 mL/kg total blood volume of the fetoplacental circulation is in the fetus.[39] Preterm infants commonly experience rapid cord clamping resulting in a decreased blood volume. This occurs because of the urgency in initiating resuscitative measures.

Fetomaternal Hemorrhage

Maternal and fetal circulating cells may at various times cross the placental barrier. Fetal contamination of the maternal circulation can occur before delivery, as evidenced by studies of maternal blood group immunization. About 50% to 75% of pregnancies are associated with some degree of fetomaternal hemorrhage (FMH). This event is uncommon in the first trimester. Volumes of fetal transplacental transfer are relatively small, usually on the order of 0.01 to 0.1 mL, but occasionally are much greater. About 1 pregnancy in 400 is associated with a fetal transplacental hemorrhage of 30 mL or greater, and about 1 pregnancy in 2000 is associated with a fetal transplacental hemorrhage of 100 mL or more.[40]

The overall risk of Rh immunization occurring in an Rh-incompatible pregnancy is 16% if the fetus is Rh positive and ABO compatible with its mother. This risk decreases to 1.5% if the fetus is Rh positive and ABO incompatible. Fetal transfer of cells to the mother occurs during abortions as well (about a 2% incidence of such transfer with spontaneous abortion and a 4% to 5% rate if induced).[41]

Because fetal hemoglobin is resistant to acid elution, cells containing fetal hemoglobin can be distinguished from cells containing hemoglobin A (Hb A). The Kleihauer-Betke stain (KB stain) of peripheral maternal blood uses this characteristic of fetal hemoglobin to detect fetal cells in the maternal circulation.[42] Results from mothers with increased fetal hemoglobin synthesis (i.e., sickle cell disease, thalassemia, and hereditary persistence of fetal hemoglobin) are not reliable, and other measures should be taken to detect FMH in these cases.

The diagnosis of FMH can also be missed when the mother and infant are ABO incompatible. In these cases, the fetal cells are rapidly cleared from the maternal circulation by maternal anti-A or anti-B antibodies.

Severe FMH occurs in 1 of 1000 deliveries and has been associated with decreased fetal movements and a fetal sinusoidal heart rate pattern.[43] Giacoia reviewed these variables to determine if they correlated with the volume of FMH.[44] Fetal movements for a period ranging between 24 hours and 7 days were absent in 17 of 134 cases evaluated. In this group, six infants survived, five were stillborn, and five died in the neonatal period. A sinusoidal heart rate pattern was reported in 21 cases and was associated with decreased fetal movement in 40% of the cases. No significant difference was found between the cases with a FMH of more than 200 mL and those with hemorrhage of less than 200 mL.

Low neonatal red cell volumes are associated with a maternal history of vaginal bleeding, placenta previa or abruption, nonelective cesarean section, and deliveries associated with cord compression.[35] Significant FMH has been described after trauma,[45] and fetal hemorrhage into the placenta has been associated with placental chorioangioma.[46]

Infants in whom a significant hemorrhage is suspected need rapid evaluation and treatment. The infant with massive hemorrhage presents with pallor and tachypnea, although usually without an oxygen requirement. Hemoglobin concentrations can be extremely low at birth, between 4 and 6 g/dL.[43] A significant metabolic acidosis is often present as a result of hypoperfusion.

Other causes of pallor in the newborn period can be excluded after the infant is stable. Infants with asphyxia and infants with chronic anemia due to hemolysis can also present with pallor. These diagnoses can be distinguished from acute hemorrhage based on differences in clinical signs and symptoms (Table 8–3). The clinical picture of an infant with chronic blood loss is usually mild, and infants respond to conserva-

Table 8–3. **Differentiation of Asphyxia, Hemorrhage, and Hemolysis in a Pale Newborn Infant**

Affected Organ System	Asphyxia	Severe Acute Hemorrhage	Hemolysis
Neurologic	Abnormal transition period; hypotonic, decreased arousal state; seizures in first days of life	Normal or hyperalert or hyperirritable ("catecholamine response")	Normal
Respiratory	Respiratory distress, O_2 requirement	Tachypnea; no O_2 requirement	Normal (respiratory distress with hydrops)
Cardiovascular	Normal to bradycardia	Tachycardia, hypotension	May vary from normal to presence of congestive heart failure and hydrops, depending on the degree of anemia
Hematologic	Hematocrit and hemoglobin levels remain stable over time; may develop thrombocytopenia and disseminated intravascular coagulation from hypoxic injury to marrow	Drop in hematocrit or hemoglobin level	Anemic from birth Hepatosplenomegaly Jaundice Positive Coombs' test

tive therapy with iron alone. Asphyxiated infants are pale and floppy, and they may have poor peripheral circulation. The hemoglobin concentration is stable but may decrease if DIC and internal bleeding occur.

Twin-to-Twin Transfusion Syndrome

Twin-to-twin transfusion syndrome (TTS) is a complication of monochorionic twin gestations, occurring in 5% to 30% of these pregnancies.[47] The perinatal mortality rate can be as high as 70% to 100%, depending on severity and timing of presentation. TTS involves placental anastomoses that allow transfer of blood from one twin to the other.

Four types of placentas can occur with twin gestations: diamnionic-dichorionic, fused diamnionic-dichorionic, fused diamnionic-monochorionic, and fused monoamnionic-monochorionic. Monochorionic twins are monozygous, and 70% of monozygous twin pregnancies have monochorionic placentas.[48] Vascular anastomoses are present in almost all instances of monochorionic placentas, but not all of those develop TTS.

Acute TTS generally results in twins of similar size, although with hemoglobin concentrations that vary by more than 5 g/dL.[49] In the chronic form of TTS, one twin becomes progressively anemic and growth retarded, whereas the recipient twin becomes polycythemic, macrosomic, and sometimes hypertensive. Both infants can develop hydrops fetalis; the donor twin becomes hydropic from profound anemia, whereas the recipient twin becomes hydropic from congestive heart failure and hypervolemia. Because of significant differences in blood volume, renal blood flow, and urine output, the donor twin experiences oligohydramnios, and the recipient twin experiences polyhydramnios.

The diagnosis of chronic TTS can be made by serial prenatal ultrasound scans measuring cardiomegaly, discordant amniotic fluid production, and fetal growth discrepancy of more than 20% and by measuring hemoglobin concentration differences of greater than 5 g/dL between infants.[47] After birth, the donor twin often requires transfusions and can experience neutropenia, hydrops from severe anemia, growth retardation, congestive heart failure, and hypoglycemia. The recipient twin is often sicker and can suffer from hypertrophic cardiomyopathy, congestive heart failure, polycythemia, hyperviscosity, respiratory difficulties, hypocalcemia, and hypoglycemia. The risk of antenatally acquired neurologic cerebral lesions is 20% to 30% in both twins,[47] and the incidence of neurologic morbidities after the intrauterine death of one of the fetuses averages 20% to 25%. Morbidities include multiple cerebral infarctions, hypoperfusion syndromes from hypotension, and periventricular leukomalacia. Long-term neurologic follow-up is indicated for all TTS survivors.

Treatment consists of close monitoring and reduction amniocenteses to decrease uterine stretch and prolong the pregnancy. The average survival rates with serial reduction amniocenteses range from 40% to 70%.[50] Selective feticide of the hydropic twin has also resulted in the survival of the healthier twin in some studies.[51] Treatment in utero has occurred during some pregnancies using laser surgery to ablate bridging vessels, resulting in improved survival rates of up to 50%, with approximately 70% of the pregnancies having at least one survivor.[52, 53] In pregnancies in which one of the twins dies, the survival rate without morbidity in the surviving twin is approximately 50%.[54]

Obstetric Accidents and Placental Anomalies

Obstetric accidents occur infrequently but can be a significant source of blood loss. Obstetric complications include placenta previa and placental abruption, incision or tearing of the placenta during cesarean section, and cord evulsion of normal or abnormal umbilical cords. Neonates can experience significant blood loss back into the placenta (i.e., fetoplacental hemorrhage). Moreover, placental anomalies, including multilobed placenta and placental chorioangiomas, can be a source of hemorrhage during the perinatal period.[46]

Placenta Abruption and Placenta Previa

Placental abruption is premature separation of the placenta from the uterus and occurs in 3 to 6 cases per 1000 live births. Severe fetal growth restriction, prolonged rupture of membranes, chorioamnionitis, hypertension (before pregnancy and pregnancy induced), cigarette smoking, advanced maternal age, and male fetal gender are risk factors for placental abruption.[55] The incidence increases with decreasing gestation, and mortality ranges from 0.8 to 2 deaths per 1000 births,[56] which equates to 15% to 20% of deliveries in which significant abruption occurs.

Placenta previa occurs when part or all of the placenta overlies the cervical os. Women with a history of previous cesarean birth and increased parity are at increased risk of having a pregnancy complicated by placenta previa.[57] Cigarette smoking is associated with a 2.6- to 4.4-fold increased risk of placenta previa.[58]

Infants born after placental abruption may be anemic but may also present with signs of hypoxia. For these infants, it is important to monitor changes in hematocrit and neurologic signs. Infants born to mothers with placenta previa can also be anemic. The need for postnatal transfusions in the infants is generally associated with the volume of maternal hemorrhage. When there is evidence of placental abruption, placenta previa, or unusual vaginal bleeding, the infant's hemoglobin should be measured at birth and again at 12 to 24 hours. A KB stain should also be performed on maternal blood to determine if fetal hemorrhage occurred. Monitoring mothers who have a history of second- or third-trimester bleeding with Doppler flow ultrasound may decrease the incidence of anemia and fetal loss by anticipating fetal hemorrhage associated with placental abnormalities.[57]

Cord Rupture and Hematomas of the Cord

Excess traction on a shortened or abnormally formed umbilical cord can result in cord rupture, usually occurring on the fetal side. Abnormalities in cord formation include cord aneurysms, varices, and cysts. Cord infections (funisitis) can increase the risk for cord rupture by weakening the cord. Infants born precipitously may also be at increased risk for hemorrhage because of a ruptured cord.

Subamniotic hematomas can occur when chorionic vessels rupture near the cord insertion. Most subamniotic hematomas are the result of excessive traction on a normal or shortened umbilical cord and are not noticed until after delivery. Hematomas of the cord occur infrequently (1 of 5000 to 6000 deliveries) but can be a cause of fetal blood loss and can be associated with significant perinatal mortality.[59] Intrauterine death may occur because of compression of the umbilical vein and arteries by the hematoma. Cord hematomas can result from trauma from PUBS and can be associated with a high levels of maternal α-fetoprotein. Hematomas of the cord can be accurately diagnosed in utero by ultrasound and differentiated from other lesions of the placenta and cord.[60] The lesion can be associated with poor fetal growth and FMH.

Velamentous Insertion

Velamentous insertion of the umbilical cord occurs in approximately 0.5% to 2% of pregnancies.[61] In velamentous insertion, the umbilical cord enters the membranes distant from the placenta. Blood vessels are therefore unprotected by Wharton's jelly and are more likely to tear. Rupture of anomalous vessels in the absence of traction or trauma can occur even if the cord itself attaches centrally or paracentrally. The fetal mortality remains very high in this condition, often because detection by routine ultrasound is rare. Eddleman and coworkers observed that targeted sonographic examination of the placental site of umbilical cord insertion could reveal abnormal placental cord insertions but that distinguishing the specific type of abnormal insertion would likely require the use of color Doppler imaging.[62]

Vasa Previa

Prenatal diagnosis of vasa previa (i.e., anomalous vessels overlying the internal os of the cervix) can occur with transvaginal color Doppler and should be suspected in any case of antepartum or intrapartum hemorrhage. Although uncommon (1 per 3000 deliveries), the perinatal death rate is high, ranging from 33% to 100% when undetected before delivery. Infants are often stillborn.[63]

Fetoplacental Hemorrhage

Blood loss into the placenta is a common cause for anemia in neonates. A large residual volume of blood remains in the placenta, and blood continues to flow in the direction of gravity after birth. Fetoplacental hemorrhage can occur when the infant is held above the placenta after birth, and infants born by cesarean section therefore have smaller blood volumes than those born vaginally.[64]

Infants can lose 10% to 20% of their total blood volume when born with a tight nuchal cord.[65] Tight nuchal cords allow blood to be pumped through umbilical arteries while constricting flow through the umbilical vein.

Birth Trauma

Subgaleal Hemorrhage

Blood loss into the subgaleal space can occur during difficult deliveries requiring instrument assistance, such as face presentation, occiput posterior presentations, and shoulder dystocias. Subgaleal hematomas are potentially life-threatening events and must be recognized as early as possible to prevent significant morbidity or mortality. These hematomas occur when emissary or "bridging" veins are torn. Blood accumulates into a large potential space between the galea aponeurotica (i.e., epicranial aponeurosis) and the periosteum of the skull. The subgaleal space extends from the orbital ridge to the base of the skull and can easily accommodate more than 85 mL/kg of blood, or an infant's entire blood volume.

Subgaleal hematomas may form because of preexisting risk factors (e.g., coagulopathy, asphyxia), but vacuum extraction itself predisposes an infant to subgaleal bleeding. The presence of a ballotable fluid collection in dependent regions of the infant's head, coupled with signs of hypovolemia in a neonate, raise the possibility of subgaleal bleeding.[66] Treatment of symptomatic infants requires restoration of blood volume and control of bleeding. Exsanguination due to subgaleal hemorrhage has been reported, and mortality is high if the hemorrhage goes unrecognized. A formula predicting the volume of blood loss has been developed: for every 1-cm increase in head circumference that occurs, 38 mL of blood has been lost.[67]

Limiting the frequency and duration of vacuum assistance in high-risk infants may decrease the incidence of subgaleal hematomas. Of 134 infants undergoing vacuum extraction, 28 had scalp trauma, and only one had subgaleal, subdural, and subarachnoid hemorrhage.[68] The duration of vacuum application is thought to be the best predictor of scalp injury, followed by duration of second stage of labor and paramedian cup placement. In another study, of those infants with reported subgaleal hemorrhages, 80% to 90% had vacuum or instrument-assisted delivery.[69] A cesarean delivery does not preclude the use of vacuum or forceps, and significant hemorrhage can still occur with this route of delivery.

Intracranial Hemorrhage

Infants born prematurely are at risk for intraventricular hemorrhage (IVH), and the risk increases with decreasing gestation.[70] Other risk factors for IVH include duration of painful labor, duration of antibiotic therapy, and maternal age.[71] The incidence and severity of IVH and periventricular leukomalacia increase with premature rupture of membranes and preterm labor, especially if infection is present.[72]

Infants with IVH may be asymptomatic or may develop signs such as apnea and bradycardia, lethargy, seizures, hypoglycemia, acidosis, anemia, or a bulging fontanelle. The volume of blood loss can be as great as 10% to 15% of the total blood volume.[73] Treatment consists of supportive care, including maintaining adequate intravascular volume and oxygen delivery, supporting oxygenation and ventilation, and maintaining blood glucose concentrations within the normal range. Erythrocyte transfusion may be indicated for severely affected preterm infants.

Infants with alloimmune thrombocytopenia are at increased risk for intracranial hemorrhage. Alloimmune thrombocytopenia results from platelet-antigen incompatibility between the mother and fetus and occurs in 1 or 2 of 1000 live births.[74] Infants present with thrombocytopenia. Between 10% and 20% of neonates with platelet alloimmunization have intracranial hemorrhages; one half occur in utero. The risk for intracranial hemorrhage is increased in newborns with an affected sibling who had an antenatal intracranial hemorrhage, and the second affected neonate generally has more severe disease than the first.[74] Treatment includes platelet transfusions and intravenous immunoglobulin (IVIG). Treatment of fetal thrombocytopenia includes maternal IVIG administration, maternal steroid administration, and fetal platelet transfusions.[75]

Infants born to mothers using crack cocaine are at risk for anemia from abruption and intracranial hemorrhage. Prenatal cocaine exposure increases the risk of maternal hypertension, placental abruption, and spontaneous abortion. Infants can experience in utero growth retardation, cephalic hemorrhage, and fetal edema.[76] However, other workers have investigated the incidence of intracranial hemorrhage with cocaine use and found it to bc similar to a population matched for prematurity.[77]

Internal Hemorrhage

Anemia appearing after the first 24 hours of life in a nonjaundiced infant may be the result of internal hemorrhage. In addition to birth trauma causing visible hemorrhages, such as cephalohematomas, excessive bruising, and subgaleal hemorrhages, internal hemorrhage can occur after a traumatic delivery. Breech deliveries can be associated with renal, adrenal, or splenic hemorrhage into the retroperitoneal space. Delivery of large infants, such as infants born to diabetic mothers, can also result in organ damage and hemorrhage. Infants with overwhelming sepsis can develop DIC and hemorrhage into liver, adrenal glands, and lungs.

Adrenal Hemorrhage

Adrenal hemorrhage can result in anemia but may also result in circulatory collapse because of the loss of organ function. The incidence of adrenal hemorrhage is 1.7 cases per 1000 births.[78] Adrenal hemorrhage can also affect surrounding organs. Intestinal obstruction and kidney dysfunction have been reported in infants with adrenal hemorrhage.[79]

The diagnosis can be made using ultrasonography, which identifies calcifications and cystic masses. Adrenal hemorrhage can be distinguished from renal vein thrombosis by ultrasound, because renal vein thrombosis generally results in a solid mass. Occasionally, both entities can coexist.[80] Infants with renal vein thrombosis can have gross or microscopic hematuria and may develop renal failure and hypertension.

Adrenal hemorrhage can be caused by trauma. Infectious causes resulting in DIC and hemorrhage have also been reported. Mostoufizadeh and colleagues reported five cases of echovirus type 11 diagnosed in neonates born in the Boston area during a single season.[81] Four of the mothers experienced gastroenteritis with fever and abdominal cramps late in the third trimester of pregnancy. Affected infants experienced jaundice, hepatosplenomegaly, hypotonia, and progressive hepatic failure. Massive hepatic and adrenal hemorrhage and necrosis, with evidence of a consumptive coagulopathy, were found at autopsy. Echovirus type 11 was isolated from various sites before and after death.

Hepatic, Splenic, and Other Soft Tissue Hemorrhages

The neonatal liver is prone to iatrogenic rupture, resulting in a high morbidity and mortality.[82] Infants can be asymptomatic until the liver ruptures and hemoperitoneum occurs. This can occur in term and preterm infants.[83] Surgical intervention and tamponade have been reported to save some infants, but the mortality remains high.[82]

Splenic rupture can result from birth trauma or from distention by extramedullary hematopoiesis, such as that seen in erythroblastosis fetalis. Abdominal distention and discoloration, scrotal swelling, and pallor are clinical signs of splenic rupture and are seen with adrenal hemorrhage or hepatic rupture.[84]

Other rare causes of hemorrhage in the neonate include hemangiomas of the gastrointestinal tract,[85] vascular malformations of the skin, and hemorrhage into soft tumors such as giant sacrococcygeal teratomas.

Disseminated Intravascular Coagulation and Sepsis

Hemorrhage can occur because of overwhelming sepsis, and is generally the result of DIC and consumption of clotting factors. Infections caused by group B streptococci (GBS), *Escherichia coli*, and other organisms can progress to septic shock and DIC. Viral pathogens such as cytomegalovirus (CMV), toxoplasmosis, herpes simplex, and others can cause a hemolytic anemia but may also be a cause of overwhelming sepsis and DIC.[81]

Hemorrhage From Abnormal Clotting Mechanisms or Iatrogenic Causes

Infants can develop hemorrhagic anemia because of abnormalities in hemostasis. Male infants with factor 8 and 9 deficiency can bleed excessively after circumcision, and infants with factor 13 deficiency can have continual oozing of blood from the umbilical stump. These infants require further evaluation of their bleeding, which is detailed in Chapter 12.

Infants admitted to the newborn intensive care unit are at risk for external hemorrhage from accidental blood loss from central lines. Line connections in these infants should be constantly monitored to make sure that connections do not become displaced, because exsanguination can occur. Preterm infants can also develop anemia because of excessive phlebotomy losses, especially during the first few weeks of hospitalization, when losses can equal or exceed 10% of the infant's total blood volume per day. Blood removed for laboratory tests should be recorded on the infant's flow sheet, and every effort should be made to limit unnecessary laboratory tests.

Diagnosis and Management of Hemorrhage

The diagnosis of hemorrhage in the newborn infant can at times be difficult. Infants can present with a spectrum of clinical characteristics, depending on the degree of hypovolemia and anemia and on the timing of blood loss. Table 8–4 describes the differences seen in acute and chronic blood loss. Infants with acute hemorrhage are pale and tachycardic. They may be neurologically normal, hyperalert, or may appear stunned, with a wide-eyed gaze. Infants who present with hypotension usually have had significant blood loss and are at risk for shock and death. Infants are often tachypneic but do

Table 8–4. **Differentiation of Acute From Chronic Blood Loss in the Neonate**

Characteristic	Acute Blood Loss	Chronic Blood Loss
General appearance	Pale, hyperalert, "stunned" gaze	Pale, normal neurologic examination
Cardiovascular system	Tachycardic, weak pulses, low blood pressure	Normal; rarely may have congestive heart failure with hepatomegaly; normal or increased blood pressure
Respiratory system	Tachypneic, no supplemental oxygen requirement	Normal; rarely may be tachypneic with a supplemental oxygen requirement if congestive heart failure is present
Hematologic system		
Hemoglobin	May be normal; drops over 24 hours	Low at birth
Morphology	Macrocytic normochromic (normal)	Microcytic hypochromic
Iron	Normal	Low
Course	Promptly treat hypovolemia; may need rapid volume expansion to prevent shock, DIC, and death	Usually uneventful hospital course; may need treatment for congestive heart failure and hydrops
Treatment	Volume expansion with isotonic fluid and PRBCs, FFP, and platelets; iron therapy later; EPO therapy may be appropriate to enhance erythropoiesis	Initiate iron therapy; PRBC transfusion rarely needed; EPO therapy may be appropriate to enhance erythropoiesis

DIC, disseminated intravascular coagulation; EPO, erythropoietin; FFP, fresh frozen plasma; PRBCs, packed red blood cells.

not improve with oxygen administration. The tachypnea results from the metabolic acidosis seen with underperfusion. Hemoglobin concentrations may be normal initially but drop over the first 6 to 8 hours. Iron stores are normal at birth, and the RBC morphology shows typical normochromic, macrocytic newborn cells.

Rapid resuscitative measures can be lifesaving for infants with a significant acute hemorrhage. The *ABCs* of newborn resuscitation are followed, which include drying, suctioning the mouth and nose, stimulating the infant, and administering oxygen. In a neonate who has extreme pallor, further resuscitative measures are required to establish rapid intravenous access. A 5- or 8-French umbilical catheter (or orogastric tube if an umbilical catheter is not available) should be inserted into the umbilical vein until blood return occurs (usually 4 to 6 cm). A sample of blood is sent for hemoglobin determination, blood type, and crossmatch. Volume resuscitation with available fluid, generally normal saline, is given as a 20 mL/kg bolus. The volume can be given even if the cause of the pallor has not yet been determined, because some infants present with anemia and asphyxia, such as infants born after placental abruption. Infants with acute blood loss often show dramatic improvement, whereas those with internal hemorrhage, DIC, or subgaleal hemorrhage may remain limp and unresponsive.

After the diagnosis of hypovolemia due to acute blood loss has been established, a repeat fluid bolus should be given. If available, type O, Rh-negative packed red blood cells (PRBCs) should be infused rapidly. Infants with acute blood loss have lost platelets and plasma clotting factors along with red cells. Further resuscitative measures should therefore include evaluation of the infant's bleeding status and replacement with fresh frozen plasma and platelets as needed.

Infants who are anemic at birth from chronic blood loss may be asymptomatic. Their hemoglobin concentration is low, and the peripheral smear often reveals microcytic, hypochromic cells, indicating iron deficiency. Infants with significant chronic blood loss (e.g., the donor twin in TTS) can present in congestive heart failure and hydrops. Therapy includes supporting cardiac function with pressors and diuretics as needed, performing pleurocenteses if significant effusions are present to improve lung expansion, and maintaining oxygen delivery to tissues.

Iron therapy is indicated for both groups of infants. Infants with acute blood loss receive iron in the form of transfused blood, but the replacement usually does not equal the amount of iron lost. Infants who have experienced chronic blood loss are iron deficient at birth, and replacement therapy should start soon at 6 mg/kg/day of ferrous sulfate. Administration of EPO to enhance erythropoiesis may be appropriate for some infants, especially those born prematurely.

HEMOLYSIS

Hemolytic anemia is commonly seen in the newborn period and can be caused by a variety of factors intrinsic and extrinsic to the RBC. Regardless of cause, the fundamental characteristic of all hemolytic anemias is a reduction in the lifespan of RBCs. The average life span for a neonatal RBC is 60 to 90 days, approximately one-half to two-thirds that of an adult RBC.[86] When neonatal red cells are transfused into adults, they exhibit a shortened life span because of alterations intrinsic to the neonatal red cell. In contrast, cells transfused from adult donors appear to survive normally in newborns.[87] Remarkably shorter red cell life spans (35 to 50 days) are found with increasing prematurity. The shortened red cell life span of the preterm and term neonate may be explained by some of the characteristics specific to newborn cells, including a rapid decline in intracellular enzyme activity and ATP, loss of membrane surface area, decreased levels of intracellular carnitine, and increased mechanical fragility and susceptibility to peroxidation.[88–91]

Hemolysis in the newborn period is most commonly accompanied by jaundice and may be associated with hepatosplenomegaly. Some of the more common causes of hemolysis in the newborn period are listed in Table 8–5. Hemolysis can be classified into three general categories: isoimmunization, congenital defects of the red cell, and acquired defects of the red cell.

Isoimmune Hemolytic Anemias

Red cell antigens in the ABO, MN, Rh, Kell, Duffy, and Vel systems are well developed in early intrauterine life.[92] They are easily demonstrated in the fifth to seventh gestational week and remain constant through the remainder of intrauterine development. Other antigens, such as the Lutheran and Xg^A systems, develop more slowly but are present at birth. Lewis antigens are lacking in the neonate. By approximately 2 years of age, the child's red cell and plasma

Table 8–5. **Causes of Hemolysis in the Newborn Period**

Immune-mediated	Congenital erythrocyte enzyme defects
Rh incompatibility (anti-D antibody)	Glucose-6-phosphate dehydrogenase (G6PD) deficiency
ABO incompatibility	Pyruvate kinase (PK) deficiency
Minor blood group incompatibility: c, C, e, G, FGya (Duffy), Kell group, Jka, MNS, Vw	Hexokinase deficiency
Drug-induced (penicillin, α-methyl DOPA, cephalothin)	Glucose phosphate isomerase deficiency
Maternal autoimmune hemolytic anemia	Pyrimidine 5′-nucleotidase deficiency
Infection	Hemoglobin defects
Bacterial sepsis (*Echerichia coli*, Group B *Streptococcus*)	Alpha-thalassemia syndromes
Parvovirus B19 (can present with hydrops fetalis)	Gamma-thalassemia syndromes
Congenital syphilis	Alpha and gamma chain structural anomalies
Congenital malaria	Macro- and microangiopathic hemolysis
Congenital TORCH infections (toxoplasmosis, cytomegalovirus, rubella, disseminated herpes)	Cavernous hemangiomas
Other congenital viral infections	Arteriovenous malformations
Disseminated intravascular coagulation	Renal artery stenosis or thrombosis
Hereditary erythrocyte membrane disorders	Other large vessel thrombi
Spherocytosis	Severe coartaction of the aorta
Elliptocytosis	Severe vavular stenoses
Stomatocytosis	Other causes
Pyropoikylocytosis	Galactosemia
Other membrane disorders	Lysosomal storage diseases
	Prolonged metabolic acidosis from metabolic disease (amino acid and organic acid disorders)
	Transfusion reactions
	TAR syndrome (thrombocytopenia with absent radii)
	Drug-induced hemolysis (valproic acid)

antigens have developed a pattern that is seen throughout the remainder of life.[93]

The A and B antigens are present early in utero, and A and B isoagglutinin production occurs much later.[94] By 30 to 34 weeks' gestation, however, about 50% of infants have some measurable anti-A or anti-B antibodies. The fetal production of such antibodies is not related to maternal ABO blood type. Intrauterine exposure to gram-negative organisms whose antigens are chemically related to those of blood groups A and B is a potent stimulus for the development of these antibodies.

Rh and ABO Isoimmunization

Isoimmunization due to Rh or ABO incompatibility is the most common cause of hemolytic disease in the newborn period and is discussed in Chapter 10. ABO incompatibility represents a spectrum of hemolytic disease in neonates, ranging from little or no evidence of erythrocyte sensitization, but evidence of hemolysis, to severe hemolytic disease in which erythrocyte sensitization is marked.[95]

Other Isoimmune Anemias

Anti-Kell anemic fetuses have lower reticulocyte counts and total serum bilirubin levels than do comparable anti-D anemic fetuses.[96] The level of hemolysis caused by anti-Kell antibodies is less than that caused by anti-D antibodies, but fetal erythropoiesis appears blunted, suggesting that Kell sensitization results in suppression of fetal erythropoiesis and in hemolysis. Vaughan and coworkers evaluated the effects of anti-Kell antibodies on erythroid progenitors.[97] They found the growth of Kell-positive erythroid progenitor cells from cord blood was markedly inhibited by anti-Kell antibodies in a dose-dependent fashion. Anti-D antibodies had no effect on erythroid progenitor growth. They concluded that anti-Kell antibodies cause fetal anemia by suppressing erythropoiesis at the level of erythroid progenitors. Fetuses with anti-Kell hemolytic anemia may therefore benefit from fetal blood sampling rather than amniotic fluid analyses, which may underestimate the degree of anemia.[96]

Extremely high titers of anti-C antibody have been associated with neonatal hemolytic disease.[98] However, routine screening of titers is not warranted, because antibody titers do not accurately reflect the severity of hemolytic disease.[99] Blood type is sufficient to screen for possible anti-D situations.

To determine the frequency of RBC antigen alloimmunizations that are capable of causing hemolytic disease, a study group in Syracuse, NY, identified 452 women who had a positive antibody screen during a 30-month screening period.[100] The frequencies of specific alloimmunization were reported: anti-D, 18.4%; anti-E, 14%; anti-c, 5.8%; anti-C, 4.7%; Kell group, 22%; anti-MNS, 4.7%; anti-Fya (Duffy), 5.4%; and anti-Jka, 1.5%. The study group concluded that anti-D was still a common antibody, despite the use of Rhogam. Rhesus and Kell antigen status can be determined by DNA studies, and molecular biology techniques such as polymerase chain reaction (PCR) have been used to determine fetal blood type. These methods may represent an advance in the clinical management of RhD and Kell alloimmunization in the future.[101]

Congenital Red Blood Cell Defects

Congenital defects of the red cell include enzymatic defects, membrane defects, and defects of hemoglobin synthesis. Enzyme defects such as glucose-6-phosphate dehydrogenase (G6PD) deficiency, pyruvate kinase deficiency, hexokinase deficiency, and glucose phosphate isomerase deficiency can present with hemolytic anemia in the first week of life. Membrane defects such as hereditary spherocytosis, hereditary elliptocytosis, and other hereditary disorders of the red cell cytoskeleton can also cause hemolysis in the newborn period. Neonatal red cell membranes deform more to a given shear force than do adult red cell membranes, resulting in greater susceptibility of neonatal cells to yield and fragment.[102] These mechanical properties lead to accelerated membrane loss and a decreased lifespan. The red cells of infants who have membrane abnormalities have even shorter lifespans. Defects in red cell membranes and metabolism are discussed in Chapter 11. Disorders of hemoglobin synthesis can also lead to increased hemolysis and are discussed in Chapter 16.

Acquired Red Blood Cell Defects

Acquired hemolytic anemias can be caused by infection, drugs, or toxins. Vascular pathology such as arteriovenous malformations, cavernous hemangiomas, and vascular thromboses can result in a hemolytic process.

Infection and Disseminated Intravascular Coagulation

Infants with viral or bacterial sepsis can develop hemolytic anemia. Sepsis due to bacteria such as GBS and *E. coli* may result in hemolysis, DIC, and hemorrhage. Infants are often jaundiced and have hepatosplenomegaly, although the degree of hyperbilirubinemia does not always correlate with the degree of anemia. Infants also may have an elevated direct bilirubin level, possibly because of infectious involvement of the liver. Some bacteria such as *E. coli* produce hemolytic endotoxins that result in increased red cell destruction, often associated with a microangiopathic process.[103, 104]

Congenital viral infections due to CMV, toxoplasmosis, rubella, and herpes simplex may also be associated with a hemolytic anemia. Congenital syphilis may manifest with hemolytic anemia despite negative test results for the mother. Initial negative screening for syphilis may be seen despite overwhelming infection, a condition called the *prozone effect*.[105, 106] The prozone effect occurs because a higher than optimal amount of antibody in the tested sera prevents the flocculation reaction seen in positive reagin test results. Serum dilution is necessary to make the correct diagnosis. Nontreponemal testing should be repeated using serum dilutions to prevent a missed diagnosis of syphilis in women with negative syphilis serologic results and an infant with nonimmune hydrops.[106]

Fetal and neonatal infection with parvovirus B19 can cause severe anemia, hydrops, and fetal demise.[107–109] The infant generally presents with a hypoplastic anemia,[110] but hemolysis can occur as well. The virus replicates exclusively in erythroid progenitor cells. In infants with an underlying hemolytic disorder, infection with parvovirus B19 can result in aplastic anemia. In utero transfusions for hydropic fetuses have been investigated but are not successful in all patients. Treatment with IVIG during aplastic crises leads to resolution of the anemia.

Other infections associated with neonatal anemia include malaria and human immunodeficiency virus (HIV). Congenital malaria can occur in endemic areas such as New York City,[111] where imported cases of malaria are increasing. Congenital HIV infection can be asymptomatic in newborns. Infants born to mothers on zidovudine (AZT) may have a hypoplastic anemia as a side effect of the drug.[112]

Other Causes of Hemolysis

Some maternal drugs can lead to hemolysis. Maternal ingestion of valproic acid has been reported to cause hemolytic disease in a breastfed newborn.[113] Mothers exposed to some oxidizing agents may induce hemolysis in their fetus with G6PD deficiency, and infants with G6PD deficiency are at risk for increased hemolysis when exposed to oxidizing agents such as sulfonamides, antimalarials, naphthalene, and henna.[114] Other unusual causes of hemolytic disease in the newborn infant include metabolic diseases such as galactosemia, lysosomal storage diseases, and some amino acid disorders. Prolonged metabolic acidosis, transfusion reactions, thrombocytopenia with absent radius (TAR) syndrome, and osteopetrosis[115] can all present with hemolytic anemia in the newborn. Macroangiopathic and microangiopathic hemolytic anemias can occur with vascular malformations such as severe coarctation of the aorta, atriovenous malformations, large vessel thromboses, and cavernous hemangiomas.

IMPAIRED RED BLOOD CELL PRODUCTION

Impaired erythrocyte production has many causes. Lack of an appropriate or sufficient marrow environment for growth (as seen in osteopetrosis) can cause decreased red cell production. Lack of specific substrates or their carriers, such as iron, folate, vitamin B_{12}, or transcobalamin II deficiency, can lead to deficient erythrocyte production. Lack of specific growth factors stimulating erythropoiesis, such as decreased EPO production or abnormalities in EPO receptors, can also lead to hypoproliferative anemia, such as Diamond-Blackfan syndrome or the anemia of prematurity.

Nutritional Deficiencies Causing Anemia

With the exception of iron deficiency anemia in neonates who have had chronic hemorrhage, hypoproliferative anemias due to nutritional deficiencies rarely manifest in term infants. In preterm infants, however, nutritional deficiency anemias do occur, although they generally do not become evident until after the first weeks of life. Deficiencies of iron, folate, B_{12}, vitamin E, and copper have been described and can lead to various degrees of anemia.[116]

Iron

Iron deficiency anemia can occur at various times during the newborn period in term and preterm infants. After chronic FMH or TTS, term and preterm infants can present with iron deficiency anemia manifested by hypochromic, microcytic red cells on a peripheral smear, and a low hematocrit. Because 75% to 80% of the total body iron is stored in hemoglobin, infants born with anemia have decreased iron stores. Preterm infants develop an iron-deficient state even more rapidly because of their relatively smaller total blood volumes and greater phlebotomy losses. As blood cells are destroyed, the iron from hemoglobin is recycled, becoming available for future erythropoiesis. Without adequate initial red cell volumes, the iron for new hemoglobin production is lacking, and iron deficiency anemia ensues. Table 8–6 shows the differences in iron stores present in three preterm infants born with different red cell volumes. The initial hemoglobin concentration significantly affects the ability of preterm infants to maintain normal hematologic indices during growth.

In term infants, significant iron stores in the bone marrow do not accumulate until the first month of life. Stainable marrow iron is present from 4 weeks until 20 to 24 weeks of age. Preterm infants accumulate iron during the first 4 to 8 weeks and then deplete these stores by 12 weeks of age. These infants often have serum ferritin concentrations below 50 ng/mL. Adults compensate for decreased iron by improving oral iron absorption, but this does not occur as often in preterm infants. Preterm infants regulate iron absorption poorly and often do not increase gastrointestinal absorption despite decreased serum ferritin concentrations.[117] This places preterm infants at even greater risk for iron deficiency.

Table 8–6. **Iron Endowment and Its Role in the Development of Iron Deficiency Anemia in the Low Birth Weight Infant**

	Infant A	Infant B	Infant C
Birth weight (g)	1000	1000	1000
Blood volume (ml)	100	100	100
Hemoglobin (g/dL)	13	17	22
Hemoglobin iron (mg)*	44.2	57.8	74.8
Storage iron (mg)	15	15	15
Total iron	59.2	73.8	89.8
Maximum hemoglobin value† when infant reaches a weight of 2000 g	8.7	10.9	13.2

*3.4 mg of iron are present in 1 g of hemoglobin.
†Assumes that infant has received no exogenous iron and has lost no blood.

Chronically ill preterm infants often receive multiple transfusions and may also be receiving significant nutritional support, including iron therapy. Despite this, some infants develop the anemia of bronchopulmonary dysplasia (BPD), a normocytic, normochromic, hyporegenerative anemia[118] with marrow normoblast iron stains that are distinct from those observed in the anemia of chronic disorders.[119] Infants with the anemia of BPD often have adequate stainable iron in their marrow but are not able to access the iron efficiently.

The use of parenteral iron in preterm infants has been slowly increasing. One concern about parenteral iron administration has been the reported increased risk of infection. However, studies reporting an increased incidence of infection in infants receiving parenteral iron evaluated intramuscular routes and doses greater than 100 mg/day.[120, 121]

The addition of parenteral iron to total parenteral (TPN) formulas is slowly forthcoming, and further study is needed to determine optimal doses based on erythropoietic stimuli. Friel and coworkers[122] evaluated the use of iron dextran added to the TPN of 14 very-low-birth-weight (VLBW) infants and found that, despite parenteral doses of 200 to 250 μg/kg/day (with a total enteral plus parenteral iron intake of 400 μg/kg/day), infants remained in negative iron balance during the course of study. They observed no adverse effects of this treatment and recommended an iron intake of 1000 μg/kg/day supplemented in TPN.

The use of EPO to prevent and treat the anemia of prematurity has added a new level of complexity to the iron requirements of preterm infants. Numerous studies of preterm infants receiving EPO have shown evidence of iron deficiency when iron supplementation is not adequate. Iron has been administered parenterally and enterally in published studies. Carnielli and colleagues reported no adverse effects from intravenous iron with a dosage of 20 mg/kg given once each week.[123] These infants also received vitamin E (10 mg/kg intramuscularly) twice each week. This dose of intravenous iron, although not the standard dose or typical route of administration in the United States, may have improved iron availability and resulted in a greater and more prolonged erythropoietic response than that seen in other studies.

Oral iron supplementation has ranged from 2 mg/kg/day in early studies to almost 40 mg/kg/day in later studies.[124] No evidence of hemolysis was found in either of the two EPO trials in which the greatest amounts of supplemental iron were used.[123, 125] Functional iron deficiency has been frequently reported in pediatric and adult patients receiving EPO[126–128] and probably limited the success of some of the early EPO trials in preterm infants. Two studies evaluated iron stores in EPO recipients and found increased iron requirements in infants receiving EPO, as evidenced by diminished ferritin concentrations and elevated numbers of hypochromic red cells, despite iron doses of 6 mg/kg/day.[129, 130]

Infants receiving EPO probably are at greater risk for iron deficiency than they are at risk for iron overload and increased oxidant stress. However, no studies have directly evaluated iron requirements in preterm infants receiving EPO.[131] Further evaluation is required to determine the optimal dose and route of administration of iron in preterm infants receiving EPO.

Vitamin E

Vitamin E is an antioxidant that inhibits peroxidation of polyunsaturated fatty acids (PUFAs) in the lipid bilayers of all cell membranes. Because vitamin E is transferred across the placenta to the greatest degree in the last trimester, preterm infants are born with lower stores than term infants.[116] Unlike other nutritional deficiency anemias, vitamin E deficiency does not result in a hypoproliferative anemia, but rather a hemolytic anemia, because of the functions of the compound.

Vitamin E deficiency anemia in preterm infants was first described in the 1960s and 1970s.[132] Early preterm infant formulas containing high concentrations of PUFAs and low vitamin E caused increased hemolysis and anemia. Studies in the mid-1970s showed that when preterm infants were fed diets high in PUFAs and given iron supplementation, their hemolytic anemia worsened.[133, 134] The anemia resolved with vitamin E administration. Vitamin E–deficient, hemolytic anemia has largely disappeared because of improvements in preterm infant formulas containing lower concentrations of PUFAs and adequate vitamin E supplementation.

Infants with severe fat malabsorption require greater vitamin E supplementation. Vitamin E requirements probably are increased in preterm infants receiving increased iron supplementation, because iron promotes oxidation of cellular membranes and also inhibits intestinal absorption of vitamin E. Preterm infants receiving EPO require greater iron supplementation and should therefore receive vitamin E supplementation as well. The optimal dose of vitamin E in preterm infants receiving EPO has not been determined, but oral doses in some studies ranged 15 to 25 IU per day.

Folate

Folate is stored in the fetal liver late in gestation, and infants can become deficient if born prematurely.[116] Infants fed diets low in folate, those with malabsorption, and infants receiving goat's milk or milk that has been boiled are at risk for becoming folate deficient. Red cell folate concentrations represent total body folate stores, and serum folate concentrations reflect recent folate intake. Serum and RBC folate concentrations are greater in preterm and term infants than in adults. RBC folate concentrations decrease rapidly after birth and are generally lower than adult concentrations by 1 to 3 months of life.

Folate deficiency results in a megaloblastic anemia, with mean cell volumes (MCV) generally greater than 110 fL. Preterm infants with lower folate stores need supplementation in situations where erythropoiesis is increased, such as infants with hemolytic anemia or infants receiving EPO. General requirements for term and preterm infants are 25 to 50 μg taken orally each day.

Vitamin B_{12}

Vitamin B_{12} (or cobalamin) must be obtained through dietary intake because only microorganisms are able to synthesize the compound. B_{12} is actively transported across the placenta and stored in the fetal liver. B_{12} deficiency is rare in preterm infants but can sometimes be seen in breast-fed infants of vegetarian mothers who are B_{12} deficient or in infants with gastrointestinal abnormalities such as short gut syndrome, necrotizing gastroenteritis (NEC), or post-NEC stenoses.[116]

The hematologic characteristics of B_{12} deficiency anemia are similar to those seen in folate deficiency anemia. Erythroid hyperplasia occurs, and the decreased myeloid to erythroid ratio is in the range of 2:1 to 1:1. Megaloblastic proerythroblasts have a shortened survival, and remaining cells have an increased MCV. Reticulocytosis occurs rapidly with B_{12} supplementation.

Copper

Copper deficiency anemia can occur when supplemental copper is not given in some circumstances: low-birth-weight premature infants fed milk only, protracted total parenteral nutrition without trace mineral supplements, and chronic diarrhea with severe malnutrition. Severe neutropenia generally precedes the onset of sideroblastic, hypochromic anemia. Serum iron concentrations are usually low, but iron therapy is ineffective in resolving the anemia. The diagnosis is established by detecting low serum copper concentrations, the presence of fractures or periosteal reaction on radiographs, and a dramatic reticulocytosis in response to copper therapy. The recommended intake of copper for term infants is 0.4 to 0.6 mg per day.

Congenital Anemias

Diamond-Blackfan Syndrome

Diamond-Blackfan anemia (DBA) consists of a group of congenital pure RBC aplasias diagnosed usually within the first year of life (Table 8–7). The syndrome represents a phenotypic expression of multiple genotypic abnormalities affecting erythropoiesis.[135, 136] Up to 25% of patients are anemic at birth.[137] Hydrops fetalis associated with severe anemia has been reported but is rare. Most cases are sporadic, but 10% to 15% of cases are familial, and more cases of autosomal dominant inheritance have been reported.[137–139]

Physical abnormalities are present in about one third of DBA patients.[140] Abnormalities include short stature, triphalangeal or duplicated thumbs, cleft palate, ocular anomalies, short or webbed neck, and congenital heart disease. Patients can be profoundly anemic and reticulocytopenic, but other cell lineages are normal in number and function. The bone marrow reflects hypoproliferative erythropoiesis, showing a very low number of erythropoietic precursors and a reduction of erythroid progenitor cells. Proliferation and differentiation of the other lineages are normal.

Most DBA patients have elevated EPO concentrations, but the very high EPO levels are usually not proportionate to the level of anemia. Erythroid progenitors from some DBA patients show a defective or incomplete response to other erythropoietic growth factors, such as interleukin (IL)-3, IL-6, or stem cell factor (Fig. 8–1).[141] Other patients show a significant response in vitro to stem cell factor and IL-9.[142, 143]

Defective erythropoiesis in DBA patients ap-

Table 8–7. **Genetic Disorders Associated With Anemia**

Syndrome	Genetic Characteristics	Hematologic Phenotype
Diamond-Blackfan syndrome	Autosomal recessive (AR); sporadic mutations and autosomal dominant (AD) inheritance have been described.	Steroid-responsive hypoplastic anemia after 5 months of age
Fanconi pancytopenia	AR, probably abnormalities in multiple genes (at least five genetic subtypes have been identified)	Steroid-responsive hypoplastic anemia some macrocytic red blood cells, shortened Cells are hypersensitive to DNA
Aase syndrome	AR, possible AD	Steroid-responsive hypoplastic anemia that improves with age
Pearson's syndrome	Mitochondrial DNA abnormalities, X-linked or AR	Hypoplastic sideroblastic anemia unresponsive to pyridoxine
Lethal osteopetrosis	AR, caused by defective resorption of immature bone	Hypoplastic anemia due to marrow
Congenital dyserythropoietic anemias (CDA)	AR	Type I: megaloblastoid erythroid and nuclear chromitin bridges between cells Type II: erythroblastic multinuclearity and positive acidified serum test results (HEMPAS) Type III: erythroblastic multinuclearity and macrocytosis
Peutz-Jeghers syndrome	AD	Iron deficiency anemia from chronic blood loss
Dyskeratosis congenita	X-linked recessive, locus on Xq28, some cases with AD inheritance	Hypoplastic anemia usually present between 5 and 15 years of age
X-linked α-thalassemia/ mental retardation (ATR-X and ATR-16) syndromes	ATR-X: X-linked recessive, mapped to Xq13.3; ATR-16: mapped to 16p13.3, deletions of α-globin locus	ATR-X: hypochromic, microcytic anemia mild form of hemoglobin H disease ATR-16: more significant hemoglobin H disease and anemia are present
Thrombocytopenia with absent radii (TAR) syndrome	Autosomal recessive (AR)	Hemorrhagic anemia, possibly hypoplastic anemia as well
Osler hemorrhagic telangiectasia syndrome	AD, mapped to 9q33–34	Hemorrhagic anemia

pears to involve EPO receptor binding and processing of EPO,[144] although studies of some family cohorts show no abnormalities of EPO receptor sequencing.[145] Potential defects include erythroid growth factors and growth factor receptors[146] and *trans*-acting proteins that regulate their expression. Other defects responsible for the syndrome have been postulated, including a defective bone marrow microenvironment[147] and abnormalities in number and function of erythroid progenitors.[148]

Gustavsson and coworkers performed linkage analyses with chromosome 19 markers in DBA families of Swedish, French, Dutch, Arabic, and Italian origin.[149] They established significant linkage to chromosome 19q13 for dominant and recessively inherited DBA. Other such analyses of cohorts of DBA patients are forthcoming and may add clues to the genetic basis of this disease.

Many patients respond clinically to corticosteroids, and some develop hematologic remissions (spontaneous and after corticosteroid therapy). Patients who do not respond to corticosteroids and those who have to discontinue treatment because of side effects must rely on chronic transfusion and are exposed to the associated complications. Janov and coworkers described the natural history of 76 patients with DBA treated at the Children's Hospital in Boston between 1931 and 1992.[150] They found that the MCV in infants younger than 5 months of age rarely exceeded the normal range and was of little diagnostic value but that macrocytosis was evident in older infants. Nine of their 16 patients who never received steroids experienced remissions, sometimes after years of transfusions. Of the 56 patients receiving corticosteroids, 31 responded. Thirteen of the steroid responders experienced remissions, 11 re-

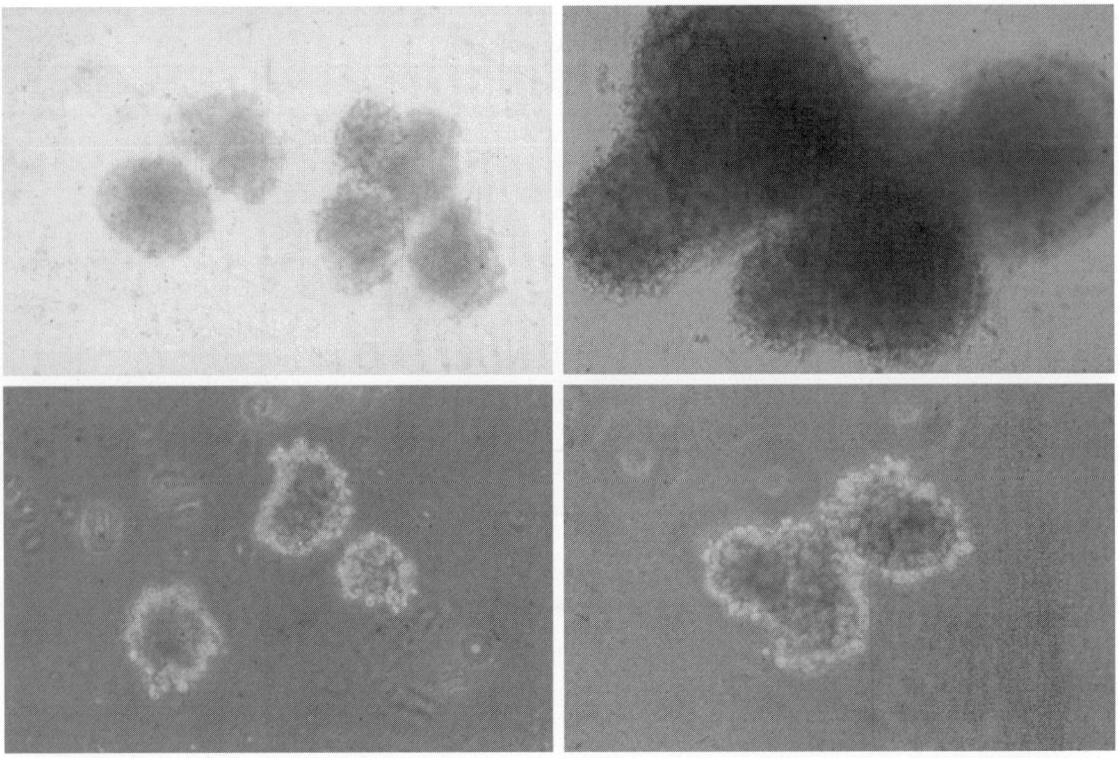

Figure 8–1. Changes in erythroid progenitor colony (BFU-E) morphology. BFU-E from normal adults stimulated with interleukin-3 and granulocyte macrophage colony–stimulating factor is shown in the *upper left panel.* BFU-E from a patient with Diamond-Blackfan syndrome stimulated with the same growth factors is shown in the *lower left panel.* The effects of stem cell factor on BFU-E from normal adults can be seen in the *upper right panel.* The effects of stem cell factor on BFU-E from a patient with Diamond Blackfan syndrome are shown in the *lower right panel.* Addition of stem cell factor greatly increased the size and density of BFU-E in normal adults but did not change the morphology of BFU-E in Diamond-Blackfan patients.

mained steroid dependent, and 7 later required transfusions. The median survival was 38 years, probably reflecting the complications of multiple transfusions (most commonly hemosiderosis) and increased risk for leukemia (RR = 200; 95% CI, 54.5–512.1).

New treatment strategies are being investigated that involve the administration of growth factors such as IL-3, granulocyte-macrophage colony-stimulating factor (GM-CSF), and stem cell factor.[151] Successful bone marrow transplantation has been performed in some individuals,[144] suggesting a normal marrow microenvironment in those patients.

Congenital Dyserythropoietic Anemia

Congenital dyserythropoietic anemia (CDA) is a rare disorder marked by ineffective erythropoiesis, megaloblastic anemia, and characteristic abnormalities of the nuclear membrane and cytoplasm seen on electron microscopy. Autosomal dominant and autosomal recessive inheritance patterns have been reported. Three types of congenital dyserythropoietic anemia have been described. Type I CDA shows megaloblastoid erythroid hyperplasia and nuclear chromatin bridges between cells and has been linked to chromosome 15q15.1-15.3 in a large cohort.[152] Type II CDA is the most common form, characterized by erythroblastic multinuclearity and positive acidified serum test results (i.e., HEMPAS anemia). This form appears to result from enzymatic defects in the cellular glycosylation pathway that affect band 3 anion transport activity.[153, 154] Type III CDA is marked by erythroblastic multinuclearity and macrocytosis.

CDA can manifest in the newborn period with megaloblastic anemia, early jaundice, hepatosplenomegaly, and intrauterine growth retardation. Infants with type 1 CDA may have bony abnormalities and syndactyly.[155] Fetuses with hydrops fetalis and CDA have been reported.[156] Although rare, this disorder should be included in the differential of newborns with anemia, jaundice, and hepatosplenomegaly. In one study, one half of the patients with CDA I presented in the neonatal period, although macrocytosis did not become evident until later in the course of disease.[155] Treatment for this disorder consists of supportive therapy and close observation for side effects of chronic transfusions. Splenectomy in some patients with severe anemia has been helpful.

Aase Syndrome

Aase syndrome is another congenital hypoplastic anemia syndrome involving marrow and skeletal anomalies.[157] The syndrome is characterized by hypoplastic anemia and abnormally digitalized thumbs and may also be associated with growth failure. Bony abnormalities have been reported in these patients as well.[158] Similar to DBA, bone marrow cultures reveal decreased production of erythropoietic precursors. The inheritance pattern is thought to be comparable to that seen in DBA, because autosomal dominant and autosomal recessive conditions have been reported.[159]

Osteopetrosis

Osteopetrosis is a rare autosomal recessive disorder characterized by defects in osteoclastic function, resulting in a decreased bone marrow space.[160] Developmental delay, ocular involvement, and neurodegenerative findings are associated with hypoplastic anemia, although patients may also present with hemolytic anemia.

Longitudinal studies in the United States and Europe have shown variability in outcome, although the survival rate beyond 5 to 6 years is less than 30%.[160, 161] Patients presenting with early hematologic and visual impairment had an even shorter life expectancy. The limited treatment options for this disorder include marrow transplantation and administration of calcitriol and interferon-γ.[161]

Fanconi's Anemia

Fanconi's anemia (FA) is an autosomal recessive disorder characterized by marrow failure and congenital anomalies, including abnormalities in skin pigmentation, gastrointestinal anomalies, renal anomalies, and upper limb anomalies.[162] Approximately one third of patients have no obvious congenital anomalies. Five genetic phenotypes of FA have been reported, and two of the genes have been cloned.[163] Cells are hypersensitive to DNA cross-linking agents such as diepoxybutane and mitomycin C. The diepoxybutane tests represents a sensitive and specific diagnostic test for FA.

Most patients present in early childhood, but newborn infants with FA have been reported, usually when obvious congenital anomalies are present.[164] Patients generally have a steroid-responsive hypoplastic anemia, reticulocytopenia, macrocytic RBCs on peripheral smear, and shortened RBC life span.[165] EPO concentrations are usually elevated, and hemoglobin F production is increased. A significant percentage of these patients develop myelodysplastic syndrome or acute myelogenous leukemia later in life. Treatment of FA is similar to that for DBA, and marrow transplantation has been successful.

Pearson's Syndrome

Pearson's marrow-pancreas syndrome is a disorder involving the hematopoietic system, exocrine pancreas, liver, and kidneys.[166] Patients present in infancy with macrocytic anemia that is sometimes associated with neutropenia and thrombocytopenia. Marrow samples have normal cellularity but show abnormalities, including vacuolization of erythroid and myeloid precursors, hemosiderosis, and ringed sideroblasts. The disorder appears to involve defects in oxidative phosphorylation caused by mitochondrial DNA abnormalities.[167, 168] The anemia is unresponsive to pyridoxine supplementation. Bone marrow transplantation has not been reported in these patients, and the disorder is considered fatal.

Oxygen Delivery in Preterm Infants

In low-birth-weight infants, the amount of oxygen released by hemoglobin can be determined based on an unloading from a normal arterial oxygen tension adjusted for age to an arbitrary central venous oxygen tension of 40 mm Hg.[169] Although oxygen-carrying capacity (hemoglobin concentration × percent of oxygen saturation × 1.36 mL oxygen per 1 g of hemoglobin) decreases over the first 2.5 months of life as a consequence of a decline in hemoglobin concentration, the amount of oxygen capable of being delivered to tissues actually increases. For example, a neonate weighing 1000 g with a hemoglobin concentration of 15 g/dL, a P_{50} of 19, and a central venous oxygen tension of 40 mm Hg unloads 1 mL of oxygen to tissues for every 100 mL of blood that passes through the capillary bed. At 10 weeks of age, the P_{50} has shifted to the right, and is 24 mm Hg. The same infant then delivers 2.1 mL of oxygen per 100 mL of blood, even though the hemoglobin concentration has declined to 8 g/dL. These calculations emphasize the importance of understanding an infant's P_{50} before administering an erythrocyte transfusion.

Transfusions significantly affect erythropoiesis in neonates, and the decision to transfuse should not be based on hemoglobin concentration alone.[170] For infants who undergo exchange transfusion or multiple transfusions, erythropoietin concentrations and reticulocyte counts are lower at any given hemoglobin concentration.[169] It is often assumed that oxygen delivery is decreased in newborns because of the presence of a high-affinity hemoglobin. A leftward shift in the hemoglobin-oxygen dissociation curve because of high levels of fetal hemoglobin may better maintain oxygen delivery during episodes of severe hypoxemia.

Anemia of Prematurity

In preterm infants, adaptive mechanisms to the extrauterine environment are incomplete. EPO concentrations in anemic preterm infants are still significantly lower than those found in adults, given the degree of their anemia.[32, 33] This normocytic, normochromic anemia, called the *anemia of prematurity*, commonly affects infants ≤ 32 weeks' gestation. The anemia of prematurity is "nutritionally insensitive" and therefore not responsive to the addition of iron, folate, or vitamin E. Some infants are asymptomatic, and others demonstrate signs of anemia, which are alleviated by transfusion. The signs include tachycardia, increased episodes of apnea and bradycardia, poor weight gain, an increased oxygen requirement, and elevated serum lactate concentrations that decrease after transfusion.[171–174]

Shulman first described the anemia of prematurity in 1959, dividing it into three clinical phases.[175] The early phase was marked by an initial fall in hemoglobin concentration. The second phase was characterized by maintenance of low hemoglobin concentrations for a period of 1 to 3 weeks. The third phase was the only period of "true" anemia (hemoglobin concentrations below those needed to meet the oxygen demands of the tissues) and was marked by hemoglobin concentrations that continued to fall despite signs and symptoms attributed to anemia. The anemia of prematurity resolved spontaneously by 3 to 6 months of life.

Infants with the anemia of prematurity have a decreased ability to increase serum EPO concentrations, despite diminished "available oxygen" to tissues[32, 33] and the appearance of signs of anemia.[171] However, erythroid progenitors are highly sensitive to EPO,[176, 177] and concentrations of other erythropoietic growth factors responsible for erythrocyte production (e.g., IL-3, GM-CSF) appear to be normal.[178]

The molecular and cellular mechanisms responsible for the anemia of prematurity remain undefined. Possible explanations include the transition from fetal to adult hemoglobin, shortened erythrocyte survival, and hemodilution associated with a rapidly increasing body mass.[179–181] It is unknown whether preterm infants rely on EPO produced by the liver (the source of EPO in utero), that produced by the kidney, or a combination of the two. However, macrophages from preterm infants generate EPO mRNA and protein as effectively as do those from term infants and adults.[182] The anemia of prematurity probably involves a delay in shifting the anatomic site of EPO production from the liver to peritubular cells in the kidney.

Clinical trials published in the last 8 years evaluating EPO administration to preterm infants to prevent or treat the anemia of prematurity have reported a variety of results.[124] Initial studies used "adult" doses and reported little or no effect. Pharmacokinetic studies in newborn monkeys and sheep indicated that neonates have a larger volume of distribution and a more rapid elimination of EPO,[183, 184] necessitating the use of higher doses per kilogram of body weight than required for adults. These pharmacokinetic differences were found to apply to preterm infants as well.[185, 186] A variety of EPO doses and dosing schedules have since been evaluated in preterm infants (Table 8–8).

The "erythrokinetics" of EPO in preterm infants are unknown. In a study giving EPO continuously over 24 hours to preterm infants for 10 days (versus a daily subcutaneous injection), EPO concentrations and reticulocyte responses were similar in both groups.[186] Peak concentrations in both groups declined from day 3 to day 10. It appears that higher doses (ranging from 750 to 1400 U/kg/week) result in an adequate clinical response, but it remains to be determined if high peak EPO concentrations are more efficacious than lower, more constant EPO levels.

Carnielli and coworkers were the first to evaluate the use of EPO in preventing the anemia of prematurity.[123] They randomized 22 VLBW preterm infants in the first 2 days of life to receive 400 U of EPO/kg three times a week or receive no treatment. Infants receiving EPO were also given 20 mg/kg iron intravenously once each week. The EPO recipients had a significant increase in reticulocytes and required fewer transfusions (0.8 ± 1.5 transfusions and 14.2 ± 25.9 mL/kg volume transfused in the EPO group versus 3.1 ± 2.1 transfusions and 48.4 ± 34.0 mL/kg volume transfused in the control group).

In a European multicentered trial, Maier and colleagues evaluated the effect of EPO on the need for transfusions in preterm infants 750 to 1499 g.[129] Infants who were stable (off mechanical ventilation by day 6 of life) were randomized on day 3 of life to receive EPO (250 U/kg three times per week) or no treatment. A total of 241 infants were evaluated, 177 of whom completed the study according to protocol. EPO recipients received fewer transfusions (1.2 versus 0.8) and had a greater success rate (defined as maintaining hematocrit above 32% without transfusions) than placebo recipients. The same study group evaluated low (750 U/kg/week) and high (1500 U/kg/week) weekly doses in 184 infants with birth weights of 500 to 1000 g who were treated from day 3 of life until 37 weeks' postconceptional age.[187] One third of the infants in each group did not receive any transfusions during the treatment period, and the volume of PRBCs transfused was similar. The success rate, defined as no transfusion needed and hematocrit value 0.30 L/L or greater, was similar between groups (27.6% in the low-dose and 29.5% in the high-dose group). They concluded that increasing the EPO dose from 750 U/kg/week to 1500 U/kg/week was not indicated in infants with birth weights of less than 1000 g.

A multicentered trial performed in the United States by Shannon and coworkers evaluated the efficacy of EPO to treat the anemia of prematurity.[188] Infants with birth weights of $\leq$ 1250 g and less than 31 weeks' gestation were randomized to receive EPO (100 U/kg) or placebo subcutaneously, 5 days each week, for a total of 6 weeks. Infants were receiving enteral feedings of at least 60 kcal/kg/day, had hematocrits less than 40%, and had minimal phlebotomy losses at the time of study entry. Infants in both groups received oral iron and vitamin E supplementation, and uniform transfusion criteria were followed by all participating centers. Infants were 24 days of age at the time of study and had received an average of 3.5 transfusions before study entry. EPO recipients required fewer number (1.1 versus 1.6) and volume of transfusions (16 mL/patient versus 24 mL/patient) than did placebo recipients, and no adverse effects were observed. Other trials have shown similar positive results.[125, 130, 189–193]

After the study by Carnielli and colleagues, other groups evaluated the efficacy of treating VLBW infants with EPO in the first weeks of life. In one study,[194] preterm infants randomized to receive EPO (200 units/kg/day) had higher reticulocyte counts and received fewer number and volume of transfusions than infants randomized to placebo (0.2 versus 1.4 transfusions per patient; 2.7 versus 22.3 mL/kg/patient). When compared with other infants in the intensive care unit who met all of the study eligibility criteria, the placebo recipients were given fewer transfusions than "nonstudy" infants (2.8 transfusions per patient during the same period). This finding was confirmed by Bifano and colleagues,[195] who observed that instituting standardized transfusion guidelines decreased the transfusion requirements of VLBW infants.

Other studies evaluating the use of EPO in smaller preterm infants reported a decreased number and volume of transfusions in the first weeks of life.[196, 197] In one study, 28 infants $\leq$

Table 8–8. **Clinical Studies of Erythropoietin Therapy in Preterm Infants**

Study	Population	Recombinant Human Erythropoietin Treatment Regimen (Number of Patients)	Transfusions per Patient	Volume of Blood Transfused
Carnielli et al.[123]	22 preterm infants <1500 g	400 U/kg IV/SC 3 times/wk from day 2 until discharge (11)	0.8	14.2 mL/kg*
		Control (11)	3.1	48.4 mL/kg
Donato et al.[197]	114 infants <1250 g	801–1250 g: 1250 U/kg/wk × 2 wk, then 750 U/kg/wk × 6 wk (57)	1.8 ± 2.3	
	(29 infants ≤800 g, with	≤800 g: 1250 U/kg/wk × 2 wk, then 750 U/kg/wk × 6 wk (15/29)	3.4 ± 1.1	51 ± 35
	blood out ≥30 mL/kg)	801–1250 g: placebo × 2 wk, then 750 U/kg/wk × 6 wk (57)	1.8 ± 2.5	
		≤800 g: placebo × 2 wk, then 750 U/kg/wk × 6 wk (14/29)	5.4 ± 3	84 ± 55
Kumar et al.[193]	30 infants ≤1250 g	300 U/kg 2 ×/wk (15)	0.07 ± 0	1.0 ± 3.9 mL/patient*
		Placebo (15)	0.8 ± 0.8	11.7 ± 11.1 mL/patient
Maier et al.[129]	241 infants ≤1500 g	250 U/kg 3 ×/wk SC for 4 wk (15)	0.8	0.09 mL/kg/day*
		Control (15)	1.2	0.41 mL/kg/day
Meister et al[189]	30 infants ≤1500 g	300 U/kg 3 ×/wk SC for 4 wk (15)	NR	0
		Control (15)	NR	0.86 mL/kg/day
Messer et al.[192]	51 infants <1500 g	100 U/kg SC 3 times/wk for 6 wk (10)	0	0 mL/kg
		200 U/kg SC 3 times/wk for 6 wk (11)	0.2	16 mL/kg
		300 U/kg SC 3 times/wk for 6 wk (10)	0.3	26 mL/kg
		Control (20)	0.7	40 mL/kg
Meyer et al.[130]	80 preterm infants ≤1500 g, at least 2 weeks old	200 U/kg SC 3 times/wk for 6 wk (40)	0.18	148 mL total*
		Placebo (40)	0.53	438 mL total
Obladen et al.[191]	83 infants	30 U/kg SC 3 times/wk from day 4 to day 25 (43)	NR	14.1 mL/kg
		Control (50)	NR	16.5 mL/kg
Ohls et al.[194]	28 infants ≤750 g	200 U/kg/day IV for 14 days (15)	4.7 ± 0.7*	70 ± 11 mL/kg*
		Placebo (13)	7.5 ± 1.1	112 ± 17 mL/kg
Ohls et al.[194]	20 infants <1500 g	200 U/kg/day IV for 14 days (10)	0.2*	2.7 mL/kg*
		Placebo (10)	1.4	22.3 mL/kg
Shannon et al.[188]	157 preterm infants ≤1250 g	100 IU/kg SC 5 times/wk for 6 wk (77)	1.1 ± 1.5	17 ± 23 mL/patient
		Placebo (80)	1.6 ± 1.7	24 ± 26 mL/patient
Soubasi et al.[190]	Com. and uncom. preterm infants ≤1500 g	150 IU/kg SC 2 times/wk for 6 wks (9 uncom†)	0.4‡	5.5 mL/patient
		150 IU/kg SC 2 times/wk for 6 wk (16 com‡)	8.25	83.3 mL/patient
		Control (7 uncom†)	1.28	26.4 mL/patient
		Control (12 com‡)	7.75	84.8 mL/patient

IV, intravenous; NR, not reported; SC, subcutaneous.
*P <0.05 versus control (or placebo); **P <.05 versus day 1; †P = .013 versus control; ‡P <.01 versus control (or placebo).
†Uncomplicated, defined as infants with minimal or no signs of respiratory distress and with no signs of sepsis.
‡Complicated, defined as infants requring mechanical ventilation (for respiratory distress syndrome, apnea or sepsis).

750 g were randomized to EPO or placebo for 2 weeks.[196] EPO recipients had 4.7 ± 0.7 transfusions and 70 ± 11 mL/kg blood transfused, whereas placebo recipients had 7.5 ± 1.1 transfusions and 112 ± 17 mL/kg blood transfused ($P<0.05$). A study performed in Argentina evaluated infants $\leq$ 1250 g who received EPO for 8 weeks, compared with infants who received placebo for 2 weeks followed by EPO for 6 weeks.[197] Of the 114 infants evaluated, 29 were $\leq$ 800 g with phlebotomy losses $\geq$ 30 mL/kg. There was an initial difference in the number and volume of transfusions in the smallest infants, but the differences did not carry through to the end of the study. It appears that EPO therapy is effective in preterm infants, but the degree of effectiveness varies with the volume of phlebotomy losses and the transfusion criteria used.

The side effects of EPO administration in adults include hypertension, bone pain, rash, and rarely, seizures. None of these side effects has been reported for any of the preterm infants involved in clinical trials. Transient neutropenia was seen in EPO recipients in some studies.[198–200] The neutropenia was not associated with depletion of neutrophil reserves or colony-forming unit–granulocyte-macrophage concentrations but appeared to involve reduced production of neutrophils from granulocytic progenitors[201, 202] and resolved after discontinuation of the EPO. The cause may involve depletion of the total number of progenitors in slightly older preterm infants or may involve down-modulation of granulocyte colony-stimulating factor receptors on pluripotent progenitors. A study reported no differences in circulating granulocyte progenitors in preterm infants receiving EPO.[189]

Neutropenia was not reported in any of the EPO trials evaluating administration to preterm infants starting in the first days of life. EPO recipients did not experience any increase in morbidity or adverse outcome measures when compared with the placebo recipients. One study reported a decreased incidence in symptomatic patent ductus arteriosus (PDA).[194] One possibility for this side effect involves interactions between EPO and endothelin-1 production,[203] although Cogar and colleagues observed no significant increase in serum endothelin-1 or blood pressure in preterm infants receiving EPO.[204] The effect of EPO on the incidence of symptomatic PDAs is still being evaluated.

Anemia of Bronchopulmonary Dysplasia

Alverson observed the development of anemia in patients with BPD and reported that repeated transfusions usually were required for management of anemia.[205] Christensen and coworkers subsequently characterized the anemia of BPD as a normocytic, normochromic, hyporegenerative anemia,[118] with marrow normoblast iron stains that are distinct from those observed in the anemia of chronic disorders[119] and the anemia of prematurity.[171] Patients with the anemia of BPD differ from infants with the anemia of prematurity in that not all of the patients with the anemia of BPD are born prematurely and their average age usually is greater than that of the anemia of prematurity group.[198] Preliminary results show EPO to be effective as treatment for the anemia of BPD.[206]

Further study is needed to determine the explanation for the reduced EPO production in patients with BPD, including the evaluation of factors that may create a relatively "EPO-resistant" environment, such as IL-1, tumor necrosis factor, interferon-γ,[207] and common medications used in infants with BPD, such as methylxanthines and corticosteroids.[208–210] Larger trials are needed to assess adverse effects and to compare the long-term benefits with the risks of EPO treatment in this population.

Late Anemia of Rh Disease

Infants with Rh hemolytic disease often have an early (congenital) anemia because of ongoing, antibody-mediated hemolysis and can develop a "late" (age, 1 to 3 months) anemia because of diminished erythrocyte production. The incidence of late anemia appears to be much higher in infants who receive intrauterine transfusions.[211] This anemia is characterized by low serum concentrations of EPO but erythroid progenitors that remain highly responsive to recombinant EPO in vitro.[212] Infants with the late anemia of Rh hemolytic disease routinely receive transfusions until their anemia spontaneously resolves, generally by the third or fourth month of life.

During the period of decreased circulating antibody and delayed endogenous EPO production, administration of exogenous EPO may serve as an alternative to erythrocyte transfusion. EPO administration may also diminish or eliminate the need for rehospitalization for transfusions. Preliminary studies evaluating the use of recombinant EPO as treatment for the late anemia of Rh hemolytic disease have shown it to be effective in stimulating erythropoiesis.[213, 214]

Other Erythropoietin-Responsive Anemias

In an attempt to decrease transfusion requirements and possibly decrease the incidence of graft rejection, infants with congenital heart disease awaiting transplantation received daily EPO (200 U/kg/day).[215] These infants had a significant increase in their hematocrits and a decrease in transfusions. Additional trials evaluating the use of EPO to decrease transfusion requirements of newborns with congenital heart disease are needed to evaluate hematopoietic and nonhematopoietic effects. EPO has been used to successfully treat anemia in newborns with end-stage renal disease.[216] Phase I trials evaluating combinations of EPO plus other growth factors with erythroid activity (e.g., GM-CSF) are ongoing.[217]

It could be argued that, given the risks of transfusion transmission of hepatitis, CMV, and HIV and the possible development of graft-versus-host disease,[218] treatment of anemic neonates using recombinant EPO might be cost effective. EPO administration, in combination with instituting more rigorous and standardized transfusion criteria and diminishing the volume of blood lost through phlebotomy, probably has the greatest impact in decreasing transfusion requirements in term and preterm infants. Regardless of treatment strategy, a critical understanding of the physiologic influences affecting oxygen delivery in term and preterm infants is required before altering the hematocrit through an erythrocyte transfusion or administration of EPO.

Guidelines for Erythrocyte Transfusions

A discussion of blood banking and transfusion practices is provided in Chapter 18. Guidelines for administering an erythrocyte transfusion are different for term and preterm infants and depend on the cause and duration of blood loss. Regardless of cause, an infant should never be transfused based on hemoglobin concentration alone. Transfusions after acute blood loss are discussed in the previous section on hemorrhage. Factors such as heart rate, blood pressure, oxygen requirements, neurologic status, metabolic status, and hemoglobin concentration should all be considered to determine the immediate need for erythrocytes.[219]

Indications for transfusions in preterm infants have been gradually changing in the past decade, primarily because of clinical studies of EPO administration in this population. The impact of instituting strict transfusion guidelines has been as great as the impact of decreasing phlebotomy losses or beginning EPO therapy.[194, 195] This is most beneficial to preterm infants in a practical sense, because it can be implemented in newborn intensive care units throughout the world, without additional cost and without using new medications. An example of specific transfusion criteria used in an EPO study is presented in Table 8–9.

Neonatologists must determine their individual level of comfort in following specific transfusion criteria, but general guidelines can be recommended. Phlebotomy losses should be minimized to the greatest extent possible without compromising patient care. Hemoglobin or hematocrit values should be determined shortly after birth and then followed at 1- to 2-week intervals during hospitalization (less frequently as the infant grows older). During the first week of life, replacing the volume of blood out with an alternative isotonic colloid or crystalloid may benefit extremely-low-birth-weight infants in maintaining adequate intravascular volume.[194] This can be especially important when daily phlebotomy losses exceed 10% of the infant's total blood volume. Supplementation with iron as soon as possible (intravenously if available) can prevent iron deficiency and maintain adequate iron stores. Optimizing nutrition and ensuring adequate vitamin and mineral supplements can improve RBC production and

Table 8–9. **Transfusion Guidelines for Preterm Infants**

Hematocrit/ Hemoglobin*	Ventilator Requirement and/or Symptoms	Transfusion Volume
Hct≤35/Hgb≤11	Infants requring moderate or signficant mechanical ventilation (MAP >8 cm H_2O and FiO_2 >40%)	15 mL/kg PRBCs over 2–4
Hct≤30/Hgb≤10	Infants requiring minimal mechanical ventilation (any mechanical ventilation, or CPAP >6 cm H_2O and FiO_2≤40%)	15 mL/kg PRBCs over 2–4 h
Hct≤25/Hgb≤8	Infants on supplemental oxygen who are not requiring mechanical ventilation and one or more of the following is present: • ≤24 hours of tachycardia (HR >180) or tachypnea (RR >80) • An increased oxygen requirement from the previous 48 hours, defined as ≤four-fold increase in nasal canula flow (i.e., 1/4 L/min to 1 L/min) or an increase in nasal CPAP ≤20% from the previous 48 hours (i.e. 10 cm to 12 cm H_2O) • An elevated lactated concentration (≤2.5 mEq/L) • Weight gain <10 g/kg/d over the previous 4 days while receiving ≤100 kcal/kg/d • An increase in the episodes of apnea and bradycardia (>9 episodes in 24 h or ≤2 episodes in 24 h requiring bag-mask ventilation) while receiving therapeutic doses of methylxanthines • Undergoing surgery	20 mL/kg PRBCs over 2–4 h (divide into two 10 mL/kg volumes if fluid sensitive)
Hct≤20/Hgb≤7	Infant without any symptoms and an absolute reticulocyte count <100,000 cells/μL (RBC × % uncorrected retics)	20 mL/kg PRBCs over 2–4 h (divide into two 10 mL/kg volumes if fluid sensitive)

CPAP, continuous positive airway pressure; FiO_2, fractional inspired oxygen; HR, heart rate; MAP, mean airway pressure; PRBCs, packed red blood cells; RBC, red blood cells; RR, respiratory rate.

*Hematocrit values are percentages; hemoglobin values are given in units of grams per deciliter.

decrease red cell destruction, whether or not the infant is receiving recombinant EPO.

DIFFERENTIAL DIAGNOSIS OF ANEMIA

The diagnosis of anemia in the newborn period often requires rapid investigation and laboratory evaluation. Infants presenting in shock from anemia have likely suffered massive hemorrhage, and patient stabilization is of utmost importance to avoid organ damage and death. Initial steps include stabilizing the airway, administering oxygen if needed, and determining the cardiovascular and intravascular volume status. Immediate volume expansion should begin with normal saline when acute hemorrhage is suspected, followed by 5% albumin or available colloid. An immediate transfusion of type O, Rh-negative blood is needed in the first hour if massive hemorrhage has occurred, and repeat transfusions of crossmatched PRBCs may be necessary to treat lactic acidosis if oxygen delivery to the tissues is significantly compromised.

After the infant is stable, information can be gathered to determine the cause of anemia. One example of a strategy for obtaining information in a progressive fashion is shown in Figure 8–2. Information should first be gathered from the maternal chart. Any family history of anemia, bleeding, "low blood" counts, transfusions, jaundice, or unusual hematologic indices should be noted. Ethnicity of both parents should be obtained, because some inherited disorders (e.g., G6PD deficiency, thalassemias, sickle cell disease) are more prevalent in specific ethnic groups.

A thorough maternal history should be obtained and should include information on vaginal bleeding, trauma, infection or exposure to infected individuals, and any prescribed or illicit drug use during the pregnancy. Exposure to substances that increase oxidative stress and hemolysis in G6PD-deficient mothers include naphthalene (mothballs) and fava beans. The maternal use of cocaine or crack before delivery increases the potential for placental abruption, fetal infarction, and postinfarction hemorrhage. Important maternal laboratory values to record include blood type and antibody screen, maternal hepatitis, syphilis, and rubella status.

Information regarding labor and delivery can sometimes be difficult to obtain, especially in

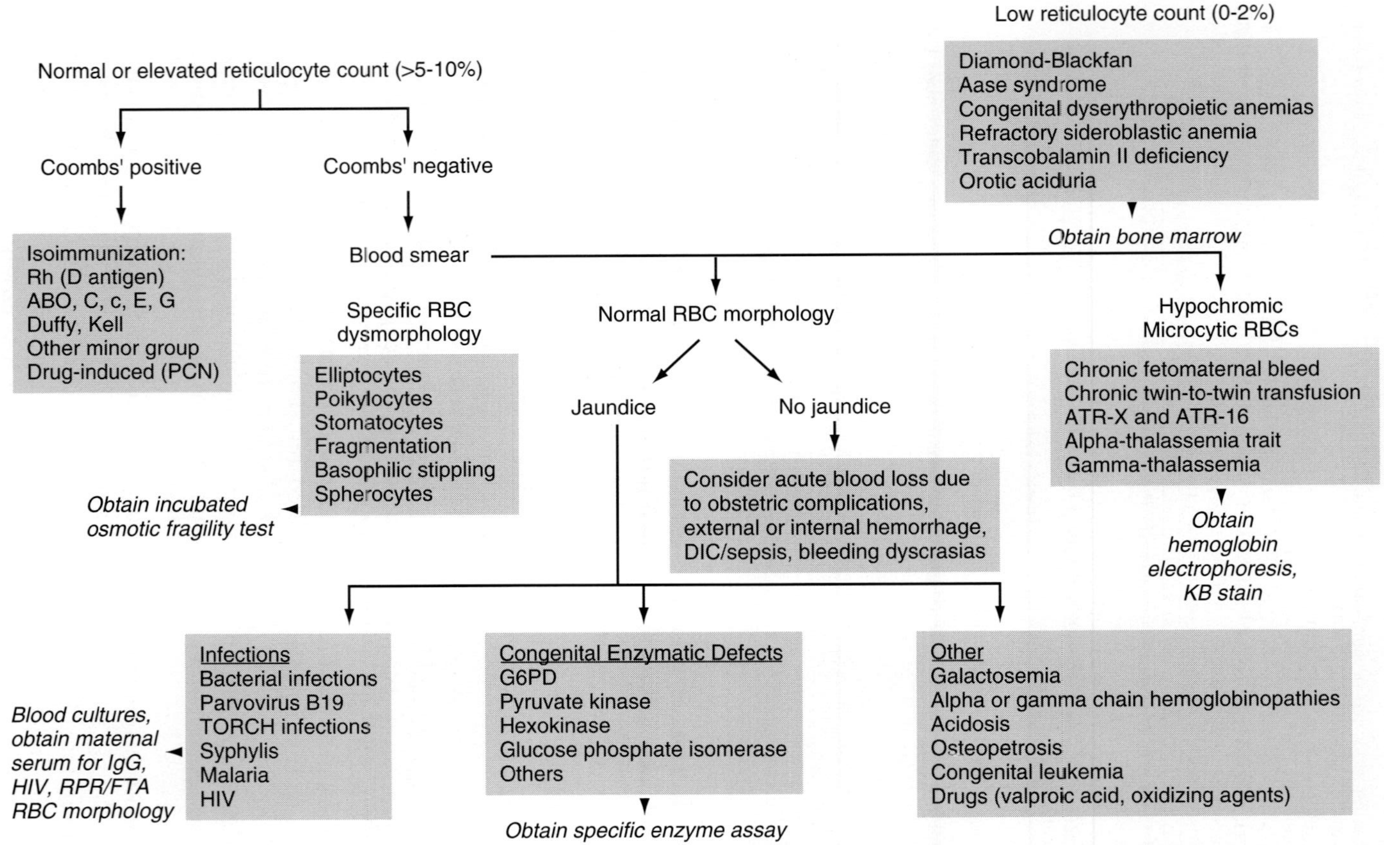

Figure 8–2. Differential diagnosis of neonatal anemia. The physician first seeks information from the family, maternal, and labor and delivery histories and then obtains initial laboratory tests: hemoglobin, reticulocyte (retic) count, blood type, direct Coombs' test, peripheral smear, red blood cell (RBC) indices, and bilirubin concentration. Results are used to navigate the diagnostic flow chart. DIC, disseminated intravascular coagulation; HIV, human immunodeficiency virus; PCN, penicillin; RPR, rapid plasma reagin test; FTA, fluorescent treponemal antibody test; G6PD, glucose-6-phosphate dehydrogenase.

an emergent cesarean section for fetal distress. The length of labor, vaginal bleeding, evidence of placenta previa, vasa previa, or placental abruption, and route of delivery should be noted. Information regarding the placenta (e.g., cord hematoma, cord rupture, chorioangioma, velamentous insertion of the cord) should be gathered and the placenta examined if possible. The use of forceps, vacuum, or other manipulations should documented. It is important to document the presence of multiple gestations, especially when discordant growth is present.

The timing of presentation of anemia is important. Infants with significant acute blood loss before or during delivery may be anemic and hypovolemic at birth, but infants with chronic FMH, TTS, or hemolysis from isoimmunization may not be symptomatic for 24 to 48 hours. Infants with internal hemorrhage (adrenal, renal, splenic, or hepatic) may not become symptomatic for 48 to 72 hours and then can rapidly decompensate. The initial laboratory evaluation of the anemic infant includes a complete blood count with RBC indices and peripheral smear, a reticulocyte count, a direct Coombs' test, and a bilirubin determination if jaundice is evident. A KB stain of maternal blood is helpful in identifying fetal cells in the maternal circulation. With minimal laboratory tests, a thorough history, and a physical examination, most causes of anemia in the newborn period can be determined.

Anemic infants with low reticulocyte counts have decreased erythropoiesis. Although the peripheral blood smear may present clues to the diagnosis, in most cases, a bone marrow aspiration is required to diagnosis hypoproliferative anemias presenting in the newborn period. These anemias include Diamond-Blackfan syndrome, Aase syndrome, Pearson's syndrome, osteopetrosis, congenital dyserythropoietic anemia, and transcobalamin II deficiency.

Anemic infants with elevated reticulocyte counts (>5% to 8%) have stimulated erythropoiesis; their anemia is often caused by hemolysis or hemorrhage. A positive Coombs' test result is evidence of immune-mediated hemolytic anemia. A blood type should be obtained on the infant, and maternal serum should be evaluated for antibodies. A negative Coombs' test result (or matching blood types) does not completely exclude immune-mediated hemolysis, and minor blood group incompatibilities should be considered.

A negative Coombs' test result associated with jaundice is common in nonimmune hemolytic anemias, and further work-up is required to determine a specific cause. Infants may have normal or elevated reticulocyte counts and may not present with symptomatic anemia at birth. The major causes of hemolysis in the newborn period are listed in Table 8–4. Abnormalities in RBC morphology such as spherocytosis and elliptocytosis can be determined by evaluating the peripheral smear. The presence of microcytic, hypochromic anemia can be evidence for iron deficiency anemia caused by chronic FMH or TTS. The obstetric history should be evaluated and the maternal blood screened with a KB stain for fetal hemoglobin. Anemias with an MCV less than 95 fL are associated with iron deficiency of hemoglobinopathies, such as α-thalassemia. Further work-up includes hemoglobin electrophoresis (see Chapter 16).

Anemic infants with normocytic, normochromic RBCs need further evaluation. If jaundice is excluded, acute blood loss should be suspected. The obstetric history should be reviewed and the infant evaluated for internal hemorrhage, sepsis, and DIC. Infants may present simply with pallor or may be in shock. Infants with continued active bleeding should be evaluated for deficiencies in clotting factors.

Intrinsic RBC defects may present with hemolytic anemia and jaundice in the first days to weeks of life. Red cell enzyme deficiencies such as G6PD, pyruvate kinase, and hexokinase deficiencies may lead to increased hemolysis. Male infants of Mediterranean or Asian descent are at increased risk for G6PD deficiency.

Bacterial and viral infections can cause hemolytic anemia in the newborn period and can cause marrow suppression if present for some time before delivery. Hepatosplenomegaly, jaundice, and DIC can result from viral or bacterial sepsis. Appropriate antibiotic therapy should be instituted when these symptoms are present and continued until a cause is determined or until it becomes clear that the infant does not have a bacterial infection. Systemic viral infections caused by toxoplasmosis, CMV, herpes simplex, or parvovirus can be associated with various degrees of anemia. Hydrops fetalis may be present in cases of *in utero* infection and may be severe enough to result in fetal demise.

If a cause for hemolytic anemia has not been determined, other unusual causes of hemolytic disease in the newborn should be evaluated. Unusual causes of hemolytic anemia include galactosemia, lysosomal storage diseases, and amino acid disorders. Prolonged metabolic acidosis, transfusion reactions, TAR syndrome, and osteopetrosis can manifest with hemolytic anemia in the newborn. Macroangiopathic and microangiopathic hemolytic anemias can occur with vascular malformations such as coarctation, hemangiomas, and large vessel thromboses.

Knowledge about the various proven and experimental therapies is required to determine the best treatment strategy for each anemic infant. Would the infant benefit from recombinant EPO? Is nutritional support with iron, vitamin E, folate, or B_{12} needed? Will repeated erythrocyte transfusions be required with the attendant risk of iron overload? Are steroids or IVIG indicated? Will bone marrow transplantation give the best chance for long-term survival? Although a few infants with anemia presenting in the newborn period go undiagnosed despite vigorous evaluation, most can be diagnosed and treated successfully.

References

1. Zanjani ED, Pixley JS, Slotnick N, et al: Erythropoietin does not cross the placenta into the fetus. Pathobiology 1993;61:211.
2. Malek A, Sager R, Eckardt KU, et al: Lack of transport of erythropoietin across the human placenta as studied by an *in vitro* perfusion system. Pflugers Arch 1994;427:157.
3. Widness JA, Sawyer ST, Schmidt RL, et al: Lack of maternal to fetal transfer of ^{125}I-erythropoietin in sheep. J Dev Physiol 1991;15:139.
4. Matoth Y, Zaizov R: Regulation of erythropoiesis in the fetal rat. Proceedings of the Tel Aviv University Conference on Erythropoiesis, Petak Tikva. New York: Academic Press, 1970, p 24.
5. Jacobsen LO, Marks EK, Gaston EO: The effect of transfusion-induced polycythemia in the mother on the fetus. Blood 1959;4:644.
6. Goldberg MA, Dunning SP, Bunn HF: Regulation of the erythropoietin gene: evidence that the oxygen sensor is a heme protein. Science 1988;242:524.
7. Peschle C, Marone G, Genovese A, et al: Erythropoietin production by the liver in fetal-neonatal life. Life Sci 1975;17:1325.
8. Fried W: The liver as a source of extrarenal erythropoietin production. Blood 1972;40:671.
9. Erslev AJ, Caro J, Kansu E, et al: Renal and extrarenal erythropoietin production in anemic rats. Br J Haematol 1980;45:65.
10. Naughton VA, Dornfest BS, Preti RA, et al: Hepatic and renal erythropoietin production during various intervals of short-term hypoxia. J Med 1984;15:45.
11. Beru N, McDonald J, Lacombe C, Goldwasser E: Expression of erythropoietin gene. Mol Cell Biol 1986;6:2571.
12. Arnaud S, Blanchet JP: Mouse serum enables CFU-E to grow under physiologic concentration of erythropoietin in vitro. Exp Hematol 1986;14:143.
13. DeWitte T, Holdrinet R, Raymakers J, et al: Influence of peripheral blood admixture on the number of hematopoietic progenitor cells (CFU-GM and BFU-E) in human bone marrow aspirates. Acta Haematol 1985;70:74.
14. Zanjani ED, Banisadre M: Hormonal stimulation of erythropoietin production and erythropoiesis in anephric sheep fetuses. J Clin Invest 1979;64:1181.
15. Udupa KB, Crabtree HM, Lipschitz DA: In vitro culture of proerythroblasts: characterization of proliferative response to erythropoietin and steroids. Br J Haematol 1986;62:705.
16. Zanjani ED, Gormus BJ, Bhakthavathsalan A, et al: Effects of thyroid hormone on erythropoiesis and the switch from fetal to adult hemoglobin synthesis in fetal sheep. In Stamatoyannopoulos G, Nienhuis AW (eds): Cellular and Molecular Regulation of Hemoglobin Switching. New York: Grune & Stratton, 1979, pp 169–178.
17. Datta MC: Prostaglandin E_2-mediated effects on synthesis of fetal and adult hemoglobin in blood erythroid bursts. Prostaglandins 1985;29:561.
18. Drake JR, Fitch CD: Status of vitamin E as an erythropoietic factor. Am J Clin Nutr 1980;33:2386.
19. Konwalinka G, Breier C, Peschle C, et al: Effect of human plasma lipoproteins on the erythropoietic progenitor cells in serum-free cultures. Blut 1986;52:191.
20. Zanjani ED, Poster J, Burlington H, et al: Liver as primary site of erythropoietin formation in the fetus. J Lab Clin Med 1977; 89:640.
21. Widness JA, Phillips AF, Clemons GK: Erythropoietin levels and erythropoiesis at birth in infants with Potter's syndrome. J Pediatr 1990;117:155.
22. Halvorsen S, Finne PH: Erythropoietin production in the human fetus and newborn. Ann N Y Acad Sci 1968;149:576.
23. Meberg A: Hemoglobin concentration and erythropoietin levels inappropriate in small for gestational age infants. Scand J Haematol 1980;24:162.
24. Thomas RM, Canning CE, Cotes PM, et al: Erythropoietin in cord blood hemoglobin and the regulation of fetal erythropoiesis. Br J Obstet Gynaecol 1983;90:795.
25. Widness JA, Clemons GK, Garcia JF, et al: Increased immunoreactive erythropoietin in cord blood after labor. Am J Obstet Gynecol 1984;148:194.
26. Stevenson DK, Bucalo LR, Cohen RS, et al: Increased immunoreactive erythropoietin in cord blood and neonatal bilirubin production in normal term infants after labor. Obstet Gynecol 1986;67:69.
27. Finne PH: Erythropoietin levels in cord blood as an indicator of intrauterine hypoxia. Acta Paediatr Scand 1986;55:478.
28. Widness JA, Teramok A, Clemons GK, et al: Correlation of the interpretation of fetal heart rate records with cord plasma erythropoietin levels. Br J Obstet Gynaecol 1985;92:326.
29. Erslev AJ, Wilson J, Caro J: Erythropoietin titers in anemic, nonuremic patients. J Lab Clin Med 1987;109:429.
30. Kling PJ, Schmidt RL, Roberts RA, et al: Serum erythropoietin levels during infancy: associations with erythropoiesis. J Pediatr 1996;128:791.

31. Stockman JA, Oski FA: Red blood cell values in low birth weight infants during the first seven weeks of life. Am J Dis Child 1980;134:945.
32. Brown MS, Garcia JF, Phibbs RH, et al: Decreased response of plasma immunoreactive erythropoietin to "available oxygen" in anemia of prematurity. J Pediatr 1984;105:793.
33. Stockman JA, et al: Anemia of prematurity: determinants of the erythropoietin response. J Pediatr 1984;105:786.
34. Stockman JA: Anemia of prematurity: current concepts in the issue of when to transfuse. Pediatr Clin North Am 1986;33:111.
35. Faxelius G, Raye J, Gutberlet R, et al: Red cell volume measurements and acute blood loss in high-risk newborn infants. J Pediatr 1977;90:273.
36. Oski FA: The erythrocyte and its disorders. In Oski FA, Nathan DG (eds): Hematology of Infancy and Childhood. Philadelphia: WB Saunders, 1993, pp 18–43.
37. Oh W, Lind J: Venous and capillary hematocrit in newborn infants and placental transfusion. Acta Paediatr Scand 1966;55:38.
38. Linderkamp O, Nelle M, Kraus M, Zilow EP: The effect of early and late cord-clamping on blood viscosity and other hemorheological parameters in full-term neonates. Acta Paediatr 1992;81:745.
39. Wardrop CA, Holland BM: The roles and vital importance of placental blood to the newborn infant. J Perinat Med 1995;23:139.
40. Scott JR, Warenski JC: Tests to detect and quantitate fetal maternal bleeding. Clin Obstet Gynecol 1982;25:277.
41. Bowman JM: Maternal blood group immunization. In Eden RD, Boehm FH (eds): Assessment and Care of the Fetus: Physiologic, Clinical and Medicolegal Principles. Norwalk, CT: Appleton & Lange, 1989, pp 749–772.
42. Kleihauer E, Stein G, Schmidt G: Demonstration of fetal hemoglobin in the erythrocytes of the blood of a newborn. Klin Wochenschr 1957;35:637.
43. Kosasa TS, Ebesugawa I, Nakayama RT, et al: Massive fetomaternal hemorrhage preceded by decreased fetal movement and a nonreactive fetal heart rate pattern. Obstet Gynecol 1993;82:711.
44. Giacoia GP: Severe fetomaternal hemorrhage: a review. Obstet Gynecol Surv 1997;52:372.
45. Rose PG, Strohm PL, Zuspan FP: Fetomaternal hemorrhage following trauma. Am J Obstet Gynecol 1985;153:844.
46. Stiller AG, Skafish PR: Placental chorioangioma: a rare cause of fetomaternal transfusion with maternal hemolysis and fetal distress. Obstet Gynecol 1986;67:296.
47. Lopriore E, Vandenbussche FP, Tiersma ES, et al: Twin-to-twin transfusion syndrome: new perspectives. J Pediatr 1995;127:675.
48. Benirschke, K: Accurate recording of twin placenta. Obstet Gynecol 1961;18:334.
49. Tan KL, Tan R, Tan SH, et al: The twin transfusion syndrome. Clinical observations on 35 affected pairs. Clin Pediatr 1979;18:111.
50. Dennis LG, Winkler CL: Twin-to-twin transfusion syndrome: aggressive therapeutic amniocentesis. Am J Obstet Gynecol 1997;177:342.
51. Dommergues M, Mandelbrot L, Delezoide AL, et al: Twin-to-twin transfusion syndrome: selective feticide by embolization of the hydropic fetus. Fetal Diagn Ther 1995;10:26.
52. De Lia JE, Kuhlmann RS, Harstad TW, et al: Fetoscopic laser ablation of placental vessels in severe previable twin-twin transfusion syndrome. Am J Obstet Gynecol. 1995;172(4 Pt 1):1202.
53. Ville Y, Hyett J, Hecher K, et al: Preliminary experience with endoscopic laser surgery for severe twin-twin transfusion syndrome. N Engl J Med 1995;332:224.
54. van Heteren CF, Nijhuis JG, Semmekrot BA, et al: Risk for surviving twin after fetal death of co-twin in twin-twin transfusion syndrome. Obstet Gynecol 1998;92:215.
55. Kramer MS, Usher RH, Pollack R, et al: Etiologic determinants of abruptio placentae. Obstet Gynecol 1997;89:221.
56. Rasmussen S, Irgens LM, Bergsjo P, et al: Perinatal mortality and case fatality after placental abruption in Norway, 1967–1991. Acta Obstet Gynecol Scand 1996;75:229.
57. McMahon MJ, Li R, Schenck AP, et al: Previous cesarean birth. A risk factor for placenta previa? J Reprod Med 1997;42:409.
58. Chelmow D, Andrew DE, Baker ER: Maternal cigarette smoking and placenta previa. Obstet Gynecol 1996;87(5 Pt 1):703.
59. Schreier R, Brown S: Hematoma of the umbilical cord: report of a case. Obstet Gynecol 1962;20:798.
60. Deans A, Jauniaux E: Prenatal diagnosis and outcome of subamniotic hematomas. Ultrasound Obstet Gynecol 1998;11:319.
61. Benirschke K: Obstetrically important lesions of the umbilical cord. J Reprod Med 1994;39:262.
62. Eddleman KA, Lockwood CJ, Berkowitz GS, et al: Clinical significance and sonographic diagnosis of velamentous umbilical cord insertion. Am J Perinatol 1992;9:123.
63. Chen KH, Konchak P: Use of transvaginal color Doppler ultrasound to diagnose vasa previa. J Am Osteopath Assoc 1998;98:116.
64. Kleinberg F, Phibbs R, Dong L: Lack of placenta to infant transfusion with delayed cord clamping after cesarean section delivery. Pediatr Res 1973;7:403.
65. Cashore WJ, Usher RH: Hypovolemia resulting from a tight nuchal cord at birth. Pediatr Res 1973;7:399.
66. Benaron DA: Subgaleal hematoma causing hypovolemic shock during delivery after failed vacuum extraction: a case report. J Perinatol 1993;13:228.
67. Robinson RJ, Rossiter MA: Massive subaponeurotic haemorrhage in babies of African origin. Arch Dis Child 1968;43:684.
68. Teng FY, Sayre JW: Vacuum extraction: does duration predict scalp injury? Obstet Gynecol 1997;89:281.
69. Chadwick LM, Pemberton PJ, Kurinczuk JJ: Neonatal subgaleal haematoma: associated risk factors, complications and outcome. J Paediatr Child Health 1996;32:228.
70. Papile LA, Burstein J, Burstein R, et al: Incidence and evolution of subependymal and intraventricular hemorrhage: a study of infants with birth weights less than 1,500 gm. J Pediatr 1978;92:529.
71. Thorp JA, Poskin MF, McKenzie DR, et al: Perinatal factors predicting severe intracranial hemorrhage. Am J Perinatol 1997;14:631.
72. Verma U, Tejani N, Klein S, et al: Obstetric antecedents of intraventricular hemorrhage and periventricular leukomalacia in the low-birth-weight neonate. Am J Obstet Gynecol 1997;176:275.
73. Korobkin R: The relationship between head circumference and the development of communicating hydrocephalus in infants following intraventricular hemorrhage. Pediatrics 1975;56:74.
74. Bussel JB, Zabusky MR, Berkowitz RL, et al: Fetal alloimmune thrombocytopenia. N Engl J Med 1997;337:22.

75. Bussel JB. Immune thrombocytopenia in pregnancy: autoimmune and alloimmune. J Reprod Immunol 1997;37:35.
76. Church MW, Crossland WJ, Holmes PA, et al: Effects of prenatal cocaine on hearing, vision, growth, and behavior. Ann N Y Acad Sci 1998;21;846:12.
77. Behnke M, Davis Eyler F, Conlon M, et al: Incidence and description of structural brain abnormalities in newborns exposed to cocaine. J Pediatr 1998;132:291.
78. Felc Z: Ultrasound in screening for neonatal adrenal hemorrhage. Am J Perinatol 1995;12:363.
79. Pinto E, Guignard JP: Renal masses in the neonate. Biol Neonate 1995;68:175.
80. Levine C: Intestinal obstruction in a neonate with adrenal hemorrhage and renal vein thrombosis. Pediatr Radiol 1989;19:477.
81. Mostoufizadeh M, Lack EE, Gang DL, et al: Postmortem manifestations of echovirus 11 sepsis in five newborn infants. Hum Pathol 1983;14:818.
82. Davies MR: Iatrogenic hepatic rupture in the newborn and its management by pack tamponade. J Pediatr Surg 1997;32:1414.
83. Emma F, Smith J, Moerman PH: Subcapsular hemorrhage of the liver and hemoperitoneum in premature infants: report of 4 cases. Eur J Obstet Gynecol Reprod Biol 1992 21;44:161.
84. Miele V, Galluzzo M, Patti G, et al: Scrotal hematoma due to neonatal adrenal hemorrhage: the value of ultrasonography in avoiding unnecessary surgery. Pediatr Radiol 1997;27:672.
85. Nagaya M, Kato J, Niimi N, et al: Isolated cavernous hemangioma of the stomach in a neonate. J Pediatr Surg 1998;33:653.
86. Wranne L: Studies on erythrokinetics in infancy. Acta Paediatr Scand 1967;56:381.
87. Mollison PL: The survival of transfused erythrocytes in hemolytic disease of the newborn. Arch Dis Child 1943;18:161.
88. Komazawa M, Oski FA: Biochemical characteristics of "young" and "old" erythrocytes of the newborn infant. J Pediatr 1975;87:102.
89. Schmidt-Sommerfield E, Penn D: Carnitine and total parenteral nutrition of the neonate. Biol Neonate 1990;58:81.
90. Bracci R, Martini G, Buonocore G, et al: Changes in erythrocyte properties during the first hours of life: electron spin resonance of reacting sulfhydryl groups. Pediatr Res 1988;24:391.
91. Bohler T, et al: Mechanical fragility of erythrocyte membrane in neonates and adults. Pediatr Res 1992;32:92.
92. Toivanen B, Hirvonen T: Iso- and heteroagglutinins in human fetal and neonatal sera. Scand J Haematol 1969;6:42.
93. Marsh WL, Allen FH: Erythrocyte blood groups in humans. In Nathan DG, Oski FA (eds): Hematology of Infancy and Childhood, 3rd ed. Philadelphia: WB Saunders, 1987, pp 1497–1521.
94. Thomaidis T, Agathopoules A, Matsaniotis N: Natural isohemagglutinin production by the fetus. J Pediatr 1969;74:39.
95. Zipursky A, Pollock J, Neeland P, et al: The transplacental passage of foetal red blood cells and the pathogenesis of Rh immunisation during pregnancy. Lancet 1963;2:489.
96. Weiner CP, Widness JA: Decreased fetal erythropoiesis and hemolysis in Kell hemolytic anemia. Am J Obstet Gynecol 1996;174:547.
97. Vaughan JI, Manning M, Warwick RM, et al: Inhibition of erythroid progenitor cells by anti-Kell antibodies in fetal alloimmune anemia. N Engl J Med 1998;338:798.
98. Kozlowski CL, Lee D, Shwe KH, et al: Quantification of anti-c in haemolytic disease of the newborn. Transfus Med 1995;5:37.
99. van Dijk BA, Dooren MC, Overbeeke MA. Red cell antibodies in pregnancy: there is no "critical titre." Transfus Med 1995;5:199.
100. Geifman-Holtzman O, Wojtowycz M, Kosmos E, et al: Female alloimmunization with antibodies known to cause hemolytic disease. Obstet Gynecol 1997;89:272.
101. Lipitz S, Many A, Mitrani-Rosenbaum S, et al: Obstetric outcome after RhD and Kell testing. Hum Reprod 1998;13:1472.
102. Linderkamp O, Stadler AA, Zilow EP: Blood viscosity and optimal hematocrit in preterm and full-term neonates in 50- to 500 μm tubes. Pediatr Res 1992;32:97.
103. Cleary TG, Lopez EL: The Shiga-like toxin-producing *Escherichia coli* and hemolytic uremic syndrome. Pediatr Infect Dis J 1989;8:720.
104. Bokete TN, O'Callahan CM, Clausen CR, et al: Shiga-like toxin-producing *Escherichia coli* in Seattle children: a prospective study. Gastroenterology 1993;105:1724.
105. Levine Z, Sherer DM, Jacobs A, et al: Nonimmune hydrops fetalis due to congenital syphilis associated with negative intrapartum maternal serology screening. Am J Perinatol 1998;15:233.
106. Berkowitz K, Baxi L, Fox HE: False-negative syphilis screening: the prozone phenomenon, nonimmune hydrops, and diagnosis of syphilis during pregnancy. Am J Obstet Gynecol 1990;163:975.
107. Vogel H, Kornman M, Ledet SC, et al: Congenital parvovirus infection. Pediatr Pathol Lab Med 1997;17:903.
108. Sheikh AU, Ernest JM, O'Shea M: Long-term outcome in fetal hydrops from parvovirus B19 infection. Am J Obstet Gynecol 1992;167:337.
109. Cameron AD, Swain S, Patrick WJ: Human parvovirus B19 infection associated with hydrops fetalis. Aust N Z J Obstet Gynaecol 1997;37:316.
110. Brown KE, Young NS: Parvovirus B19 infection and hematopoiesis. Blood Rev 1995;9:176.
111. McNeely DF, Chu A, Lowe S, et al: Malaria surveillance in New York City: 1991–1996. Int J Infect Dis 1998;2:132.
112. Ferrazin A, De Maria A, Gotta C, et al: Zidovudine therapy of HIV-1 infection during pregnancy: assessment of the effect on the newborns. J Acquir Immune Defic Syndr 1993;6:376.
113. Stahl MM, Neiderud J, Vinge E: Thrombocytopenic purpura and anemia in a breast-fed infant whose mother was treated with valproic acid. J Pediatr 1997;130:1001.
114. Zinkham WH, Oski FA: Henna: a potential cause of oxidative hemolysis and neonatal hyperbilirubinemia. Pediatrics 1996;97:707.
115. Gerritsen EJ, Vossen JM, van Loo IH, et al: Autosomal recessive osteopetrosis: variability of findings at diagnosis and during the natural course. Pediatrics 1994;93:247.
116. Gallagher PG, Ehrenkranz RA: Nutritional anemias in infancy. Clin Perinatol 1995;22:671.
117. Ehrenkranz RA, Gettner PA, Nelli C, et al: Iron absorption and incorporation into red blood cells by very low birthweight infants: studies with the stable isotope ^{58}Fe. J Pediatr Gastroenterol Nutr 1992;15:270.
118. Christensen RD, Hunter DD, Goodell H, et al: Evaluation of the mechanism causing anemia in infants with bronchopulmonary dysplasia. J Pediatr 1992;120:593.

119. Lee RE: The anemia of chronic disorders. Semin Hematol 1973;20:61.
120. Barry DMJ, Reeve AW: Increased incidence of gram-negative neonatal sepsis with intramuscular iron administration. Pediatrics 1977;60:908.
121. Becroft DMO, Dix MR, Farmer K: Intramuscular iron-dextran and susceptibility of neonates to bacterial infections. Arch Dis Child 1977;52:778.
122. Friel AK, Andrews WL, Hall MS, et al: Intravenous iron administration to very-low-birth-weight newborns receiving total and partial parenteral nutrition. J Parenteral Enteral Nutr 1995;19:114.
123. Carnielli V, Montini G, Da Riol R, et al: Effect of high doses of human recombinant erythropoietin on the need for blood transfusions in preterm infants. J Pediatr 1992;121:98.
124. Ohls RK: Recombinant human erythropoietin to prevent and treat the anemia of prematurity. Erythropoiesis 1995;6:35.
125. Bechensteen AG, Håagåa P, Halvorsen S, et al: Erythropoietin, protein, and iron supplementation and the prevention of anaemia of prematurity. Arch Dis Child 1993;69:19.
126. Eschbach JW, Egrie JC, Downing MR, et al: Correction of the anemia of end stage renal disease with recombinant human erythropoietin. N Engl J Med 1987;310:73.
127. Eschbach JW, Kelly MR, Haley RN, et al: Treatment of the anemia of progressive renal failure with recombinant human erythropoietin. N Engl J Med 1989;321:158.
128. Winearls CG, Oliver DO, Pippard MJ, et al: Effect of human erythropoietin derived from recombinant DNA on the anemia of patients maintained by chronic haemodialysis. Lancet 1986;2:1175.
129. Maier RF, Obladen M, Scigalla P, et al: The effect of epoetin beta (recombinant human erythropoietin) on the need for transfusion in very low birth weight infants. N Engl J Med 1994;330:1173.
130. Meyer MP, Meyer JH, Commerford A, et al: Recombinant human erythropoietin in the treatment of the anemia of prematurity: results of a double-blind, placebo-controlled study. Pediatrics 1994;93:918.
131. Ehrenkrantz RA, Sherwonit EA, Nelli CM, et al: Recombinant human erythropoietin (r-HuEPO) stimulates incorporation of absorbed iron (Fe) into RBCs in VLBW infants (Abstract). Pediatr Res 1994;35:311A.
132. Oski FA, Barness LA: Vitamin E deficiency: a previously unrecognized cause of hemolytic anemia in premature infants. J Pediatr 1967;79:569.
133. Williams ME, Shott RJ, Oski FA: Role of dietary iron and fat on vitamin E deficiency anemia of infancy. N Engl J Med 1975;292:887.
134. Melhorn DK, Gross S: Vitamin E dependent anemia in the preterm infant: effects of large doses of medicinal iron. J Pediatr 1971;79:569.
135. Diamond LK, Blackfan KD. Hypoplastic anemia. Am J Dis Child 1938;56:464.
136. Diamond LK, Wang WC, Alter BP. Congenital hypoplastic anemia. Adv Pediatr 1976;22:349.
137. Rogers BB, Bloom SL, Buchanan GR: Autosomal dominantly inherited Diamond-Blackfan anemia resulting in nonimmune hydrops. Obstet Gynecol 1997;89(5 Pt 2):805.
138. McLennan AC, Chitty LS, Rissik J, et al: Prenatal diagnosis of Blackfan-Diamond syndrome: case report and review of the literature. Prenat Diagn 1996;16:349.
139. Gojic V, van't Veer-Korthof ET, Bosch LJ, et al: Congenital hypoplastic anemia: another example of autosomal dominant transmission. Am J Med Genet 1994;50:87.
140. Alter BP, Nathan DG: Red cell aplasia in children. Arch Dis Child 1979;54:263.
141. Ohls RK, Liechty KW, Schibler KR, et al: Assessment of stem cell factor as a candidate defect for Diamond Blackfan anemia in a Utah kindred (Abstract). Pediatr Res 1992;31:144A.
142. Abkowitz JL, Sabo KM, Nakamoto B, et al: Diamond-Blackfan anemia: in vitro response of erythroid progenitors to the ligand for c-kit. Blood 1991;78:2198.
143. Dianzani I, Garelli E, Crescenzio N, et al: Diamond-Blackfan anemia: expansion of erythroid progenitors in vitro by IL-9, but exclusion of a significant pathogenetic role for the IL-9 gene and the hematopoietic gene cluster on chromosome 5q. Exp Hematol 1997;25:1270.
144. Dianzani I, Garelli E, Ramenghi U: Diamond-Blackfan anemia: a congenital defect in erythropoiesis. Haematologica 1996;81:560.
145. Dianzani I, Garelli E, Dompe C, et al: Mutations in the erythropoietin receptor gene are not a common cause of Diamond-Blackfan anemia. Blood 1996;87:2568.
146. Visckochil DH, Carey JC, Glader BE, et al: Congenital hypoplastic (Diamond-Blackfan) anemia in seven members of one kindred. Am J Med Genet 1990;35:251.
147. Nathan DG, Clarke BJ, Hillman DG, et al: Erythroid precursors in congenital hypoplastic (Diamond-Blackman) anemia. J Clin Invest 1978;61:489.
148. Lipton JM, Kudish M, Gross R, et al: Defective erythroid progenitor differentiation system in congenital hypoplastic (Diamond Blackfan) anemia. Blood 1986;7:962.
149. Gustavsson P, Willing TN, van Haeringen A, et al: Diamond-Blackfan anaemia: genetic homogeneity for a gene on chromosome 19q13 restricted to 1.8 Mb. Nat Genet 1997;16:368.
150. Janov AJ, Leong T, Nathan DG, et al: Diamond-Blackfan anemia: natural history and sequelae of treatment. Medicine (Baltimore) 1996;75:77.
151. Sieff C, Guinan E: In vitro enhancement of erythropoiesis by steel factor in Diamond-Blackfan anemia and treatment of other congenital cytopenias with recombinant interleukin 3/granulocyte-macrophage colony stimulating factor. Stem Cells (Dayt) 1993;11:113.
152. Tamary H, Shalmon L, Shalev H, et al: Localization of the gene for congenital dyserythropoietic anemia type I to a <1-cM interval on chromosome 15q15.1.3. Am J Hum Genet 1998;62:1062.
153. De Franceschi L, Turrini F, del Giudice EM, et al: Decreased band 3 anion transport activity and band 3 clusterization in congenital dyserythropoietic anemia type II. Exp Hematol 1998;26:869.
154. Marks PW, Mitus AJ: Congenital dyserythropoietic anemias. Am J Hematol 1996;51:55.
155. Shalev H, Tamary H, Shaft D, et al: Neonatal manifestations of congenital dyserythropoietic anemia type I. J Pediatr 1997;131(1 Pt 1):95.
156. Cantu-Rajnoldi A, Zanella A, Conter U, et al: A severe transfusion-dependent congenital dyserythropoietic anaemia presenting as hydrops fetalis. Br J Haematol 1997;96:530.
157. Aase JM, Smith DW: Congenital anemia and triphalangeal thumbs: a new syndrome. J Pediatr 1969;74:471.
158. Hing AV, Dowton SB: Aase syndrome: novel radiographic features. Am J Med Genet 1993;45:413.
159. Hurst JA, Baraitser M, Wonke B: Autosomal dominant

transmission of congenital erythroid hypoplastic anemia with radial abnormalities. Am J Med Genet 1991;40:482.
160. Charles JM, Key LL: Developmental spectrum of children with congenital osteopetrosis. J Pediatr 1998;132:371.
161. Gerritsen EJ, Vossen JM, Fasth A, et al: Bone marrow transplantation for autosomal recessive osteopetrosis: a report from the Working Party on Inborn Errors of the European Bone Marrow Transplantation Group. J Pediatr 1994;125(6 Pt 1):896.
162. Alter BP: Fanconi's anaemia and its variability. Br J Haematol 1993;85:9.
163. D'Andrea AD, Grompe M: Molecular biology of Fanconi anemia: implications for diagnosis and therapy. Blood 1997;90:1725.
164. Perel Y, Butenandt O, Carrere A, et al: Oesophageal atresia, VACTERL association: Fanconi's anaemia related spectrum of anomalies. Arch Dis Child 1998;78:375.
165. Butturini A, Gale RP, Verlander PC, et al: Hematologic abnormalities in Fanconi anemia: an International Fanconi Anemia Registry Study. Blood 1994;84:1650.
166. Pearson HA, Lobel JS, Kocoshis SA, et al: A new syndrome of refractory sideroblastic anemia with vacuolization of marrow precursors and exocrine pancreatic dysfunction. J Pediatr 1979;95:976.
167. Toth T, Bokay J, Szonyi L, et al: Detection of mtDNA deletion in Pearson syndrome by two independent PCR assays from Guthrie card. Clin Genet 1998;53:210.
168. Rotig A, Cormier V, Blanche S, et al: Pearson's marrow-pancreas syndrome: a multisystem mitochondrial disorder in infancy. J Clin Invest 1990;86:1601.
169. Stockman JA, Garcia JF, Oski FA: The anemia of prematurity: factors governing the erythropoietin response. N Engl J Med 1977;296:647.
170. Erslev AJ, Caro J, Schuster SJ: Is there an optimal hemoglobin level? Trans Med Rev 1989;3:237.
171. Ross MP, Christensen RD, Rothstein G, et al: A randomized trial to develop criteria for administering erythrocyte transfusions to anemic preterm infants 1 to 3 months of age. J Perinatol 1989;9:246.
172. Bifano EM, Smith F, Borer J: Relationship between determinants of oxygen delivery and respiratory abnormalities in preterm infants with anemia. J Pediatr 1992;120:292.
173. Keyes WG, Donohue PK, Spivak JL, et al: Assessing the need for transfusion of premature infants and the role of hematocrit, clinical signs, and erythropoietin level. Pediatrics 1989;84:412.
174. Izraeli S, Ben-Sira L, Harell D, et al: Lactac acid as a predictor for erythrocyte transfusion in healthy preterm infants with the anemia of prematurity. J Pediatr 1993;122:629.
175. Schulman I: The anemia of prematurity. J Pediatr 1959;54:663.
176. Shannon KM, Naylor GS, Torkildson JC, et al: Circulating erythroid progenitors in the anemia of prematurity. N Engl J Med 1987;31:728.
177. Rhondeau SM, Christensen RD, Ross MP, et al: Responsiveness to recombinant human erythropoietin of marrow erythroid progenitors from infants with the "anemia of prematurity." J Pediatr 1988;112:935.
178. Ohls RK, Liechty KW, Turner MC, et al: Erythroid "burst promoting activity" in the serum of patients with the anemia of prematurity. J Pediatr 1990;116:786.
179. Delivoria-Papadopoulos M, Roncevic NP, Oski FA: Postnatal changes in oxygen transport of term, preterm and sick infants: the role of red cell 2,3-diphosphoglycerate in adult hemoglobin. Pediatr Res 1971;5:235.
180. Pearson HA: Life-span of the fetal red blood cell. J Pediatr 1967;70:166.
181. Bratteby LE: Studies on erythrokinetics in infants. IX. Prediction of red cell volume from venous haematocrit in early infancy. Acta Pediatr Scand 1968;57:125.
182. Ohls RK, Li Y, Trautman MS, et al: Erythropoietin production by preterm macrophages: implications regarding the anemia of prematurity. Pediatr Res 1994;35:169.
183. George JW, Bracco CA, Shannon KM, et al: Age-related differences in erythropoietic response to recombinant human erythropoietin: comparison in adult and infant Rhesus monkeys. Pediatr Res 1990;28:567.
184. Widness JA, Pedersen PV, Modi NB, et al: Developmental changes in erythropoietin (Epo) pharmacokinetics in fetal and neonatal sheep. Pediatr Res 1990;28:284.
185. Brown MS, Jones MA, Ohls RK, et al: Single-dose pharmacokinetics of recombinant human erythropoietin in preterm infants after intravenous and subcutaneous administration. J Pediatr 1993;122:655.
186. Ohls RK, Veerman MW, Mandell L, et al: Pharmacokinetics of recombinant erythropoietin administered to preterm infants by continuous infusion in parenteral nutrition solution. J Pediatr 1996;128:518.
187. Maier RF, Obladen M, Kattner E, et al: High- versus low-dose erythropoietin in extremely low birth weight infants. J Pediatr 1998;132:866.
188. Shannon KM, Keith JF, Mentzer WC, et al: Recombinant human erythropoietin stimulates erythropoiesis and reduces erythrocyte transfusions in very low birth weight preterm infants. Pediatrics 1995;95:1.
189. Meister B, Maurer H, Simma B, et al: The effect of recombinant human erythropoietin in circulating hematopoietic progenitor cells in anemic premature infants. Stem Cells (Dayt) 1997;15:359.
190. Soubasi V, Kremenopoulos G, Diamandi E, et al. In which neonates does early recombinant human erythropoietin treatment prevent anemia of prematurity? Results of a randomized, controlled study. Pediatr Res 1993;34:675.
191. Obladen M, Maier R, Segerer H, et al: Efficacy and safety of recombinant human erythropoietin to prevent the anaemias of prematurity. European randomized multicenter trial. Contrib Nephrol 1991;88:314.
192. Messer J, Haddad J, Donato L, et al: Early treatment of premature infants with recombinant human erythropoietin. Pediatrics 1993;92:519.
193. Kumar P, Shankaran S, Krishnan RG: Recombinant human erythropoietin therapy for treatment of anemia of prematurity in very low birth weight infants: a randomized, double-blind, placebo-controlled trial. J Perinatol 1998;18:173.
194. Ohls RK, Osborne KA, Christensen RD: Efficacy and cost analysis of treating very low birth weight infants with erythropoietin during their first two weeks of life: a randomized, placebo controlled trial. J Pediatr 1995;126:421.
195. Bifano EM, Miggiani WP, Parker PR: Impact of transfusion guidelines on transfusion practices in premature infants (Abstract). Pediatr Res 1994;35:216A.
196. Ohls RK, Harcum J, Schibler KR, et al: The effect of erythropoietin on the transfusion requirements of preterm infants $\leq$ 750 grams: a randomized, double-blind, placebo-controlled study. J Pediatr 1997; 131:661.

197. Donato H, Vivas N, Vain L, et al: Early vs. late recombinant human erythropoietin (rHuEPO) in anemia of prematurity: results of randomized, placebo-controlled, multicentric trial (Abstract). Pediatr Res 1998;43:236A.
198. Ohls RK, Christensen RD: Recombinant erythropoietin compared with erythrocyte transfusion in the treatment of anemia of prematurity. J Pediatr 1991;119:781.
199. Halpérin DS, Wacker P, Lacourt G, et al: Effects of recombinant human erythropoietin in infants with the anemia of prematurity: a pilot study. J Pediatr 1990;116:779.
200. Beck D, Masserey E, Meyer M, et al: Weekly intravenous administration of recombinant human erythropoietin in infants with the anaemia of prematurity. Eur J Pediatr 1991;150:767.
201. Christensen RD, Liechty KW, Koenig JM, et al: Administration of erythropoietin to newborn rats results in diminished neutrophil production. Blood 1991;78:1241.
202. Christensen RD, Rothstein G: Erythropoietin affects the maturation pattern of fetal G-CSF–responsive progenitors. Am J Hematol 1992; 39:108.
203. Katoh K, Mizuno K, Hashimoto S, et al: Direct evidence for erythropoietin-induced release of endothelin from peripheral vascular tissue. Life Sci 1994;54:253.
204. Cogar AA, Ohls RK: Endothelin concentrations in preterm infants treated with human recombinant erythropoietin (Abstract). Pediatr Res 1997;41:215A.
205. Alverson DC, Isken VA, Cohen RS: Effect of booster blood transfusions on oxygen utilization in infants with bronchopulmonary dysplasia. J Pediatr 1988;113:722.
206. Ohls RK, Hunter DD, Christensen RD: A randomized, placebo-controlled trial of recombinant erythropoietin as treatment for the anemia of bronchopulmonary dysplasia. J Pediatr 1993;123:996.
207. Koury MJ: Investigating erythropoietin resistance. N Engl J Med 1993;328:205.
208. Bakris GL, Sauter ER, Hussey JL, Fisher JW, Gaber AO, Winsett R: Effects of theophylline on erythropoietin production in normal subjects and in patients with erythrocytosis after renal transplantation. N Engl J Med 1990;323:86.
209. Gonzalez MT, Sherwood J, Brion LP, Schulman M: Erythropoietin (EPO) levels during theophylline treatment in low birth weight (BW) infants (Abstract). Pediatr Res 1993;33:213A.
210. Roodman GD, Lee J, Gidari AS: Effects of dexamethasone on erythroid colony formation from fetal liver and adult marrow. Br J Hematol 1983;53:621.
211. Millard DD, Gidding SS, Socol ML, et al: Effects of intravascular, intrauterine transfusion on prenatal and postnatal hemolysis and erythropoiesis in severe fetal isoimmunization. J Pediatr 1990;117:447.
212. Koenig, JM, Ashton DR, De Vore GR, et al: Late hyporegenerative anemia in Rh hemolytic disease. J Pediatr 1989;115:315.
213. Ohls RK, Wirkus PE, Christensen RD: Recombinant erythropoietin as treatment for the late hyporegenerative anemia of Rh hemolytic disease. Pediatrics 1992;90:678.
214. Scaradavou A, Inglis S, Peterson P, et al: Suppression of erythropoiesis by intrauterine transfusions in hemolytic disease of the newborn: use of erythropoietin to treat the late anemia. J Pediatr 1993;123:279.
215. Shaddy RE, Bullock EA, Tani LY, et al: Epoetin alpha therapy in infants awaiting heart transplantation. Arch Pediatr Adolesc Med 1995;149:322.
216. Kling PJ, Widness JA, Guillery EW, et al: Pharmacokinetics and pharmacodynamics of erythropoietin therapy in an infant with renal failure. J Pediatr 1992;121:822.
217. Christensen RD, Hunter DD, Ohls RK: A pilot study comparing recombinant erythropoietin alone with erythropoietin plus recombinant granulocyte-macrophage colony-stimulating factor for treatment of the anemia of prematurity. J Perinatol 1994;14:110.
218. DePalma L, Luban NLC: Blood component therapy in the perinatal period: guidelines and recommendations. Semin Perinatol 1990;14:403.
219. Alverson DC: The physiologic impact of anemia in the neonate. Clin Perinatol 1995;22:609.

CHAPTER 9

Evaluation and Treatment of Polycythemia in the Neonate

Rolf Lindemann, M.D., Ph.D., and Per Hågå, M.D., Ph.D.

In the first edition of *Hematologic Problems in the Newborn*, published in 1966, the subject of neonatal polycythemia was discussed on only one page. In the third edition, published in 1982, the subject was covered on 8 pages. Since then, surprisingly few new studies on this relatively common disorder have appeared.

Living in a relatively hypoxic environment, the fetus compensates with an increased erythropoietic activity. The red blood cell mass of the newborn infant is therefore significantly increased compared with the level later in life. The red blood cell mass can be pathologically increased by primary (e.g., increased fetal erythropoietic activity) or secondary (e.g., transfusion of red blood cells) causes, or reduced plasma volume, leading to the syndrome of polycythemia and hyperviscosity.[1–5]

FETAL AND NEONATAL ERYTHROPOIESIS

The fetus adapts to the relatively hypoxic intrauterine environment by increased erythropoiesis.[6] Fetal erythropoiesis develops through three stages. As detailed in Chapters 1 and 2, the process begins in the yolk sac. The liver is the main erythropoietic organ from the third to the sixth month of gestation and continues to produce erythrocytes until right after birth. The bone marrow is the major production site during the last 3 months of gestation.[6, 7] By the beginning of the third trimester, hematocrit levels are nearly stable and only slightly lower than those of term neonates.[8, 9]

Fetal erythrocytes are fundamentally different from red blood cells produced later in life in their membrane proteins, surface antigens, and metabolic enzyme patterns.[7] They also have a larger mean cell volume and mean cell hemoglobin than adult erythrocytes.[10] Fetal hemoglobin has a higher oxygen affinity and produces a rightward shift of the hemoglobin-oxygen dissociation curve. It also binds less strongly to 2,3-diphosphoglycerate (2,3-DPG) than hemoglobin A, rendering it less subject to 2,3-DPG's reduction of hemoglobin's oxygen affinity.[7]

Fetal hemoglobin is the predominant hemoglobin during fetal life and remains so in early infancy. The switch from fetal to adult hemoglobin production appears to be determined by gestation and takes place at around 40 weeks of gestation.[11] By the end of the first year of life, erythropoiesis is similar to that of the adult.

POLYCYTHEMIA AND HYPERVISCOSITY

Polycythemia and hyperviscosity are not synonymous terms. Most researchers define neonatal polycythemia as a peripheral venous hematocrit greater than 65%. Factors that should be considered when interpreting hematocrit levels in the newborn include the age of the newborn infant (hours and days), the site of collection, and the method of analysis (see Chapter 7).

Polycythemia

Polycythemia can occur as a result of increased red blood cell mass, decreased plasma volume, or both. In some cases of primary neonatal polycythemia, the red blood cell mass is increased, whereas the plasma volume is normal, resulting in an increased blood volume.[12] Significant changes in the hematocrit take place from cord blood through the first 24 hours of life. The hematocrit peaks at 2 hours of age and then progressively decreases, with significant changes observed at 6 and 24 hours of age.[13, 14] This condition is probably caused by transudation of fluid out of the intravascular space. Capillary hematocrit measurements are highly subject to variations in blood flow. Numerous studies have shown that capillary hematocrits are significantly higher than venous values,[15] a difference even more apparent in infants receiving large placental transfusions.[16] For the diagnosis of polycythemia, capillary hematocrits may be used as a screening test but should be verified with a venous specimen.

The method of analyzing the hematocrit can play a significant role. An automated hematology analyzer, which calculates the hematocrit from direct measurements of the mean cell volume and the hemoglobin, shows slightly lower values than hematocrits determined in a microcentrifuge. Villalta and colleagues[17] showed, in a study of 10 symptomatic, polycythemic infants, that none of the automated counter hematocrits was greater than 65%, whereas 8 of 10 infants had spun hematocrits above this value.

Hyperviscosity

Three major factors determine the viscosity of blood: the hematocrit, the deformability of the red blood cells, and the plasma viscosity. Plasma proteins, platelets, and endothelial factors are major determinants of plasma viscosity.[18]

$$\text{Viscosity (centipoise)} = \text{Shear stress (dynes/cm}^2\text{)/Shear rate}$$

Shear stress refers to the frictional forces within a fluid, and the *shear rate* is defined by the velocity of flow at a given radius. The shear rate in the aorta is approximately 230 seconds^{-1} and only 11.5 seconds^{-1} in the small arterioles and venules. The viscosity increases as the shear rate declines. At low shear rates, such as those in the microcirculation, blood with a high hematocrit may virtually cease flowing.

The relationship between viscosity and hematocrit has been suggested to be almost linear up to a hematocrit of 65% and exponential thereafter.[19, 20] There are, however, indications that this exponential relationship begins at hematocrits as low as 42% in neonates (Fig. 9–1).[13, 14]

Clinical symptoms correlate better with blood viscosity than with hematocrit.[21] The neonatal polycythemia-hyperviscosity syndrome is nevertheless largely confined to infants with hematocrits higher than the normal range or at the upper end of that range. Because instruments to measure viscosity are not available for most nurseries, neonatal hyperviscosity is diagnosed by the combination of clinical symptoms and an abnormally high venous hematocrit.

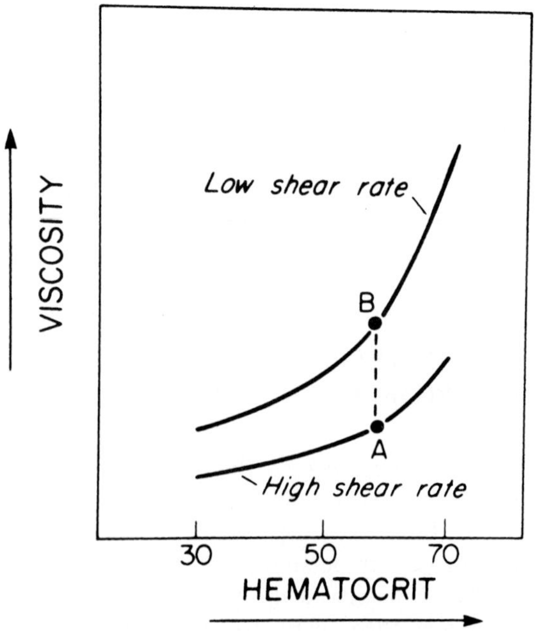

Figure 9–1. Relation of viscosity to hematocrit at high and low shear rates. (From Phibbs RH: Neonatal polycythemia. In Rudolph AD (ed): Pediatrics, 16th ed. New York: Appleton-Centry-Crofts, 1997.)

INCIDENCE

The hemoglobin and hematocrit values rise during the first 4 to 12 hours of life, particularly in infants who have received a large placental transfusion. The hematocrit varies somewhat as a function of gestational age, the size of the infant, and the altitude at which the studies have been performed.[4, 22–26] In Denver, Colorado, which is approximately 1600 meters above sea level, the incidence of polycythemia was found to be 4%,[22] in contrast to values of 2.2%[4] and 1.8%[24] in studies performed at sea level. One study reported an incidence as high as 12.3% based on a venous hematocrit of 65% or higher.[27]

Infants who are small for gestational age, who have been affected by maternal gestational diabetes, or who have suffered perinatal asphyxia, intrauterine hypoxia, or hypoglycemia are at high risk for polycythemia, hyperviscosity, or both. The incidence of polycythemia is highest among small-for-gestational-age and large-for-gestational-age infants. In contrast, polycythemia is not likely to occur in infants born before 34 weeks of gestation.[22] Because of these variables, the incidence of neonatal polycythemia has varied from study to study (Figs. 9–2 and 9–3).

Although the polycythemia-hyperviscosity syndrome is reasonably common, with an incidence of 1% to 5%, significant symptoms occur less frequently.[25] The symptoms are nonspecific and may be attributed more to the predisposing

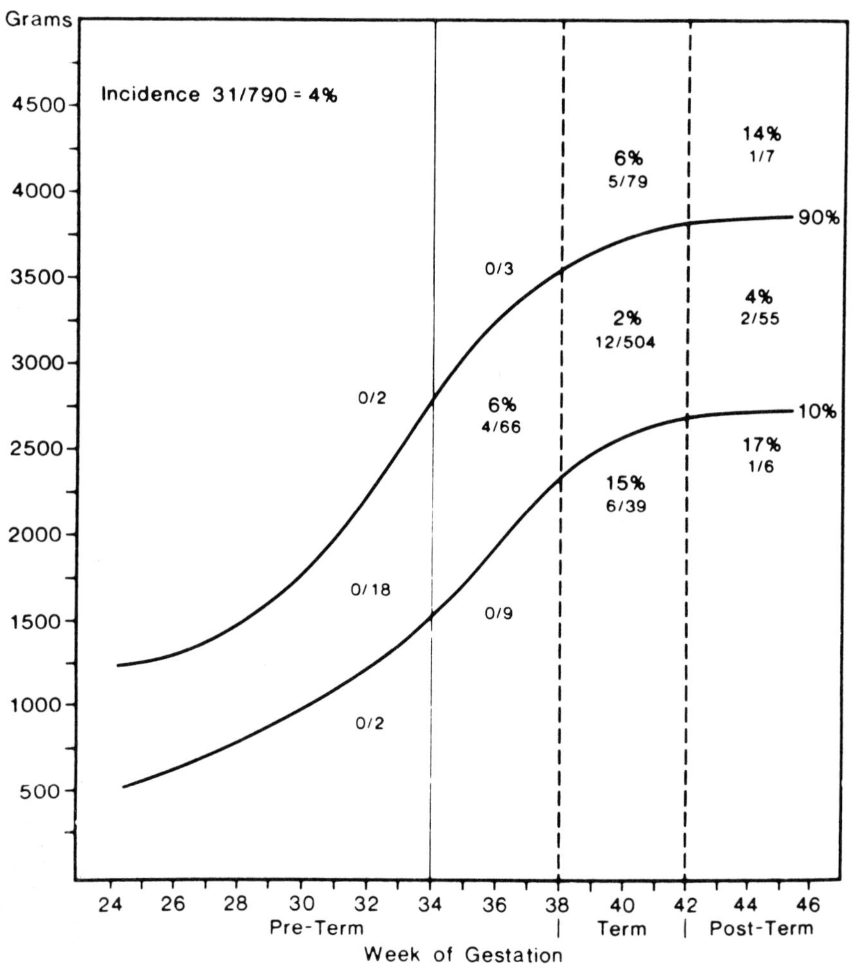

Figure 9–2. The incidence of venous polycythemia (i.e., hematocrit ≥65%) is shown by birth weight and gestational age groupings. (From Wirth FH, Goldberg KE, Lubchenco LO: Neonatal hyperviscosity: I. Incidence. Pediatrics 1979;63:833.)

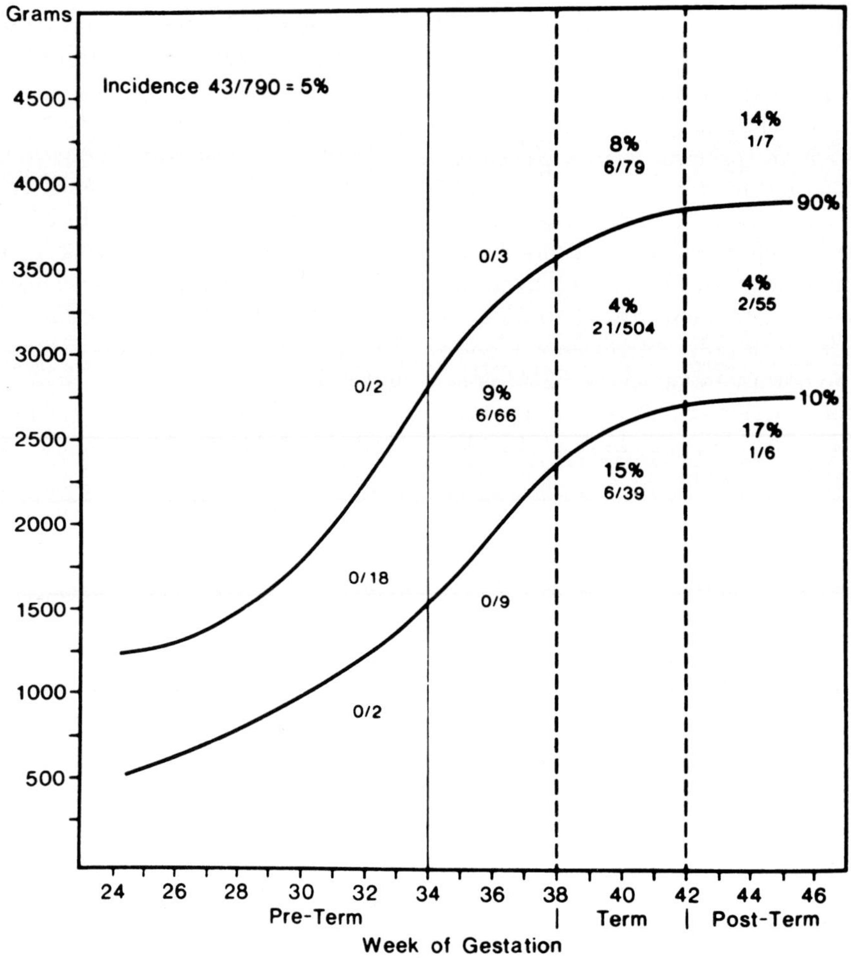

Figure 9–3. The incidence of hyperviscosity (i.e., viscosity >2 SD above mean) for newborn infants is shown by birth weight and gestational age groupings. (From Wirth FH, Goldberg KE, Lubchenco LO: Neonatal hyperviscosity: I. Incidence. Pediatrics 1979;63:833.)

factors (e.g., placental insufficiency, insulin-dependent diabetic mother, intrauterine asphyxia) than to the polycythemia itself.

DIAGNOSIS

The definition of neonatal polycythemia has been based on a peripheral venous hematocrit and has varied from a low of 60%[28] to a high of 70%,[21] although most modern researchers define neonatal polycythemia as a hematocrit of 65% or higher. The difference between a capillary and venous hemoglobin is illustrated in Figure 9–4 from the study of Oettinger and Mills.[15] Venous hematocrits correlate significantly with arterial hematocrits (r = 0.95, $P < .001$).[29]

The upper limit of the normal hematocrit at the age of 2 hours is 71% and at the age of 6 hours is 68%.[16] Regardless of the time of sampling, most researchers define neonatal polycythemia as a peripheral venous hematocrit of 65% or greater. However, our experience of more than 20 years is that symptoms of polycythemia rarely occur unless the venous hematocrit exceeds 70%. If a symptomatic infant has a capillary hematocrit higher than 70%, a peripheral venous hematocrit should be checked for confirmation of polycythemia: a peripheral venous hematocrit higher than 65% or, preferably, higher than 70%.

ETIOLOGY

Figure 9–5 and Tables 9–1 and 9–2 show the etiologic factors affecting development of the

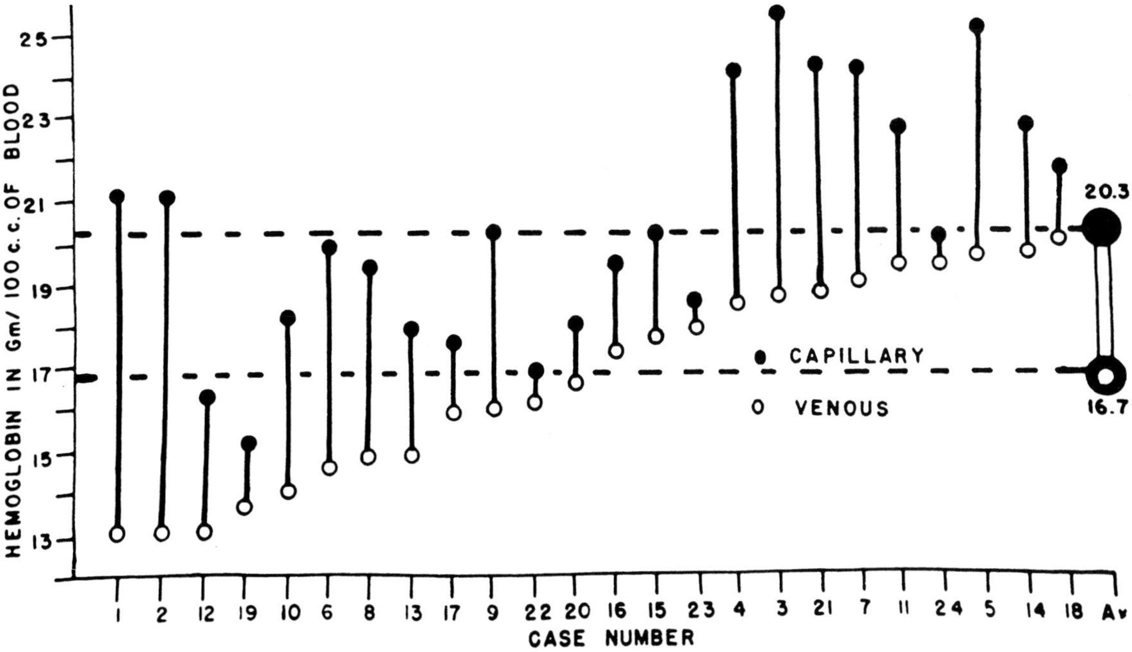

Figure 9–4. Simultaneous capillary and venous hemoglobin determinations for 24 newborn infants. (From Oettinger L Jr, Mills WB: Simultaneous capillary and venous hemoglobin determinations in newborn infants. J Pediatr 1949;35:362.)

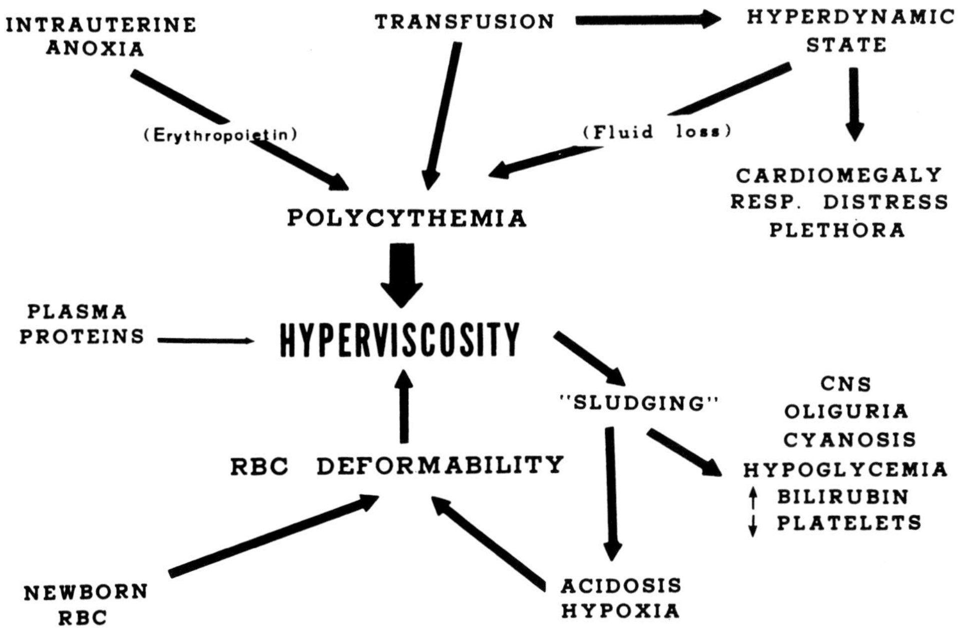

Figure 9–5. Proposed schema for the etiology and pathogenesis of symptomatic hyperviscosity states in neonate. (RBC, red blood cells.) (From Gross GP, Hathaway WE, McGaughey HR: Hyperviscosity in the neonate. J Pediatr 1973;82:1004.)

Table 9–1. **Causes of Primary Neonatal Polycythemia**

Intrauterine hypoxia
Placental insufficiency
Small for gestational age, growth retardation
Preeclampsia
Severe maternal heart disease
Maternal smoking
Maternal insulin-dependent diabetes
Neonatal thyrotoxicosis
Congenital adrenal hyperplasia
High-altitude conditions
Chromosome abnormalities
Trisomy 13
Trisomy 18
Trisomy 21
Hyperplastic viceromegaly (Beckwith-Wiedemann syndrome)
Decreased erythrocyte deformability

neonatal polycythemia and hyperviscosity syndrome.[30] Erythropoietin does not cross the human placenta.[31, 32] Primary polycythemia is caused by increased fetal production of erythropoietin, leading to an increased red blood cell mass (see Fig. 9–5).

Intrauterine Growth Retardation

Reduced fetal growth can have a maternal or placental origin; both usually give rise to chronic intrauterine hypoxia. The major maternal factors are hypertension and chronic renal diseases. Fetal causes can also lead to intrauterine growth retardation, although usually without polycythemia.

An increased number of circulating nucleated red blood cells reflects active erythropoiesis.[33] In one study, a high hemoglobin level (>21 g/dL) was found in 7.5% of average-for-gestational-age infants, increasing to 9.5% of infants with mild growth retardation and to 41.5% of those with severe growth retardation.[34] The risk of polycythemia in average-for-gestational-age infants of hypertensive mothers has been shown to be more than 12-fold greater than the risk in the general population,[35] indicating that intrauterine growth retardation and maternal hypertension can lead to neonatal polycythemia.

Infants of Mothers with Insulin-Dependent Diabetes

Macrosomia and hypoglycemia characterize infants of diabetic mothers. As many as 22% to 29% of such infants also have polycythemia[36, 37] Several mechanisms for the development of polycythemia in these infants are possible. Maternal hemoglobin A_{IC} levels correlate with fetal erythropoietin levels.[38, 39] An increased production of erythropoietin may result from increased oxygen consumption caused by fetal hyperinsulinism and hyperketonemia.[36, 38] Insulin has been shown in vitro to promote the expansion of erythroid colonies.[40] Placental vascular abnormalities are found in maternal diabetes and can lead to placental insufficiency and fetal hypoxia.[41] The level of glucose control of the maternal diabetes correlates with the incidence of fetal hypoglycemia and macrosomia. However, increased fetal erythropoiesis and polycythemia can occur despite good maternal glucose control.[37]

Maternal Smoking

Maternal smoking can cause increased fetal erythropoiesis and neonatal polycythemia.[42, 43] Elevated umbilical cord blood erythropoietin levels have been reported in neonates of smoking mothers.[44] Maternal cigarette use correlates with fetal hemoglobin, hematocrit, and hemoglobin P_{50} levels.[43] A smaller placenta with decreased oxygen delivery is presumed to be the principal mechanism. A reduction in oxygen carrying capacity of fetal hemoglobin by carbon monoxide may also play a role.[44]

Fetal Disorders

Increased erythropoiesis appears to be responsible for neonatal polycythemia in fetal conditions such as trisomies 13, 18, and 21; congenital hypothyroidism; neonatal thyrotoxicosis; congenital adrenal hyperplasia; and Beckwith-Wiedemann syndrome.[5] Lappalainen and Kouvalainen[45] observed that infants with Down syndrome had elevated capillary hematocrit values. Increased erythropoietin concentrations with concomitant reticulocytosis correlated with a 19-fold increased risk of polycythemia in infants with Down syndrome compared with normal newborns.[46, 47]

Secondary Polycythemia

Secondary polycythemia indicates a transfer of erythrocytes to the fetus during delivery or in utero through twin-twin or maternal-fetal transfusion. The condition can also result from reduced plasma volume.

Placental Transfusion and Delayed Cord Clamping

The most common cause of secondary neonatal polycythemia is a placental transfusion, usually resulting from delayed clamping of the umbilical cord, which can increase the postnatal blood volume by as much as 60%.[48] Within 6 to 12 hours, the average hematocrit can be 10% higher than that observed in infants with early cord clamping.[49] A study of early (<10 seconds) and late (>3 minutes) cord clamping showed that the hematocrit decreased 24 hours after birth in the early group (from 48% to 43%) and that it increased in the late group (from 50% to 59%).[50] Blood viscosity increased only in the late group (40% within the 2 first hours) and then did not change during the next 5 days. Plasma viscosity and red blood cell aggregation, however, increased in both groups because of a significant increase in total plasma protein and fibrinogen concentrations.[50]

Erkkola and associates[51] observed that delayed cord clamping (>3 minutes) resulted in significantly lower Po_2 and pH values and higher plasma lactate levels. Intrauterine asphyxia increases the neonatal blood volume through increased placental transfusion.[52] If, however, an infant is severely asphyxiated, the amount of placental transfusion is often reduced. One reason for this is that the infant's condition necessitates immediate cord clamping, and the infant becomes slightly hypovolemic. In premature infants, a placental transfusion can be advantageous, because the incidence of respiratory distress syndrome appears to be lower with late clamping.[53]

The difference between early and late cord clamping can result in an almost 30% increase in blood volume and red blood cell mass delivered to the infant. Positioning of the infant is also important. Transfusion is augmented when the infant is held below the introitus, but holding the infant above this level prevents transfusion.[54] A placental transfusion can also be responsible for the increased incidence of polycythemia observed in large-for-gestational-age infants (i.e., larger infants, larger placentas, and larger placental transfusions).[22]

On the basis of several studies, positioning the infant at the level of introitus and postponing cord clamping for approximately 30 seconds are recommended. A secondary advantage of delayed cord clamping is the transfer of the blood iron that may prevent iron deficiency anemia and improve cognitive development. A considerable transfer of immunoglobulins also occurs, which may be particularly important in developing countries.[55]

Twin-Twin Transfusion

In approximately one third of cases of monochorionic twins, transfusion of blood occurs from one twin into the other, defined as a discrepancy of hemoglobin concentration greater than 5 g/dL. As many as 75% of recipient twins have symptomatic polycythemia.[56] The recipient, polycythemic twin is larger and is prone to cardiorespiratory failure and hyperbilirubinemia, whereas the anemic donor is smaller and at risk for congestive heart failure.[56]

Maternal-Fetal Transfusion

Transfer of a significant volume of maternal erythrocytes to the fetus during pregnancy is a rare cause of polycythemia. This diagnosis is usually one of exclusion and can be confirmed by differential agglutination techniques.[57]

Reduced Plasma Volume

A reduction of the plasma volume in the neonatal period gives rise to an elevated hema-

Table 9–2. **Causes of Secondary Neonatal Polycythemia**

Delayed cord clamping
Twin-to-twin transfusion
Maternal-fetal transfusion
Dehydration
Perinatal asphyxia

tocrit and the same symptoms as polycythemia. Reduced fluid intake or increased water loss make the condition iatrogenic in most cases. Severe diarrhea that manifests in the first days of life may be caused by rare metabolic disorders such as glucose-galactose malabsorption or may have an infectious origin.

CLINICAL SYMPTOMS

A wide range of symptoms involving several organ systems can suggest polycythemia or hyperviscosity (Table 9–3). In severe cases (i.e., hematocrit >75%), the infant usually appears more red than blue (rubeosis instead of cyanosis) and plethoric, with slow refilling of the capillaries after anemization. Of infants with a central venous hematocrit greater than 65%, about one half are symptomatic.[25] Using hyperviscosity as a criterion, symptoms are found in at least 50% of the infants.[30]

The most consistent clinical findings in infants with polycythemia or hyperviscosity are lethargy, tachypnea, hypotonia, poor suck, difficulty in arousal to an alert state, irritability when aroused, poor response to light, vomiting, jitteriness, and easy startle ability.[2, 25] As many as 61% of affected infants feed poorly.[58] Many of the symptoms may be attributable to the underlying condition, such as hypoglycemia in infants born to diabetic mothers, and not to hyperviscosity.

Table 9–3. **Clinical Symptoms and Laboratory Abnormalities of Neonatal Polycythemia**

Clinical Symptoms
Weak suck (i.e., feeding difficulties)
Plethora
Lethargy
Rubeosis-like cyanosis
Tachypnea (i.e., respiratory distress)
Jitteriness or tremulousness
Difficult to arouse
Irritable when aroused
Hypotonia
Easily startled
Myoclonic jerks
Vomiting
Cardiomegaly (heart murmur)
Hepatomegaly
Jaundice
Laboratory Abnormalities
Hypoglycemia
Hypocalcemia
Thrombocytopenia

Cardiorespiratory System

As many as 50% of neonates with polycythemia have cardiopulmonary symptoms such as tachypnea, cyanosis, and tachycardia.[30] The cyanotic appearance (actually rubeosis) may suggest a diagnosis of cyanotic congenital heart disease. Infants may be cyanotic at rest, but skin color is often normal until they are aroused or crying. With activity, the skin can appear very blue or reddish. Radiologic findings include pulmonary vascular congestion, hyperaeration, pleural effusions, and various degrees of cardiomegaly.[1]

Central Nervous System

The most common organ system involved in the polycythemia-hyperviscosity syndrome is the central nervous system. Lethargy, poor feeding, tremors, and jitteriness are common findings. Some infants have seizures.[30, 59] Cerebral blood flow is reduced significantly and can return to normal with partial-exchange transfusion.[60, 61] Cerebrovascular events have only rarely been attributed to the condition.

Metabolism

Hypoglycemia occurs in 12% to 40% and hypocalcemia in 1% to 11% of polycythemic infants.[25, 30] Calcitonin gene-related peptide, which modulates vascular tone by stimulating local vasodilation and which produces hypocalcemia, has been found in higher concentrations in polycythemic newborns, suggesting a role for this peptide in the response to polycythemia.[62]

It has been suggested that the hypoglycemia is a consequence of increased cerebral extraction of glucose or reduced endogenous glucose production caused by a sluggish hepatic circulation.[63] In either case, a partial-exchange transfusion often corrects the hypolycemia.[64]

Thrombocytopenia

Primary polycythemia is often associated with thrombocytopenia, and thrombocytopenia is a common finding for infants with neonatal polycythemia. The platelet levels are seldom so low as to pose a risk of hemorrhage.

Circulation

Blood is normally concentrated in the postglomerular efferent arteriole. In hyperviscosity, kidney function may be affected. The glomerular filtration rate and urinary sodium excretion can be reduced but return to normal after partial-exchange transfusion.[65]

Necrotizing enterocolitis, usually an event in sick premature infants, has been associated with the polycythemia-hyperviscosity syndrome in 16% to 44% of term infants[66, 67] and in 58% of infants weighing more than 2000 g.[68] The cause may be reduced blood flow in the mesenteric vessels. Necrotizing enterocolitis is, however, multifactorial, and several other features associated with the development of necrotizing enterocolitis may also cause polycythemia and hyperviscosity.[69] For example, necrotizing enterocolitis is rare in Norway, although polycythemia is not uncommon. A possible etiologic factor may be the treatment; necrotizing enterocolitis has been associated with umbilical venous catheters, reflecting vasospasm in the mesenterial vessels.[70, 71] Another possibility is a change in viscosity caused by partial-exchange transfusion if adult plasma is used. Adult plasma significantly raises viscosity when mixed with fetal erythrocytes.[18]

TREATMENT

The goal of therapy with a partial-exchange transfusion is to lower the hematocrit and reduce the viscosity. The treatment should also include correction of any accompanying metabolic abnormalities, such as aberrant glucose, calcium, and oxygen levels.

Partial Exchange Transfusion

A partial-exchange transfusion is most easily performed through the umbilical vein. The aim is to achieve a hematocrit of approximately 60%. The volume exchanged is calculated from this formula:

$$\text{Blood volume} = \frac{(\text{Observed hematocrit} - \text{Desired hematocrit [60\%]})}{\text{Observed Hematocrit}}$$

The blood volume in the newborn infant is usually estimated at 80 to 100 mL/kg body weight. It may be higher in polycythemic infants, especially those of low birth weight.[12, 72] For example, an infant weighing 3500 g has a venous hematocrit of 75%. Using the previous equation, the needed volume is calculated as 3.5 kg × 100 mL/kg × (75 − 60)/75 = 70 mL. *Our practical approach to such an infant has been to prepare four 20-mL syringes, three filled with 20 mL of 4% albumin, Ringer's lactate, or saline solution and the fourth with 10 mL of the chosen solution. An empty 20-mL syringe is attached to the umbilical vein catheter, and then 20 mL of blood is withdrawn and discharged. A 20-mL syringe with albumin, Ringer's lactate, or saline solution is then connected, and the solution is infused, followed by withdrawing 20 mL of blood using the same syringe. The process is continued until only 10 mL is withdrawn and the last 10 mL is infused. For a preterm infant, the syringe sizes used would be 15, 10, or 5 mL, gauged according to the birth weight.*

The results obtained after a partial-exchange transfusion following this formula may vary but usually are in the range of 55% to 60%. Partial-exchange transfusion has reversed the clinical symptoms and increased capillary perfusion,[73] cerebral blood flow,[61] and cardiac function.[74] It is, however, questionable whether the long-term outcome is improved.[75–77] One reason may be that damage from reduced microcirculation in the various organs already has occurred, but it is important to reduce any risk of further damage by a partial-exchange transfusion.

Plasma, Albumin, and Crystalloid Solutions

Diluents used for partial-exchange transfusion have included fresh frozen plasma, albumin, and crystalloid solutions. No studies have shown an advantage for any of these diluents. However, plasma may contain infectious materials even if the donor has passed the controls of blood bank testing.

Crystalloid solutions are easily available and less expensive, but the physician must be aware of the amount of electrolytes being transfused before the renal function has normalized. Saline and Ringer's solutions have been found to be safe and effective for partial-exchange transfusion.[78–82] As in the previous example, 70 mL of albumin, Ringer's lactate, or saline solution would give a sodium load of 3 mmol/kg to the infant weighing 3500 g.

Increased Fluid Intake

If the long-term outcome effect of a partial-exchange transfusion compared with an expectant approach is questionable, secured fluid intake is a reasonable and less invasive choice. Using an umbilical vein catheter may have disadvantages, as mentioned earlier. Increased fluid intake delivered enterally (i.e., gavage feeding because polycythemic infants are poor feeders) or parenterally may be an alternative. However, our experience is that a partial-exchange transfusion is fast and safe, resolving the clinical symptoms and allowing the infants to be breast-fed more rapidly.

COMPLICATIONS AND SEQUELAE

Complications such as tachypnea, congestive heart failure, seizures, priapism, gangrene of an extremity, testicular infarction, retinopathy of prematurity, necrotizing enterocolitis, abdominal distention, ileus, distal bowel obstruction, hyperbilirubinemia, and acute renal failure have been ascribed to polycythemia and hyperviscosity (Table 9–4).[69] Most of these complications are reversible after an exchange transfusion. The most important question is whether the infants have developed damage leading to delayed psychomotor development.

Table 9–4. **Complications Associated with Neonatal Polycythemia**

Respiratory distress syndrome
Congestive heart failure
Convulsions
Peripheral gangrene
Priapism
Necrotizing enterocolitis
Ileus
Acute renal failure
Abnormal electroencephalographic pattern

Short-term and long-term follow-up have shown significantly more neurologic abnormalities in infants with neonatal polycythemia-hyperviscosity syndrome than in nonpolycythemic controls.[76] Spastic diplegia, hemiparesis, and developmental delay have been found in 38% of affected infants, compared with approximately 11% of matched controls.[75] Concurrent hypoglycemia increased the risk of a poor outcome in as many as 55% of the infants. The children also appear to have lower spelling and arithmetic achievement scores by 7 years of age.[77] However, some studies have not shown developmental abnormalities during follow-up.[83] Because these infants were asymptomatic, it is possible that perinatal etiologic factors, not polycythemia, played the most significant role in their long-term neurologic complications.

PREVENTION

Some cases of polycythemia can be prevented by avoiding late clamping of the cord (i.e., delay of 3 minutes), which is routine according to the Leboyer method.[84] The infant's position after delivery and before the cord is clamped is also important.[54] Ideally, the infant should be kept at the level of the introitus or preferably 20 cm beneath, and the cord clamping should be postponed for approximately 30 seconds, allowing a suitable amount of blood to be transfused (Fig. 9–6).[85]

The neonatal polycythemia-hyperviscosity syndrome should be suspected in every newborn infant who has the symptoms of tachypnea, congestive heart failure, seizures, priapism, gangrene of an extremity, testicular infarction, necrotizing enterocolitis, abdominal distention, ileus, distal bowel obstruction, hyperbilirubinemia, or acute renal failure. If the capillary hematocrit is 70% or higher, a venous or central hematocrit should be obtained to confirm the diagnosis.

It is our practice and teaching that a symptomatic polycythemic-hyperviscotic infant should receive a partial-exchange transfusion. We intervene for a symptomatic infant when the peripheral venous hematocrit is higher than 70% using a crystalloid replacement. Because they are at high risk for sequelae, every symp-

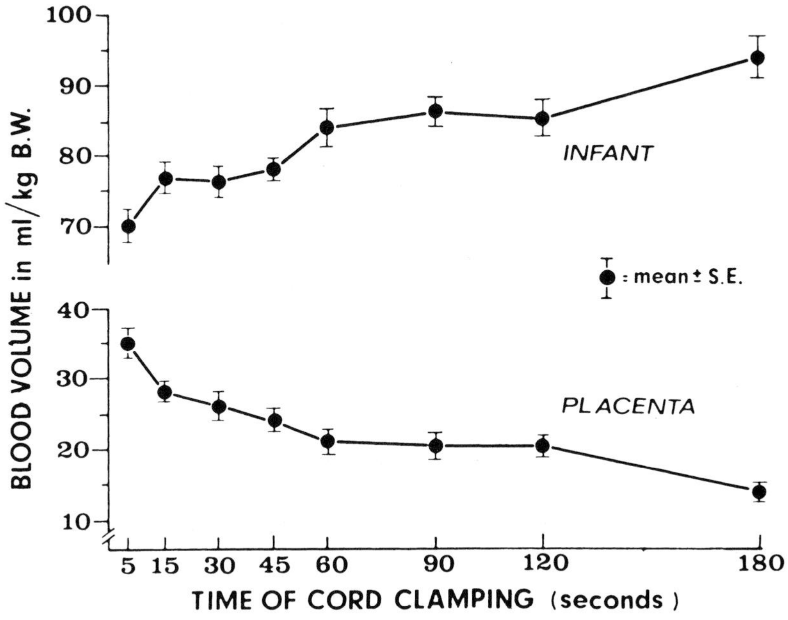

Figure 9–6. Relation between an infant's blood volume and placental residual blood volume at various times of cord clamping. (From Yao, AC, Moinian M, Lind J: Distribution of blood between infant and placenta after birth. Lancet 1969;2:871.)

tomatic polycythemic infant should be followed with psychomotor evaluation.

References

1. Wesenberg RL, Rumack CM, Lubchenco LO, et al: The thick blood syndrome. Radiology 1977;125:181.
2. Wesenberg RL: Neonatal "thick blood" syndrome. Hosp Pract 1978;13:137.
3. Mentzer WC: Polycythemia and the hyperviscosity syndrome. Clin Hematol 1978;7:63.
4. Ramamurthy RS: Neonatal polycythemia and hyperviscosity: state of the art. Perinatol Neonatol 1979;3:38.
5. Werner EJ: Neonatal polycythemia and hyperviscosity. Clin Perinatol 1995;22:693.
6. Finne PH, Halvorsen S: Regulation of erythropoiesis in the fetus and newborn. Arch Dis Child 1972;47:683.
7. Brugnara C, Platt OS: The neonatal erythrocyte and its disorders: the neonatal erythrocyte. In Nathan DG, Oski FA (eds): Nathan and Oski's Hematology of Infancy and Childhood, 5th ed. Philadelphia: WB Saunders, 1998, p 19.
8. Meberg A: Haemoglobin concentrations and erythropoietin levels in appropriate and small for gestational age infants. Scand J Haematol 1980;24:162.
9. Haque KN, Bahakim HM: Percentile curves for various hematologic measurements at birth in Arab preterm babies of different gestational ages. Am J Dis Child 1991;145:645.
10. Forestier F, Daffos F, Galactéros F, et al: Hematological values of 163 normal fetuses between 18 and 30 weeks of gestation. Pediatr Res 1986;20:342.
11. Refsum HE, Bechensteen AG, Lindemann R: The shift from HbF- to HbA-production in a premature infant after an exchange transfusion: a quantitative approach. Eur J Pediatr Hematol Oncol 1998;15:431.
12. Brans YW, Shannon DL, Ramamurthy RS: Neonatal polycythemia. II. Plasma, blood and red cell volume estimates in relation to hematocrit levels and quality of intrauterine growth. Pediatrics 1981;68:175.
13. Shohat M, Merlob P, Reisner SH: Neonatal polycythemia. I. Early diagnosis and incidence relating to time of sampling. Pediatrics 1984;73:7.
14. Shohat M, Reisner SH, Mimouni F, et al: Neonatal polycythemia. II. Definition related to time of sampling. Pediatrics 1984;73:11.
15. Oettinger L Jr, Mills WB: Simultaneous capillary and venous hemoglobin determinations in newborn infants. J Pediatr 1949:35:362.
16. Oh W, Lind J: Venous and capillary hematocrit in newborn infants and placental transfusion. Acta Paediatr Scand 1966;55:38.
17. Villalta IA, Pramanik AK, Diaz-Blanco J, et al: Diagnostic errors in neonatal polycythemia based on method of hematocrit determination. J Pediatr 1989;115:460.
18. Linderkamp O, Versomld HT, Riegel KP, et al: Contribution of red cells and plasma to blood viscosity in preterm and full-term infants and adults. Pediatrics 1984;74:45.
19. Macintosh TF, Walker CHM: Blood viscosity in the newborn. Arch Dis Child 1973;48:537.
20. Phibbs RH: Neonatal polycythemia. In Rudolph AD (ed): Pediatrics, 16th ed. New York: Appleton-Century-Crofts, 1997, p 179.
21. Ramamurthy RD, Brans YW: Neonatal polycythemia: I. Criteria for diagnosis and treatment. Pediatrics 1981;68:168.
22. Wirth FH, Goldberg KE, Lubchenco LO: Neonatal hyperviscosity. I. Incidence. Pediatrics 1979;63:833.
23. Hakanson DO, Oh W: Hyperviscosity in the small-for-gestational age infant. Biol Neonate 1980;37:109.
24. Stevens K, Wirth FH: Incidence of neonatal hyperviscosity at sea level. J Pediatr 1980;97:118.
25. Wiswell TE, Cornish MC, Northam RS: Neonatal polycythemia: frequency of clinical manifestations and other associated findings. Pediatrics 1986;78:26.
26. Drew JH, Guaran RL, Grauer S, et al: Cord whole blood hyperviscosity: measurement, definition, incidence and clinical features. J Paediatr Child Health 1991;27:363.

27. Reisner SH, Mor N, Levy Y, et al: Incidence of neonatal polycythemia. Isr J Med Sci 1983;19:848.
28. Kontras SB: Polycythemia and hyperviscosity syndromes in infants and children. Pediatr Clin North Am 1972;19:919.
29. Teng RJ, Chang HS, Ling CH, et al: Diagnostic value of arterial hematocrits in neonatal polycythemia. Acta Paediatr Sin 1990;31:81.
30. Gross GP, Hathaway WE, McGaughey HR: Hyperviscosity in the neonate. J Pediatr 1973;82:1004.
31. Finne PH: On placental transfer of erythropoietin. Acta Paediatr Scand 1967;56:233.
32. Wu H, Liu X, Jaenisch R, et al: Generation of committed erythroid BFU-E and CFU-E progenitor does not require erythropoietin or the erythropoietin receptor. Cell 1995;83:59.
33. Philip AGS, Tito AM: Increased nucleated red blood cell counts in small for gestational for age infants with very low birth weight. Am J Dis Child 1989;143:164.
34. Kramer MS, Olivier M, McLean FH, et al: Impact of intrauterine growth retardation and body proportionality on fetal and neonatal outcome. Pediatrics 1990; 86:707.
35. Kurlat I, Sola A: Neonatal polycythemia in appropriately grown infants of hypertensive mothers. Acta Paediatr 1992;81:662.
36. Mimouni F, Miodovnik M, Siddiqi TA, et al: Neonatal polycythemia in infants of insulin-dependent diabetic mothers. Obstet Gynecol 1986;68:370.
37. Hod M, Merlob P, Friedman S, et al: Prevalence of congenital anomalies and neonatal complications in the offspring of diabetic mothers in Israel. Isr J Med Sci 1991;27:498.
38. Widness JA, Susa JB, Garcia JF, et al: Increased erythropoiesis and elevated erythropoietin in infants born to diabetic mothers and in hyperinsulinemic rhesus fetuses. J Clin Invest 1981;67:637.
39. Green DW, Khoury J, Mimouni F: Neonatal hematocrit and maternal glycemic control in insulin-dependent diabetes. J Pediatr 1992;120:302.
40. Perrine SP, Green MF, Lee PDK, et al: Insulin stimulates cord blood erythroid progenitor growth: evidence of an aetiological role in neonatal polycythaemia. Br J Haematol 1986;64:503.
41. Georgieff MK, Landon MB, Mills MM, et al: Abnormal iron distribution in infants of diabetic mothers. J Pediatr 1990;117:455.
42. Meberg A, Hågå P, Sande H, et al: Smoking during pregnancy: haematological observations in the newborn. Acta Paediatr Scand 1979;68:731.
43. Bureau MA, Shapcott D, Berthiaume Y, et al: Maternal cigarette smoking and fetal oxygen transport: a study of p50, 2,3-diphosphoglycerate, total hemoglobin, hematocrit and type F hemoglobin in fetal blood. Pediatrics 1983;72:22.
44. Bili H, Mamapoulos M, Tsantali MD, et al: Elevated umbilical erythropoietin levels during labor in newborns of smoking mothers. Am J Perinatol 1996;13:85.
45. Lappalainen J, Kouvalainen K: High hematocrits in newborns with Down's syndrome. Clin Pediatr 1972;11:472.
46. Weinberger MM, Oleinick A: Congenital marrow dysfunction in Down's syndrome. J Pediatr 1970;77:273.
47. Naveh D, Schwart JM, Pang KW, et al: Neonatal polycythemia and elevated plasma erythropoietin (ESF) in Down's syndrome. Prog Am Soc Hematol 1971; p 142.
48. User R, Shepard M, Lind J: The blood volume of the newborn infant and placental transfusion. Acta Paediatr Scand 1963;52:497.
49. Oh W, Lind J, Gessner IH: The circulatory and respiratory adaptation to early and late cord clamping in newborn infants. Acta Paediatr Scand 1966;55:197.
50. Linderkamp O, Nelle M, Kraus M, et al: The effect of early and late cord-clamping on blood viscosity and other hemorheological parameters in full-term neonates. Acta Paediatr 1992;81:745.
51. Erkkola R, Kero P, Kanto J, et al: Delayed cord clamping in cesarean section with general anesthesia. Am J Perinatol 1984;1:165.
52. Linderkamp O, Versmold HT, Strohhacker I, et al: The effect of intra-partum and intra-uterine asphyxia on placental transfusion in premature and full-term infants. Eur J Pedaitr 1978;127:91.
53. Hohmann M: Früh oder spätabnabelung? Frage nach dem optimalen Zeitpunkt. Wien Klin Wochenschr 1985;97:497.
54. Yao AC, Lind J: Placental transfusion. Am J Dis Child 1974;127:128.
55. Grajeda R, Perez-Escamilla R, Dewey KG: Delayed clamping of the umbilical cord improved haemtologic status of Guatemalan infants at 2 mo of age. Am J Clin Nutr 1997;65:425.
56. Tan KL, Tan R, Tan SH, et al: The twin transfusion syndrome: clinical observations on 35 affected pairs. Clin Pediatr 1979;18:111.
57. Michael AF Jr, Mauer AM: Maternal-fetal transfusion as a cause of plethora in the neonatal period. Pediatrics 1961;28:458.
58. Black VD, Rumack CM, Lubchenco LO, et al: Gastrointestinal injury in polycythemic term infants. Pediatrics 1985;76:225.
59. Humbert JR, Abelson H, Hathaway WE: Hyperviscosity in small for gestational age infants. J Pediatr 1969;75:812.
60. Bada HS, Korones SB, Kolni HW, et al: Partial plasma exchange transfusion improves cerebral hemodynamics in symptomatic neonatal polycythemia. Am J Med Sci 1986;29:157.
61. Rosenkrantz TS, Oh W: Cerebral blood flow velocity in infants with polycythemia and hyperviscosity: effects of partial exchange transfusion with Plasmanate. J Pediatr 1982;101:94.
62. Sagasse G, Bertelloni S, Baroncelli GI, et al: Elevated calcitonin gene-related peptide in polycythemic newborn infants. Acta Paediatr 1992;81:966.
63. Leake RD, Chan G, Zakaudden S, et al: Glucose utilization in hyperviscosity. Pediatr Res 1976;10:412.
64. Leake RD, Chan G, Zakaudden S, et al: Glucose perturbation in experimental hyperviscosity. Pediatr Res 1980;14:1320.
65. Aperia A, Bergquist G, Broberger O, et al: Renal function in newborn infants with high haematocrit values before and after isovolaemic haemodilution. Acta Paediatr Scand 1974;63:878.
66. Polin RA, Pollack PF, Barlow B, et al: Necrotizing enterocolitis in term infants. J Pediatr 1976;89:460.
67. Kliegman RM, Fanaroff AA: Neonatal necrotizing enterocolitis: a nine year experience: epidemiology and uncommon observations. Am J Dis Child 1981;135: 603.
68. Wilson R, del Portillo M, Schmidt E, et al: Risk factors for necrotizing enterocolitis in infants weighing more than 2,000 grams at birth: a case-control study. Pediatrics 1983;71:19.
69. Wiswell TE, Robertson CF, Jones TA, et al: Necrotizing enterocolitis in full term infants: a case-control study. Am J Dis Child 1988;142:532.
70. Livaditis A, Wallgren G, Faxelius G: Necrotizing enterocolitis after catheterization of the umbilical vessels. Acta Paediatr Scand 1974;63:277.

71. Shah KJ, Corkery JJ: Necrotizing enterocolitis following umbilical vein catheterization. Clin Radiol 1978;29:295.
72. Rawlings JS, Pettrett G, Wiswell TE, et al: Estimated blood volumes in polycythemic neonates as a function of birthweight. J Pediatr 1982;101:594.
73. Norman M, Fafrell B, Herin P: Effects of neonatal polycythemia and hemodilution on capillary perfusion. J Pediatr 1992;121:103.
74. Murphy DJ Jr, Reller MD, Meyer RA, et al: Effects of neonatal polycythemia and partial exchange transfusion on cardiac function: an echocardiographic study. Pediatrics 1985;76:909.
75. Black VD, Lubchenco LO, Luckey DW, et al: Developmental and neurologic sequelae of neonatal hyperviscosity syndrome. Pediatrics 1982;69:426.
76. Goldberg K, Wirth FH, Hathaway WE, et al: Neonatal hyperviscosity. II. Effect of partial plasma exchange transfusion. Pediatrics 1982;69:419.
77. Delaney-Black V, Camp BW, Lubchenco LO, et al: Neonatal hyperviscosity association with lower achievement and IQ scores at school age. Pediatrics 1989;83:662.
78. Deorari AK, Paul VK, Shreshta L, et al: Symptomatic neonatal polycythemia: comparison of partial exchange transfusion with saline versus plasma. Indian Pediatr 1995;32:1167.
79. Roithmaier A, Arlettaz R, Bauer K, et al: Randomized controlled trial of Ringer solution versus serum for partial exchange transfusion in neonatal polycythaemia. Eur J Pediatr 1995;154:53.
80. So KW, Fok TF, Ng PC, et al: Randomised controlled trial of colloid or crystalloid in hypotensive preterm infants. Arch Dis Child 1997;76:F43.
81. Wong W, Fok TF, Ng PC, et al: Randomised controlled trial: comparison of colloid or cristalloid for partial exchange transfusion for treatment of neonatal polycythaemia. Arch Dis Child 1997;77:F115.
82. Hope P: Pump up the volume? The routine early use of colloid in very preterm infants. Arch Dis Child 1998;78:F163.
83. Bada HS, Korones SB, Pourcyrous M, et al: Asymptomatic syndrome of polycythemic hyperviscosity: effect of partial exchange transfusion. J Pediatr 1992;120:579.
84. Nelle M, Zilow EP, Kraus M, et al: The effect of Leboyer delivery on blood viscosity and other hemorheologic parameters in term neonates. Am J Obstet Gynecol 1993; 169:189.
85. Kinmond S, Aitchison TC, Holland BM, et al: Umbilical cord clamping and preterm infants: a randomized trial. BMJ 1993;306:172.

CHAPTER 10

Evaluation and Treatment of Erythroblastosis Fetalis in the Neonate

Joyce M. Koenig, M.D.

HISTORICAL BACKGROUND

In 1932, Diamond and colleagues first described the relationship of fetal hydrops, jaundice, anemia, and erythroblasts in the circulation, a condition later called *erythroblastosis fetalis.*[1] Eight years later, Landsteiner and Weiner, using rhesus monkeys, discovered the Rh antigen.[2] They observed that red blood cells from 85% of human subjects agglutinated in the presence of rhesus monkey red blood cell antiserum, whereas the 15% of subjects who lacked the antigen on their red blood cells did not. This antigen was shown to be the source of most transfusion reactions.[3] In a later study, Levine and coworkers suggested a role for the Rh antigen in the pathophysiology of hemolytic disease in newborn infants,[4] which was subsequently confirmed by Chown.[5] Before the establishment of modern therapy, nearly 1% of all pregnant women developed alloimmunization.[6] Since the advent of routine prophylaxis of at-risk women with Rh immune globulin, this number has diminished to 11 cases per 10,000 total births,[7, 8] and of these Rh-sensitized fetuses, 9% require intrauterine transfusion.[9] Despite modern advances, hemolytic disease of the newborn continues to be a public health issue with a significant economic impact.

PATHOGENESIS OF ALLOIMMUNIZATION

In 1948, Race proposed that Rh antigens exist in three gene loci: Cc, Dd, and Ee.[10] Because the d antigen has not been identified, it is the absence of the D antigen that confers Rh-negative status. Of individuals who are Rh positive, 45% are homozygous, and 55% are heterozygous.[11] In instances of maternal Rh negativity, the paternal zygosity determines the likelihood of an Rh-positive child; all offspring will be Rh-positive when the father is homozygous for the D locus, and there is a 50% chance that a child will be Rh negative if the father is heterozygous.

Chown[5] showed that Rh alloimmunization results from the passage of fetal red blood cells that express surface Rh (D) antigen across the placenta into the circulation of a mother whose red blood cells lack that antigen. This passage of fetal Rh antigen into the maternal circulation occurs as the result of transplacental hemorrhage. Bowman and associates used the Kleihauer acid elution test[12] to determine the proportion of fetal red blood cells in the maternal circulation.[13] In 60% of these pregnancies, the amount of fetal blood was less than 0.1 mL. More than 5 mL and more than 30 mL were found in 1% and 0.25% of these women, respectively. The incidence and degree of such hemorrhage appears to increase with gestation: whereas up to 15% of women in the second trimester have detectable fetal red blood cells in their circulation, 45% of women in the third trimester have evidence of fetal red blood cell contamination, and the volume can be large. The risk of transplacental hemorrhage is increased in pregnancies complicated by placental abruption and toxemia and after cesarean section, spontaneous or therapeutic abortion, and ectopic pregnancy.[14, 15] Procedures such as amniocentesis, chorionic villus sampling, and cordocentesis also increase the subsequent risk of alloimmunization.[15–17] However, because the degree of transplacental hemorrhage in most pregnancies is less than 0.1 mL, most women are sensitized to the Rh antigen as a result of small or undetectable fetomaternal hemorrhage.[15]

After the initial, or primary, exposure to a foreign antigen in the maternal circulation, the maternal immune system produces antibodies of the IgM isotype, which do not cross the placenta because of their size. The weak IgM response is followed by production of IgG antibodies that can traverse the placental barrier. In the secondary immune response, a repeat exposure of an Rh-negative woman to the Rh antigen rapidly induces the production of anti-D antibodies, most of which are IgG (Fig. 10–1). This response can be induced with as little as 0.03 mL of D-positive red blood cells.[15]

The overall risk of Rh sensitization to a nonimmunized primiparous Rh-negative woman after delivery of her first ABO-compatible, Rh-positive child ranges from 11% to 16%,[18] and this risk increases with subsequent pregnancies. In the event of ABO incompatibility between the mother and child, this risk drops to approximately 2%.[19] The ABO blood group antigens usually are expressed in tissues and cells. As a result, fetal ABO-incompatible red blood cells are rapidly destroyed in the maternal circulation, which diminishes the opportunity of the Rh antigen to induce an immune response.[20] However, after a primary immune response to the Rh antigen has been mounted, ABO incompatibility between the mother and the fetus offers no protection against a secondary immune response.

The degree of Rh sensitization of the maternal immune system is proportionately related to the dose of antigen exposure. As a result of a small volume of transplacental hemorrhage (<0.1 mL), 3% of nonimmunized Rh-negative women are sensitized.[21] In contrast, more than 0.1 mL increases that incidence to nearly 22%.[19] The isotype of the IgG antibody also has a role in the severity of hemolytic disease. The avidity with which the antibody-coated erythrocyte binds to the Fc receptor of the monocyte is greater for the IgG3 subclass of antibody than for IgG1, and fewer molecules of IgG3 anti-D antibody induce clearance of Rh-positive erythrocytes than do IgG1 antibodies.[22] The combination of IgG1 and IgG3 is associated with a greater risk for severe alloimmunization than either antibody alone.[23, 24]

Prevention of Rh sensitization in the developed world has been undertaken to a relatively successful degree since the licensure of Rh immune globulin in 1968.[25] Before its routine use, approximately 1 of every 100 pregnancies re-

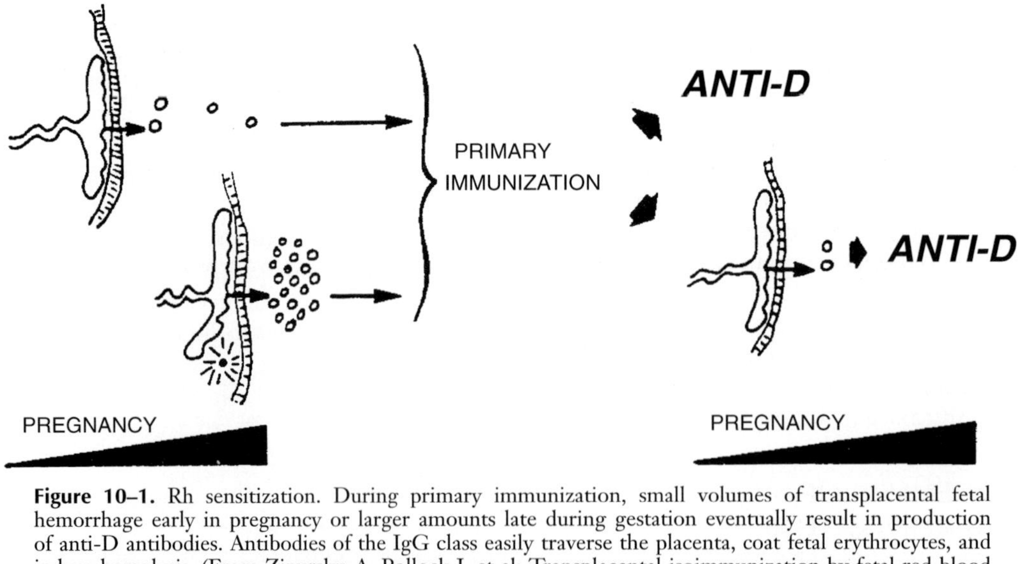

Figure 10–1. Rh sensitization. During primary immunization, small volumes of transplacental fetal hemorrhage early in pregnancy or larger amounts late during gestation eventually result in production of anti-D antibodies. Antibodies of the IgG class easily traverse the placenta, coat fetal erythrocytes, and induce hemolysis. (From Zipursky, A, Pollock J, et al: Transplacental isoimmunization by fetal red blood cells. In Bergsma D. [ed]: Symposium on the Placenta. Birth Defects Original Article Series. Vol. 1. The National Foundation. New York: Wiley-Liss, 1965, p 87.)

sulted in Rh alloimmunization, but that incidence has dropped by a factor of 10.[8] Despite these encouraging statistics, it is of continued concern that 9% of alloimmunized fetuses require intrauterine transfusion. Recommendations for prophylaxis include the administration of a polyclonal antibody, Rh immune globulin, to Rh-negative women at 28 weeks of gestation and within 72 hours of delivery of an Rh-positive infant.[26] Prophylaxis at 28 weeks reduces the incidence of Rh sensitization to 0.11%.[27] Prophylaxis is also recommended after abortion and after invasive procedures, including amniocentesis and chorionic villus sampling. The dosage of Rh immunoglobulin administered depends on the degree of transplacental hemorrhage. Problems in the prevention of Rh immunization remain, including failure to give prophylactic therapy when indicated, failed immunity after a massive transplacental hemorrhage, and rare allergic reactions to Rh immune globulin.[28]

The prophylactic antibody is derived from anti-D antibodies produced by immunized donors. As a result of the success of immunization programs, supplies of the polyclonal anti-D antibody may become limited. Developments in the prophylaxis of anti-D alloimmunization include the use of monoclonal antibodies against the Rh (D) antigen, for which clinical trials are under way.[29, 30]

PATHOPHYSIOLOGY OF HEMOLYTIC DISEASE IN THE FETUS AND NEONATE

Certain blood groups, such as ABH, are expressed in a wide spectrum of tissues, including those of the erythroid lineage.[31, 32] In contrast, expression of the Rh antigen is restricted to red blood cells,[33] with an increasing antigen density during their development into mature cells.[34] However, the Rh antigen is not expressed on the red blood cell progenitors, burst-forming unit–erythroid and colony-forming unit–erythroid.[35]

After sensitization, maternal anti-D antibodies, which cross the placenta into the fetal circulation, attach to surface Rh (D) antigen on fetal red blood cells. Antibody-coated fetal red blood cells form adherent rosettes on macrophages in the reticuloendothelial system, especially in the spleen.[36] The antibody-coated erythrocytes undergo lysis by lysosomal enzymes released by cytotoxic macrophages or natural killer lymphocytes.[37, 38] Destruction of these red blood cells does not appear to involve activation of the complement system.[39] Prolonged hemolysis results in severe anemia in the fetus, which stimulates fetal erythropoietin production[40] and subsequently accelerates erythropoiesis in the liver, spleen, and bone marrow.[41] Extramedullary erythropoiesis has also been observed in the skin and in the placenta.[42, 43] In severe cases, destruction of hepatocytes and distortion of normal parenchyma can result from an overabundance of erythropoietic cells, eventually leading to hepatic dysfunction and hypoproteinemia.

This process has been thought to contribute to the pathogenesis of hydrops in severe alloimmunization.[44] Destruction of red blood cells also liberates heme. The enzymatic degradation of heme ultimately results in the production of unconjugated bilirubin and its byproducts, a subject that has been reviewed elsewhere.[45–47] However, because the placenta normally metabolizes bilirubin,[48] hyperbilirubinemia is of consequence only to the delivered newborn.

Alloimmunization can occur to a variety of other fetal red blood cell surface antigens (Table 10–1). Included among these are other antigens of the Rh blood-group system (c, C, e, E, cc and Ce) and those belonging to the Kell (K and k), Duffy (Fya), Kidd (Jk[a] and Jk[b]), and MNSs (M,N,S, and s) systems.[49] Among antigens of the Rh group, alloimmunization with E and c occurs most frequently after anti-D sensitiza-

Table 10–1. **Association of Neonatal Hemolytic Disease with Atypical Maternal Blood Group Antigen**

Frequency of Disease	Maternal Antigen
Common	c, Kell, E
Uncommon	e, C, Ce, Kp[a], Kp[b], cE, k, s, Wr[a], Fy[a]
Rare	S, U, M, Fy[b], N, Do[a], Co[a], Di[a], Di[b], Lu[a], Yt[a], Jk[a], Jk[b]
No occurrence	Le[a], Le[b], P

From Bowman JM: Hemolytic disease (erythroblastosis fetalis). In Creasy RK, Cresnik R (eds): Maternal-Fetal Medicine: Principles and Practice, 2nd ed. Philadelphia: WB Saunders, 1989, p 650.

tion.[50] In rare circumstances, hemolytic disease can occur in neonates delivered to Rh-positive D^u variant mothers.[50] Alloimmunization as a result of sensitization to the Kell antigen is seen infrequently. Maternal antibodies to Kell are commonly associated with prior transfusion and are observed 60% as often as antibodies to the Rh antigen.[51] However, because of the low frequency of the paternal gene for K:1, the risk of hemolytic disease in the fetus and newborn as a result of maternal Kell sensitization is less than 5%. Of these, one half require neither intrapartum nor neonatal intervention, but the remainder can develop severe hemolysis.[52, 53] Alloimmunization to the Kell antigen or its subgroups accounts for up to 10% of severely affected fetuses. Hemolytic disease of the newborn as a result of Kell sensitization differs from that caused by anti-D in that the Kell antigen is expressed on the surfaces of erythroid progenitors,[54] whereas the D antigen is not. Kell sensitization, in addition to causing hemolysis, results in suppression of fetal erythropoiesis.[55]

PRENATAL DIAGNOSIS AND MANAGEMENT OF THE ALLOIMMUNIZED GESTATION

Optimal management of the newborn infant with Rh incompatibility begins with prenatal diagnosis and careful management of the sensitized pregnancy, as has been extensively reviewed elsewhere.[49, 56–58] Women at risk for alloimmunization should have an indirect Coombs' test obtained during the first prenatal visit, followed by a titer and paternal blood type and genotype if the test result is positive. If the paternal genotype is homozygous for the Rh antigen, serial maternal titers are obtained on a frequent basis until a titer indicating a high risk for fetal hydrops, usually 1:16, is obtained. However, with paternal heterozygosity, it may be necessary to determine the fetal blood type. Available methods for determining genotype in the fetus use polymerase chain reaction–based testing of fetal cells in the amniotic fluid or from chorionic villi.[59–62] Alternatively, the fetal blood type can be directly established from a cordocentesis sample.[63]

If alloimmunization has been established or is strongly suspected, serial monitoring is required during gestation. Several parameters are associated with the severity of fetal hemolytic disease.[6] These include previous children with hemolytic disease of the newborn; rising maternal antibody titers; rising bilirubin concentrations in amniotic fluid as determined by optical density (OD) readings; ultrasonographic evidence of fetal ascites, edema, or worsening biophysical profile; and decreasing hemoglobin concentration. In general, frequent serial amniocenteses are obtained, and deviations in linearity from the optical density reading at a wavelength of 450 nm (ΔOD_{450}) are plotted on a Liley curve[64] (Fig. 10–2). For gestations of less than 24 weeks, the modified Liley curve (Fig. 10–3) is used to correct for the fact that unaffected fetuses normally produce bilirubin with levels that peak at 23 to 25 weeks of gestation.[65] Eleva-

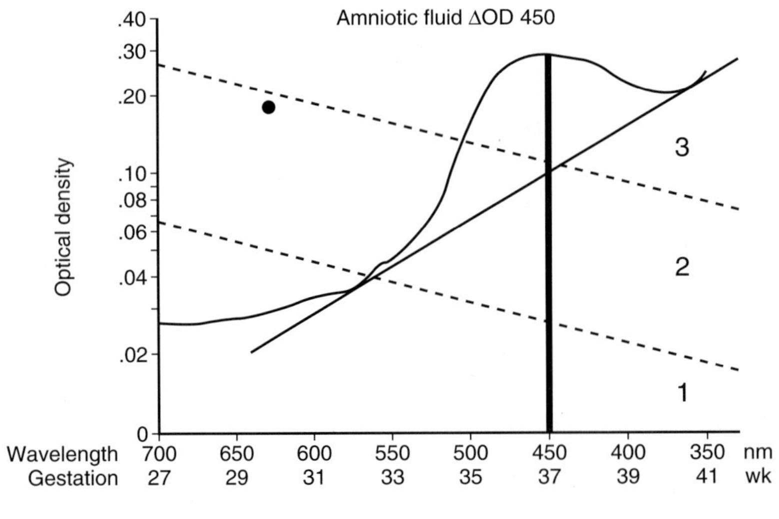

Figure 10–2. Liley curve. At 29 weeks' gestation, the amniotic fluid spectrophotometric reading at 450 nm, 0.200 in this example, falls close to zone 3, indicating severe hemolytic disease. The curved line indicates optical density (OD) readings on patient's amniotic fluid; the solid, straight line represents the OD baseline. (From Bowman JM: Haemolytic disease of the newborn (erythroblastosis fetalis). In Roberton NRC [ed]: Textbook of Neonatology. Edinburgh: Churchill Livingstone, 1986, p 473.)

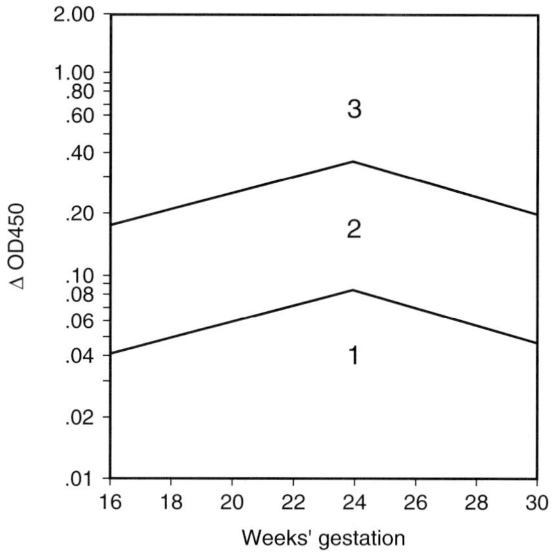

Figure 10–3. Liley curve modified for gestations of less than 24 weeks. This modification reflects the observation that bilirubin levels in amniotic fluid peak at 23 to 24 weeks' gestation in normal pregnancies. (From Bowman JM, Pollock JM, Manning FA, et al: Maternal Kell blood group alloimmunization. Reprinted with permission from the American College of Obstetricians and Gynecologists (*Obstetrics and Gynecology*, 1992; 79:239.)

tion of ΔOD_{450} values greater than the 65th percentile of zone 2 is a usual indication for more direct fetal monitoring by cordocentesis. Generally, a fetal hematocrit of less than 30% is considered an indication for intrauterine transfusion. For a woman who has had a severely affected fetus or newborn, frequent ultrasonographic monitoring is preferred over serial maternal antibody titers.[57]

Kell sensitization can result in fetal hydrops in the presence of very low maternal antibody titers,[66] a reflection of the diminished effective erythropoiesis associated with this type of alloimmunization. Diminished production of red blood cells is associated with decreased numbers of hemolyzed cells. The ΔOD_{450} values therefore are unreliable in determining disease severity.[55]

There are many excellent reviews on the subject of intrauterine transfusion.[57, 58, 67, 68] Methods for transfusing red blood cells into anemic fetuses include intraperitoneal and intravascular routes. Liley[69] first described intraperitoneal transfusion (IPT) in 1963. However, because of higher complication rates with IPT,[70] the intravascular route has become the preferred method of fetal transfusion. The use of IPT also is contraindicated if the infant is hydropic or moribund or when the placenta is anteriorly placed.[57]

Direct intravascular transfusion (IVT) was first successfully performed by Rodeck and colleagues[71] in 1981. In many centers, IPT is performed in addition to IVT to provide a slowly absorbed reservoir of red blood cells; absorption is usually complete in 8 to 10 days.[72] The goal when only IVT is performed is a hematocrit of 60%, whereas a hematocrit of 40% is desired when combined IPT and IVT are used. Survival of hydropic or severely anemic fetuses is better if the post-transfusion hematocrit is less than 25% or if the final hematocrit represents no more than a fourfold increase over pretransfusion values.[73] Donor cells typically are cross-matched against the maternal blood type and packed to a hematocrit of 80% to attain a fetal hematocrit of 40%. Most centers use fresh red blood cells from type O Rh-negative donors. However, several centers have successfully used washed maternal erythrocytes as the donor source.[74]

The survival of adult erythrocytes transfused into the fetal circulation appears to be similar to their survival in adult recipients.[75] Studies of four children after intrauterine transfusion showed the persistence of donor lymphocytes for up to 2 years.[76]

IVT immediately places a stress on the cardiovascular system of the fetus by increasing intravascular volume, as reflected by increased umbilical venous pressures in the first 24 hours after transfusion.[77] In the long term, intrauterine transfusion benefits the anemic fetus by decreasing the cardiac work load, as evidenced by decreased stroke volume and heart rate.[78] The replacement of fetal hemoglobin with adult hemoglobin increases oxygen release to the tissues, a result of greater binding of 2,3-diphosphoglycerate (2,3-DPG) to hemoglobin A than to hemoglobin F. Erythrocyte 2,3-DPG concentrations in normal fetuses, regardless of the gestational age, are higher than are those in normal adults.[79] Infants with erythroblastosis fetalis have even higher 2,3-DPG concentrations, which vary inversely with hemoglobin concentrations. After intrauterine transfusion, adult erythrocytes in the fetal circulation increased their 2,3-DPG levels to a degree similar to that expected for fetal erythrocytes. These observations suggest that the fetal environment promotes oxygen delivery to fetal tissues in the presence of anemia.

Another potential benefit of IVT is a decrease in the rate of hemolysis and a subsequent decreased release of glutathione into the circulation. As a result, the development of fetal hyperinsulinemia, associated with increased serum glutathione levels, is diminished.[80] In addition to improving overall fetal survival, intrauterine IVT reverses the progression of hydrops fetalis in severely affected fetuses.[81] Intrauterine transfusion also accelerates appropriate fetal weight gain,[82] a benefit to severely alloimmunized but nonhydropic fetuses, who are often growth retarded.[83]

In centers that frequently perform intrauterine transfusions, the risk of fetal loss ranges from 1% to 3%.[57] One complication associated with this procedure (Table 10–2) is the potential for significant fetomaternal hemorrhage, which increases the risk for more severe alloimmunization in subsequent pregnancies.[84] Another potential, although rare, risk for the fetus is that of iron overload and subsequent hepatic dysfunction.[85] A more common observation in infants who were transfused in utero has been the occurrence of a "late" hyporegenerative anemia in the first few months of life.[86, 87] Intracranial hemorrhage has been associated with intrauterine transfusion, although it has also been reported in cases of severe hemolytic disease of the newborn without intrauterine transfusion.[88]

Table 10–2. **Complications of Intrauterine Transfusion**

Procedure	Maternal Complications	Fetal Complications
IPT	Infection, tissue trauma	Over-transfusion Exsanguination Cardiac tamponade Infection Induction of labor Graft-versus-host disease Radiation damage
IVT	Fetomaternal TPH	Over-transfusion Exsanguination Umbilical vein compression

IPT, intraperitoneal transfusion; IVT, intravascular transfusion; TPH, transplacental hemorrhage.

Adapted from Bowman JM: Hemolytic disease (erythroblastosis fetalis). In Creasy RK, Cresnik R (eds): Maternal-Fetal Medicine: Principles and Practice, 2nd ed. Philadelphia: WB Saunders, 1989, p 650.

Neurologic outcome studies of alloimmunized infants who received intrauterine transfusions have shown conflicting results. Turner and coworkers[89] observed that only 50% of survivors were considered normal in long-term follow-up, but their observations may reflect relative inexperience in the early years of intrauterine transfusion. Others have reported that most survivors are neurologically intact.[90, 91] Janssens and associates[92] observed that neurologic abnormalities were closely correlated with the severity of the hemolytic disease, as evidenced by anemia at birth and perinatal hypoxia.

During the period when intrauterine transfusion by the peritoneal route was the usual means of treating the alloimmunized gestation, newborns were routinely delivered at 32 weeks.[57] This practice resulted in a high incidence of hyaline membrane disease and exchange transfusions in these premature infants. Since the advent of IVT in utero, the general approach to the severely alloimmunized gestation is to perform intrauterine transfusion as required until 34 to 35 weeks' gestation, with delivery planned at term.[58] Establishment of fetal lung maturity to determine timing of delivery can be difficult for these patients, because the accuracy of certain tests can be influenced by residual blood in the amniotic fluid after intrauterine transfusion.[93]

Alloimmunized fetuses are at risk for the development of hydrops before and after the 34th week of gestation. Early in gestation, before 20 to 22 weeks, is a period during which fetuses can succumb to severe anemia.[58] Unfortunately, the size of the fetus at that time limits the utility of intrauterine transfusion. Since it was first reported by Berlin and colleagues,[94] multiple studies have found at least a partially beneficial effect of intravenous immunoglobulin (IVIG) administration to mothers in the early treatment of severe fetal alloimmunization.[95–98] The mechanism of action of IVIG in alloimmune hemolytic disease appears to involve blockage of Fc receptors on macrophages in the fetal reticuloendothelial system. However, IVIG does not inhibit maternal anti-D antibody production or its passage across the placenta.[96] The beneficial effect of IVIG administration to the fetus appears to be directly related to the amount administered[99] and to the timing of its administration before the development of severe anemia. Its use in combination with intrauterine transfusion in one study showed that fetal survival was 36% higher when high-dose IVIG treatment preceded intrauterine transfusion than when transfusion alone was instituted.[98]

DIAGNOSIS OF THE SENSITIZED FETUS AND NEONATE

Various prenatal factors are important in determining the severity of the disease in the neonate, and knowledge of the maternal and gestational history is critical to the diagnosis and management of the alloimmunized neonate. The infant delivered after an alloimmunized gestation exhibits clinical characteristics that depend on the severity of the disease. Typical clinical signs of the neonate with hemolytic disease include jaundice, pallor, and hepatosplenomegaly.

Diagnostic Findings

Jaundice

Most neonates develop some degree of jaundice in the first few days of life because of the delayed capacity of the liver to process bilirubin resulting from normal red blood cell degradation. This *physiologic jaundice* usually peaks after the second or third day of life in term infants and generally requires no intervention. Jaundice that is present at birth or occurs at less than 24 hours of life with rapidly rising unconjugated bilirubin serum levels is pathologic and is most commonly caused by hemolytic disease.[100] In hemolytic disease of the newborn, the severity of the jaundice correlates with the degree of hemolysis. Occasionally, an infant with severe hemolysis presents with elevated serum levels of directly conjugated bilirubin. The mechanism appears to be related to placental or hepatic dysfunction as a result of extensive hemolysis.[101–103]

In the absence of a positive direct Coombs' test result other causes of pathologic jaundice that should be considered include hemolysis due to infection, especially that of viral origin; erythrocyte membrane defects such as spherocytosis; and red blood cell enzyme deficiencies, such as glucose-6-phosphate dehydrogenase deficiency (Table 10–3). Nonhemolytic causes of jaundice include polycythemia and degradation of red blood cells after "enclosed hemorrhages" such as cephalhematoma or generalized bruising.[104] Hyperbilirubinemia has also been associ-

Table 10–3. **Causes of Jaundice During the First Week of Life**

Hemolysis–isoimmune	Rh or ABO incompatibility
Hemolysis–inherited defects	Spherocytosis
	Enzyme deficiencies (glucose-6-phosphate dehydrogenase, pyruvate kinase)
Hemolysis–other causes	Drugs and toxins (naphthalene, oxytoxin)
Infections	Bacterial (sepsis, syphilis)
	Viral (cytomegalovirus, herpes simplex virus, congenital rubella)
	Protozoal (toxoplasmosis)
Enclosed hemorrhage	Cephalhematoma
Polycythemia	Infant of diabetic mother
	Intrauterine growth retardation
Metabolic disorders	α_1-Antitrypsin deficiency
	Breast milk jaundice
	Crigler-Najjar syndrome
	Familial neonatal hyperbilirubinemia
	Galactosemia
	Hypothyroidism
	Hypopituitarism
Increased enterohepatic absorption	Bile stasis from upper gastrointestinal obstruction
	Swallowed blood
Miscellaneous	Asphyxia
	Reduced caloric intake
Neonatal giant cell hepatitis	
Physiologic jaundice	

Adapted from Naiman JL: Erythroblastosis fetalis. In Oski FA, Naiman JL (eds): Hematologic Problems in the Newborn, 3rd ed. Philadelphia: WB Saunders, 1982, p 294.

ated with renal vein thrombosis[105] and hypothyroidism. After feedings have been initiated, vomiting in association with jaundice can indicate gastrointestinal obstruction or galactosemia. Suspicion of galactosemia should prompt the testing of the urine for reducing substances.

Kernicterus

Volpe[106] reviewed the pathogenesis and clinical features of acute bilirubin encephalopathy, or kernicterus. In brief, kernicterus is the result of bilirubin staining of regions of the basal ganglia and associated neuronal necrosis. Its development in neonates with hemolytic disease due to Rh incompatibility is related to the severity of the hemolytic process, which influences the degree of accumulation of unconjugated bilirubin in the serum. Factors that potentiate the risk of kernicterus in the absence of marked hyperbilirubinemia include prematurity, low birth weight, sepsis, and hypoxic-ischemic encephalopathy. Neurologic deficits resulting from kernicterus, including those of the extrapyramidal system, gaze abnormalities, and deafness, may not become apparent until after the first year of life. Fortunately, since the advent of modern management of the alloimmunized fetus and newborn, kernicterus in the newborn as a result of hemolytic disease has become rare.[107]

Anemia

Anemia is the kinetic result of increased destruction or decreased production of erythrocytes. Both mechanisms can be operative in patients with erythroblastosis fetalis. The usual anemia resulting from anti-D hemolytic disease in the neonate is the result of the destruction of antibody-coated red blood cells by the reticuloendothelial system or, in certain cases, intravascular destruction. However, the intrauterine transfusion of red blood cells to anemic fetuses, especially by the intravascular route, can suppress subsequent erythropoiesis and induce a hypogenerative anemia.[86, 87, 108] Kell alloimmunization is also associated with diminished erythroid production by virtue of the destruction of erythroid progenitors in the bone marrow.[54, 55]

The greatest risk to the alloimmunized fetus is that of severe anemia. Development of anemia is associated with an increase in plasma volume while the total blood volume remains normal.[109] With the progression of anemia, congestive heart failure can develop, leading to diminished tissue perfusion and metabolic acidosis. Severely anemic fetuses can develop hydrops or, in extreme cases, be delivered as stillbirths. The advent of intrauterine transfusion has minimized the development of these complications and can reverse hydrops in some cases.[81] However, a fetus who is hydropic before this procedure has a decreased chance of survival compared with nonhydropic fetuses.[57]

Late hyporegenerative anemia has been observed in infants after hemolytic disease in the newborn period, especially in association with intrauterine or exchange transfusions.[86, 108, 110] Another type of a delayed anemia can occur in infants who had milder forms of hemolytic disease treated with phototherapy alone. This anemia, associated with persistently elevated circulating maternal antibody titers, appears to be the result of continued red blood cell destruction.[111] One study found that the mean half-life of maternal anti-D antibody in the neonatal circulation was 14 days and that evidence of hemolysis could be detected at up to 6 weeks of age.[112]

The more common type of late anemia has been observed in neonates who received one or more intrauterine transfusions.[87, 113] This anemia may be caused by a diminished hypoxic stimulus to the kidneys followed by suppression of erythropoiesis, the result of transfusion with adult hemoglobin.[114] This hyporegenerative anemia is characterized by reticulocytopenia, decreased circulating concentration of erythropoietin, and diminished numbers of erythroid precursors in the bone marrow.[86]

Hydrops

Severe anemia is not the sole cause of hydrops in alloimmunized fetuses. Hydrops has been observed despite normal hemoglobin values, and fetuses with hemoglobin concentrations as low as 3 g/dL are not necessarily hydropic.[115] The elevated venous pressures observed in some cases of hydrops appear to be more closely related to fetal hypoxia and metabolic acidosis.[116] Fetal hydrops is also associated with increased placental weight and edema of the chorionic villi, a situation that can interfere with placental transport. Another contributory factor may be the excessive extramedullary erythropoiesis in the liver with severe hemolysis, which can cause portal and umbilical venous obstruction and diminished placental perfusion due to edema.[15] Diminished albumin production associated with hepatic dysfunction decreases intravascular oncotic pressure, in severe cases resulting in anasarca, ascites, and pleural and pericardial effusions.[44, 117]

The causes of fetal hydrops include disorders other than severe alloimmunization. Among these are nonimmune hematologic disorders associated with severe anemia; cardiovascular abnormalities, especially those involving dysrhythmias; and infectious agents, including those of viral origin such as syphilis, cytomegalovirus, and parvovirus infections. A detailed discussion is provided in several excellent reviews.[44, 118–122]

Hepatosplenomegaly

An infant with mild hemolytic disease usually has no hepatic or splenic enlargement, whereas with severe disease, the organomegaly can be significant, especially in the presence of hydrops. In the presence of ascites, hepatosplenomegaly can be difficult to appreciate by palpation. The causes of these findings include venous engorgement, portal hypertension resulting from excessive extramedullary hematopoiesis,[102] and congestive heart failure from severe anemia.

Hemorrhage

Infants with hemolysis and thrombocytopenia can present with petechiae and purpuric lesions, especially in the presence of perinatal asphyxia. These findings are associated with a poor prognosis.[100] Infants with severe hemolytic disease sometimes develop a hemostatic disorder consistent with disseminated intravascular coagulation.[123] Intracranial hemorrhage has been associated with thrombocytopenia in infants with severe hemolytic disease in the absence of or after intrauterine transfusion.[88]

Laboratory Findings

Hematologic Abnormalities

The severity of hematologic abnormalities in alloimmunized neonates varies directly with the severity of hemolysis and the compensatory ability of the bone marrow. These are summarized in Table 10–4.

Hemoglobin Concentration

The degree of anemia in the fetus is most accurately determined by direct measurement of the umbilical cord blood hemoglobin concentration during cordocentesis.[124] In the neonate, central venous or arterial samples more accurately reflect the hemoglobin concentration than do capillary samples.[125] Values below 13.5 g/dL are considered abnormal in the term neonate. A hemoglobin concentration can be normal despite a degree of hemolysis causing significant hyperbilirubinemia. This situation may reflect adequately increased production of erythrocytes by the marrow to compensate for the hemolysis or be the result of intrauterine transfusion shortly before delivery.[117] Relatively normal hemoglobin concentrations have been described in certain hydropic infants.[115] After the initial hemoglobin determination, subsequent serial measurements are not helpful in evaluating the need for the initial or subsequent exchange transfusions. Hemoglobin concentrations in infants at risk for developing a late anemia should be monitored closely in the first 6 to 8 weeks of life.[86]

Table 10–4. **Common Hematologic Findings in Hemolytic Disease of the Newborn**

Anemia
Reticulocytosis
Reticulocytopenia
Increased nucleated red blood cell concentration
Polychromasia, anisocytosis
Spherocytosis (ABO incompatibility)
Cell fragmentation (disseminated intravascular coagulation [DIC])
Neutropenia
Neutrophilia
Thrombocytopenia (± DIC)
Increased serum erythropoietin concentration
Decreased serum erythropoietin concentration

Reticulocytes, Nucleated Red Blood Cells, and Peripheral Smears

The reticulocyte count can be as high as 30% to 40% in infants with Rh hemolytic disease who did not receive an intrauterine transfusion.[100] In contrast, neonates who received an intrauterine transfusion, especially if given shortly before delivery, can have an initial reticulocyte count of zero. Infants who have been alloimmunized with the Kell antigen can have a reticulocytopenia at delivery despite severe anemia.[55] Neonates who receive exchange transfusions can develop reticulocytopenia,[126] and reticulocytopenia is characteristic of the hyporegenerative anemia observed in infants with the late anemia of hemolytic disease.[86]

A nucleated red blood cell count of up to 24 per 100 white blood cells is not unusual in the umbilical cord blood of the normal infant.[127] Nucleated cell counts are variable during significant anemia, and like the reticulocyte count, they reflect the state of erythropoiesis. However, the presence of the offending antigen on these cells can result in their destruction, yielding unexpectedly low nucleated cell counts. In the presence of a high concentration of nucleated red blood cells, the automated leukocyte count may be falsely elevated and require correction by a factor proportionate to the fraction of nucleated red blood cells.

The peripheral blood smear of an alloimmunized infant with hemolysis typically shows polychromasia and anisocytosis. Spherocytes are more commonly seen in cases of ABO incompatibility and in certain red blood cell membrane disorders.[128] In more severe cases of hemolytic disease with elements of disseminated intravascular coagulation, cell fragmentation is observed on the smear.

Neutrophil Count

Neutropenia has been reported in alloimmunized neonates.[126] It is occasionally caused by exchange transfusion with leukocyte-poor blood.[129] In the absence of exchange transfusion, the cause of neutropenia appears to be a diversion of hematopoiesis away from myeloid production in favor of erythropoiesis.[130] Neutrophilia has also been described in fetuses after intrauterine transfusion with leukocyte-poor blood.[131] The researchers ascribed their findings to possible increases in circulating cytokines, resulting in demargination of fetal neutrophils. In support of this possibility, fetal cytokines are elevated in Rh alloimmunization, and serum levels of granulocyte-macrophage colony-stimulating factor appear to correlate with fetal white blood cell counts.[132]

Platelet Count

Thrombocytopenia (platelet count $<150{,}000/mm^3$) is common in neonates with severe alloimmunization,[133] especially after intrauterine or exchange transfusions.[126] It can be caused by the use of platelet-depleted red blood cells, but other factors appear to be involved. For example, bilirubin toxicity as a cause of thrombocytopenia has been entertained.[133] Thrombocytopenia has also been described in alloimmunized fetuses and neonates in the absence of intrauterine transfusion[133] and can be of prolonged duration.[126] The possibility that platelet production, like neutrophil production, is down-regulated in favor of red blood cell production remains to be tested. Thrombocytopenia also occurs in cases of disseminated intravascular coagulation associated with severe hemolytic disease.

Erythropoietin

Erythropoietin levels in anemic alloimmunized fetuses of more than 20 weeks' gestation do not increase above those of normal adults until the hemoglobin level is substantially decreased.[10, 134] Intrauterine transfusion suppresses erythropoiesis, resulting in a hyporegenerative anemia and low levels of erythropoietin in the first months of life.[113, 135] In other infants, the erythropoietin levels increase as the hemoglobin falls, independently of whether they received an intrauterine transfusion.[134] Levels of erythropoietin do not always correlate with circulating numbers of nucleated red cells, perhaps reflecting their destruction by persistent maternal antibody.

Metabolic Abnormalities

Symptomatic hypoglycemia is common in neonates with severe hemolytic disease. The cause of this form of hypoglycemia appears to be hyperinsulinism, a result of pancreatic islet cell hyperplasia.[136] Although the mechanism is unclear, it has been postulated that metabolic byproducts of lysed erythrocytes stimulate insulin secretion directly or in response to glucagon.[137] Hypoglycemia can also occur in infants after exchange transfusion, possibly the result of increased insulin secretion.[138]

Other metabolic abnormalities are associated with exchange transfusion. Hyperkalemia can be related to the use of erythrocytes older than several days of age.[139] It is recommended that only blood less than 1 or 2 days old be used for transfusion and that the potassium content of the donor blood be checked. Hypocalcemia can result after the binding of serum calcium by citrated anticoagulant preservatives. Falling parathormone levels can also contribute to diminished serum calcium levels.[140]

Serologic Abnormalities

In the indirect Coombs' test, Rh (D)–negative maternal serum is combined with Rh (D)–positive red blood cells, and the cells are washed.[141] Coating of the test cells with the anti-D antibody contained in the maternal serum results in their agglutination by antihuman globulin (Coombs') serum, which yields a positive indirect Coombs' test result. The maternal antibody titer is the highest dilution of maternal serum at which a positive test result is still obtained. A high titer parallels a high content of anti-D antibody in the maternal serum. The direct Coombs' test is used to detect antibody-coated red blood cells in the fetal or neonatal circulation, and the magnitude of the titer correlates with the amount of circulating maternal antibody.

MANAGEMENT OF THE SENSITIZED NEONATE

Mild Hemolytic Disease

Up to 50% of neonates who have a positive result for the direct Coombs' test are only mildly affected. Serum bilirubin levels are only mildly elevated, and the hemoglobin concentration is normal. Although phototherapy is occasionally necessary, neither erythrocyte transfusion nor exchange transfusion are required to treat this group of infants.

Moderate Hemolytic Disease

Approximately 25% to 30% of affected neonates have moderate hemolytic disease. These infants are usually healthy at birth but develop detectable jaundice shortly afterward. Because the placenta efficiently removes serum bilirubin produced by hemolyzed erythrocytes,[103] jaundice is not a problem for the fetus. However, once delivered, the neonate must depend on the liver to metabolize bilirubin. In the first days of life of a normal neonate, the liver has a diminished capacity to efficiently metabolize bilirubin.[142] When the liver is presented with even greater amounts of bilirubin, as occurs after extensive hemolysis, serum concentrations of unconjugated bilirubin can increase markedly. The toxicity of this water-insoluble unconjugated bilirubin is based on its attraction to tissues, such as neurons, that contain a high lipid content. Toxic neural effects are heightened when the integrity of the blood-brain barrier is compromised, as occurs after perinatal asphyxia, during certain types of sepsis, and in premature infants.[106] The lethal staining of neurons with bilirubin is characteristic of kernicterus (i.e., bilirubin encephalopathy). Infants who survive kernicterus are afflicted with a variety of long-term neurologic insults, including deafness and, in severe cases, cerebral palsy.[106, 107]

Phototherapy

Several reviews offer in-depth discussions of bilirubin metabolism and the indications for various therapeutic modalities.[143–145] In brief, the initial treatment of abnormally elevated serum levels of indirect bilirubin is phototherapy. Indications for initiating phototherapy in term infants with hemolytic disease are summarized in Table 10–5. During phototherapy, which is most effective in the wavelength of blue light, indirect bilirubin is isomerized into a water-soluble form, which can then be excreted by the gastrointestinal tract and the kidneys.[146] However, in the presence of severe hemolysis, serum

Table 10–5. **Indications for Phototherapy in the Term Infant with Hemolytic Disease of the Newborn**

Age	Serum Bilirubin (mg/dL)
Cord blood	>3.5
<12 h	>10
<18	>12
<24	>14
2–3 d	>15

bilirubin levels continue to increase despite phototherapy treatment. When dangerously elevated levels of indirect serum bilirubin are approached, the excess bilirubin must be removed from the circulation by means of exchange transfusion.

Exchange Transfusion

The criteria used to determine the need for an exchange transfusion are controversial,[56] although severe anemia and the presence of a rapidly increasing bilirubin level despite optimal phototherapy in the first 12 hours of life indicate the need for earlier intervention. Evidence of hemolysis, especially in the presence of factors that can affect the integrity of the blood-brain barrier, lowers the threshold of acceptable serum bilirubin levels.[106] Suggested guidelines for considering exchange transfusion in neonates with hemolytic disease are summarized in Table 10–6. These guidelines depend on clinical status and gestational age and must be weighed against the risks inherent in the procedure.

Table 10–6. **Guidelines for Exchange Transfusion in Neonates with Hemolytic Disease of the Newborn**

Severe anemia (Hb < 10 gm/dL)
Rate of bilirubin rise >0.5 mg/dL/h (optimal phototherapy)
Increase in serum bilirubin, indirect fraction
>20 mg/dL (healthy, >2500 g)
>18 mg/dL (septic, >2500 g)
>17 mg/dL (2000–2499 g)
>15 mg/dL (1500–1999 g)
>13 mg/dL (1250–1499 g)
>9–12 mg/dL (<1250 g)

Adapted from Peterec SM: Management of neonatal Rh disease. Clin Perinatol 1995;22:571.

The exchange of an infant's blood with an amount of donor blood equal to twice its circulating volume (double-volume exchange) removes approximately 70% to 90% of fetal erythrocytes.[147] However, most of the body's bilirubin is found not in the circulation but in the extravascular space. Only about 25% of total bilirubin is removed by an exchange transfusion, and a rapid rebound of serum bilirubin levels after equilibration may mandate additional exchange transfusions. An overview of the exchange transfusion procedure is presented in Tables 10–7, 10–8, and 10–9.

Exchange transfusion is not without risk,[45, 100] as reviewed in Table 10–10. A variety of hematologic abnormalities have been associated with this procedure, including neutropenia and thrombocytopenia, which can be prolonged. Exchange transfusion can suppress innate erythropoiesis, as has been observed after intrauterine transfusion. In these cases, infants may develop a late anemia in the first months of life that can be of sufficient severity to warrant one or more blood transfusions or a course of erythropoietin.[86, 108] Metabolic abnormalities, most commonly hypoglycemia, can also complicate exchange transfusion. An association between exchange transfusion and subsequent bowel perforation has been reported.[148] Cerebral blood volume changes have been observed in term and preterm infants undergoing exchange transfusion.[149] Death has been associated with exchange transfusion,[150] and several infants have developed fatal graft-versus-host disease after exchange transfusion.[151] The diminished need for this procedure, a result of improved prenatal management, has created a void in expertise among pediatricians and neonatologists for performing exchange transfusions.

Intravenous Immunoglobulin

The maternal administration of high-dose IVIG during the sensitized gestation has proven effective in modulating the severity of hemolytic disease in the fetus. Several investigators have reported some degree of success in minimizing the need for exchange transfusion in hemolytic infants by instituting therapy with IVIG.[97, 152–154] Its administration to the neonate with hemolytic disease from alloimmunization appears to be an effective adjunct to phototherapy. The mecha-

Table 10–7. **Exchange Transfusion: Preparation**

Equipment

Preassembled disposable set with four-way stopcock
20-mL syringes
Waste receptacle
Intravenous connection tubing
Oxygen, suction, emergency resuscitation equipment available
Calcium gluconate

Precautions

Monitor vital signs closely throughout procedure
Use fresh blood (<5 days old)
Use appropriately warmed blood
Perform only in presence of adequate personnel:
  One person to perform procedure
  One person to monitor and record each pass
Clear line with heparinized saline if procedure is interrupted

Preparation

Anticipate need for exchange
Notify blood bank of need for exchange before bilirubin level approaches exchange level
Donor blood must be compatible with both infant and maternal blood
  Same ABO group: use group specific blood
  Different ABO group: use group compatible blood
  For A, B, or AB infant: use washed O cells reconstituted in AB plasma
Determine amount of donor blood to be given:
  Double-volume exchange: infant blood volume (BV) (80 mL/kg) × 2
  Anemia: $\text{volume exchanged (mL)} = (\text{BV}) \times \frac{(\text{Hct desired} - \text{Hct initial})}{(\text{Hct pRBCs} - \text{Hct initial})}$
Donor blood reconstituted in saline or plasma for a final hematocrit ~40%
Pre-exchange laboratory tests
  Hemoglobin, hematocrit, platelets
  Electrolytes, ionized calcium
  Glucose
  Serum bilirubin (indirect fraction)
  Coagulation profile
Determine rate of exchange procedure
  Average time per pass: 3–5 min (2–3 mL/kg/min)
  Total duration of procedure: 90–120 min

BV, blood volume; Hct, hematocrit; pRBCs, packed red blood cells.
Adapted from Edwards MC, Fletcher MA: Exchange transfusions. In Fletcher MA, MacDonald MG, Avery GB (eds): Atlas of Procedures in Neonatology. Philadelphia: JB Lippincott, 1983.

nism of action of IVIG in modulating hemolysis is not clear but appears to be related to blockage of Fc receptors in the neonatal reticuloendothelial system.[155]

Hara and colleagues[156] reported the successful use of IVIG in treating a late anemia from maternal anti-E sensitization. In that study, a dose of 250 mg/kg/d of IVIG was administered for a total of 3 days. The reversal of hyperbilirubinemia due to hemolytic disease has been reported after administration of IVIG given over several days or as a single dose.[152, 153] The results of a multicenter trial designed to evaluate the use of IVIG in Rh hemolytic anemia was reported by Rubo and colleagues in 1992.[97] In that trial, neonates who were Coombs' test positive were randomized to receive phototherapy with or without adjunctive IVIG (500 mg/kg). Of 16 patients who received IVIG, only 2 (12.5%) required exchange transfusion. In contrast, a significant number of nontreated controls, 11 (69%) of 16, required exchange transfusion. Delaying the administration of IVIG appeared to be related to the requirement for exchange transfusion in at least one of the two patients who failed treatment. Overall, the use of IVIG was associated with lower serum bilirubin levels. No adverse effects were reported with its use. In a later trial, Voto and associates observed that administration of IVIG (800 mg/kg/d for 3 days) to neonates with Rh hemolytic disease resulted in lower serum bilirubin levels and fewer hospital days.[157] Subsequent clinical trials have shown that administration of IVIG

Table 10–8. **Exchange Transfusion: Procedure**

Preparation of Infant

Open warmer
No oral intake for at least 4 hours before exchange
Peripheral intravenous line for continuous dextrose infusion
Continuous monitors: oxygen saturation, heart rate, blood pressure

Preparation of Blood

Verify identification of blood product
Check that hematocrit is 35–45%
Allow blood to pass through blood warmer

Procedure: Isovolumetric Exchange

Mask, cap, sterile gown, and gloves
Line placement for infant blood withdrawal
- UAC
- Peripheral arterial line
- (UVC; less desirable)
- Prime line with heparinized saline (5 units heparin/mL saline)
- Line placement for donor blood administration
- UVC, 8 French
- Peripheral intravenous line
- Prime line with blood
- X-ray documentation of appropriate position of umbilical lines
- UVC is *not* radiopaque if from exchange tray
- Start recording in exchange-transfusion record sheet (included in exchange tray)
- Time of each pass
- Vital signs
- Blood volume

Attach tubing to withdrawal (arterial) line per instructions included in exchange tray
Begin venous infusion of donor blood (length of infusion should approximate the total time planned for blood removal)
Gently withdraw blood from arterial line over a period equaling 2–3 mL/kg/min (*no faster* than 5 min per pass)
Intermittently flush arterial line with heparinized saline to avoid clotting of line
Monitor
- Blood glucose every 30 min
- ABG before exchange, then as needed
- Vital signs continuously
- Administer calcium (100 mg/kg calcium gluconate) only if
- Documented hypocalcemia (ionized calcium)
- Electrocardiographic changes (prolonged QT interval)

ABG, arterial blood gas determination; UAC, umbilical artery catheter; UVC, umbilical venous catheter.
Adapted from Edward MC, Fletcher MA: Exchange transfusions. In Fletcher MA, MacDonald MG, Avery GB (eds): Atlas of Procedures in Neonatology. Philadelphia: JB Lippincott, 1983.

to neonates with hemolytic disease results in diminished hemolysis, as measured by carboxyhemoglobin levels.[154, 158] In one trial of IVIG administration to neonates with ABO isoimmunization, 5 of 23 treated infants were considered treatment failures based on their ultimate requirement for exchange transfusion.[159] These five nonresponders also had the highest carboxyhemoglobin levels, consistent with a greater severity of hemolysis.

The use of IVIG in conjunction with phototherapy appears to be warranted in the treatment of neonates with significant hemolytic disease from Rh or ABO incompatibility. Because the results of multiple studies indicate that the efficacy of IVIG treatment depends on the timing of administration, duration of treatment, and severity of the hemolysis, this therapy will need further investigation before solid recommendations can be made. However, the administration of 500 to 1000 mg/kg IVIG in the first few hours of life to a neonate suspected of having significant hemolytic disease is a reasonable consideration.

Severe Hemolytic Disease

In one fourth of alloimmunized gestations, severe hemolytic disease (fetal hydrops) devel-

Table 10–9. **Exchange Transfusion: Follow-up**

Obtain blood for laboratory tests
- Blood glucose
- Arterial blood gases
- Indirect serum bilirubin
- Ionized calcium, electrolytes
- Re-crossmatching (in case further transfusion required)

Document vital signs
Monitor vital signs hourly for at least 4–6 h
Repeat laboratory tests approximately 4–6 h after exchange
No oral intake for infant for 12–24 h after exchange

Adapted from Edwards MC, Fletcher MA: Exchange transfusions. In Fletcher MA, MacDonald MG, Avery GB (eds): Atlas of Procedures in Neonatology. Philadelphia: JB Lippincott, 1983.

ops before or after 34 weeks.[15] The incidence of hydrops fetalis due to alloimmunization has been significantly reduced as a result of improvements in prenatal management,[57] but fetal hydrops still occurs despite optimal therapy. Stabilization of an infant with hydrops requires a high level of intensive management, and adequate preparation for a possibly affected infant is of the utmost importance. Many excellent reviews have been written on this subject.[44, 56, 160, 161] In general, intubation followed by drainage of pleural effusions and ascites can result in immediate benefit to the hydropic infant by significantly improving respiratory capacity. Because most infants have elevated central venous pressures and normal blood volumes,[116] cautious correction of the often severe anemia with packed erythrocytes or by exchange transfusion is necessary to avoid contributing to congestive heart failure (Fig. 10–4). Careful attention also should be given to the correction of the infant's metabolic status.

Treatment of the Infant with Late Anemia

Infants who had hemolytic disease of the newborn are at risk for developing anemia in the first few months of life.[86, 135, 162] The severity of this hyporegenerative anemia frequently necessitates treatment with erythrocyte transfusion. Recombinant human erythropoietin (rh-EPO) has been shown to have some efficacy in decreasing the need for transfusion in these patients. Ohls and colleagues reported the successful use of rh-EPO in averting transfusion in two infants with late anemia after a 10-day course of therapy (200 U/kg/d).[108] In contrast, using a modified regimen of 150 to 200 U/kg/d of rh-EPO three times each week for up to 3 weeks, Bussel and associates observed a hemato-

Table 10–10. **Potential Hazards of Exchange Transfusion**

Type of Problem	Problem Encountered
Cardiac	Arrhythmias
	Volume overload, congestive heart failure
	Arrest
Hematologic	Overheparinization
	Neutropenia
	Thrombocytopenia
	Graft-versus-host disease
	Sickling (donor blood)
Infection	Bacteremia
	Virus (hepatitis, cytomegalovirus, human immunodeficiency virus)
	Malaria
Metabolic	Acidosis
	Hyperkalemia
	Hypernatremia
	Hypocalcemia
	Hypoglycemia
Vascular	Embolization with air, clots
	Thrombosis
	Necrotizing enterocolitis with perforation
Other	Perforation of umbilical vessel
	Hypothermia

Modified from Naiman JL: Erythroblastosis fetalis. In Oski FA, Naiman JL (eds): Hematologic Problems in the Newborn, 3rd ed. Philadelphia: WB Saunders, 1982, p 316.

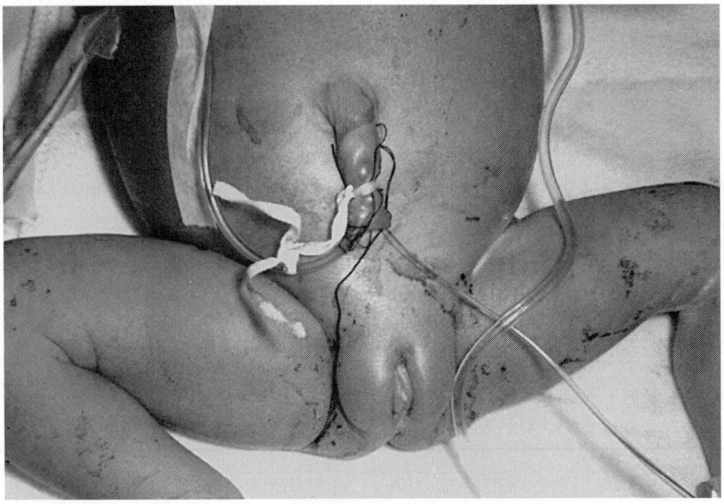

Figure 10–4. Hydropic infant with umbilical vessels in place. Stabilization of the critically ill hydropic neonate is critical for survival. Exchange transfusion may be necessary to correct severe anemia due to extensive hemolysis.

poietic response that was insufficient to prevent transfusion in two of three infants studied.[163] Scardavou and coworkers treated four infants with 200 U/kg/d of rh-EPO, administered three times per week.[164] Onset of therapy ranged from 1 to 7.5 weeks of life. All four patients showed a hematopoietic response as evidenced by reticulocytosis and increased hemoglobin concentration. In a larger pilot study, 20 infants were randomized to receive rh-EPO (600 U/kg/wk for 6 weeks) or placebo.[110] Although the treatment group of infants received fewer total transfusions than the control infants (1.8 versus 4.2, $P<.05$), treatment prevented the need for transfusion in only two infants. The results of these studies indicate an ability of these anemic neonates to respond to rh-EPO therapy. Larger trials are needed to determine appropriate dosage, scheduling, and timing of rh-EPO administration before its routine use in these infants can be advocated.

The infant diagnosed with hemolytic disease in the newborn period should have weekly hematocrit determinations in the first several months of life, especially after an intrauterine or exchange transfusion. Reticulocytopenia can be consistent with a hyporegenerative anemia or can indicate continued destruction of reticulocytes from the persistence of high titers of circulating maternal antibody. Indications for transfusion of an anemic infant[114, 162] include poor weight gain, ineffective feeding, persistent tachypnea, and tachycardia associated with cardiomegaly.

ABO INCOMPATIBILITY AND HEMOLYTIC DISEASE OF THE NEWBORN

Pathogenesis

In 1944, Halbrecht described an association between hemolytic disease in newborn infants and ABO incompatibility.[165] Incompatibility between maternal erythrocytes that lack the A or B antigen and fetal erythrocytes that have that antigen induces the production of maternal antibody against that antigen. Anti-A and anti-B antibodies are naturally present in the serum of mothers who are group O, B, and A. However, in mothers who are group A or group B, these “natural” antibodies are usually of the IgM isotype, and most are of the IgG class in mothers who are group O.[166] Because only antibodies of the IgG class can cross the placenta, hemolytic disease of the newborn is usually only clinically observed when mothers are group O. The presence of these naturally occuring antibodies in the maternal serum explains the frequent occurrence of ABO hemolytic in first-born infants, in contrast to the greater incidence of Rh hemolytic disease in subsequent gestations.

The interaction between anti-A or anti-B antibody and the corresponding antigen on the fetal red blood cell usually produces a weakly positive direct Coombs' test result. The hemolysis resulting from maternal-fetal ABO incompatibility is rarely clinically significant. Several explanations have been offered for this phenomenon. Because A and B antigens are expressed on a wide variety of cells, the absorption of anti-A or anti-B antibodies can diminish the amount of antibody left to interact with fetal erythrocytes.[167] Alternatively, fetal erythrocytes appear to have less surface expression of A or B antigen, resulting in fewer reactive sites.[168] Hemolysis of fetal erythrocytes as a result of ABO incompatibility is typically not intravascular and does not involve complement activation.[169]

Incidence

The incidence of ABO mismatch between a blood group O mother and her fetus is approximately 15%. However, only 10% to 20% of these neonates become significantly jaundiced, and most can be managed with phototherapy alone. Rarely, erythrocyte transfusions or exchange transfusions are required. Factors associated with severity of hemolytic disease resulting from ABO incompatibility include race, immunization with bacterial vaccines, and the antigenicity of the A or B antigens.[170–173] There appears to be no difference in the severity of hemolytic disease caused by B-O or A-O incompatibility.[174, 175]

Clinical Presentation

Clinically significant jaundice occurs on the first day of life in 10% to 20% of ABO-incompatible infants. Serum bilirubin levels are a reflection of the degree of hemolysis. Mild hemolysis contributes to some degree of jaundice in the remainder of these infants. In one large study, the cord blood of infants with blood group A or B antigen who were born to blood group O mothers had lower hemoglobin concentrations and higher serum bilirubin concentrations compared with the cord blood of group O infants.[175] The presence of jaundice prompted suspicion of ABO incompatibility in only 4% of the infants studied, although most of the 680 infants tested had at least a weakly positive direct Coombs' test result. These results led one researcher to comment that jaundice associated with ABO incompatibility is "the tip of the iceberg" in this type of hemolytic disease.

Pallor is an unusual finding in these infants, because anemia is rarely observed in ABO alloimmunization, and severe hemolytic disease, such as hydrops, is extremely uncommon. In the presence of marrow compensation for anemia,[176] the blood smear can show polychromasia, reticulocytosis (10% to 30%), and increased numbers of nucleated erythrocytes. Spherocytosis (≤40%) is a common finding in the blood smear of infants with ABO hemolytic disease.[109] This finding can be confused with hereditary spherocytosis, because increased osmotic fragility and autohemolysis characterize both disorders. However, glucose does not correct the autohemolysis due to ABO incompatibility, whereas it normalizes autohemolysis in hereditary spherocytosis.[177] When there is doubt regarding the diagnosis, the parents should be examined for their carrier status, especially if the hemolytic anemia persists. A delayed anemia in the first few months of life does not usually occur in ABO hemolytic disease unless the infant has required exchange transfusion.[174]

Because of the nature of the antigen-antibody interaction, the direct Coombs' test is positive in only 20% to 40% of ABO-incompatible infants, and the test is usually only weakly positive, even in the presence of significant hemolysis. However, nearly all infants with ABO incompatibility have antibody on their erythrocytes, although most at a level undetectable by the usual testing methods.[168] A positive direct Coombs' test result is a risk factor for clinically significant hemolytic disease. Infants of blood group A born to group O mothers normally have circulating anti-B antibodies but not anti-A antibodies. Conversely, blood group B infants have antibodies to group A but not to group B. However, in the presence of hemolytic disease due to ABO alloimmunization, anti-A antibodies are found in the serum of group A infants, and anti-B antibodies are in the serum of group B infants. Antibody to group A or B antigen in the alloimmunized group O mother is composed of immunoglobulins of types IgG, IgM, and IgA. However, only antibodies of the IgG subclasses cross the placenta to induce hemolysis in the newborn. Determination of antibody to anti-A or anti-B in the maternal serum is difficult, as false positives are common.[49] Determination of these maternal antibodies may be of limited usefulness when the risk of severe hemolysis in the newborn is low.

Clinical Management

Control of hyperbilirubinemia is the major goal in managing infants who have ABO hemolytic disease. For most affected infants, phototherapy is the only therapy necessary. However, in rare cases, significant elevation of serum bilirubin levels may necessitate exchange transfusion. Indications for exchange transfusion are similar to those used in cases of Rh alloimmunization.

Sn-Porphyrins

Tin (Sn) porphyrin is a potent inhibitor of heme oxygenase, the enzyme that catalyzes the rate-limiting step in the degradation of heme to bilirubin.[178] This process has been reviewed elsewhere.[47] Studies investigating the use of heme oxygenase inhibitors to obviate the need for exchange transfusion and to decrease the duration of phototherapy have met with some degree of success. Over the past 5 years, clinical trials have shown a beneficial effect of Sn-protoporphyrin and Sn-mesoporphyrin administration on the reduction of maximal serum bilirubin levels and the need for phototherapy in jaundiced newborns.[179] These options can diminish the need for medical intervention in neonates with ABO incompatibility. The use of metalloporphyrins in neonates with hemolytic disease due to Rh incompatibility has not been reported.

Reported toxic effects of metalloporphyrins include skin photosensitization, iron deficiency after prolonged use, and possible inhibition of carbon monoxide production.[178, 180] Although initial data appear encouraging, further information regarding the clinical efficacy and long-term effects of metalloporphyrins are necessary before the routine use of metalloporphyrins can be recommended.

Intravenous Immunoglobulin

IVIG has been used in the treatment of hemolytic disease due to Rh incompatibility. One study suggested a possible role for IVIG in the treatment of significant hemolytic disease of the newborn due to ABO incompatibility.[159]

Prenatal Management

The low risk for the development of severe hemolytic disease in the fetus with ABO incompatibility[175] has resulted in no specific guidelines

Table 10–11. **Comparison of Rh and ABO Incompatibility**

Characteristic	Rh	ABO
Blood group set-up		
Mother	Negative	O
Infant	Positive	A or B
Clinical aspects		
First born	5%	40–50%
Later pregnancies	More severe	No increased severity
Stillbirth/hydrops	Frequent	Rare
Severe anemia	Frequent	Rare
Degree of jaundice	Moderate to severe	Mild
Laboratory findings		
Direct Coombs' test	Positive	Positive or negative
Spherocytes	Rare	Frequent
Treatment		
Antenatal measures	Yes	No
Phototherapy	Yes	Yes
Exchange transfusion	Sometimes	Rare
Late anemia		
Incidence	Frequent	Rare

Modified from Naiman JL: Erythroblastosis fetalis. In Oski FA, Naiman JL (eds): Hematologic Problems in the Newborn, 3rd ed. Philadelphia: WB Saunders, 1982, p 333.

for the management of the pregnancy known or suspected to be ABO incompatible.

Overview of Therapeutic Strategies

Hemolytic disease of the newborn is caused by alloimmunization with a fetal erythrocyte antigen of maternal erythrocytes lacking that antigen. The degree to which the fetus is affected correlates with the amount of maternal antibody that crosses the placenta. The severity of the disease can be mild, requiring minimal therapy in the delivered newborn. Such is usually the case when hemolysis is caused by ABO incompatibility. In contrast, hemolysis can be severe enough to cause fetal hydrops or, rarely, intrauterine death. Hemolytic disease from Rh or ABO incompatibility is compared in Table 10–11. Optimal management of the alloimmunized gestation depends on close monitoring for increasing severity of fetal disease, a finding that may necessitate therapy with high-dose IVIG and intrauterine transfusion. Management of the neonate with hemolytic disease is an extension of the management during gestation and is a function of the severity of hemolysis. Phototherapy, especially in conjunction with IVIG administration, is usually effective in treating hyperbilirubinemia due to hemolysis, and the need for exchange transfusion has become increasingly uncommon. A frequent late complication of neonatal hemolytic disease due to Rh incompatibility is a hyporegenerative anemia that may be responsive to treatment with recombinant erythropoietin.

References

1. Diamond LK, Blackfan KD, Baty JM: Erythroblastosis fetalis and its association with universal edema of the fetus, icterus gravis neonatorum and anemia of the newborn. J Pediatr 1932;1:269.
2. Landsteiner K, Wiener AS: An agglutinable factor in human blood recognized by immune sera for rhesus blood. Proc Soc Exp Biol Med 1940;43:223.
3. Wiener AS, Peters HR: Hemolytic reactions following transfusions of blood of the homologous group, with three cases in which the same agglutinogen was responsible. Ann Intern Med 1940;13:2306.
4. Levine P, Katzin EM, Burnham L: Isoimmunization in pregnancy: its possible bearing on the etiology of erythroblastosis fetalis. JAMA 1941;116:825.
5. Chown B: Anemia from bleeding of the fetus into the mother's circulation. Lancet 1954;1:1213.
6. Bowman JM: Hemolytic disease (erythroblastosis fetalis). In Creasy RK, Resnick R (eds): Maternal-fetal medicine: principles and practice. Philadelphia: WB Saunders, 1994, pp 711–743.
7. van Dijk B: Preventing RhD haemolytic disease of the newborn (Editorial; comment). BMJ 1997;315:1480.
8. Chavez GF, Mulinare J, Edmonds LD: Epidemiology of Rh hemolytic disease of the newborn in the United States. JAMA 1991;265:3270.
9. Briegel K, Bartunek P, Stengl G, et al: Regulation and function of transcription factor GATA-1 during red blood cell differentiation. Development 1996; 122:3839.
10. Race RR: The Rh genotype and Fisher's theory. Blood 1948;3:27.
11. Lewis M, Kaita H, Chown B: The inheritance of the Rh blood groups. I. Frequencies in 1000 unrelated Caucasian families consisting of 2000 parents and 2806 children. Vox Sang 1971;20:502.
12. Kleihauer E, Braun H, Betke K: Demonstration von Fetalem Haemoglobin in den Erythrozyten eines Blutausstriches. Klin Wochenschr 1957;35:637.
13. Bowman JM, Pollock JM, Penston LE: Fetomaternal transplacental hemorrhage during pregnancy and after delivery. Vox Sang 1986;51:117.
14. Queenan JT, Gadow EC, Lopes AC: Role of spontaneous abortion in Rh immunization. Am J Obstet Gynecol 1971;110:128.
15. Bowman JM: Immune hemolytic disease. In Nathan DG (ed): Hematology of Infancy and Childhood. Philadelphia: WB Saunders, 1997, pp 53–78.
16. Peddle LJ: Increase of antibody titer following amniocentesis. Am J Obstet Gynecol 1986;100:567.
17. MacGregor SN, Silver RK, Sholl JS: Enhanced sensitization after cordocentesis in a rhesus-isoimmunized pregnancy. Am J Obstet Gynecol 1991;165:382.
18. Nevanlinna HR: Factors affecting maternal Rh immunization. Ann Med Exp Biol 1953;31:1.
19. Woodrow JC: Rh immunization and its prevention: the immune response in the mother. In Jensen KG, Killmann SA (eds): Copenhagen: Munksgaard, 1970, p 3.
20. Bowman JM: Fetomaternal ABO incompatibility and erythroblastosis fetalis. Vox Sang 1986;50:104.
21. Zipursky A, Israels LG: The pathogenesis and prevention of Rh immunization. Can Med Assoc J 1967;97:1245.
22. Fletcher A, Thomson A: The introduction of human monoclonal anti-D for therapeutic use. Transfus Med Rev 1995;9:314.
23. Zupanska B, Brojer E, Richards Y, et al: Serological and immunological characteristics of maternal anti-Rh(D) antibodies in predicting the severity of haemolytic disease of the newborn. Vox Sang 1989;56:247.
24. Pollock JM, Bowman JM: Anti-Rh(D) IgG subclasses and severity of Rh hemolytic disease of the newborn. Vox Sang 1990;59:176.
25. Wegmann A, Gluck R: The history of rhesus prophylaxis with anti-D. Eur J Pediatr 1996;155:835.
26. Urbaniak SJ: Consensus conference on anti-D prophylaxis, April 7 & 8, 1997: final consensus statement. Royal College of Physicians of Edinburgh/Royal College of Obstetricians and Gynaecologists. Transfusion 1998;38:97.
27. Bowman JM: Suppression of Rh isoimmunization. Obstet Gynecol 1978;52:385.
28. Bowman JM, Pollock JM: Failures of intravenous Rh immune globulin prophylaxis: an analysis of the reasons for such failures. Transfus Med Rev 1987;1:101.

29. Hadley AG, Kumpel BM: The role of Rh antibodies in haemolytic disease of the newborn. Baillieres Clin Haematol 1993;6:423.
30. Kumpel BM: Monoclonal anti-D for prophylaxis of RhD haemolytic disease of the newborn. Transfus Clin Biol 1997;4:351.
31. Hershko C, Gale RP, Ho W, Fitchen J: ABH antigens and bone marrow transplantation. Br J Haematol 1980;44:65.
32. Karhi KK, Andersson LC, Vuopio P, Gahmberg CG: Expression of blood group A antigens in human bone marrow cells. Blood 1981;57:147.
33. Rearden A, Masouredis SP: Blood group D antigen content of nucleated red blood cell precursors. Blood 1977;50:981.
34. Hughes-Jones NC, Gardner B, Lincoln PJ: Observations of the number of available c, D, and E antigens on red cells. Vox Sang 1971;21:210.
35. Rearden A, Chiu P: Lack of rhesus antigen expression by human committed erythroid progenitors. Blood 1983;61:525.
36. Lobuglio AF, Cotran RS, Jandl JH: Red cells coated with immunoglobulin G: binding and sphering by mononuclear cells in man. Science 1967;158:1582.
37. Engelfriet CP, von dem Borne AE, Fleer A, et al: In vivo destruction of erythrocytes by complement-binding and non–complement-binding antibodies. Prog Clin Biol Res 1980;43:213.
38. Urbaniak SJ, Stewart GM: ADCC activity of monoclonal anti-D antibodies. Rev Fr Transfus Immunohematol 1988;31:237.
39. Poorkhorsandi ME, Gupte SC: Role of C1q in rhesus haemolytic disease of the newborn. Indian J Med Res 1996;104:208.
40. Thilaganathan B, Salvesen DR, Abbas A, et al: Fetal plasma erythropoietin concentration in red blood cell-isoimmunized pregnancies. Am J Obstet Gynecol 1992;167:1292.
41. Gilmour JR: Erythroblastosis fetalis. Arch Dis Child 1944;19:1.
42. Pizarro A, Elorza D, Gamallo C, et al: Neonatal dermal erythropoiesis associated with severe rhesus immunization: amelioration by high-dose intravenous immunoglobulin (Letter). Br J Dermatol 1995; 133:334.
43. Bouissou H, Kanoun T, Bierme S, Bierme R: Liver and placenta during hemolytic disease due to Rh isoimmunization (histologic study and deductions). Pathol Biol 1969,17.109.
44. Gest AL, Moise KJJ: Hydrops fetalis. In Pomerance J, Richardson J (eds): Neonatology for the Clinician. East Norwalk: Appleton & Lange, 1993, pp 395–410.
45. Maisels MJ: Neonatal jaundice. Clin Perinatol 1990;17:245.
46. Gartner LM: Neonatal jaundice. Pediatr Rev 1994;15:422.
47. Yao TC, Stevenson DK: Advances in the diagnosis and treatment of neonatal hyperbilirubinemia. Clin Perinatol 1995;22:741.
48. Schier RW, Dilts PV Jr, Conger WL, Hamrin CE Jr: Bilirubin transfer across the human placenta. Am J Obstet Gynecol 1971;111:677.
49. Mollison PL, Engelfriet CP, Contreras M: Hemolytic disease of the newborn. In Mollison PL (ed): Blood Transfusion in Clinical Medicine. Oxford: Blackwell Scientific Publications, 1987, p 639.
50. Bowell PJ, Brown SE, Dike AE, Inskip MJ: The significance of anti-c alloimmunization in pregnancy. Br J Obstet Gynaecol 1986;93:1044.
51. Wenk RE, Goldstein P, Felix JK: Kell alloimmunization, hemolytic disease of the newborn, and perinatal management. Obstet Gynecol 1985;66:473.
52. Giannacopoulou CH, Relakis K, Kalmanti M: Severe anemia due to Kell alloimmunization. Haematologia (Budap) 1997;28:173.
53. Parilla BV, Socol ML: Hydrops fetalis with Kell isoimmunization. Obstet Gynecol 1996;88:730.
54. Vaughan JI, Manning M, Warwick RM, et al: Inhibition of erythroid progenitor cells by anti-Kell antibodies in fetal alloimmune anemia. N Engl J Med 1998;338:798.
55. Vaughan JI, Warwick R, Letsky E, et al: Erythropoietic suppression in fetal anemia because of Kell alloimmunization. Am J Obstet Gynecol 1994;171:247.
56. Peterec SM: Management of neonatal Rh disease. Clin Perinatol 1995;22:561.
57. Schumacher B, Moise KJJ: Fetal transfusion for red blood cell alloimmunization in pregnancy. Obstet Gynecol 1996;88:137.
58. Bowman J: The management of hemolytic disease in the fetus and newborn. Semin Perinatol 1997;21:39.
59. Fisk NM, Bennett P, Warwick RM, et al: Clinical utility of fetal RhD typing in alloimmunized pregnancies by means of polymerase chain reaction on amniocytes or chorionic villi. Am J Obstet Gynecol 1994;171:50.
60. Le Van KC, Mouro I, Brossard Y, et al: PCR-based determination of Rhc and RhE status of fetuses at risk of Rhc and RhE haemolytic disease. Br J Haematol 1994;88:193.
61. Lynen R, Neuhaus R, Schwarz DW, et al: Flow cytometric analyses of the subclasses of red cell IgG antibodies. Vox Sang 1995;69:126.
62. Noble AL, Poole GD, Anderson N, et al: Predicting the severity of haemolytic disease of the newborn: an assessment of the clinical usefulness of the chemiluminescence test. Br J Haematol 1995;90:718.
63. Nicolaides KH, Soothill PW, Rodeck CH, Clewell W: Rh disease: intravascular fetal blood transfusion by cordocentesis. Fetal Ther 1986;1:185.
64. Liley AW: Liquor amnii analysis in management of pregnancy complicated by rhesus immunization. Am J Obstet Gynecol 1961;82:1359.
65. Nicolaides KH, Rodeck CH, Mibashan RS, Kemp JR: Have Liley charts outlived their usefulness? Am J Obstet Gynecol 1986;155:90.
66. Bowman JM, Harman FA, Manning CR, Pollock JM: Erythroblastosis fetalis produced by anti-k. Vox Sang 1989;56:187.
67. Queenan JT: Fetal transfusion. Fetal Ther 1986;1:59.
68. Goodrum LA, Saade GR, Belfort MA, et al: The effect of intrauterine transfusion on fetal bilirubin in red cell alloimmunization. Obstet Gynecol 1997;89:57.
69. Liley AW: Intrauterine transfusion of foetus in haemolytic disease. BMJ 1963;2:1107.
70. Harman CR, Bowman JM, Manning FA, Menticoglou SM: Intrauterine transfusion—intraperitoneal versus intravascular approach: a case-control comparison. Am J Obstet Gynecol 1990;162:175.
71. Rodeck CH, Kemp JR, Holman CA, et al: Direct intravascular fetal blood transfusion by fetoscopy in severe rhesus isoimmunisation. Lancet 1981;1:625.
72. Moise KJ Jr, Carpenter RJ Jr, Kirshon B, et al: Comparison of four types of intrauterine transfusion: effect on fetal hematocrit. Fetal Ther 1989;4:126.
73. Radunovic N, Lockwood CJ, Alvarez M, et al: The severely anemic and hydropic isoimmune fetus: changes in fetal hematocrit associated with intrauterine death. Obstet Gynecol 1992;79:390.
74. Gonsulin WJ, Moise KJ, Milam JD, et al: Serial ma-

ternal blood donations for intrauterine transfusion. Obstet Gynecol 1990;75:158.
75. Pattison N, Roberts A: The management of severe erythroblastosis fetalis by fetal transfusion: survival of transfused adult erythrocytes in the fetus. Obstet Gynecol 1989;74:901.
76. Hutchinson DL, Turner JH, Schlesinger ER: Persistence of donor cells in neonates after fetal and exchange transfusion. Am J Obstet Gynecol 1971; 109:281.
77. Weiner CP, Pelzer GD, Heilskov J, et al: The effect of intravascular transfusion on umbilical venous pressure in anemic fetuses with and without hydrops. Am J Obstet Gynecol 1989;161:1498.
78. Moise KJ, Mari G, Fisher DJ, et al: Acute fetal hemodynamic alterations after intrauterine transfusion for treatment of severe red blood cell alloimmunization. Am J Obstet Gynecol 1990;163:776.
79. Soothill PW, Lestas AN, Nicolaides KH, et al: 2, 3-Diphosphoglycerate in normal, anaemic and transfused human fetuses. Clin Sci 1988;74:527.
80. Socol ML, Dooley SL, Ney JA, et al: Absence of hyperinsulinemia in isoimmunized fetuses treated with intravascular transfusion. Am J Obstet Gynecol 1991;165:1737.
81. Grannum PA, Copel JA, Moya FR, et al: The reversal of hydrops fetalis by intravascular intrauterine transfusion in severe isoimmune fetal anemia. Am J Obstet Gynecol 1988;158:914.
82. Roberts A, Grannum PA, Belanger K, et al: Fetal growth and birthweight in isoimmunized pregnancies after intravenous intrauterine transfusion. Fetal Diagn Ther 1993;8:407.
83. Binks AS, Lind T, McNay RA: Effect of rhesus haemolytic disease upon birthweight. J Obstet Gynaecol Br Commonw 1973;80:301.
84. Bowman JM, Pollock JM, Peterson LE, et al: Fetomaternal hemorrhage following funipuncture: increase in severity of maternal red-cell alloimmunization. Obstet Gynecol 1994;84:839.
85. Lasker MR, Eddleman K, Toor AH: Neonatal hepatitis and excessive hepatic iron deposition following intrauterine blood transfusion. Am J Perinatol 1995;12:14.
86. Koenig JM, Ashton RD, De VG, Christensen RD: Late hyporegenerative anemia in Rh hemolytic disease. J Pediatr 1989;115:315.
87. Thorp JA, O'Connor T, Callenbach J, et al: Hyporegenerative anemia associated with intrauterine transfusion in rhesus hemolytic disease. Am J Obstet Gynecol 1991;165:79.
88. Grant EG, Schellinger D, Grosso MA, et al: Intracranial hemorrhage in neonates with erythroblastosis fetalis: sonographic and CT findings. AJNR Am J Neuroradiol 1984;5:259.
89. Turner JH, Hutchinson DL, Hayashi TT, et al: Fetal and maternal risks associated with intrauterine transfusion procedures. Am J Obstet Gynecol 1975;123:251.
90. Stewart G, Day RE, Del PC, et al: Developmental outcome after intravascular intrauterine transfusion for rhesus haemolytic disease. Arch Dis Child Fetal Neonatal Ed 1994;70:F52.
91. White CA, Goplerud CP, Kisker CT, et al: Intrauterine fetal transfusion, 1965–1976, with an assessment of the surviving children. Am J Obstet Gynecol 1978;130:933.
92. Janssens HM, de HM, van Kamp IL, et al: Outcome for children treated with fetal intravascular transfusions because of severe blood group antagonism. J Pediatr 1997;131:373.
93. Tait JF, Franklin RW, Simpson JB, Ashwood ER: Improved fluorescence polarization assay for use in evaluating fetal lung maturity. I. Development of the assay procedure. Clin Chem 1986;32:248.
94. Berlin G, Selbing A, Ryden G: Rhesus haemolytic disease treated with high-dose intravenous immunoglobulin. Lancet 1985;1:1153.
95. Chitkara U, Bussel J, Alvarez M, et al: High-dose intravenous gamma globulin: does it have a role in the treatment of severe erythroblastosis fetalis? Obstet Gynecol 1990;76:703.
96. Gottvall T, Selbing A: Alloimmunization during pregnancy treated with high dose intravenous immunoglobulin: effects on fetal hemoglobin concentration and anti-D concentrations in the mother and fetus. Acta Obstet Gynecol Scand 1995;74:777.
97. Rubo J, Albrecht K, Lasch P, et al: High-dose intravenous immune globulin therapy for hyperbilirubinemia caused by Rh hemolytic disease. J Pediatr 1992;121:93.
98. Voto LS, Mathet ER, Zapaterio JL, et al: High-dose gammaglobulin (IVIG) followed by intrauterine transfusions (IUTs): a new alternative for the treatment of severe fetal hemolytic disease. J Perinat Med 1997;25:85.
99. Dooren MC, van Kamp IL, Scherpenisse JW, et al: No beneficial effect of low-dose fetal intravenous gammaglobulin administration in combination with intravascular transfusions in severe Rh D haemolytic disease. Vox Sang 1994;66:253.
100. Naiman JL: Erythroblastosis fetalis. In Oski FA, Naiman JL (eds): Hematologic Problems in the Newborn. Philadelphia: WB Saunders, 1982, pp 283–346.
101. Harris LE, Farrell FJ, Shorter RG, et al: Conjugated serum bilirubin in erythroblastosis fetalis: an analysis of 38 cases. Mayo Clin Proc 1962;37:574.
102. Dunn PM: Obstructive jaundice and haemolytic disease of the newborn. Arch Dis Child 1963;38:54.
103. Shenker S, Dawber NH, Schmid R: Bilirubin metabolism in the fetus. J Clin Invest 1964;43:32.
104. Rausen AR, Diamond LK: Enclosed hemorrhage and neonatal jaundice. Am J Dis Child 1961;101:164.
105. Walters TR, Holder TM: Neonatal hyperbilirubinemia and renal vein thrombosis. Am J Dis Child 1966;111:433.
106. Volpe JJ: Bilirubin and brain injury. In Volpe JJ (ed): Neurology of the Newborn. Philadelphia: WB Saunders, 1987, pp 386–408.
107. Cashore WJ: The neurotoxocity of bilirubin. Clin Perinatol 1990;17:437.
108. Ohls RK, Wirkus PE, Christensen RD: Recombinant erythropoietin as treatment for the late hyporegenerative anemia of Rh hemolytic disease. Pediatrics 1992;90:678.
109. Zipursky A: Isoimmune hemolytic diseases. In Nathan DG, Oski FA (eds): Hematology of Infancy and Childhood. Philadelphia: WB Saunders, 1987, pp 44–73.
110. Ovali F, Samanci N, Dagoglu T: Management of late anemia in rhesus hemolytic disease: use of recombinant human erythropoietin (a pilot study). Pediatr Res 1996;39:831.
111. Weiner CP, Wenstrom KD: Outcome of alloimmunized fetuses managed solely by cordocentesis but not requiring antenatal transfusion. Fetal Diagn Ther 1994;9:233.
112. Hayde M, Widness JA, Pollak A, et al: Rhesus isoimmunization: increased hemolysis during early infancy. Pediatr Res 1997;41:716.
113. Millard DD, Gidding SS, Socol ML, et al: Effects of intravascular, intrauterine transfusion on prenatal and postnatal hemolysis and erythropoiesis in severe fetal isoimmunization. J Pediatr 1990;117:447.

114. Stockman JA III, Garcia JF, Oski FA: The anemia of prematurity: factors governing the erythropoietin response. N Engl J Med 1977;296:647.
115. Parkin J, Walker W: Peritoneal dialysis in severe hydrops fetalis. Lancet 1968;2:283.
116. Phibbs RH, Johnson P, Kitterman JA, et al: Cardiorespiratory status of erythroblastotic newborn infants. III. Intravascular pressures during the first hours of life. Pediatrics 1976;58:484.
117. Phibbs RH, Johnson P, Tooley WH: Cardiorespiratory status of erythroblastotic newborn infants. II. Blood volume, hematocrit, and serum albumin concentration in relation to hydrops fetalis. Pediatrics 1974;53:13.
118. Jauniaux E: Diagnosis and management of early nonimmune hydrops fetalis. Prenat Diagn 1997;17:1261.
119. Arcasoy MO, Gallagher PG: Hematologic disorders and nonimmune hydrops fetalis. Semin Perinatol 1995;19:502.
120. Barron SD, Pass RF: Infectious causes of hydrops fetalis. Semin Perinatol 1995;19:493.
121. Knilans TK: Cardiac abnormalities associated with hydrops fetalis. Semin Perinatol 1995;19:483.
122. Norton ME: Nonimmune hydrops fetalis. Semin Perinatol 1994;18:321.
123. Chessells JM, Wigglesworth JS: Haemostatic failure in babies with Rh isoimmunization. Arch Dis Child 1971;46:38.
124. Nicolaides KH, Soothill PW, Clewell WH, et al: Fetal haemoglobin measurement in the assessment of red cell isoimmunisation. Lancet 1988;1:1073.
125. Moe PJ: Umbilical cord blood and capillary blood in the evaluation of anemia in erythroblastosis fetalis. Acta Paediatr Scand 1967;56:391.
126. Koenig JM, Christensen RD: Neutropenia and thrombocytopenia in infants with Rh hemolytic disease. J Pediatr 1989;114:625.
127. Anderson GW: Studies on nucleated red cell count in chorionic capillaries and cord blood of various ages of pregnancy. Am J Obstet Gynecol 1941;42:1.
128. Zipursky A, Chintu C, Brown E, et al: The quantification of spherocytes in ABO hemolytic disease. J Pediatr 1979;94:965.
129. Phibbs RH: Response of newborn infants to leukocyte depletion during exchange transfusion. Biol Neonate 1970;15:112.
130. Christensen RD, Koenig JM, Viskochil DH, Rothstein G: Down-modulation of neutrophil production by erythropoietin in human hematopoietic clones. Blood 1989;74:817.
131. Yankowitz J, Weiner CP: Blood transfusion for haemolytic disease as a cause of leukocytosis in the fetus. Prenat Diagn 1996;16:719.
132. Westgren M, Ek S, Remberger M, et al: Cytokines in fetal blood and amniotic fluid in Rh-immunized pregnancies. Obstet Gynecol 1995;86:209.
133. Ekert H, Mathew RY: Platelet counts and plasma fibrinogen levels in erythroblastosis foetalis. Med J Aust 1967;2:844.
134. Dallacasa P, Ancora G, Miniero R, et al: Erythropoietin course in newborns with Rh hemolytic disease transfused and not transfused in utero. Pediatr Res 1996;40:357.
135. Thorp JA, O'Connor T, Callenbach J, et al: Hyporegenerative anemia associated with intrauterine transfusion in rhesus hemolytic disease. Am J Obstet Gynecol 1991;165:79.
136. Barrett CT, Oliver TK Jr: Hypoglycemia and hyperinsulinism with erythroblastosis fetalis. N Engl J Med 1968;278:1260.
137. Vidnes J, Finne PH: Immunoreactive insulin in amniotic fluid from Rh-immunized women. Biol Neonate 1977;31:1.
138. Schiff D, Aranda JV, Chan G, et al: Metabolic effects of exchange transfusion. I. Effect of citrated and heparinized blood on glucose, nonesterified fatty acids, 2-(4 hydroxybenzenazo)-benzoic acid binding, and insulin. J Pediatr 1971;78:603.
139. Miller G, McCoord AB, Joos HA, et al: Studies of serum electrolyte changes during exchange transfusion. Pediatrics 1954;13:412.
140. Wieland P, Duc G, Binswanger U: Parathyroid hormone response in newborn infants during exchange transfusion with blood supplemented with citrate and phosphate: effect of i.v. calcium. Pediatri Res 1979;13:963.
141. Coombs RRA, Mourant AE, Race RR: A new test for the detection of weak and "incomplete" Rh agglutinins. Br J Exp Pathol 1945;26:255.
142. Gartner LM, Lee KS, et al: Development of bilirubin transport and metabolism in the newborn rhesus monkey. J Pediatr 1977;90:513.
143. Muraca M, Rubaltelli FF, Blanckaert N, Fevery J: Unconjugated and conjugated bilirubin pigments during perinatal development. II. Studies on serum of healthy newborns and of neonates with erythroblastosis fetalis. Biol Neonate 1990;57:1.
144. Gartner LM, Catz CS, Yaffe SJ: Neonatal bilirubin workshop. Pediatrics 1994;94:537.
145. Blackburn S: Hyperbilirubinemia and neonatal jaundice. Neonat Netw 1995;14:15.
146. Ennever JF: Blue light, green light, white light, more light: treatment of neonatal jaundice. Clin Perinatol 1990;17:467.
147. Valaes T: Bilirubin distribution and dynamics of bilirubin removal by exchange transfusion. Acta Paediatr 1963;52(Suppl 149):1.
148. Castor WR: Spontaneous perforation of the bowel in the newborn following exchange transfusion. Can Med Assoc J 1968;99:934.
149. van de Bor M, Benders MJ, Dorrepaal CA, et al: Cerebral blood volume changes during exchange transfusions in infants born at or near term. J Pediatr 1994;125:617.
150. Keenan WJ, Novak KK, Sutherland JM, et al: Morbidity and mortality associated with exchange transfusion. Pediatrics 1985;75:417.
151. Weinberg K, Parkman R: Age, the thymus, and T lymphocytes (Editorial; comment). N Engl J Med 1995;332:182.
152. Kubo S, Ariga T, Tsumeta H, Ishii T: Can high-dose immunoglobulin therapy be indicated in neonatal rhesus haemolysis: a successful case of haemolytic disease due to rhesus (c + E) incompatibility. Eur J Pediatr 1991;150:507.
153. Sato K, Hara T, Kondo T, et al: High-dose intravenous gammaglobulin therapy for neonatal immune haemolytic jaundice due to blood group incompatibility. Acta Paediatr Scand. 1991;80:163.
154. Hammerman C, Vreman HJ, Kaplan M, Stevenson DK: Intravenous immune globulin in neonatal immune hemolytic disease: does it reduce hemolysis? Acta Paediatr 1996;85:1351.
155. Besalduch J, Forteza A, Duran MA, et al: Rh hemolytic disease treated with high-dose intravenous immunoglobulin. Transfusion 1991;31:380.
156. Hara T, Mizuno Y, Kawano M, et al: Treatment of immune hemolytic anemia with gammaglobulin. J Pediatr 1987;110:817.
157. Voto LS, Sexer H, Ferreiro G, et al: Neonatal administration of high-dose intravenous immunoglobulin in

rhesus hemolytic disease (See comments). J Perinat Med 1995;23:443.
158. Ergaz Z, Gross D, Bar-Oz B, et al: Carboxyhemoglobin levels in neonatal immune hemolytic jaundice treated with intravenous gammaglobulin. Vox Sang 1995;69:95.
159. Hammerman C, Kaplan M, Vreman HJ, Stevenson DK: Intravenous immune globulin in neonatal ABO isoimmunization: factors associated with clinical efficacy. Biol Neonate 1996;70:69.
160. Forouzan I: Hydrops fetalis: recent advances. Obstet Gynecol Surv 1997;52:130.
161. McMahan MJ, Donovan EF: The delivery room resuscitation of the hydropic neonate. Semin Perinatol 1995;19:474.
162. Oski FA, Stockman JA: Anaemia in early infancy. Br J Haematol 1974;27:195.
163. Bussel JB, Inglis SR, Chervenak FA: Erythropoietin (EPO) treatment for anemia in Rh disease (Abstract). Pediatr Res 1992;31:265A.
164. Scaradavou A, Inglis S, Peterson P, et al: Suppression of erythropoiesis by intrauterine transfusions in hemolytic disease of the newborn: use of erythropoietin to treat the late anemia. J Pediatr 1993;123:279.
165. Halbrecht I: Role of hemagglutinins anti-A and anti-B in pathogenesis of jaundice of the newborn (icterus neonatorum precox). Am J Dis Child 1944;64:248.
166. Abelson NM, Rawson AJ: Studies of blood group antibodies. V. Fractionation of examples of anti-B, anti-A, anti-P, anti-JK[a], anti-Le[a], anti-D, anti-CD, anti-K, anti-Fy[a], anti-S and anti-Good. Transfusion 1961;1:116.
167. Voak D, Williams MA: An explanation of the failure of the direct antiglobulin test to detect erythrocyte sensitization in ABO hemolytic disease of the newborn and observations on pinocytosis of IgG anti-A antibodies by infant (cord) red cells. Br J Haematol 1971;20:9.
168. Romano EL, Hughes-Jones NC, Mollison PL: Direct antiglobulin reaction in ABO-haemolytic disease of the newborn. Br Med J 1973;1:524.
169. Wang MYFW, Desforges JF: Complement in ABO-hemolytic disease of the newborn. Pediatrics 1971;48:650.
170. Grundbacher FJ: The etiology of ABO hemolytic disease of the newborn. Transfusion 1980;20:563.
171. Gupte SC, Kothari J, Bhatia HM: Influence of birth weight on the severity of hemolytic disease of the newborn due to ABO incompatibility. Indian J Pediatr 1975;12:477.
172. Huntley CC, Lyerly AD, Littlejohn MP, et al: ABO hemolytic disease in Puerto Rico and North Carolina. Pediatrics 1976;57:875.
173. Kirkman HN: Further evidence for a racial difference in frequency of ABO hemolytic disease. J Pediatr 1977;90:717.
174. Kanto WP Jr, Marino B, Godwin AS, Bunyapen C: ABO hemolytic disease: a comparative study of clinical severity and delayed anemia. Pediatrics 1978;62:365.
175. Desjardins L, Blajchman MA, Chintu C, et al: The spectrum of ABO hemolytic disease of the newborn. J Pediatr 1979;95:447.
176. Boineau FG, Hallock JA: Two examples of severe fetal disease due to ABO incompatibility. Clin Pediatr (Phila) 1971;10:180.
177. Kostinas JE, Cantow EF, Wetzel RA: Autohemolysis of cord blood in congenital spherocytosis and ABO incompatibility. J Pediatr 1967;70:273.
178. Drummond GS, Valaes T, Kappas A: Control of bilirubin production by synthetic heme analogs: pharmacologic and toxicologic considerations. J Perinatol 1996;16:S72.
179. Kappas A, Drummond GS, Henschke C, Valaes T: Direct comparison of Sn-mesoporphyrin, an inhibitor of bilirubin production, and phototherapy in controlling hyperbilirubinemia in term and near-term newborns. Pediatrics 1995;95:468.
180. Kappas A, Drummond GS, Galbraith RA: Prolonged clinical use of a heme oxygenase inhibitor: hematological evidence for an inducible but reversible iron-deficiency state. Pediatrics 1993;91:537.

CHAPTER 11

Disorders of Erythrocyte Metabolism and Shape

Patrick G. Gallagher, M.D.

The mature erythrocyte differs from all other cells in the body. It lacks a nucleus, DNA, RNA, and ribosomes. It has no ability to synthesize RNA, DNA, or protein, and it cannot divide (Table 11–1). It has no mitochondria, it cannot perform the Krebs cycle, and it lacks an electron transport system for oxidative phosphorylation. After enucleation, the reticulocyte, the precursor of the mature erythrocyte, leaves the marrow and enters the circulation with a complete collection of enzymes, cofactors, and other proteins necessary to perform all the essential functions of the red blood cell during its life span.

The principal functions of erythrocyte metabolism include maintenance of adequate supplies of adenosine triphosphate (ATP), production of reducing substances to act as antioxidants, and control of the oxygen affinity of hemoglobin by production of adequate amounts of 2,3-diphosphoglycerate (2,3-DPG). Because the mature erythrocyte has lost its ability to perform oxidative phosphorylation, its energy is supplied by anaerobic glycolysis through the Embden-Meyerhof pathway, by oxidative glycolysis through the hexose monophosphate (HMP) shunt, and through nucleotide salvage pathways.

Table 11–1. **Differences Among Erythrocytes at Various Stages of Maturation**

Characteristic	Nucleated Red Blood Cell	Reticulocyte	Mature Erythrocyte
Replication	+	0	0
DNA synthesis	+	0	0
RNA synthesis	+	0	0
RNA present	+	+	0
Lipid synthesis	+	+	0
Heme synthesis	+	+	0
Protein synthesis	+	+	0
Cytochrome and electron transfer system	+	+	0
Carbohydrate metabolism			
Krebs cycle	+	+	0
Embden-Meyerhof pathway	+	+	+
Pentose phosphate pathway	+	+	+

+, present; 0, absent.

The erythrocyte membrane plays an important role in maintenance of the cell's homeostasis by means of several mechanisms, including retention of vital compounds and removal of metabolic waste, regulation of erythrocyte metabolism and pH, and importation of iron required for hemoglobin synthesis. The membrane maintains a slippery exterior so that erythrocytes do not aggregate or adhere to endothelial cells. The membrane skeleton, a network of proteins on the inner surface of the red blood cell, provides the strength and flexibility needed to maintain the normal shape and deformability of the erythrocyte, allowing it to survive the shear stresses of circulation.

This chapter reviews the principal metabolic processes of the erythrocyte and their disorders, as well as the structure and function of the erythrocyte membrane and its disorders. Historically, inherited disorders of erythrocyte metabolism and erythrocyte shape have been considered together, even though the underlying fundamental defects are quite different. For years, the spherocytosis syndromes were considered disorders of erythrocyte metabolism, as documented in Dacie's treatise on hemolytic anemias: "In hereditary spherocytosis, the hemoglobin itself is normal, and the abnormality seems to depend on a subtle defect in erythrocyte metabolism."[1]

ERYTHROCYTE METABOLISM

The primary function of the erythrocyte, gas transport and exchange, is maintained without a net change in energy state. However, several critical functions of the erythrocyte depend on the production and expenditure of energy: initiation and maintenance of glycolysis, synthesis of glutathione and related antioxidants, maintenance of hemoglobin in its functional reduced ferrous state, protection of hemoglobin proteins from oxidative damage, pumping of cations against electrochemical gradients, nucleotide salvage reactions, and maintenance of membrane phospholipids.

As the erythrocyte ages, glucose use and ATP levels fall, leading to decreased membrane deformability and ultimately to a shortened life span. Lower potassium levels, higher sodium levels, and decreased membrane lipids are also seen in ATP-deficient aging erythrocytes.

The erythrocyte assimilates glucose from the plasma through facilitated transfer, with erythrocyte glucose levels rapidly equilibrating with changes in blood glucose levels. Although glucose is the preferred carbohydrate of the erythrocyte, fructose or mannose are metabolized almost as readily. Inside the cell, glucose is converted to glucose-6-phosphate or to fructose through sorbitol. Glucose-6-phosphate may follow one of three pathways:

1. It may enter the Embden-Meyerhof pathway (90%), where it is eventually converted into lactate, pyruvate, and ATP.
2. It may enter the hexose monophosphate shunt (5% to 10%) to produce reduced intermediates and ribulose-5-phosphate. Ribulose-5-phosphate eventually enters the Embden-Meyerhof pathway.
3. Less than 1% of glucose-6-phosphate is converted to glucose-1-phosphate, which is converted to glycogen.

Embden-Meyerhof Pathway

The erythrocyte generates most of its energy by glycolysis through the Embden-Meyerhof pathway (Fig. 11–1), with storage as high-energy phosphates such as ATP or as reducing energy in the form of glutathione or pyridine nucleotides (NADH and NADPH).[2–4] The Embden-Meyerhof pathway is the major supplier of ATP to the erythrocyte. Approximately 90% of erythrocyte glucose is converted through this pathway, with the catabolism of 1 mole of glucose yielding 2 moles of ATP and 2 moles of lactate. However, approximately 20% of metabolized glucose traverses the 2,3-DPG cycle (i.e., the Rapoport-Luebering shunt), bypassing generation of ATP by phosphoglycerate kinase (PGK). Two moles of ATP per mole of metabolized glucose seems insignificant compared with the Krebs cycle of intermediary metabolism, in which 1 mole of glucose metabolized produces 38 moles of ATP. However, this ATP production is adequate to renew red blood cell ATP to 150% to 200% of the total red blood cell ATP every hour.

The Embden-Meyerhof pathway is also the primary source of NADH. NADH is a necessary cofactor for NADH methemoglobin reductase, which maintains heme iron in the reduced state. Without this reaction, heme iron would be oxidized to methemoglobin, which does not transport oxygen. The Rapoport-Luebering shunt of the Embden-Meyerhof pathway produces 2,3-DPG, a compound found in high concentrations in erythrocytes but in low concentrations in other cells. 2,3-DPG decreases the oxygen affinity of hemoglobin and increases oxygen delivery to peripheral tissues.

Neonatal and adult erythrocytes have several metabolic differences (Table 11–2).[5, 6] Neonatal erythrocytes contain higher levels of ATP than adult erythrocytes, with the highest levels occurring in preterm infants. Fetal and neonatal erythrocytes consume more glucose than adult cells. They also consume more galactose than adult cells and exhibit higher levels of galactokinase activity. In fetal and neonatal cells, the activity of PGK and enolase is increased, and the activity of phosphofructokinase (PFK) is decreased. These enzymes exhibit a developmentally regulated change in values in the first year of life that is independent of erythrocyte age and that appears to reflect the transition from fetal to adult hematopoiesis. Decreased activity of PFK, a rate-limiting enzyme in glycolysis, results in alterations of glucose metabolism and may have functional significance.

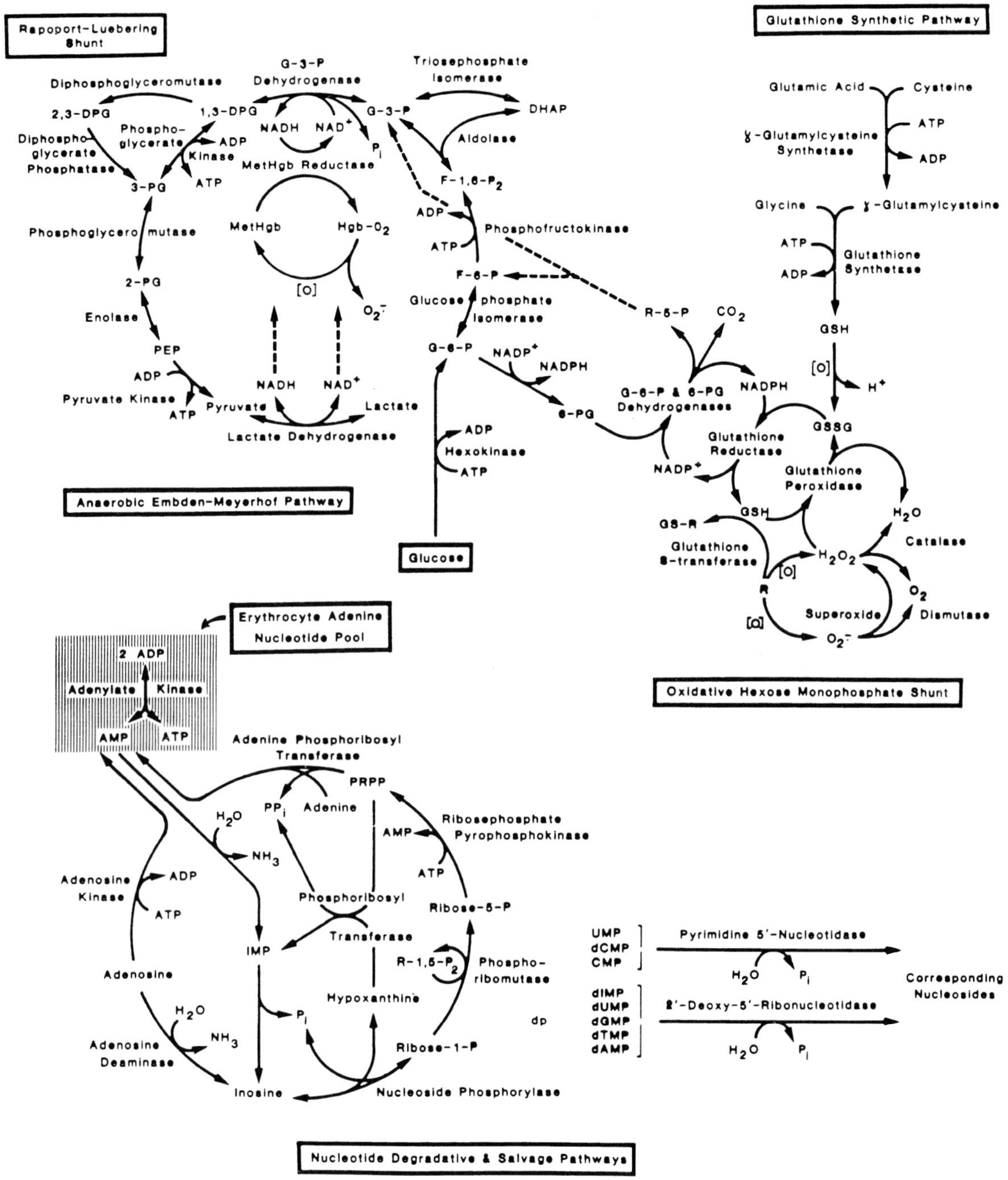

Figure 11–1. Pathways of energy metabolism in the erythrocyte. Glucose-6-phosphate may be degraded anaerobically to lactate through the Embden-Meyerhof pathway or oxidatively through the hexose monophosphate shunt. Pentose phosphates (R-5-P) can reenter anaerobic glycolysis as fructose-6-phosphate (F-6-P) and glyceraldehyde-3-phosphate (G-3-P) after conversion by enzymes of the terminal pentose phosphate pathway or as a product of adenosine or inosine degradation. 2,3-Diphosphoglycerate (2,3-DPG) may be generated instead of ATP by diversion of triose through the Rapoport-Luebering shunt. Glutathione may be synthesized directly from constituent amino acids; its cycling from oxidized (GSSG) to reduced forms (GSH) depends on reduced pyridine cofactor (NADPH) generation. (From Tanaka KR, Paglia DE: Pyruvate kinase and other enzymopathies of the erythrocyte. In Scriver CR, Beaudet AL, Sly WS, Valle D (eds): The Metabolic and Molecular Bases of Inherited Disease, 7th ed. Vol III. New York: McGraw-Hill, 1995, pp 3485–3511; copyright © by McGraw-Hill, Inc. Used by permission of McGraw-Hill Book Company.)

Table 11–2. **Metabolic Characteristics of Neonatal Erythrocytes**

Carbohydrate Metabolism

Glucose consumption increased
Galactose more completely used as substrate under normal circumstances and for methemoglobin reduction*
Decreased activity of sorbitol pathway*
Decreased triokinase activity*

Glycolytic Enzymes

Increased activity of hexokinase, phosphoglucose isomerase,* aldolase, glyceraldehyde-3-phosphate dehydrogenase,* phosphoglycerate kinase,* phosphoglycerate mutase, enolase,* pyruvate kinase, lactate dehydrogenase, glucose-6-phosphate dehydrogenase, 6-phosphogluconic dehydrogenase, galactokinase, and galactose-1-phosphate uridyl-transferase
Decreased activity of phosphofructokinase*
Distribution of hexokinase isoenzymes differs from that of adults*

Nonglycolytic Enzymes

Increased activity of glutamic oxaloacetic transaminase and glutathione reductase
Decreased activity of NADP-dependent methemoglobin reductase catalase,* glutathione peroxidase, carbonic anhydrase,* adenylate kinase,* and glutathione synthetase*
Presence of α-glycerol-3-phosphate dehydrogenase*

Adenosine Triphosphate (ATP) and Phosphate Metabolism

Decreased phosphate uptake,* slower incorporation into ATP and 2,3-diphosphoglycerate*
Accelerated decline of 2,3-diphosphoglycerate during red blood cell incubation*
Increased ATP levels
Accelerated decline of ATP during brief incubation

Storage Characteristics

Increased potassium efflux and greater degrees of hemolysis during short periods of storage
More rapid assumption of altered morphologic forms during storage or incubation*

Membrane Characteristics

Decreased ouabain-sensitive ATPase*
Decreased potassium influx*
Decreased permeability to glycerol and thiourea*
Decreased membrane filterability*
Increased sphingomyelin, decreased lecithin content of stromal phospholipids
Decreased content of linoleic acid*
Increase in lipid phosphorus and cholesterol per cell
Greater affinity for glucose*

Other Characteristics

Increased methemoglobin content*
Increased affinity of hemoglobin for oxygen*
Glutathione instability*
Increased tendency for Heinz body formation in presence of oxidant compounds*

*Appears to be a unique characteristic of the newborn's erythrocytes and not merely a function of the presence of young red cells.

Rapoport-Luebering Shunt and 2,3-Diphosphoglycerate Metabolism

A variety of influences can change the affinity of hemoglobin for oxygen. 2,3-DPG is a highly charged organic phosphate anion that binds to deoxyhemoglobin but not to oxyhemoglobin, effectively decreasing the affinity of hemoglobin for oxygen. 2,3-DPG is generated by the Rapoport-Luebering shunt of the Embden-Meyerhof pathway (see Fig. 11–1). Under physiologic conditions of pH and solute concentrations, 2,3-DPG binds reversibly to tetramers of deoxyhemoglobin. The affinity of 2,3-DPG for fetal deoxyhemoglobin is lower than its affinity for adult deoxyhemoglobin, and it therefore does not bind fetal deoxyhemoglobin as tightly. This difference leads to a leftward shifted hemoglobin oxygen dissociation curve, indicating relatively less sensitivity to higher levels of 2,3-DPG. As the amount of fetal hemoglobin declines, there is a rightward shift in the hemoglobin oxygen dissociation curve, with increasing amounts of adult hemoglobin and 2,3-DPG altering the position of the hemoglobin oxygen dissociation curve. The oxygen half-saturation pressure of hemoglobin, the P_{50} value, of fetal blood is 20 ± 1 mm Hg, approximately 7 mm Hg less than adult blood. Neonates who have been transfused with high levels of adult hemoglobin but relatively lower 2,3-DPG levels may have the same P_{50} value as infants with high levels of fetal hemoglobin and 2,3-DPG.

Hexose Monophosphate Shunt

Approximately 5% to 10% of erythrocyte glucose is consumed in the hexose monophosphate shunt (HMP), also called the pentose phosphate pathway (see Fig. 11–1).[2] In this pathway, the first product of glucose phosphorylation, glucose-6-phosphate, undergoes oxidation, followed by a series of rearrangements that eventually yield fructose-6-phosphate and glyceraldehyde-3-phosphate. Both compounds are intermediates in the glycolytic pathway. The HMP shunt is the primary source of NADPH in erythrocytes, with 2 moles of NADPH produced for each mole of glucose metabolized. NADPH is required for the reduction of oxidized glutathione and some protein sulfhydryl groups.

Mature erythrocytes synthesize relatively high concentrations of reduced glutathione (GSH) (Fig. 11–2). GSH protects erythrocytes from oxidants such as hydrogen peroxide (H_2O_2), superoxide anions (O_2^-), and hydroxyl radicals (OH), which are produced as byproducts of the oxidation of heme by oxygen (Fig. 11–3). Oxidants are also produced by activated phagocytes (i.e., during infection) and by erythrocytes after exposure to certain agents. If these oxidants are allowed to accumulate, they can damage cellular proteins and lipids. The detoxification of H_2O_2 is markedly enhanced by glutathione peroxidase. GSH is converted to oxidized glutathione (GSSG) and to mixed disulfides with protein thiols. GSH levels are restored by glutathione reductase. In this process, NADPH is oxidized to NADP, which stimulates the HMP shunt, regenerating NADPH. After oxidant exposure, hypoxia, or acidosis, erythrocytes can increase the amount of glucose metabolized through the HMP shunt up to 10-fold to 20-fold to generate increased amounts of reduced glutathione. This tight coupling of the HMP shunt with glutathione metabolism protects the erythrocyte from oxidative stress.

The HMP shunt also produces ribose-5-phosphate. Ribose-5-phosphate is a constituent of the purine nucleotides, ADP and ATP, and the pyridine nucleotides, NAD and NADP. Although the mature erythrocyte has no capacity for de novo purine or pyrimidine formation, it does maintain the ability to form some nucleotides through salvage pathways. Ribose-5-phosphate is a vital component of these salvage pathways.

Differences in the HMP shunt exist between neonatal and adult erythrocytes. The activity of

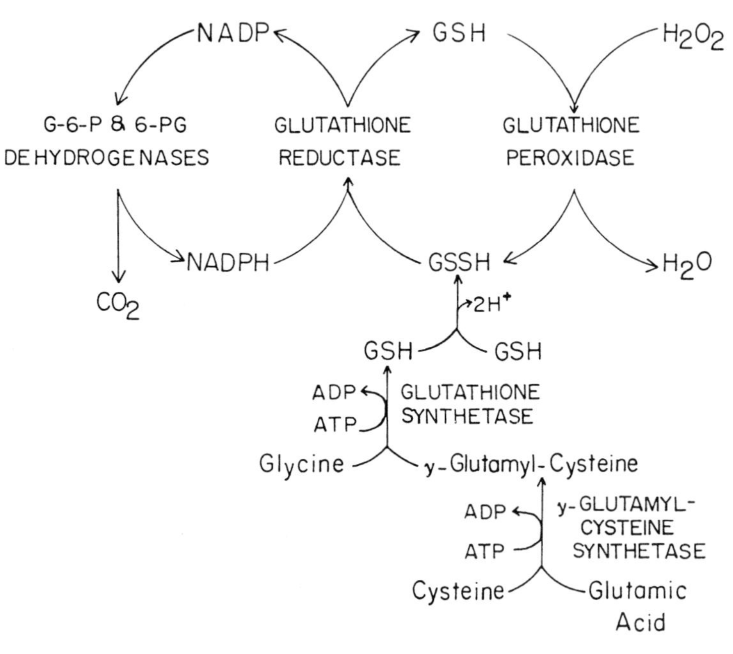

Figure 11–2. Pathway of glutathione synthesis and reduction in the mature red blood cell. (G-6-P; glucose-6-phosphate; GSH, reduced glutathione; GSSH, oxidized glutathione.)

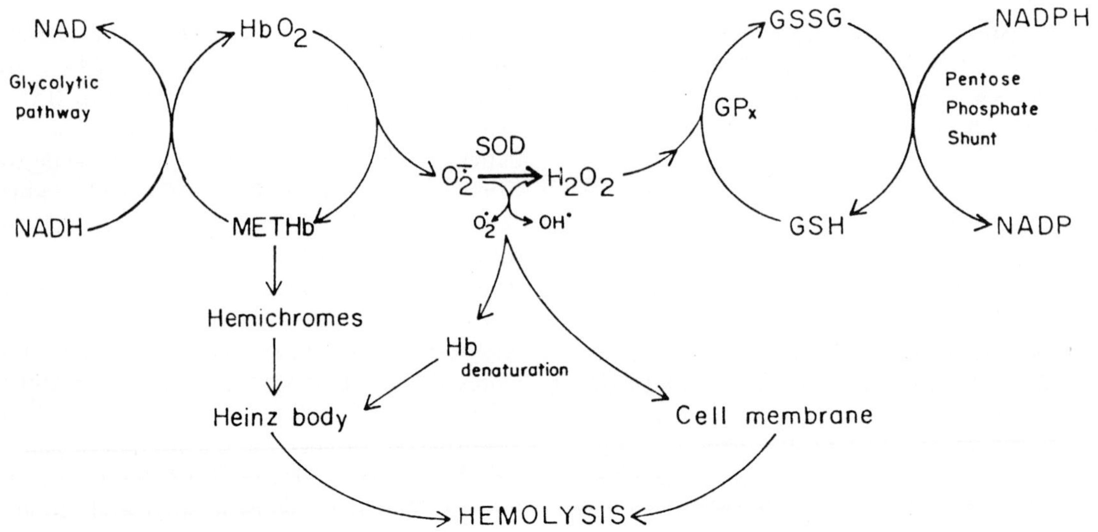

Figure 11–3. Production and reduction of activated oxygen (O_2). The accumulation of activated oxygen and free radical species (O_2^1 OH^1.) can cause hemolysis by denaturing hemoglobin or injuring the red blood cell membrane. (SOD, supraoxide dismutase; GPx, glutathione peroxidase; GSH, reduced form of glutathione; GSSH, oxidized form of glutathione; Hb, hemaglobin.)

two components of the HMP shunt, glucose-6-phosphate dehydrogenase (G6PD) and 6-phosphogluconic acid dehydrogenase, are found at higher levels in neonatal erythrocytes. Differences in the HMP shunt have been suggested to be the cause of increased susceptibility of neonatal erythrocytes to oxidant injury. However, other factors may be involved in the increased oxidative susceptibility of the neonatal red blood cell, including decreased glutathione peroxidase levels and, in some infants, decreased levels of superoxide dismutase. Other factors, such as decreased plasma antioxidant capacity and increased erythrocyte membrane sulfhydryl groups leading to increased susceptibility to Heinz body formation, have also been implicated.

DISORDERS OF ERYTHROCYTE METABOLISM

Congenital nonspherocytic hemolytic anemia (CNSHA) traditionally includes disorders not attributable to immune-mediated disorders, defects of hemoglobin, defects of the red blood cell membrane, or other disorders such as paroxysmal nocturnal hemoglobinuria and is therefore considered a diagnosis of exclusion. It is a heterogeneous group of disorders caused by a variety of metabolic abnormalities of the red blood cell, including enzymopathies of glucose, glutathione, and nucleotide metabolism. Clinical, biochemical, and genetic heterogeneity are typical within individual enzymopathies. Hemolysis can develop as a result of enzyme or antioxidant deficiency and as a result of impaired enzyme function, such as abnormal substrate or cofactor binding, altered activation or inhibition characteristics, or decreased stability or specific activity.

Peripheral blood smears from persons with CNSHA, except in cases of pyrimidine 5′-nucleotidase deficiency, are unremarkable. Osmotic fragility of fresh erythrocytes is normal, and response to splenectomy is variable. In most cases, except G6PD and PGK deficiency (X-linked) and adenosine deaminase overproduction (autosomal dominant), these disorders are inherited in an autosomal recessive fashion. A thorough family history is important and can assist in determining the diagnosis. Manifestations of the metabolic defect are usually limited to the erythrocyte but sometimes involve various nonerythroid tissues. In these cases, specific organ involvement may aid in determining the metabolic defect.

Definitive diagnosis of metabolic abnormalities of the red blood cell depend on qualitative or quantitative assays of specific enzyme activity or identification of the specific genetic mutation by DNA analysis. It is important to be cautious when reviewing the results of quantitative erythrocyte enzyme assays for many reasons. These assays only sample surviving red blood cells in the peripheral blood, and the metabolic milieu of these cells is not necessarily comparable to cells already hemolyzed. Moreover, in vitro conditions of enzyme assays may not accurately reflect the in vivo environment. Transfusions before the assay can obscure the underlying metabolic defect, and leukocyte contamination may lead to spuriously elevated assay results. The mean enzyme activity may not accurately reflect the activity in some erythrocyte populations. For example, when assays are performed for subjects with reticulocytosis, the mean enzyme activity may be artificially elevated because of higher enzyme levels found in reticulocytes.

Disorders of the Embden-Meyerhof Pathway

Defects of the Embden-Meyerhof pathway are inherited in an autosomal recessive fashion, and typically, hemolysis is seen only in homozygotes.[2–4] Heterozygotes, whose red blood cells contain less than normal amounts of the abnormal enzyme, are clinically normal. One exception is a defect in PGK, an X-linked disorder in which hemolysis is seen only in male offspring. It has been suggested that hemolysis in patients with these disorders results from insufficient levels of erythrocyte ATP.

In these disorders, hemolysis is chronic and is not usually affected by drugs or other inciting agents. Patients often have splenomegaly caused by trapping of the abnormal erythrocytes. The hostile environment of the spleen may further shorten the life span of the defective red blood cell. Definitive diagnosis usually requires specific enzyme assays performed under a variety of conditions. Measurement of glycolytic intermediates may aid in diagnosis, because concentrations of various intermediates are increased proximal to a defect and are decreased distal to a defect.

Pyruvate Kinase Deficiency

Pyruvate kinase (PK) deficiency accounts for approximately 90% of inherited defects of the Embden-Meyerhof pathway and is probably the second most common inherited erythrocyte enzymopathy associated with anemia, after G6PD deficiency. PK deficiency has a worldwide distribution, but it is most common in individuals of northern European descent.

Pathophysiology and Inheritance

PK catalyzes the conversion of phosphoenolpyruvate (PEP) to pyruvate with the generation of ATP (see Fig. 11–1). Deficiency of PK leads to decreased ATP levels in the red blood cell. There is also an increase in upstream catabolites, including a twofold to threefold increase in 2,3-DPG, which enhances tissue oxygenation and may help minimize some of the physiologic effects of anemia (Fig. 11–4).

PK deficiency is inherited in an autosomal recessive manner. Affected individuals are homozygous or compound heterozygotes for PK defects. Heterozygotes are clinically normal or exhibit very slight hemolysis.

Clinical Syndromes

The clinical severity of PK deficiency is quite variable. Usually, patients present in the neonatal period or in early childhood with anemia and jaundice.[7–14] Neonatal hyperbilirubinemia is common in PK-deficient individuals, and exchange transfusion may be required. Kernicterus has been reported.[7, 10, 15] Severe cases have presented with significant anemia in utero or in the first few days of life. Cases of nonimmune hydrops fetalis due to PK deficiency have been reported.[11, 16] Occasionally, patients may escape detection until later in life, when complications related to anemia and chronic hemolysis occur or the diagnosis is made serendipitously when the patient is evaluated for another condition.[7, 10, 15]

Diagnosis, Treatment, and Outcome

The peripheral blood smear demonstrates normocytic, normochromic erythrocytes, frequently with spiculations (Fig. 11–5*A*). Poikilocytes and acanthocytes may also be seen. Reticulocytosis is common. Osmotic fragility of fresh and incubated erythrocytes is usually normal,

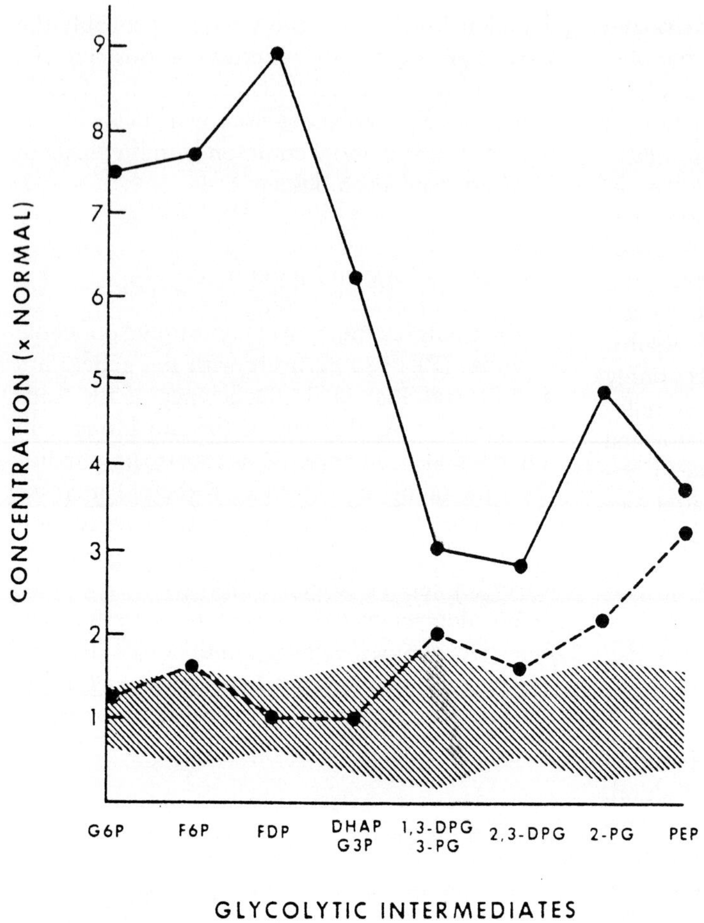

Figure 11–4. Accumulation of glycolytic intermediates in pyruvate kinase (PK) deficiency. Results, shown in multiples of normal values, are provided for a patient with severe PK deficiency *(solid line)* and a patient with mild PK deficiency *(hatched line)*. (G6P, glucose-6-phosphate; F6P, fructose-6-phosphate; FDP, fructose-1,6-diphosphate; G3P, glyceraldehyde-3-phosphate; DPG, diphosphoglycerate; PEP, phosphoenolpyruvate.) (From Mentzer WC: Pyruvate kinase deficiency and disorders of glycolysis. In Nathan D, Orkin S (eds): Hematology of Infancy and Childhood, 5th ed. Philadelphia: WB Saunders, 1997, pp 665–703.)

with a few patients exhibiting a population of fragile cells after incubation.

The fluorescence of NADH under ultraviolet light is the screening test for PK deficiency employed by many laboratories. After phosphoenolpyruvate, lactate dehydrogenase, and NADH are mixed with the patient's blood, incubated, and spotted on filter paper, the fluorescence is measured. Direct enzyme assay, which uses phosphoenolpyruvate as substrate for PK, can be performed on leukocyte-free hemolysate to confirm abnormal fluorescence tests. Leukocytes contain more than 300 times the PK activity of erythrocytes.

In severe cases of PK deficiency, splenectomy typically leads to a decrease in hemolysis. In some cases, postsplenectomy reticulocytosis is marked, up to 50% to 70%. This paradoxical reticulocytosis is caused by increased reticulocyte survival after removal of the hostile splenic environment.

Other Disorders of the Embden-Meyerhof Pathway

Other abnormalities of the Embden-Meyerhof pathway have manifested during infancy.[17] *Hexokinase deficiency* is uncommon, with great phenotypic variability reported for cases. Severely affected patients have suffered from neonatal hyperbilirubinemia or anemia requiring blood transfusion.

Glucose phosphate isomerase deficiency is the third most common hemolytic enzymopathy, and it frequently manifests during the first year of life with significant anemia. Severe neonatal anemia and hyperbilirubinemia have been described, as have nonimmune hydrops fetalis and neonatal death.[17, 18]

Phosphofructokinase deficiency may involve erythrocytes, muscle, or both tissues. It usually manifests during adolescence with exertional

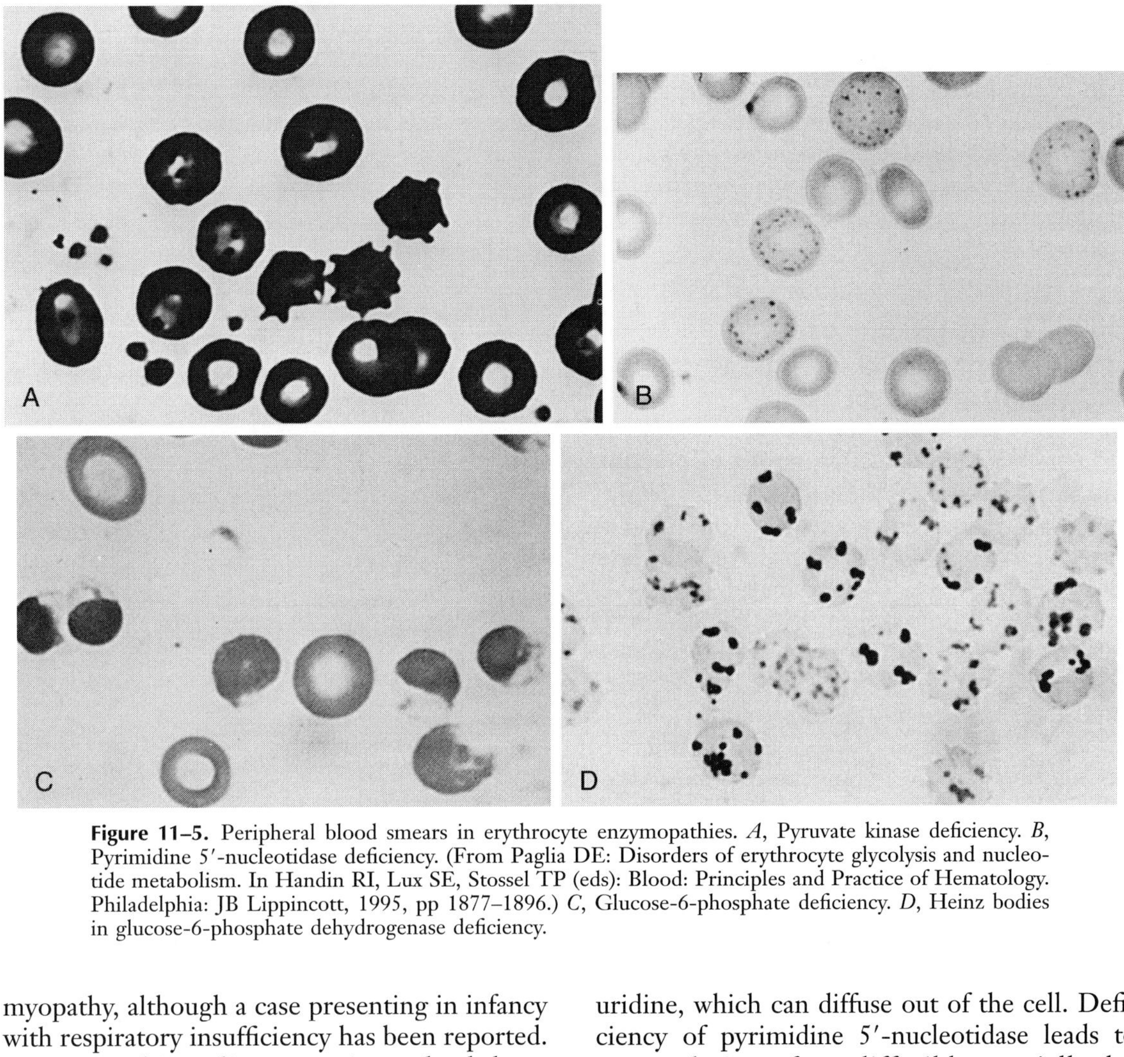

Figure 11–5. Peripheral blood smears in erythrocyte enzymopathies. *A*, Pyruvate kinase deficiency. *B*, Pyrimidine 5′-nucleotidase deficiency. (From Paglia DE: Disorders of erythrocyte glycolysis and nucleotide metabolism. In Handin RI, Lux SE, Stossel TP (eds): Blood: Principles and Practice of Hematology. Philadelphia: JB Lippincott, 1995, pp 1877–1896.) *C*, Glucose-6-phosphate deficiency. *D*, Heinz bodies in glucose-6-phosphate dehydrogenase deficiency.

myopathy, although a case presenting in infancy with respiratory insufficiency has been reported.

Neonatal jaundice, anemia, or both have been described in isolated cases of *2,3-bisphosphoglycerate mutase deficiency* and *phosphoglycerate kinase* deficiency. Other glycolytic defects have rarely been associated with manifestations in the neonatal period.

Disorders of Nucleotide Metabolism

The mature erythrocyte lacks the ability to synthesize purine and pyrimidine nucleotides de novo. However, it is able to form some nucleotides through salvage pathways.[2]

Pyrimidine 5′-Nucleotidase Deficiency

Pyrimidine 5′-nucleotidase degrades the pyrimidine nucleotides of RNA to cytidine and uridine, which can diffuse out of the cell. Deficiency of pyrimidine 5′-nucleotidase leads to accumulation of nondiffusible, partially degraded RNA, producing the marked basophilic stippling characteristic of erythrocytes deficient in this enzyme (see Fig. 11–5*B*). These accumulated pyrimidine nucleotides inhibit the transport of GSSG out of red blood cells, which probably accounts for the high levels of glutathione seen in erythrocytes from these patients. Patients have moderately severe hemolytic anemia. The cause of the hemolysis is unknown. Splenomegaly is common, but splenectomy typically does little to ameliorate the condition.

Adenosine Deaminase Overactivity

A disorder characterized by very high levels of adenosine deaminase activity (up to 100 times normal values) in erythrocytes but not in other tissues associated with a chronic hemolytic anemia has been described. The high level of adenosine deaminase activity presumably depletes the red blood cell of its adenine nucleotides and impairs nucleotide metabolism. The genetic mechanism causing this disorder, which is inherited in an autosomal dominant fashion, is unknown.

Disorders of the Hexose Monophosphate Shunt and Associated Pathways

Disorders of the HMP shunt or the glutathione metabolic pathways compromise the ability of the red blood cell to adequately respond to oxidative stress.[2, 19] In the normal erythrocyte, GSH detoxifies oxidants produced by various agents, such as infectious organisms. In G6PD deficiency, GSH levels are inadequate because of the inability to generate NADPH, leaving oxidants free to damage the vital proteins of the cell. Oxidation of the sulfhydryl groups of hemoglobin produces functionless methemoglobin and intracellular precipitates of hemoglobin called Heinz bodies.

Heinz bodies, which are not visible on Wright-stained peripheral blood smears but are seen with supravital stains such as methyl violet, attach to and damage the red blood cell's membrane. They cause clustering of immunoglobulins and membrane protein band 3, marking the erythrocyte for opsonization by phagocytes. Heinz bodies are "pitted" from circulating cells by the spleen and are more commonly seen in patients who have been splenectomized. *Bite cells,* erythrocytes with localized invaginations, possibly at the site of Heinz body damage or removal, are seen during acute hemolytic episodes. In addition to damage from Heinz bodies, GSH-deficient erythrocytes also undergo peroxidation of membrane phospholipids and oxidative cross-linking of spectrin, decreasing membrane deformability and promoting splenic trapping.[20, 21]

Glucose-6-Phosphate Dehydrogenase Deficiency

G6PD deficiency is the most common inherited enzyme defect, affecting more than 400 million persons worldwide (Fig. 11–6).[19, 22, 23] The high prevalence of G6PD deficiency is probably the result of genetic selection. Heterozygotes enjoy a selective advantage against invasion by the malaria parasite *Plasmodium falciparum.*[24]

Pathophysiology

Glucose-6-phosphate is a ubiquitous enzyme found in all cells of the body. In the red blood cell, G6PD action is the first and rate-limiting step in the HMP shunt that coverts NADP into reduced NADP. NADP is necessary for the generation of glutathione, a critical component in the control of oxidative damage to the cell. Patients with G6PD deficiency may develop acute hemolytic anemia after exposure to an oxidative stress. Erythrocytes are particularly susceptible to oxidative stress because the HMP shunt is the red blood cells' only source of NADPH.

Hundreds of G6PD variants have been described, but only a few are common (Table 11–3).[23] These variants are classified on the basis of electrophoretic mobility, biochemical characteristics, ability to use the substrate analogue, the K_m for NADP and G6PD, the pH activity profile, and thermal stability. The normal enzyme, Gd^B, is present in 99% of Caucasian Americans and 70% of African-Americans. A normal variant, Gd^{A+}, found in 20% of African-Americans, has a faster electrophoretic mobility than Gd^B. Gd^{A-}, the most common variant associated with hemolysis, is found in about 10% of African-Americans and in many African populations. Gd^{A-} has the same electrophoretic mobility as Gd^{A+}, but its catalytic ability is decreased. Gd^{Med}, the second most common abnormal variant, is common in the Mediterranean area, in India, and in southeast Asia, with a prevalence between 5% and 50% in certain populations. Its electrophoretic mobility is normal, but its catalytic activity is greatly decreased. Gd^{Canton}, a common variant in East Asian populations, produces a clinical syndrome similar to Gd^{A-}.

As normal cells age, the activity of Gd^B decreases, with a half-life of approximately 60 days. Despite the absence of active G6PD, older cells preserve the ability to produce NADPH and maintain GSH in response to oxidative stress. The Gd^{A-} variant has a half-life of only 13 days; young cells have a normal amount of

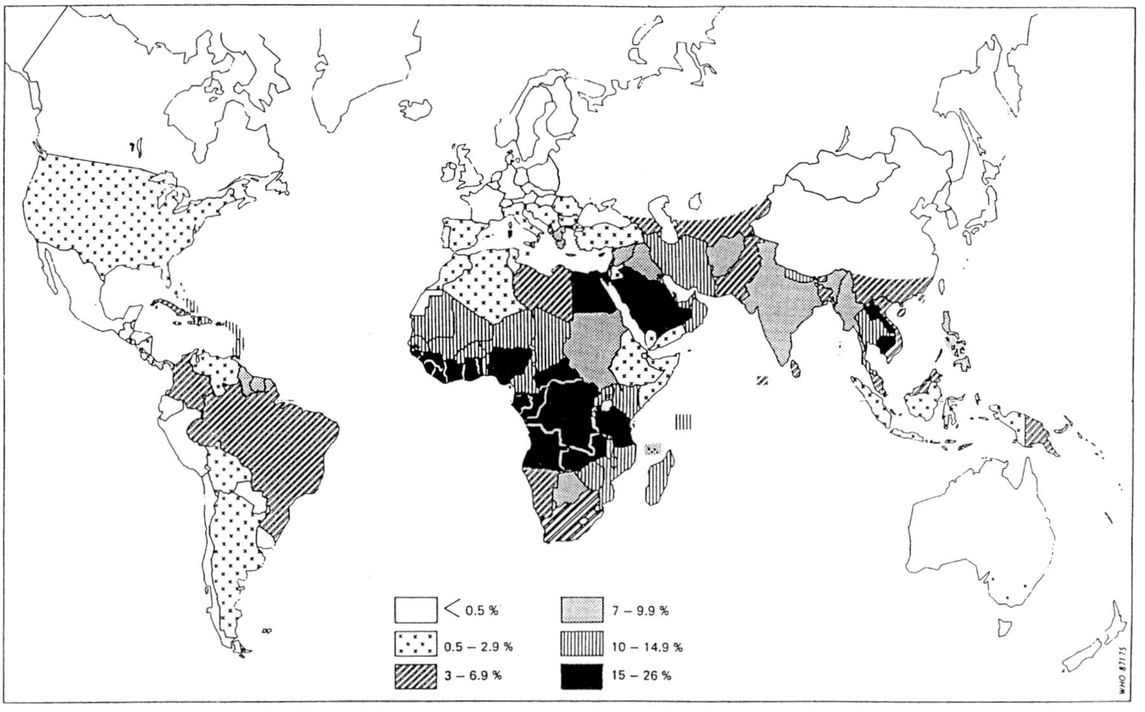

Figure 11–6. Worldwide distribution of glucose-6-phosphate dehydrogenase (G-6-PD) deficiency. The values shown by the different shadings are frequencies in the populations of G-6-PD–deficient males, which are also gene frequencies, because the gene is X linked. (From WHO Working Group: Glucose-6-phosphate dehydrogenase deficiency. Bull World Health Organ 1989;67:601.)

enzyme activity, but older red blood cells are grossly deficient. Because of this heterogeneity in G6PD levels, Gd^{A-} individuals experience only limited hemolysis after oxidant exposure.

More than 100 mutations in the G6PD gene have been described. Most mutations result from amino acid substitutions that affect enzyme kinetics, stability, or both. A few rare dele-

Table 11–3. **Examples of Glucose-6-Phosphate Dehydrogenase Variants**

Class	Example	Clinical Features	G6PD activity (% of normal)	Electrophoretic Mobility	K_m of G6P (μmol/L)	Population Frequency
IV	B	None	100	Normal	70	Worldwide
IV	A	None	110	Fast	70	Polymorphic in Africa
III	Seattle	Rarely AHA	25	Slow	20	Polymorphic, widespread
III	A^-	AHA, NNJ	110	Fast	70	Polymorphic in Africa, southern Europe, and Middle East
II	Mediterranean	AHA, NNJ	3	Normal	25	Polymorphic in southern Europe, Middle East, India
I	Santiago de Cuba	CNSHA	2	Slow	45	Rare
I	Barcelona	CNSHA and frequent bacterial infection	2	Fast	40	Rare

AHA, acute hemolytic anemia; NNJ, neonatal jaundice; CNSHA, chronic nonspherocytic hemolytic anemia; G6PD, glucose-6-phosphate dehydrogenase.

From Luzzatto L: Glucose-6-phosphate dehydrogenase deficiency and the pentose phosphate pathway. In Handin RI, Lux SL, Stossel TP (eds): Blood: Principles and Practice of Hematology. Philadelphia: JB Lippincott, 1995, pp 1897–1923.

tions and splicing mutations have also been described.

Inheritance

The G6PD gene has been localized to Xq28. G6PD deficiency is an X-linked disorder affecting primarily male offspring. Boys have only one type of G6PD; girls can have two. According to the Lyon hypothesis, only one X chromosome is active in any given cell, and any given cell in a heterozygous female subject is normal or deficient. In girls who are heterozygous for G6PD deficiency, average G6PD activity may be normal, moderately reduced, or significantly reduced, depending on the degree of lyonization. G6PD deficient cells in heterozygous girls are just as susceptible to oxidant stress as those in boys, but the overall degree of hemolysis generally is less because the vulnerable population of cells is smaller.

Clinical Syndromes

G6PD deficiency has been divided into five classes based on clinical severity and the degree of enzyme deficiency. Class I is characterized by CNSHA without precipitating cause. Patients in classes II and III, which constitute more than 90% of G6PD variants, experience hemolysis after oxidant stress. The class IV and V variants are typically clinically harmless. The most significant clinical syndromes of G6PD deficiency are acute hemolytic anemia (AHA), neonatal jaundice (NNJ), and, rarely, CNSHA.

AHA is the most dramatic clinical presentation of G6PD deficiency, with acute intravascular hemolysis after exposure to an oxidative stress. These stresses include ingestion of certain drugs such as primaquine or sulfa-containing compounds, exposure to naphthalene (i.e., mothballs), ingestion of fava beans, or infection, the most common cause of hemolysis. Children typically present with irritability, fever, nausea, abdominal pain, and diarrhea within 48 hours of oxidant exposure. Hemoglobinuria, jaundice, and anemia then appear. The spleen and liver may be enlarged and tender. In severe cases, congestive heart failure may occur. Laboratory findings include a normochromic, normocytic anemia with anisocytosis and reticulocytosis (see Fig. 11–5*C*). Poikilocytes and bite cells may be seen. Heinz bodies, a classic finding in G6PD deficiency (see Fig. 11–5*D*),[25] may be seen with supravital staining, but this is an inconsistent finding, because these cells are rapidly cleared from the circulation by the spleen. In neonates, the discovery of Heinz bodies in the peripheral blood is uncommon. However, Heinz body preparations remain part of the diagnostic evaluation of the child with acute hemolysis because of its relative ease, speed, and low cost. Additional laboratory findings include hemoglobinuria and the presence of free hemoglobin in the blood.

Several cases of presumed or documented G6PD deficiency have been associated with severe neonatal anemia and nonimmune hydrops fetalis.[26–28] In these cases, there was prior maternal ingestion of an oxidant agent such as a sulfa drug, ascorbic acid, or fava beans.

Another significant clinical syndrome of G6PD deficiency is NNJ (Table 11–4).[29–37] Jaundice is rarely present at birth, and the peak incidence of onset is between the second and third day of life (Fig. 11–7). The degree of hyperbilirubinemia is quite variable. It may be severe, resulting in kernicterus or, in some cases, death. Occasionally, exchange transfusions are necessary. In most cases, however, the hyperbilirubinemia is adequately treated with phototherapy.[38–41] In cases of NNJ, the anemia is rarely severe.

The pathophysiology of NNJ has not been precisely elucidated, and its cause remains controversial.[42–46] It has been hypothesized that decreased hepatic elimination of bilirubin is the critical determinant of NNJ. Others believe that hemolysis is the cause of the jaundice and that, outside the normal immaturity of neonatal bilirubin conjugating ability, there is no need to blame the liver. Although in some cases the hyperbilirubinemia is the result of an identifiable oxidant, the jaundice persists even when there is no contact with causative agents. NNJ is increased in G6PD-deficient infants who also carry a polymorphism of the uridine diphosphoglucuronosyltransferase gene *(UDPGT1)* associated with Gilbert syndrome.[47, 48]

Chronic nonspherocytic hemolytic anemia has been associated with rare variants of G6PD deficiency. NNJ may manifest during the neonatal period and be accompanied by anemia in a male patient. In a few cases, exchange transfu-

Table 11–4. Glucose-6-Phosphate Dehydrogenase Deficiency and Neonatal Jaundice

Population*	Incidence of G6PD Deficiency	Incidence of NNJ Among G6PD Deficient Individuals	Incidence of NNJ in Control Groups	Incidence of G6PD Deficiency in NNJ Patients
Africa				
West Africa	21	26	10	31
South Africa	1.3			3.1 (All)
Bantu				10 (Term)
America				
Jamaica	14.7			20.5
United States	7.2	6	11.6	12.5
	11.2			
Asia				
China/Hong Kong	3.6		1.2	15–30
Thailand	7.5	30	3.0	30–60
Singapore	1.3	20	25	
Europe				
Greece	3	30	9.1	15
Sardinia	8.8	20–30	10	8.5

G6PD, glucose-6-phosphate dehydrogenase; NNJ, neonatal jaundice.
*All figures are percentage values in males only.
From Luzzatto L: Glucose-6-phosphate dehydrogenase deficiency and hemolytic anemia. In Nathan D, Orkin S (eds): Hematology of Infancy and Childhood. Philadelphia: WB Saunders, 1997, pp 704.

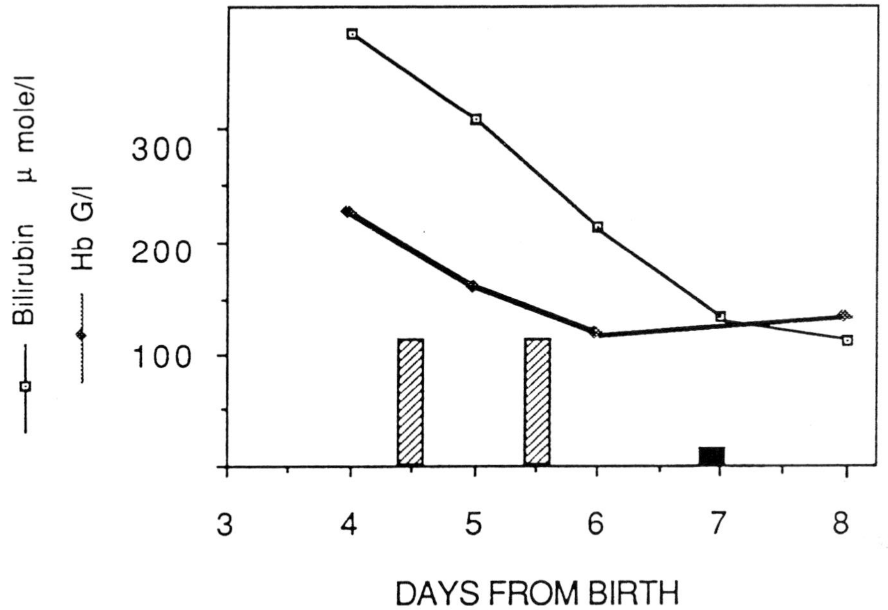

Figure 11–7. Clinical course of a neonate with glucose-6-phosphate dehydrogenase deficiency. Jaundice was found in this 3200-g (birth weight) term male infant on day 3 of life. His grandfather was known to have suffered from favism. The hatched bars represent double-volume exchange transfusions, and the filled bar indicates a packed red blood cell transfusion. The infant did not develop significant anemia until after the exchange transfusions. (From Luzzatto L: Glucose-6-phosphate dehydrogenase deficiency and hemolytic anemia. In Nathan D, Orkin S (eds): Hematology of Infancy and Childhood. Philadelphia: WB Saunders, 1997, pp 704–726.)

sions have been required. The degree of chronic anemia in cases of CNSHA due to G6PD deficiency has been variable. These cases have usually been associated with variant enzymes that are unable to maintain basal NADPH production.

Diagnosis

Simple screening tests for G6PD deficiency have been developed, including the dye decolorization test, the methemoglobin reduction test, and the fluorescence spot test.[49] These tests are semiquantitative and classify a sample as normal or deficient. Screening tests must be properly run by experienced individuals and their limitations understood. These tests are unreliable after an acute hemolytic episode and do not usually detect female heterozygotes. Positive screening test results should be confirmed by spectrophotometric assay.

Definitive assay of the enzyme depends on direct spectrophotometric measurement of NADPH production. Although more sensitive than screening tests, this still requires 20% to 30% G6PD-deficient cells to obtain an abnormal result. Sensitivity can be increased by comparing the level of G6PD deficiency to levels of other age-dependent red blood cell enzymes, especially when testing is done in proximity to an acute hemolytic episode. The cyanide-ascorbate test measures the ability of erythrocytes to prevent the oxidation of hemoglobin by ascorbate. Because this test employs intact erythrocytes, as few as 10% to 15% deficient cells can be detected, making it useful in detecting female heterozygotes and in males after a hemolytic episode. This test can also be used to detect other abnormalities of the HMP shunt or glutathione metabolism.

Treatment and Outcome

The best treatment for the individual with AHA is careful prescription of medications (Table 11–5) and avoidance of inciting agents (Table 11–6). Outside of acute hemolytic episodes, these patients do not require any special therapy. AHA episodes should be managed with particular attention to hematologic, cardiopulmonary, and renal complications of hemolysis. The management of NNJ does not differ from that recommended for other causes of neonatal hyperbilirubinemia.[38] In cases of CNSHA, management is expectant. Exposure to oxidant stresses should be avoided. Blood transfusions may be necessary during acute hemolytic episodes. In rare severe cases, splenectomy has produced some amelioration of the anemia.

Hemolysis after transfusion or exchange transfusion with G6PD-deficient red blood cells in neonates has been described.[50–53] It has been recommended that, in areas endemic for G6PD

Table 11–5. **Agents That Can Safely Be Administered in Therapeutic Doses to Glucose-6-Phosphate Dehydrogenase–Deficient Patients**

Acetaminophen (paracetamol, Tylenol, Tralgon, hydroxyacetanilid)	Phenylbutazone
	Phenytoin
Acetylsalicylic acid (aspirin)	Probenecid (Benemid)
Aminopyrine (Pyramidon, amidopyrine, aminophenazone)	Procainamide hydrochloride (Pronestyl)
Actazoline (Anistine)	Pyrimethamine (Daraprim)
Antipyrine	Quinidine
Ascorbic acid (vitamin C)*	Quinine
Benzhexol (Artane)	Streptomycin
Chloramphenicol	Sulfacytine
Chlorguanidine (proguanil, Paludrine)	Sulfadiazine
Chloroquine	Sulfaguanidine
Colchicine	Sulfamerazine
Diphenhydramine (Benadryl)	Sulfamethoxypyridazine (Kynex)
Isoniazid	Sulfisoxazole (Gantrisin)
L-Dopa	Tiaprofenic acid
Menadione sodium bisulfite (Hykinone)	Trimethoprim
Menaphthone	Tripelennamine (pyribenzamine)
p-Aminobenzoic acid	Vitamin K

*Very high "therapeutic" doses (~80 g-administered intravenously) have precipitated severe, even fatal, hemolysis.
From Beutler E: G6PD deficiency. Blood 1994;84:3613.

Table 11–6. **Agents To Be Avoided by Glucose-6-Phosphate Dehydrogenase–Deficient Patients**

Antimalarials	**Analgesics**
Primaquine (persons with the African A⁻ variant may take it at reduced dosage, 15 mg/d or 45 mg twice weekly under surveillance)*	Acetylsalicylic acid (aspirin): moderate doses can be used
Pamaquine*	Safe alternative: paracetamol
Chloroquine (may be used under surveillance when required for prophylaxis or treatment of malaria)	**Anthelmintics**
Sulfonamides and Sulfones	β-Naphthol*
Sulfanilamide*	Stibophen*
Sulfapyridine*	Niridazole*
Sulfadimidine*	**Miscellaneous Agents**
Sulfacetamide (albucid)*	Vitamin K analogues (1 mg of menaphthone can be given to babies)*
Sulfafurazole	Naphthalene (mothballs)*
Salicylazosulfapyridine (Salazopyrin, Azulfidine)*	Probenecid*
Dapsone*	Dimercaprol (British antilewisite [BAL])*
Sulfoxone*	Methylene blue*
Glucosulfone sodium (Promin)*	Arsine*,†
Septrin*	Phenylhydrazine*,†
Other Antibacterial Compounds	Acetylphenylhydrazine*,†
Nitrofurans-nitrofurantoin, furazolidone, nitrofurazone*	Toluldine blue*
[Nalidixic acid]	Mepacrine
Chloramphenicol	
p-Aminosalicylic acid	

*These drugs should be avoided by people with all forms of G6PD deficiency. Those not marked should be avoided, in addition, by G6PD-deficient people of Mediterranean, Middle Eastern, and Asian origin. Unmarked and items within square brackets apply only to people with the African A^- variant.

†These drugs or chemicals may cause hemolysis in normal persons if given in large doses. Many other drugs may produce hemolysis in certain individuals.

From Luzzatto L: Glucose-6-phosphate dehydrogenase deficiency and the pentose phosphate pathway. In Handin RI, Lux SL, Stossel TP (eds): Blood: Principles and Practice of Hematology. Philadelphia: JB Lippincott, 1995, pp 1897–1923.

deficiency, donor blood should be screened before neonatal transfusion or exchange transfusion. The World Health Organization has recommended neonatal screening of all infants in areas where the prevalence of G6PD deficiency exceeds 3% to 5% or more among male neonates.[51]

Disorders of Glutathione Metabolism

Defects of glutathione metabolism may be associated with hemolysis.[17, 54] Erythrocytes from patients lacking *glutathione synthetase* or γ-*glutamylcysteine synthetase*, enzymes involved in glutathione synthesis, have very low levels of GSH. Clinically, these disorders resemble G6PD deficiency. There is mild to moderate chronic hemolytic anemia with increased susceptibility to oxidant stress. Many individuals and essentially all neonates are relatively deficient in *GSH peroxidase*, but they do not exhibit hemolysis, probably because nonenzymatic reduction of peroxide by GSH occurs at very high rates.

THE ERYTHROCYTE MEMBRANE

The erythrocyte membrane has a variety of functions (Fig. 11–8).[55–57] It helps the body maintain pH in a physiologic range through chloride and bicarbonate ion exchange. It is involved in the preservation of vital compounds such as organic phosphates and reductants required to prevent corrosion by oxygen and in the excretion of various metabolic wastes. The membrane assists in the regulation of erythrocyte metabolism by selectively and reversibly binding and inactivating various glycolytic enzymes. During erythropoiesis, the membrane imports the iron required by the red blood cell for hemoglobin synthesis. The membrane helps maintain a slippery exterior so that erythrocytes do not adhere to endothelial cells or aggregate

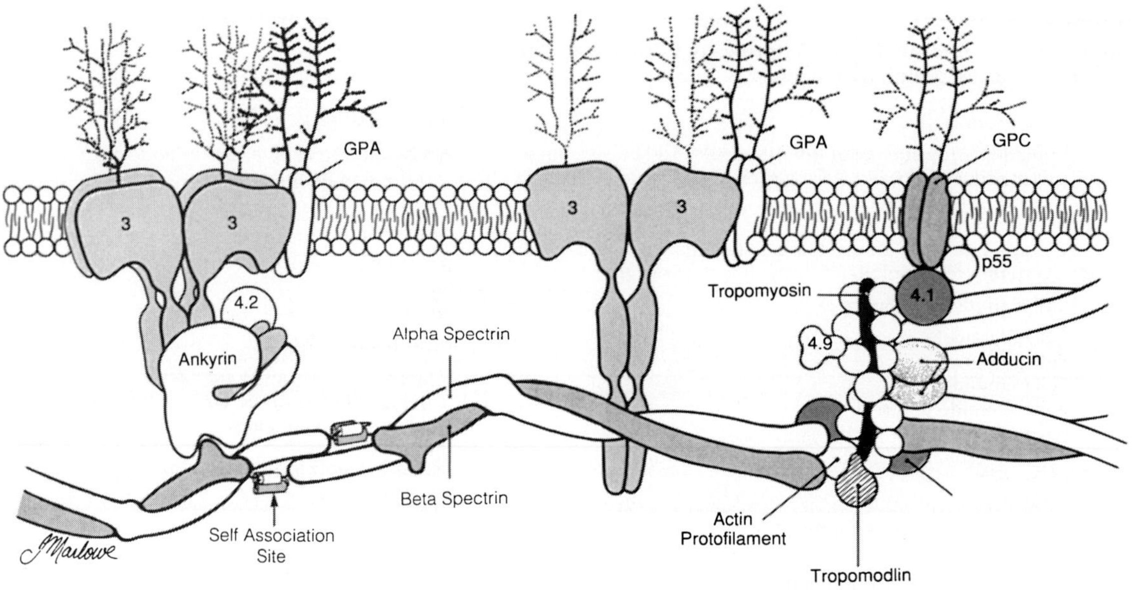

Figure 11–8. A model of the major proteins of the erythrocyte membrane shows α and β spectrin, ankyrin, band 3 (the anion exchanger), 4.1 (protein 4.1), 4.2 (protein 4.2), actin, and glycophorin. (From Lux SE, Palek J: Disorders of the red cell membrane. In Handin RI, Lux SE, Stossel TP (eds): Blood: Principles and Practice of Hematology. Philadelphia: JB Lippincott, 1995, pp 1701–1816.)

and occlude the microcirculation. The membrane skeleton confers the flexibility and deformability to the erythrocyte that allows it to maintain its integrity while enduring circulatory stresses. Defects of the membrane skeleton lead to abnormalities of erythrocyte shape.

Several features differentiate the fetal and neonatal erythrocyte from the adult red blood cell, including variations in shape and deformability. Irregularly shaped cells such as poikilocytes, acanthocytes, and burr cells are much more common in peripheral blood smears of neonates than adults.

Erythrocyte deformability, which influences several factors, including the life span of the red blood cell, blood flow in the peripheral circulation, and whole blood viscosity, is decreased in the neonatal erythrocyte. Deformability is influenced by cellular cytoplasmic viscosity, cell surface area–volume relationships, and intrinsic flexibility of the erythrocyte membrane itself. This decreased deformability of the neonatal erythrocyte is reflected in an increase in osmotic resistance, which normalizes by 4 to 6 weeks of age.

This observation has practical implications. Although it has been suggested that osmotic fragility curves are unreliable in the first month of life, when a complete osmotic fragility curve is calculated and compared with normal neonatal values, the diagnosis of hereditary spherocytosis (HS) can frequently be made. The performance of osmotic fragility testing need only be delayed in rare cases, such as when there is confusion between HS and ABO incompatibility.

Membrane Lipids

The erythrocyte membrane, which constitutes 1% of total red blood cell weight, is composed of mobile lipids and proteins that interact in a variety of ways. Red blood cell membrane lipids are asymmetrically distributed across the bilayer membrane, reflecting a steady state involving a constant exchange of phospholipids between the two bilayer hemileaflets. Glycolipids and cholesterol are intercalated between the phospholipids in the bilayer, with their long axes perpendicular to the bilayer plane.

Glycolipids are located in the external half of the bilayer, with their carbohydrate moieties extending into the aqueous phase. They carry several important red blood cell antigens, including A, B, H, Le^a, Le^b, and P, and they may serve other important functions. For example, globoside, the P glycolipid, is the cellular receptor for parvovirus B19, the causative agent of many aplastic crises. Mature erythrocytes are unable to synthesize fatty acids, phospholipids, or cholesterol de novo and depend on lipid exchange and fatty acid acylation as mechanisms for phospholipid repair and renewal.

Membrane Proteins

The red blood cell membrane contains about a dozen major proteins and hundreds of minor ones. In general, membrane proteins are classified as integral or peripheral. Integral membrane proteins penetrate or traverse the lipid bilayer and interact with the hydrophobic lipid core. They include transport proteins such as band 3, the anion exchanger, and the glycophorins, which carry membrane receptors and antigens. Peripheral proteins interact with integral proteins or lipids at the membrane surface but do not penetrate into the bilayer core. In the red blood cell, the major peripheral membrane proteins are on the cytoplasmic membrane face and include enzymes such as glyceraldehyde-3-phosphate dehydrogenase and structural proteins such as spectrin and actin.

Integral Membrane Proteins

Band 3 (i.e., AE1), the major integral protein of the red blood cell, has two primary functions: ion transport and maintenance of protein-protein interactions. It mediates chloride-bicarbonate exchange and provides a binding site for glycolytic enzymes, hemoglobin, and the skeletal proteins ankyrin, protein 4.1, and protein 4.2.

Defects of band 3 have been identified in hereditary spherocytosis, Southeast Asian ovalocytosis, rare forms of inherited acanthocytosis, type II congenital dyserythropoietic anemia, and autosomal dominant distal renal tubular acidosis. A single *N*-glycan chain is attached to an asparagine in the membrane-spanning domain of band 3. This chain is composed of *N*-acetylgalactosamine units arranged in an unbranched, linear fashion (i.e., i antigen) in fetal erythrocytes and in a branched fashion in adult cells (i.e., I antigen). Erythrocytes expressing the i antigen are not typically found after the first year of life.

The next most abundant integral membrane proteins, the *glycophorins*, provide most of the negative surface charge required by red blood cells to avoid sticking to each other and to the vascular wall. They are involved in transmembrane signaling and carry receptors for *P. falciparum*, a number of viruses and bacteria, and several blood group antigens. The red blood cell membrane contains a large number of other integral proteins, including the Rh protein, Kell antigen, glucose transporter, urea transporter, Na^+,K^+-ATPase, Ca^{2+}-ATPase, Mg^{2+}-ATPase, various kinases and phosphatases, acetylcholinesterase, decay accelerating factor, complement proteins, and receptors for transferrin, insulin, insulin-like growth factors, thyroid hormone, parathyroid hormone, α-adrenergic agonists, cholinergic agents, diphtheria toxin, ceruloplasmin, and opiates.

Peripheral Membrane Proteins

Spectrin is the major component of the membrane skeleton. Spectrin is composed of two subunits, α- and β-spectrin, that are structurally related but functionally distinct. These subunits intertwine around each other in an antiparallel fashion to form heterodimers, which self-associate head to head to form tetramers. Electron microscopy shows these to be slender, twisted, wormlike molecules that extend to a total length of about 100 nm. Spectrin is highly flexible and assumes a variety of conformations, an unusual property that may be critical for normal membrane pliancy. The spectrin membrane skeleton is linked to the plasma membrane through the actin-protein 4.1 junctional complex and through spectrin-ankyrin interactions.

Protein 4.1, a protein necessary for normal membrane stability, interacts with spectrin, actin, and other proteins of the red blood cell membrane. Patients whose red blood cells lack protein 4.1 have marked hemolysis and very fragile erythrocytes. *Ankyrin* serves as the primary linkage protein for the high-affinity binding of spectrin to the inner membrane through interactions with the cytoplasmic domain of band 3. *Protein 4.2* is a peripheral membrane protein that helps link the skeleton to the lipid bilayer through interactions with ankyrin and band 3. Other integral proteins include actin and the actin-associated proteins, the adducins, dematin, myosin, tropomyosin, and tropomodulin.

DISORDERS OF THE ERYTHROCYTE MEMBRANE

Hemolytic anemias caused by defects in the erythrocyte membrane compose an important group of hereditary anemias. HS, hereditary elliptocytosis (HE), and hereditary pyropoikilocytosis (HPP) are the most common disorders in this group. Detailed clinical studies of these disorders were completed several years ago. Advances in molecular biology have allowed further characterization of these disorders and, in many cases, detection of the precise genetic defects. Analysis of these defects has provided a better understanding of the pathogenesis of these disorders and of the structure-function relationships of the proteins of the erythrocyte membrane.

Hereditary Spherocytosis

HS refers to a group of disorders characterized by spherical, doughnut-shaped erythrocytes in the peripheral blood.[55, 56] HS affects approximately 1 in 4000 to 5000 individuals in the United States and England. It is the most common inherited anemia of individuals of northern European ancestry and is much more common among Caucasians than individuals of African ancestry. Clinical, laboratory, and genetic heterogeneity characterize this group of disorders.

Pathophysiology

The primary defect in HS is the loss of erythrocyte membrane surface area because of defects in erythrocyte membrane proteins, including α spectrin, β spectrin, ankyrin, band 3, and protein 4.2 (Fig. 11–9). Qualitative or quantitative defects of one or more of these membrane proteins lead to membrane instability, which leads to membrane loss. In some cases, the precise molecular defects have been identified. Review of the genetic defects identified in HS reveals great heterogeneity. Multiple genetic loci have been implicated and a variety of mutations identified (Table 11–7).[55–57] Except for rare instances, the mutations in HS are "private" (i.e., each individual has a unique mutation), implying no selective advantage for HS

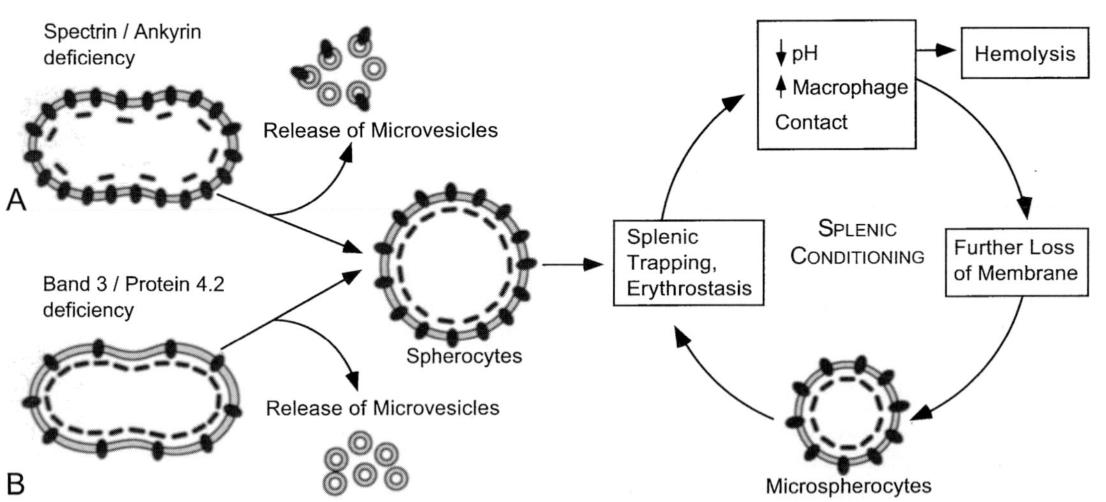

Figure 11–9. Pathophysiology of hereditary spherocytosis. The primary defect in hereditary spherocytosis is a deficiency of membrane surface area. Decreased surface area may be produced by two different mechanisms. In one, defects of spectrin, ankyrin, or protein 4.2 lead to reduced density of the membrane skeleton, destabilizing the overlying lipid bilayer and releasing band 3–containing microvesicles. In the other, defects of band 3 lead to band 3 deficiency and loss of its lipid-stabilizing effect. This results in the loss of band 3–free microvesicles. Both pathways result in membrane loss, decreased surface area, and formation of spherocytes with decreased deformability. These deformed erythrocytes become trapped in the hostile environment of the spleen, where splenic conditioning inflicts further membrane damage, amplifying the cycle of red cell membrane injury.

Table 11–7. **Erythrocyte Membrane Genetic Defects in Inherited Disorders of Red Blood Cell Shape**

Defective Gene Product	Disorder	Comment
Ankyrin	HS	Most common cause of typical dominant HS
Band 3	HS, SAO, NIHF	"Pincered" spherocytes seen on smear presplenectomy; SAO due to 9 AA deletion
Spectrin β chain	HS, HE, HPP, NIHF	"Acanthocytic" spherocytes seen on smear presplenectomy; location of mutation in spectrin determines clinical phenotype.
Spectrin α chain	HS, HE, HPP, NIHF	Location of mutation in spectrin determines clinical phenotype; α-spectrin mutations are most common cause of typical HE
Protein 4.2	HS	Common in Japanese HS
Protein 4.1	HE	
Glycophorin C	HE	Concomitant protein 4.1 deficiency is basis of HE in glycophorin C defects

AA, amino acid; HS, hereditary spherocytosis; HE, hereditary elliptocytosis; HPP, hereditary pyropoikilocytosis; NIHF, nonimmune hydrops fetalis; SAO, Southeast Asian ovalocytosis.

mutations. A surprising number of de novo mutations have been reported in the HS genes.[58, 59]

The spleen plays a secondary but important role in the pathophysiology of HS. Splenic destruction of abnormal erythrocytes with decreased deformability is the primary cause of hemolysis experienced by HS patients.[60–62] Physical entrapment of erythrocytes in the splenic microcirculation and ingestion by phagocytes have been proposed as mechanisms of destruction. The splenic environment is hostile to erythrocytes. Low pH, low glucose and ATP concentrations, and high local concentrations of toxic free radicals produced by adjacent phagocytes all contribute to membrane damage. Loss of membrane surface area is the basis for the laboratory diagnosis of HS.

Inheritance

HS is caused by defective genes for α-spectrin, ankyrin, β-spectrin, band 3 protein, and protein 4.2. In approximately 75% of HS patients, inheritance is autosomal dominant. In the remaining patients, inheritance is nondominant because of a de novo mutation or autosomal recessive inheritance. Cases with autosomal recessive inheritance are caused by defects in α spectrin or protein 4.2. A few cases of homozygous HS have been reported. This condition results in fetal death or severe hemolytic anemia manifesting in the neonatal period.

In general, affected individuals of the same kindred experience similar degrees of hemolysis. Rarely, members of the same kindred experience various degrees of hemolysis. When HS is identified in one or more siblings whose parents have no identifiable abnormalities or when there is great variability in the clinical severity of affected HS family members, a number of explanations can be sought, including variable penetrance of the genetic defect; a de novo mutation; a mild form of recessively inherited HS in the kindred; a modifier allele that influences the expression of a membrane protein, leading to the variability in clinical expression that may exist in the family; or tissue-specific mosaicism of the defect.

Clinical Syndromes

The clinical manifestations of the spherocytosis syndromes vary widely.[55–57, 63] The classic triad of anemia, jaundice, and splenomegaly is uncommon in neonates. Anemia is the most common finding in neonates with HS.[64, 65] Burman found anemia in 38 of 43 infants with HS.[64] Some patients have required blood transfusion to treat their anemia. The degree of anemia seen in the neonatal period does not predict the severity of the anemia seen in later life.[65, 66]

Jaundice is seen in about one half of HS neonates and may be severe enough to require phototherapy or exchange transfusion. Like G6PD deficiency, jaundice in HS neonates may be accentuated by the coinheritance of the Gilbert syndrome *UDPGT1* gene polymorphism.[67]

Kernicterus has been reported.[64] Later in infancy and childhood, jaundice is intermittent and is less pronounced than in adults.

Rarely, patients may have severe hemolytic anemia presenting in utero or shortly after birth, continuing through the first year of life. These patients may require multiple blood transfusions and, in a some cases, splenectomy in the first year of life.[68–71] These severe HS patients usually suffer from significant spectrin deficiency, probably because of homozygosity or compound heterozygosity for α spectrin gene defects.[72] Several cases of hydrops fetalis caused by severe anemia in HS patients have been associated with band 3 or spectrin defects.[73, 74] In a few unfortunate cases, in utero or early neonatal death has been reported.

Many HS patients escape detection in the neonatal period. For these asymptomatic patients, the diagnosis of HS may not be made until they are being evaluated for unrelated disorders later in life or when complications related to anemia or chronic hemolysis occur. Although the life span of the erythrocyte in these patients may be shortened to only 20 to 30 days, they adequately compensate for their hemolysis with increased marrow erythropoiesis.

Complications of HS include aplastic crises after virally induced bone marrow suppression and manifest with anemia, jaundice, fever, and vomiting. The most common etiologic agent in these cases is parvovirus B19. Hemolytic crises, usually associated with viral illnesses and occurring before 6 years of age, are generally mild and manifest with jaundice, increased spleen size, and a drop in hematocrit. A third, preventable, crisis is the megaloblastic crisis, which occurs in HS patients with increased folate demands, such as the pregnant patient, growing children, or patients recovering from an aplastic crisis.

Chronic hemolysis leads to the formation of bilirubinate gallstones, the most frequently reported complication in HS patients. Although gallstones have been observed in infancy, most appear in adolescents and young adults. Routine management should include interval ultrasonography to detect gallstones, because many patients with cholelithiasis and HS are asymptomatic. Uncommon manifestations of HS, including skin ulceration, gout, chronic leg dermatitis, cardiomyopathy, spinal cord dysfunction, movement disorders, and extramedullary erythropoiesis, are rare in infancy. In patients with untreated severe HS, poor growth and findings attributable to extramedullary hematopoiesis such as hand and skull deformabilities may be found.

Diagnosis

Patients with HS may present at any age, usually with anemia, hyperbilirubinemia, or an abnormal blood smear. Initial assessment should include a thorough history and physical examination. In evaluating a neonate with suspected HS, particular attention should be paid to the family history, including questions about anemia, jaundice, gallstones, and splenectomy. Initial laboratory investigation should include a complete blood count with a peripheral smear, reticulocyte count, direct antiglobulin test (Coombs' test), and serum bilirubin. When the peripheral smear or family history suggests hereditary spherocytosis, an incubated osmotic fragility determination should be obtained. Rarely, additional, specialized testing is required to confirm the diagnosis.

Similar to the clinical presentation of HS, laboratory findings for HS are heterogeneous. Erythrocyte morphology is quite variable. Typical HS patients have blood smears with easily identifiable spherocytes lacking central pallor (Fig. 11–10*A*). Less commonly, patients present with only a few spherocytes on peripheral smear or, at the other end of the spectrum, with numerous small, dense spherocytes and bizarre erythrocyte morphology with anisocytosis and poikilocytosis. Specific morphologic findings have been identified in patients with certain membrane protein defects, such as pincered erythrocytes (band 3) or spherocytic acanthocytes (β-spectrin).

When examining a smear in a case of suspected spherocytosis, it is important to have a high-quality smear with the erythrocytes well separated and some cells with central pallor in the field of examination, because spherocytes are a common artifact on peripheral blood smears. Other disorders seen in the neonatal period with prominent spherocytes on peripheral blood smear include ABO incompatibility, microangiopathic and macroangiopathic hemolytic anemias, liver disease, and clostridial sepsis.[75]

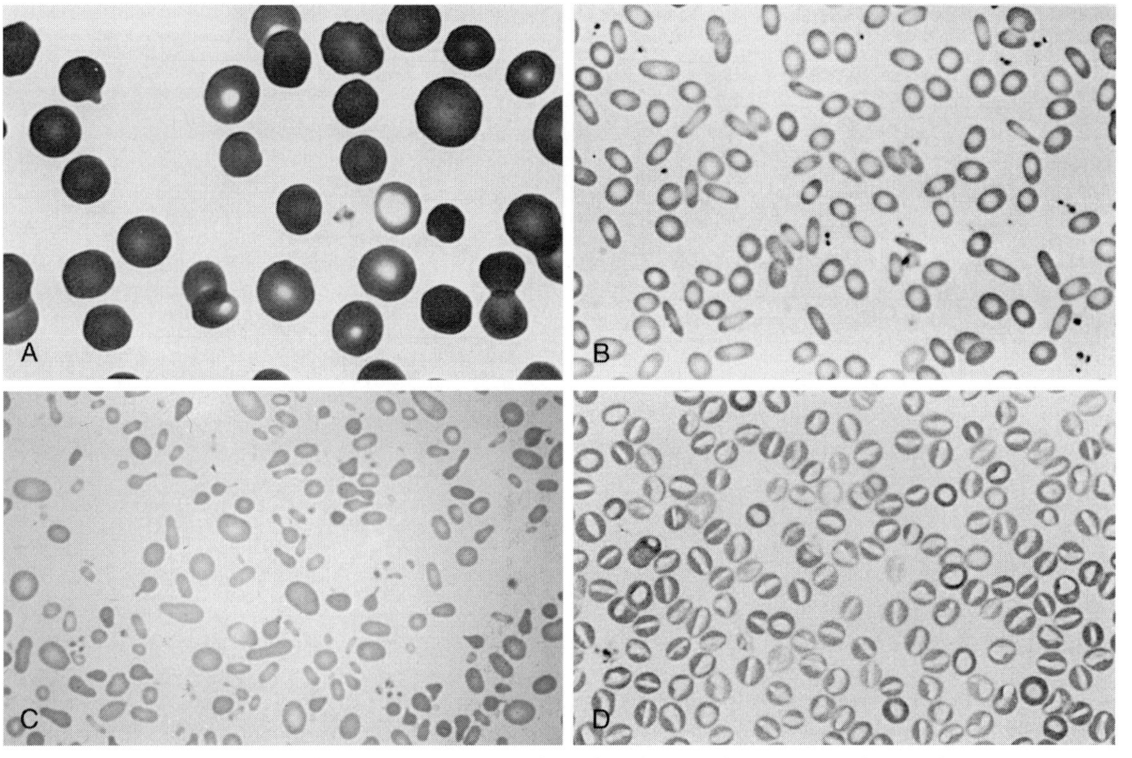

Figure 11–10. Peripheral blood smears in disorders of erythrocyte shape. *A*, Hereditary spherocytosis. Characteristic spherocytes lack central pallor. *B*, Hereditary elliptocytosis is characterized by smooth, cigar-shaped elliptocytes. *C*, Hereditary pyropoikilocytosis, with pronounced microcytosis, poikilocytosis, fragmentation of erythrocytes, and elliptocytes. *D*, Hereditary stomatocytosis.

The mean corpuscular hemoglobin concentration (MCHC) is increased (between 35 and 38) because of relative cellular dehydration. The mean corpuscular volume (MCV) is usually normal or slightly decreased. The Technicon H1 blood counter (Technicon, Tarrytown, NY) provides a histogram of MCHCs that is claimed to be accurate enough to identify nearly all HS patients.[76]

In the normal erythrocyte, a redundancy of cell membrane gives the cell its characteristic discoid shape and provides it with abundant surface area. Spherocytes have decreased surface area relative to cell volume, resulting in their abnormal shape. This change is reflected in the increased osmotic fragility found in these cells (Fig. 11–11). Osmotic fragility is tested by adding increasingly hypotonic concentrations of saline to red blood cells. The normal erythrocyte is able to increase its volume by swelling, but spherocytes, which are already at maximum volume for surface area, burst at higher saline concentrations than normal. Approximately one fourth of HS individuals have a normal osmotic fragility on freshly drawn red blood cells, with the osmotic fragility curve approximating the number of spherocytes seen on peripheral smear. However, after incubation at 37°C for 24 hours, HS red blood cells lose membrane surface area more readily than normal, because their membranes are leaky and unstable. Incubation accentuates the defect in HS erythrocytes and brings out the defect on osmotic fragility, making incubated osmotic fragility the standard test in diagnosing HS. When the spleen is intact, a subpopulation of very fragile erythrocytes that have been conditioned by the spleen form the "tail" of the osmotic fragility curve (see Fig. 11–11). This tail disappears after splenectomy.

Unfortunately, the osmotic fragility test suffers from poor sensitivity, with as many as 20% of mild cases of HS missed after incubation. The osmotic fragility test is unreliable for patients who have small numbers of spherocytes, including those who have been recently transfused. It is abnormal in other conditions in which spherocytes are present. The incubated

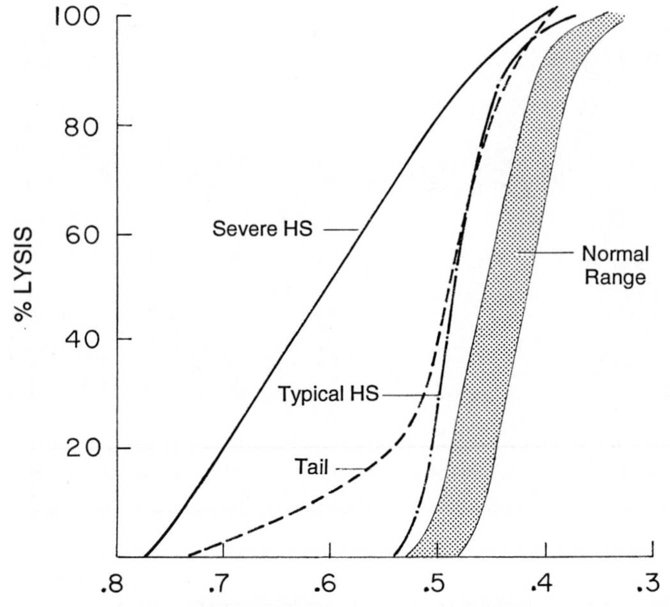

Figure 11–11. Osmotic fragility curves for hereditary spherocytosis (HS). The shaded area is the normal range. Results representative of typical and severe spherocytosis are shown. A "tail," representing very fragile erythrocytes that have been conditioned by the spleen, is common in many HS patients before splenectomy.

osmotic fragility has proven to be a reliable diagnostic test in the newborn period.[65, 66, 77] When HS is suspected and immune-mediated hemolysis is unlikely, a positive incubated osmotic fragility test is usually confirmatory of the diagnosis. For a few infants, it may be impossible to make the diagnosis in the neonatal period. This is particularly likely for the infant with isolated or concomitant ABO incompatibility. Anemia, microspherocytes, and altered osmotic fragility are found in both conditions.[75, 78] These patients should be followed closely, because the natural history of the diseases eventually differentiate the two.

Other tests such as the autohemolysis test and the acidified glycerol test suffer from lack of specificity and are cumbersome to perform. They are not widely used.

Other laboratory findings for HS are manifestations of the ongoing hemolysis. Increased serum bilirubin, increased lactate dehydrogenase, increased urinary and fecal urobilinogen, and decreased serum haptoglobin levels reflect increased erythrocyte destruction. Haptoglobin may be decreased or absent in neonates and is an unreliable marker of hemolysis in the newborn.[79]

Specialized testing is available for studying difficult cases or cases for which additional information is desired. Useful tests for these purposes include structural and functional studies of erythrocyte membrane proteins such as protein quantitation, limited tryptic digestion of spectrin, spectrin, and ion transport. Membrane frigidity and fragility may be examined using an ektacytometer. cDNA and genomic DNA analyses are available when a molecular diagnosis is desired.

After diagnosing a patient with HS, family members should be examined for the disorder. This can be of great epidemiologic importance, particularly for very old and very young patients. Prenatal diagnosis of HS has been made in a few cases, but this is rarely necessary.

Treatment and Outcome

Splenic sequestration is the primary determinant of erythrocyte survival in HS patients. Splenectomy cures or alleviates the anemia in most patients, reducing or eliminating the need for red blood cell transfusions. Eliminating the need for chronic blood transfusions has obvious implications for future iron overload. The incidence of cholelithiasis is also decreased. After splenectomy, spherocytes remain in the peripheral blood, but their life span is near normal.

In the past, splenectomy, which has a low operative mortality rate, was considered routine in HS patients. However, the risk of overwhelming post-splenectomy infections, particularly from encapsulated organisms such as *Streptococcus pneumoniae*, *Neisseria meningitidis*, and

Haemophilus influenzae, and the recent emergence of relatively penicillin-resistant pneumococci has led some to reconsider the role of splenectomy in the treatment of HS. The risk of overwhelming post-splenectomy infections is highest early in life, particularly before 5 years of age.

Before splenectomy, patients should receive vaccination for *S. pneumoniae* and *H. influenzae*. Prophylactic penicillin should be administered postsplenectomy. Other considerations before splenectomy should include the higher risk for parasitic infection such as malaria or babesiosis in the splenectomized patient.

Partial splenectomy has been advocated for infants and young children with significant anemia associated with erythrocyte membrane disorders. The goals of this procedure are to allow for the palliation of hemolysis and anemia while maintaining some residual splenic immune function. However, long-term data for this procedure are lacking.

The indications for splenectomy are controversial. Splenectomy is warranted in patients with significant hemolysis and anemia. Other factors that may influence the decision toward splenectomy include transfusion dependence, recurrent crises, failure to thrive, and skeletal anomalies due to extramedullary erythropoiesis. If possible, splenectomy should be delayed until after 5 years of age.

Patients with HS should be provided supplemental folate, particularly those with active hemolysis, to prevent megaloblastic anemia.

Hereditary Elliptocytosis, Hereditary Pyropoikilocytosis, and Related Disorders

Hereditary Elliptocytosis

HE is characterized by the presence of elliptical or oval, cigar-shaped erythrocytes seen on the peripheral blood smears of affected individuals.[55, 56] HE occurs in approximately 1 of 2000 to 4000 individuals. The true incidence of HE is unknown, because its clinical severity is heterogeneous and many patients are asymptomatic. It is common in African-Americans and persons of Mediterranean ancestry, presumably because elliptocytes confer some resistance to malaria. In parts of Africa, the incidence of HE approaches 1 in 100.

Pathophysiology

The principal defect in HE is mechanical weakness or fragility of the erythrocyte membrane skeleton. Qualitative and quantitative defects occur in a number of red blood cell membrane proteins, including α-spectrin, β-spectrin, protein 4.1, and glycophorin C (see Table 11–7).[80–85] Most defects occur in spectrin, the principal structural protein of the erythrocyte membrane skeleton. The α-β spectrin heterodimers self-associate into tetramers and higher-order oligomers that are critical for erythrocyte membrane stability and for erythrocyte shape and function. Most spectrin defects in HE impair the ability of spectrin dimers to self-associate into tetramers and oligomers, thereby disrupting the membrane skeleton (Fig. 11–12).[83, 86, 87] Structural and functional defects of protein 4.1 appear to disrupt the spectrin-actin contact in the membrane skeleton.[88] Glycophorin C variants are also deficient in protein 4.1. The precise pathobiology of how elliptocytes are formed in these syndromes is unclear.

Inheritance

Genetically, HE is heterogeneous with multiple genetic loci. A wide variety of mutations have been described in the genes for α-spectrin, β-spectrin, protein 4.1, and glycophorin C. These include point mutations, gene deletions and insertions, and mRNA processing defects.[55–57] Several mutations have been identified in a number of individuals with the same genetic background, suggesting a "founder effect" for these mutants. This observation supports the hypothesis that there has been genetic selection for elliptocytosis, because these red blood cells confer some resistance to malaria.[89, 90] In most cases, HE is inherited in an autosomal dominant pattern with rare cases of de novo mutations.

Clinical Syndromes

The clinical manifestation of HE is heterogeneous, ranging from asymptomatic carriers to patients with severe, life-threatening anemia.

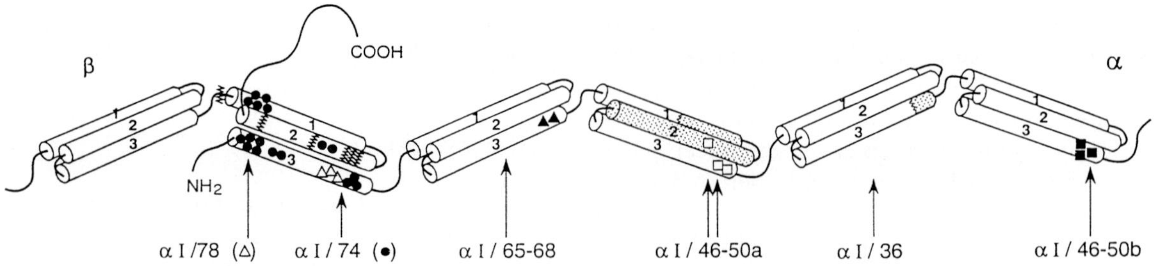

Figure 11–12. Triple helical model of the spectrin repeats that constitute the spectrin self-association site. The symbols denote positions of various genetic defects identified in patients with hereditary elliptocytosis or hereditary pyropoikilocytosis. Limited tryptic digestion of spectrin followed by two-dimensional gel electrophoresis identifies abnormal cleavage sites *(arrows)* in spectrin associated with different mutations. (Adapted from Gallagher PG, Tse WT, Forget BG: Clinical and molecular aspects of disorders of the erythrocyte membrane skeleton. Semin Perinatol 1990;14:351.)

Most patients with HE are asymptomatic. Approximately 12% of patients with HE become symptomatic from their anemia sometime during their lives. Typically, patients are diagnosed incidentally during testing for unrelated conditions. Some asymptomatic carriers posses the same molecular defect as an affected HE relative, but the carriers have normal peripheral blood smears. The erythrocyte life span is normal in most patients and decreased in only 10% of patients. It is this subset of HE patients with decreased red blood cell life span who experience hemolysis, anemia, splenomegaly, and intermittent jaundice. Many of these patients have parents with typical HE and are homozygotes or compound heterozygotes for defects inherited from each of the parents. Symptoms may vary among members of the same family and may even vary in the same individual at different times.

In newborns, anemia and jaundice may be seen, but it is uncommon to find clinical symptoms of elliptocytosis in the neonatal period.[91, 92] More typically, mild anemia appears around 4 to 6 months of age with the appearance of elliptocytes on peripheral blood smear. Occasionally, severe forms of HE may manifest with severe hemolytic anemia and jaundice requiring blood transfusions. These neonates have required exchange transfusion, splenectomy, or both early in life. Usually, even in severely affected patients, the hemolysis abates between 6 and 12 months of age, and the patient develops typical HE with mild anemia.

A few cases of hydrops fetalis are accompanied by fetal or early neonatal death because of unusually severe forms of HE.[93–95] One severely affected hydropic infant salvaged by intrauterine transfusions and early exchange transfusion has remained transfusion dependent for more than 2 years.

Diagnosis

Cigar-shaped elliptocytes on the peripheral blood smear are the hallmark of HE (see Fig. 11–10*B*). These normochromic, normocytic elliptocytes may vary in number from a few to 100% of the sample. The degree of hemolysis does not correlate with the number of elliptocytes present. Ovalocytes, spherocytes, stomatocytes, and fragmented cells may also be seen. Pyknocytes may be prominent. Elliptocytes do not typically appear in the peripheral blood of most infants with HE until 4 to 6 months of age. In older patients, elliptocytes may be associated with several disorders, including megaloblastic anemias, hypochromic microcytic anemias (i.e., iron deficiency anemia and thalassemia), myelodysplastic syndromes, and myelofibrosis; however, elliptocytes generally represent less than one third of red blood cells in these conditions. The history and additional laboratory testing usually clarify the diagnosis of these disorders.

Pseudoelliptocytosis is an artifact of blood smear preparation. Pseudoelliptocytes are found only in certain areas of the smear, usually near its tail, and the long axes of pseudoelliptocytes are parallel, whereas the axes of true elliptocytes are distributed randomly. In typical cases, the incubated osmotic fragility is normal, whereas in severe HE and in the related condition HPP, osmotic fragility is increased.

Other laboratory findings in HE are similar

to those found in other hemolytic anemias and are nonspecific markers of increased erythrocyte production and destruction. The reticulocyte count generally is less than 5%, but it may be higher when hemolysis is severe.

Hereditary Pyropoikilocytosis

HPP is a rare cause of anemia first described by Zarkowsky and colleagues.[96, 97] They described three children with severe anemia in the neonatal period who had erythrocyte morphology similar to that seen in patients suffering severe burns. The erythrocytes from these patients also exhibited increased thermal sensitivity. Subsequently, other patients, mostly of African origin, with similar clinical and laboratory findings were described.[86, 98]

There is a strong relationship between HE and HPP. Approximately one third of parents or siblings of patients with HPP have typical HE. Many patients with HPP eventually develop typical mild to moderate HE. Patients with HPP tend to experience severe hemolysis and anemia in infancy that gradually improves, evolving toward typical elliptocytosis later in life.

In HPP, in addition to the peripheral blood smear findings seen in HE, many erythrocytes have bizarre shapes with fragmentation or budding (see Fig. 11–10*C*). Pyknocytes are prominent in smears of neonates with HPP. Microspherocytosis is common, and the MCV is usually low (50 to 70 fL). The incubated osmotic fragility is increased. In cases of suspected neonatal HE or HPP, review of the family history and analysis of peripheral blood films from the parents are usually of greater diagnostic benefit than other available studies.

Like HS, specialized laboratory procedures are available to study the erythrocyte membranes of HE and HPP patients. These studies include ektacytometry, analysis of membrane proteins by one-dimensional gel electrophoresis, limited tryptic digestion of membrane spectrin followed by one- or two-dimensional gel electrophoresis, spectrin dimer self-association assays, and cDNA or genomic DNA analyses. These studies are not routinely required to make the diagnosis of HE or HPP, but they may be helpful in studying problematic cases and in elucidating the underlying molecular defects. Prenatal diagnoses of HE and HPP have been made using tryptic digestion, ektacytometry, and spectrin dimer self-association studies.[99, 100] Because these anemias are rarely life-threatening conditions, routine prenatal diagnosis is not required.

Treatment and Outcome

Therapy is rarely needed for patients with HE. In rare cases, a few red blood cell transfusions may be required. In cases of severe HE and HPP, splenectomy has been palliative, because the spleen is the site of erythrocyte sequestration and destruction. Many practitioners feel that the same indications for splenectomy in HS should be applied to patients with symptomatic HE or HPP. After splenectomy, patients with HE or HPP have increased hematocrits, decreased reticulocyte counts, and improved clinical symptoms.

Patients should be followed for signs of decompensation during acute illnesses. Interval ultrasonography to detect gallstones should be performed. In patients with significant hemolysis, folate should be administered daily.

Hereditary Stomatocytosis Syndromes

Red blood cell hydration is primarily determined by the intracellular concentration of monovalent cations. A net increase in sodium and potassium ions causes water to enter, forming *stomatocytes* or *hydrocytes*, whereas a net loss of sodium and potassium produces dehydrated red blood cells, or *xerocytes*. Numerous descriptions of congenital or familial hemolytic anemias associated with abnormal cation permeability and, in some cases, disturbed red blood cell hydration have been reported.[55, 101–104] These span the range from severe hydrocytosis to severe xerocytosis. The molecular basis of this group of disorders is unknown. Neonates with variants of hereditary stomatocytosis syndrome with severe hemolysis, hyperbilirubinemia, or hydrops fetalis have been described.[55, 105–108] An unusual characteristic of the stomatocytosis syndromes is a predisposition to thrombosis after splenectomy.[109]

Overhydrated Hereditary Stomatocytosis

Overhydrated hereditary stomatocytosis (OHST), also called hydrocytosis, is a group of disorders characterized by stomatocytes, erythrocytes with a mouth-shaped (stoma) area of central pallor on peripheral blood smear (see Fig. 11–10*D*); severe hemolysis; macrocytosis (110 to 150 fL); elevated erythrocyte sodium concentration; reduced potassium concentration; and increased total sodium plus potassium content. The excess cations elevate the cell's water concentration, producing large, osmotically fragile cells with a low MCHC (24% to 30%). The clinical severity of OHST is variable; some patients experience hemolysis and anemia, but others are asymptomatic.

Dehydrated Hereditary Stomatocytosis

Blood smears from patients with dehydrated hereditary stomatocytosis (DHST; xerocytosis) patients exhibit contracted and spiculated red blood cells, dessicytes, a variable number of stomatocytes, and target cells. Most patients have nearly normal erythrocyte morphology, with only a few target cells and an occasional echinocyte or stomatocyte. The MCHC and MCV (95 to 115 fL), are increased, and the osmotic fragility is decreased (i.e., resistance to osmotic lysis). The characteristic biochemical abnormality is a reduced potassium concentration and total monovalent cation content.

Intermediate Syndromes and Hereditary Stomatocytosis Variants

Hydrocytosis and xerocytosis represent the extremes of a spectrum of red blood cell permeability defects. Several families with features of both conditions have been reported.[55, 110] Some patients with severe permeability defects have little or no hemolysis. The proportion of stomatocytes and the degree of sodium influx do not correlate with each other, and neither correlates with the amount of hemolysis or anemia. Moreover, stomatin deficiency has not been observed in some patients with the most severe permeability defects. This suggests that hereditary stomatocytosis is a complex mixture of diseases and that factors other than sodium leak and stomatin content may be critical to the demise of the stomatocyte.

Membrane Protein Defects in the Neonatal Period

Neonates with erythrocyte membrane disorders may experience a more severe hemolysis than adults. The precise cause for this observation is unknown, but it may be caused by a combination of factors. The neonatal intraerythrocytic environment and microcirculatory effects may play a role in this increased hemolysis.[111, 112] Because of the inability of fetal hemoglobin to effectively bind 2,3-DPG, there are increased levels of free 2,3-DPG in neonatal erythrocytes. Increased 2,3-DPG levels destabilize protein interactions at the spectrin-actin–protein 4.1 junctional complex, offering a partial explanation for the increased hemolysis experienced by neonates with membrane skeletal defects.[113] Other factors implicated in the more severe hemolysis seen in HS neonates are the shortened life span of the neonatal erythrocyte and the sluggish response of the marrow to hemolytic stress seen in the first year of life.

Differences in the HMP shunt have been suggested to be the cause of increased susceptibility of neonatal erythrocytes to oxidant injury. However, other factors may be involved in the increased oxidative susceptibility of the neonatal red blood cell, including decreased glutathione peroxidase levels and, in some infants, decreased levels of superoxide dismutase. Other factors, such as decreased plasma antioxidant capacity and increased erythrocyte membrane sulfhydryl groups leading to increased susceptibility to Heinz body formation, have been implicated.

Acknowledgments

This work was supported in part by grants from the March of Dimes Birth Defects Foundation, the National Institutes of Health, and the Children's Clinical Research Center, Yale University School of Medicine.

References

1. Dacie J: Hereditary spherocytosis (HS). In Dacie J (ed): Haemolytic Anaemias, 2nd ed. New Haven: Grune & Stratton, 1960, pp 82–150.
2. Beutler E: The molecular biology of enzymes of erythrocyte metabolism. In Stamatoyannopoulos G, Nienhuis AW, Majerus PW, Varmus H (eds): The Molecular Basis of Blood Diseases, 2nd ed. Philadelphia: WB Saunders, 1994, pp 331–349.
3. Tanaka KR, Paglia DE: Pyruvate kinase and other enzymopathies of the erythrocyte. In Scriver CR, Beaudet AL, Sly WS, Valle D (eds): The Metabolic and Molecular Bases of Inherited Disease, 7th ed. Vol. III. New York: McGraw-Hill, 1995, pp 3485–3511.
4. Paglia DE: Disorders of erythrocyte glycolysis and nucleotide metabolism. In Handin RI, Lux SE, Stossel TP (eds): Blood: Principles and Practice of Hematology. Philadelphia: JB Lippincott, 1995, pp 1877–1896.
5. Oski FA: Disorders of red cell metabolism. In Oski FA, Naiman JL (eds): Hematologic Problems in the Newborn, 3rd ed. Vol. IV. Philadelphia: WB Saunders, 1982, pp 97–136.
6. Ohls RK: Developmental erythropoiesis. In Polin RA, Fox WW (eds): Fetal and Neonatal Physiology, 2nd ed. Vol. 2 Philadelphia: WB Saunders, 1997, pp 1762–1786.
7. Matthay KK, Mentzer WC: Erythrocyte enzymopathies in the newborn. Clin Haematol 1981;10:31.
8. Abu-Melha AM, Ahmed MA, Knox-Macaulay H, et al: Erythrocyte pyruvate kinase deficiency in newborns of eastern Saudi Arabia. Acta Haematol 1991;85:192.
9. Bossu M, Dacha M, Fornaini G. Neonatal hemolysis due to a transient severity of inherited pyruvate kinase deficiency. Acta Haematol 1968;40:166.
10. Bowman HS, McKusick VA, Dronamraju KR: Pyruvate kinase deficient hemolytic anemia in an Amish isolate. Am J Hum Genet 1965;17:1.
11. Gilsanz F, Vega MA, Gomez-Castillo E, et al: Fetal anaemia due to pyruvate kinase deficiency. Arch Dis Child 1993;69:523.
12. Ivey HH, Sabio H: Multiple exchange transfusions in the treatment of a newborn with pyruvate kinase deficiency. Clin Pediatr 1979;18:756.
13. Oski FA, Diamond LK: Erythrocyte pyruvate kinase deficiency: report of three cases. N Engl J Med 1963;269:763.
14. Volpato S, Vigi V, Cattarozzi G: Nonspherocytic haemolytic anaemia and severe jaundice in a newborn with partial pyruvate kinase deficiency. Acta Paediatr Scand 1968;57:59.
15. Oski F, Nathan D, Sidel V, et al: Extreme hemolysis and red cell distortion in erythrocyte pyruvate kinase deficiency. I. Morphology, erythrokinetics and family enzyme studies. N Engl J Med 1964;270:1023.
16. Hennekam RC, Beemer FA, Cats BP, et al: Hydrops fetalis associated with red cell pyruvate kinase deficiency. Genet Couns 1990;1:75.
17. Mentzer WC: Pyruvate kinase deficiency and disorders of glycolysis. In Nathan D, Orkin S (eds): Hematology of Infancy and Childhood, 5th ed. Philadelphia: WB Saunders, 1997, pp 665.
18. Ravindranath Y, Paglia DE, Warrier I, et al: Glucose phosphate isomerase deficiency as a cause of hydrops fetalis. N Engl J Med 1987;316:258.
19. Luzzatto L: Glucose-6-phosphate dehydrogenase deficiency and the pentose phosphate pathway. In Handin RI, Lux SL, Stossel TP (eds): Blood: Principles and Practice of Hematology. Philadelphia: JB Lippincott, 1995, pp 1897–1923.
20. Jarolim P, Lahav M, Liu SC, Palek J: Effect of hemoglobin oxidation products on the stability of red cell membrane skeletons and the associations of skeletal proteins: correlation with a release of hemin. Blood 1990;76:2125.
21. Snyder LM, Fortier NL, Trainor J, et al: Effect of hydrogen peroxide exposure on normal human erythrocyte deformability, morphology, surface characteristics, and spectrin-hemoglobin cross-linking. J Clin Invest 1985;76:1971.
22. Luzzatto L: Glucose-6-phosphate dehydrogenase deficiency and hemolytic anemia. In Nathan D, Orkin S (eds): Hematology of Infancy and Childhood. Philadelphia: WB Saunders, 1997, pp 704.
23. Beutler E: G6PD deficiency. Blood 1994;84:3613.
24. Ruwende C, Khoo SC, Snow RW, et al: Natural selection of hemi- and heterozygotes for G6PD deficiency in Africa by resistance to severe malaria. Nature 1995;376:246.
25. Jacob HS, Winterhalter KH: The role of hemoglobin heme loss in Heinz body formation: studies with a partially heme-deficient hemoglobin and with genetically unstable hemoglobins. J Clin Invest 1970; 49:2008.
26. Corchia C, Balata A, Meloni GF, Meloni T: Favism in a female newborn infant whose mother ingested fava beans before delivery (see comments). J Pediatr 1995;127:807.
27. Mentzer WC, Collier E: Hydrops fetalis associated with erythrocyte G-6-PD deficiency and maternal ingestion of fava beans and ascorbic acid. J Pediatr 1975;86:565.
28. Perkins RP: Hydrops fetalis and stillbirth in a male glucose-6-phosphate dehydrogenase-deficient fetus possibly due to maternal ingestion of sulfisoxazole; a case report. Am J Obstet Gynecol 1971;111:379.
29. Doxiadis SA, Valaes T: The clinical picture of glucose-6-phosphate dehydrogenase deficiency in early infancy. Arch Dis Child 1964;39:545.
30. Eshaghpour E, Oski FA, Williams M: The relationship of erythrocyte glucose-6-phosphate dehydrogenase deficiency to hyperbilirubinemia in Negro premature infants. J Pediatr 1967;70:595.
31. Fessas PH, Doxiadis SA, Valaes T: Neonatal jaundice in glucose-6-phosphate dehydrogenase deficient infants. BMJ 1962;2:1359.
32. Gibbs WN, Gray R, Lowry M: Glucose-6-phosphate dehydrogenase deficiency and neonatal jaundice in Jamaica. Br J Haematol 1979;43:263.
33. Huang CS, Hung KL, Huang MJ, et al: Neonatal jaundice and molecular mutations in glucose-6-phosphate dehydrogenase deficient newborn infants. Am J Hematol 1996;51:19.
34. Kaplan M, Abramov A: Neonatal hyperbilirubinemia associated with glucose-6-phosphate dehydrogenase deficiency in Sephardic-Jewish neonates: incidence, severity, and the effect of phototherapy. Pediatrics 1992;90:401.
35. Valaes T: Severe neonatal jaundice associated with glucose-6-phosphate dehydrogenase deficiency: pathogenesis and global epidemiology. Acta Paediatr Suppl 1994;394:58.
36. Washington EC, Ector W, Abboud M, et al: Hemolytic jaundice due to G6PD deficiency causing kernicterus in a female newborn. South Med J 1995;88:776.
37. Zarkowsky HS, Oski FA, Sha'afi R, et al: Congenital hemolytic anemia with high sodium, low potassium red cells. I. Studies of membrane permeability. N Engl J Med 1968;278:573.
38. Kopelman AE, Ey JL, Lee H: Phototherapy in new-

born infants with glucose-6-phosphate dehydrogenase deficiency. J Pediatr 1978;93:497.
39. Meloni T, Costa S, Dore A, Cutillo S: Phototherapy for neonatal hyperbilirubinemia in mature newborn infants with erythrocyte G-6-PD deficiency. J Pediatr 197485:560.
40. Tan KL: Phototherapy for neonatal jaundice in erythrocyte glucose-6-phosphate dehydrogenase-deficient infants. Pediatrics 1977;59(Suppl):1023.
41. Tan KL, Boey KW: Efficacy of phototherapy in neonatal hyperbilirubinaemia associated with glucose-6-phosphate dehydrogenase deficient status. Eur J Pediatr 1993;152:601.
42. Arese P, and De Flora A: Pathophysiology of hemolysis in glucose-6-phosphate dehydrogenase deficiency. Semin Hematol 1990;27:1.
43. Kaplan M, Rubaltelli FF, Hammerman C, et al: Conjugated bilirubin in neonates with glucose-6-phosphate dehydrogenase deficiency. J Pediatr 1996; 128:695.
44. Seidman DS, Shiloh M, Stevenson DK, et al: Role of hemolysis in neonatal jaundice associated with glucose-6 phosphate dehydrogenase deficiency. J Pediatr 1995;127:804.
45. Valaes T: Pathophysiology of spontaneous neonatal bilirubinemia associated with glucose-6-phosphate dehydrogenase deficiency. J Pediatr 1996;128:863.
46. Yu MW, Hsiao KJ, Wuu KD, Chen CJ: Association between glucose-6-phosphate dehydrogenase deficiency and neonatal jaundice: interaction with multiple risk factors. Int J Epidemiol 1992;21:947.
47. Kaplan M, Renbaum P, Levy-Lahad E, et al: Gilbert syndrome and glucose-6-phosphate dehydrogenase deficiency: a dose-dependent genetic interaction crucial to neonatal hyperbilirubinemia. Proc Natl Acad Sci U S A 1997;94:12128.
48. Sampietro M, Lupica L, Perrero L, Comino A, Martinez di Montemuros F, Cappellini MD, and Fiorelli G: The expression of uridine diphosphate glucuronosyltransferase gene is a major determinant of bilirubin level in heterozygous beta-thalassaemia and in glucose-6-phosphate dehydrogenase deficiency. Br J Haematol 1997;99:437.
49. Kaplan M, Leiter C, Hammerman C, Rudensky B: Comparison of commercial screening tests for glucose-6-phosphate dehydrogenase deficiency in the neonatal period. Clin Chem 1997;43:1236.
50. Forni GL, Napoli G, Gaetani GF, Ferraris AM: G6PD deficiency-related chronic hemolysis treated with splenectomy: a case report (Letter). Am J Hematol 1994;47:146.
51. WHO Working Group: Glucose-6-phosphate dehydrogenase deficiency. Bull World Health Organ 1989;67:601.
52. Kumar P, Sarkar S, Narang A: Acute intravascular haemolysis following exchange transfusion with G-6-PD deficient blood. Eur J Pediatr 1994;153:98.
53. Mimouni F, Shohat S, Reisner SH: G6PD-deficient donor blood as a cause of hemolysis in two preterm infants. Isr J Med Sci 1986;22:120.
54. Lo SS, Marti HR, Hitzig WH: Hemolytic anemia associated with decreased concentration of reduced glutathione in red cells. Acta Haematol 1971;46:14.
55. Gallagher PG, Forget BG, Lux SE: Disorders of the erythrocyte membrane. In Nathan D, Orkin S (eds): Hematology of Infancy and Childhood, 5th ed. Philadelphia: WB Saunders, 1997, pp 544–664.
56. Lux SE, Palek J: Disorders of the red cell membrane. In Handin RI, Lux SE, Stossel TP (eds): Blood: Principles and Practice of Hematology. Philadelphia: JB Lippincott, 1995, p 1701.
57. Gallagher PG, Ferriera JD: Molecular basis of erythrocyte membrane disorders. Curr Opin Hematol 1997;4:128.
58. Miraglia del Giudice E, Francese M, Nobili B, et al: High frequency of de novo mutations in ankyrin gene *(ANK1)* in children with hereditary spherocytosis. J Pediatr 1998;132:117.
59. Randon J, Miraglia del Giudice E, Bozon M, et al: Frequent de novo mutations of the ANK1 gene mimic a recessive mode of transmission in hereditary spherocytosis: three new ANK1 variants: ankyrins Bari, Napoli II, and Anzio. Br J Haematol 1997;96:500.
60. Lusher JM, Barnhart MI: The role of the spleen in the pathophysiology of hereditary spherocytosis and hereditary elliptocytosis. Am J Pediatr Hematol Oncol 1980;2:31.
61. Mayman D, Zipursky A: Hereditary spherocytosis: the metabolism of erythrocytes in the peripheral blood and in the splenic pulp. Br J Haematol 1974;27:201.
62. Myhre Jensen O, Kristensen J: Red pulp of the spleen in autoimmune haemolytic anaemia and hereditary spherocytosis: morphometric light and electron microscopy studies. Scand J Haematol 1986;36:263.
63. Krueger HC, Burgert EO Jr: Hereditary spherocytosis in 100 children. Mayo Clin Proc 1966;41:821.
64. Burman D: Congenital spherocytosis in infancy. Arch Dis Child 1958;33:335.
65. Trucco JI, Brown AK: Neonatal manifestations of hereditary spherocytosis. Am J Dis Child 1967;113:263.
66. Stamey C, Diamond L: Congenital hemolytic anemia in the newborn. Am J Dis Child 1957;94:616.
67. Iolascon A, Faienza MF, Moretti A, et al: UGT1 promoter polymorphism accounts for increased neonatal appearance of hereditary spherocytosis. Blood 1998;91:1093.
68. Agre P, Asimos A, Casella JF, McMillan C: Inheritance pattern and clinical response to splenectomy as a reflection of erythrocyte spectrin deficiency in hereditary spherocytosis. N Engl J Med 1986;315:1579.
69. Agre P, Casella JF, Zinkham WH, McMillan C, Bennett V: Partial deficiency of erythrocyte spectrin in hereditary spherocytosis. Nature 1985;314:380.
70. Agre P, Orringer EP, Bennett V: Deficient red-cell spectrin in severe, recessively inherited spherocytosis. N Engl J Med 1982;306:1155.
71. Tse WT, Gallagher PG, Jenkins PB, et al: Amino acid substitution in α-spectrin commonly coinherited with nondominant hereditary spherocytosis. Am J Hematol 1997;54:233.
72. Wichterle H, Hanspal M, Palek J, Jarolim P: Combination of two mutant alpha spectrin alleles underlies a severe spherocytic hemolytic anemia. J Clin Invest 1996;98:2300.
73. Whitfield CF, Follweiler JB, Lopresti-Morrow L, Miller BA: Deficiency of alpha-spectrin synthesis in burst-forming units-erythroid in lethal hereditary spherocytosis. Blood 1991;78:3043.
74. Allosio N, Texier P, Vallier A, et al: Modulation of clinical expression and band 3 deficiency in hereditary spherocytosis. Blood 1997;90:414.
75. Zipursky A, Chintu C, Brown E, Brown EJ: The quantitation of spherocytes in ABO hemolytic disease. J Pediatr 1979;94:965.
76. Pati AR, Patton WN, Harris RI: The use of the Technicon H1 in the diagnosis of hereditary spherocytosis. Clin Lab Haematol 1989;11:27.
77. Schroter W, Kahsnitz E: Diagnosis of hereditary spherocytosis in newborn infants. J Pediatr 1983;103:460.
78. Gallagher PG, Tse WT, Forget BG: Clinical and molecular aspects of disorders of the erythrocyte membrane skeleton. Semin Perinatol 1990;14:351.

79. Bergstrand C, Czar B: Serum haptoglobin in infancy. J Clin Lab Invest 1961;13:576.
80. Conboy J, Marchesi S, Kim R, et al: Molecular analysis of insertion/deletion mutations in protein 4.1 in elliptocytosis. II. Determination of molecular genetic origins of rearrangements. J Clin Invest 1990;86:524.
81. Conboy J, Mohandas N, Tchernia G, Kan YW: Molecular basis of hereditary elliptocytosis due to protein 4.1 deficiency. N Engl J Med 1986;315:680.
82. Delaunay J: Genetic disorders of the red cell membrane. Crit Rev Oncol Hematol 1995;19:79.
83. Delaunay J, Dhermy D: Mutations involving the spectrin heterodimer contact site: clinical expression and alterations in specific function. Semin Hematol 1993;30:21.
84. Maillet P, Alloisio N, Morle L, Delaunay J: Spectrin mutations in hereditary elliptocytosis and hereditary spherocytosis. Hum Mutat 1996;8:97.
85. Winardi R, Reid M, Conboy J, Mohandas N: Molecular analysis of glycophorin C deficiency in human erythrocytes. Blood 1993;81:2799.
86. Coetzer T, Palek J, Lawler J, et al: Structural and functional heterogeneity of alpha spectrin mutations involving the spectrin heterodimer self-association site: relationships to hematologic expression of homozygous hereditary elliptocytosis and hereditary pyropoikilocytosis. Blood 1990;75:2235.
87. Liu SC, Palek J, Prchal J, Castleberry RP: Altered spectrin dimer-dimer association and instability of erythrocyte membrane skeletons in hereditary pyropoikilocytosis. J Clin Invest 1981;68:597.
88. Conboy JG: Structure, function, and molecular genetics of erythroid membrane skeletal protein 4.1 in normal and abnormal red blood cells. Semin Hematol 1993;30:58.
89. Chishti AH, Palek J, Fisher D, et al: Reduced invasion and growth of *Plasmodium falciparum* into elliptocytic red blood cells with a combined deficiency of protein 4.1, glycophorin C, and p55. Blood 1996;87:3462.
90. Dluzewski AR, Nash GB, Wilson RJ, et al: Invasion of hereditary ovalocytes by *Plasmodium falciparum* in vitro and its relation to intracellular ATP concentration. Mol Biochem Parasitol 1992;55:1.
91. Austin RF, Desforges JF: Hereditary elliptocytosis: an unusual presentation of hemolysis in the newborn associated with transient morphologic abnormalities. Pediatrics 1969;44:196.
92. Baker SJ, Jacob E, Rajan KT, Gault EW: Hereditary haemolytic anaemia associated with elliptocytosis: a study of three families. Br J Haematol 1961;7:210.
93. Gallagher PG, Petruzzi MJ, Weed SA, et al: Mutation of a highly conserved residue of β spectrin associated with fatal and near-fatal neonatal hemolytic anemia. J Clin Invest 1997;99:267.
94. Gallagher PG, Weed SA, Tse WT, et al: Recurrent fatal hydrops fetalis associated with a nucleotide substitution in the erythrocyte beta-spectrin gene. J Clin Invest 1995;95:1174.
95. Sahr KE, Coetzer TL, Moy LS, et al: Spectrin Cagliari: an Ala–>Gly substitution in helix 1 of beta spectrin repeat 17 that severely disrupts the structure and self-association of the erythrocyte spectrin heterodimer. J Biol Chem 1993;268:22656.
96. Zarkowsky HS: Heat-induced erythrocyte fragmentation in neonatal elliptocytosis. Br J Haematol 1979;41:515.
97. Zarkowsky HS, Mohandas N, Speaker CB, Shohet SB: A congenital haemolytic anaemia with thermal sensitivity of the erythrocyte membrane. Br J Haematol 1975;29:537.
98. Coetzer T, Lawler J, Prchal JT, Palek J: Molecular determinants of clinical expression of hereditary elliptocytosis and pyropoikilocytosis. Blood 1987;70:766.
99. Morris SA, Ohanian V, Lewis ML, et al: Prenatal diagnosis of hereditary red cell membrane defect. Br J Haematol 1986;62:763.
100. Dhermy D, Feo C, Garbarz M, et al: Prenatal diagnosis of hereditary elliptocytosis with molecular defect of spectrin. Prenat Diagn 1987;7:471.
101. Nathan DG, Oski FA, Shaafi RI, Shohet SB: Congenital hemolytic anemia with extensive cation permeability. Blood 1966;28:976.
102. Nathan DG, Shohet SB: Erythrocyte ion transport defects and hemolytic anemia: "hydrocytosis" and "desiccytosis". Semin Hematol 1970;7:381.
103. Nolan GR: Hereditary xerocytosis. A case history and review of the literature. Pathology 1984;16:151.
104. Oski FA, Naiman JL, Blum SF, et al: Congenital hemolytic anemia with high-sodium, low-potassium red cells: studies of three generations of a family with a new variant. N Engl J Med 1969280:909.
105. Bienzle U, Bhadki S, Knufermann H, et al: Abnormality of erythrocyte membrane protein in a case of congenital stomatocytosis. Klin Wochenschr 1977;55:569.
106. Bienzle U, Niethammer D, Kleeberg U, et al: Congenital stomatocytosis and chronic haemolytic anaemia. Scand J Haematol 1975;15:339.
107. Entezami M, Becker R, Menssen HD, et al: Xerocytosis with concomitant intrauterine ascites: first description and therapeutic approach. Blood 1996; 87:5392.
108. Glader BE, Fortier N, Albala MM, Nathan DG: Congenital hemolytic anemia associated with dehydrated erythrocytes and increased potassium loss. N Engl J Med 1974;291:491.
109. Stewart GW, Amess JA, Eber SW, et al: Thromboembolic disease after splenectomy for hereditary stomatocytosis. Br J Haematol 1996;93:303.
110. Kanzaki A, Yawata Y: Hereditary stomatocytosis: phenotypical expression of sodium transport and band 7 peptides in 44 cases. Br J Haematol 1992;82:133.
111. Gross GP, Hathaway WE: Fetal erythrocyte deformability. Pediatr Res 1972;6:593.
112. Jain SK: The neonatal erythrocyte and its oxidative susceptibility. Semin Hematol 1989;26:286.
113. Mentzer WC Jr, Iarocci TA, Mohandas N, et al: Modulation of erythrocyte membrane mechanical stability by 2,3-diphosphoglycerate in the neonatal poikilocytosis/elliptocytosis syndrome. J Clin Invest 1987;79:943.

CHAPTER 12

Developmental Aspects of Blood Hemostasis and Disorders of Coagulation and Fibrinolysis in the Neonatal Period

Cynthia S. Edstrom, M.D., Robert D. Christensen, M.D., and Maureen Andrew, M.D.

Over the past two decades, significant advances have been made in the understanding of coagulation and fibrinolysis in adults. The hemostatic process is dynamic and in neonates depends on both gestational and postnatal age. Plasma concentrations of most hemostatic proteins are significantly different in fetuses, neonates, infants, and adults, and multiple reference ranges are needed to define normal values.[1, 2] The dynamic factor and protein values reflect the relative immaturity of the neonatal hemostatic system; however, they are physiologic and protect healthy infants from hemorrhagic and thrombotic complications. Adults with plasma concentrations for any single hemostatic protein similar to neonatal plasma concentrations are frequently at risk for pathologic bleeding or thrombosis. The relative immaturity of the neonatal hemostatic system places sick or stressed infants at risk for bleeding or thrombotic complications.[3]

Hemorrhagic and thrombotic problems are encountered frequently in sick neonates and present a complex challenge for neonatologists. Most severe congenital deficiencies of coagulant proteins and some congenital thrombotic disorders first present during the neonatal period, as do acquired hemorrhagic and thrombotic disorders. Neonatologists need to have an understanding of the evolution of the neonatal hemostatic system and a high index of suspicion to ensure accurate diagnoses and appropriate interventions for affected neonates.

This chapter reviews the physiology, diagnosis, and management of hemorrhagic and thrombotic problems. It emphasizes specific differences and needs of neonates and concentrates on the plasma or fluid phase of hemostasis. Issues related to platelet physiology and dysfunction are covered in Chapter 13.

COAGULATION

Principles

Coagulation was described in the 1960s as a cascade. According to the cascade model, each protein, beginning with factor XII, activates the next protein in the cascade sequence, leading ultimately to the production of fibrin.[4, 5] The cascade model of coagulation failed to explain the important role of tissue factor and factor VII, which were known to activate factor X in response to tissue damage. According to this model, coagulation could be initiated by either the "intrinsic" pathway, for which all required components were present in plasma, or the "extrinsic" pathway, for which tissue factor was required. The "intrinsic" pathway was activated by exposure to a glass surface such as a blood collection tube, and was assessed by the partial thromboplastin time. The "intrinsic" pathway was considered the primary mechanism of coagulation because deficiencies in "intrinsic" pathway factors VIII and IX resulted in severe bleeding. The "extrinsic" pathway, which was assessed by the prothrombin time, was considered less important than the "intrinsic" pathway.[6]

Although the cascade model of coagulation was useful, it did not adequately explain the following observations from known deficiency states: (1) patients with deficiencies of the contact factors (factor XII, high-molecular-weight kininogen, and prekallekrein) are asymptomatic; (2) patients with deficiencies of factor XI have much milder symptoms than patients with factor VIII or factor IX deficiency; and (3) patients with isolated factor VII deficiency bleed excessively.[7] Osterud and Rapaport[8] demonstrated that factor VII and tissue factor form a complex that then activates both factor IX and factor X. Elucidation of tissue factor/factor VIIa (activated factor VII) complex activation of factors IX and X, coupled with the recognition of tissue factor pathway inhibitor (also known as extrinsic pathway inhibitor and lipoprotein-associated inhibitor) as an important inhibitor of factor Xa (activated factor X) and the tissue factor/factor VIIa complex, suggested a more prominent role for the tissue factor/factor VII complex in the initiation of coagulation.

In a revised theory of coagulation, endothelial damage results in exposure of tissue factor to factor VII or factor VIIa. Factor VII is activated by tissue factor. Tissue factor and factor VIIa form a complex that, in the presence of ionized calcium and phospholipid, activates both factor X and factor IX. Some factor Xa then converts prothrombin to thrombin. The majority of factor Xa is rapidly bound by tissue factor pathway inhibitor, forming a tissue factor pathway inhibitor/factor Xa complex that then forms a quaternary complex with factor VIIa/tissue factor complex. The tissue factor pathway inhibitor/factor Xa/tissue factor/factor VIIa complex inhibits further activation of factor Xa by tissue factor. However, additional factor X is activated by factor IX. Thrombin activates factor XI to factor XIa, which activates factor IX. Factor IXa then converts factor X to factor Xa.[6]

Factor X, once converted to factor Xa, activates factor V by limited proteolysis. Factor Va then serves as a cofactor, in the presence of ionized calcium and a phospholipid surface, for factor Xa conversion of prothrombin to thrombin.[6, 9] Thrombin has many functions. It activates factor V by limited proteolysis[10] and activates factor XI, which enables further production of factor Xa and thrombin.[11] Thrombin contributes to its own inhibition by binding to thrombomodulin on cell surfaces. The thrombin/thrombomodulin complex activates protein C.[12] Thrombin cleaves fibrinopeptides A and B from fibrinogen in a highly complex reaction that results in the formation of fibrin. Once fibrinogen is cleaved by thrombin to form fibrin monomer, fibrin monomer rapidly polymerizes.[12] Fibrin monomer contains three domains: one central "E" domain and two "D" domains, one at each end of the molecule. Polymerization of fibrin proceeds by end-to-end association of the "D" domains and side-to-side association of the "E" domains. As polymerization progresses, a dense, insoluble fibrin "net" forms. Factor XIII stabilizes polymerized fibrin through the formation of cross-links between the "D" domains of adjacent fibrin monomers.[13] Cross-linked fibrin is resistant to fibrinolysis[13] (Fig. 12–1).

Coagulation Inhibitors

To achieve normal hemostasis, thrombin generation is regulated by a number of inhibitors. Direct plasma inhibitors of thrombin include antithrombin, α_2-macroglobulin, and heparin cofactor II. Indirect inhibitors include tissue factor pathway inhibitor, the thrombomodulin/protein C/protein S system, and fetal anticoagulant.

Antithrombin

Antithrombin is a glycoprotein serine protease inhibitor that is likely synthesized in hepato-

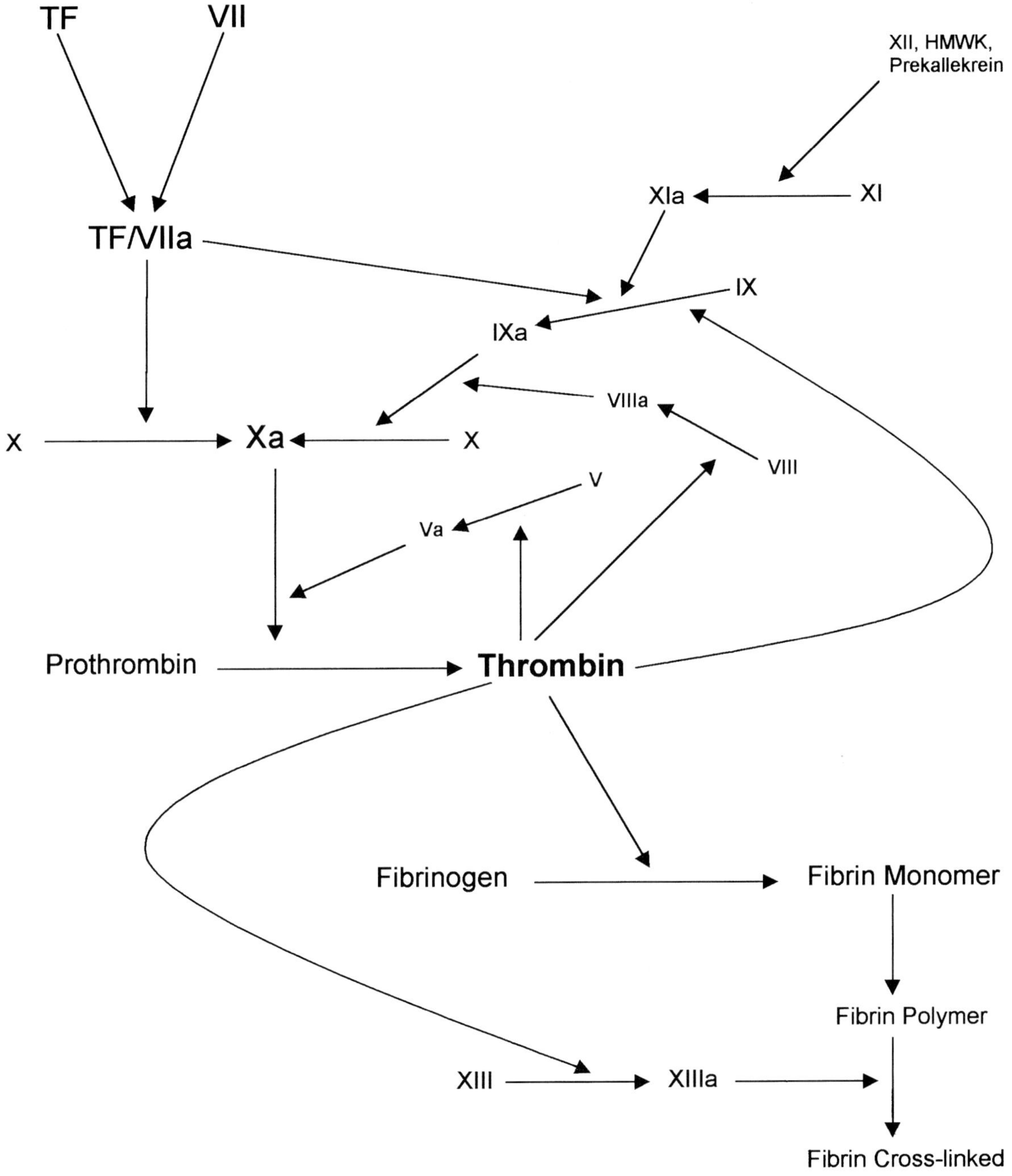

Figure 12–1. The blood coagulation system. TF, tissue factor; HMWK, high-molecular-weight kininogen; a, activated factor.

cytes and endothelial cells.[14–16] Antithrombin is the major inhibitor of the coagulation system and inhibits factor Xa, factor IXa, thrombin, and other coagulant serine proteases. In the absence of heparin, antithrombin inactivates proteases by forming 1:1 complexes relatively slowly. Heparin catalyzes antithrombin inhibition of thrombin 100,000-fold and factor Xa inhibition 3500-fold.[17] Heparin catalysis of antithrombin also blocks the conversion of tissue factor/factor VII to tissue factor/factor VIIa. Congenital deficiencies of antithrombin result in increased incidences of thromboses.[18]

Heparin Cofactor II

Heparin cofactor II is a glycoprotein serine protease inhibitor that is highly homologous with antithrombin. It inhibits thrombin directly by forming complexes that block a thrombin active site, but it does not inhibit other serine proteases. Similar to heparin catalysis of antithrombin, dermatan sulfate catalyzes the antithrombin activity of heparin cofactor II.[19, 20] Congenital deficiencies of heparin cofactor II are rare and result in increased risks of thromboses.[21–23]

α_2-Macroglobulin

α_2-Macroglobulin is a nonspecific protease inhibitor that is present in cerebrospinal fluid, the lungs, and other extravascular tissues.[24] It inhibits thrombin and other serine proteases.[25] In adults, α_2-macroglobulin is a less important inhibitor than antithrombin. In neonates, however, α_2-macroglobulin inhibits significantly more thrombin than it does in adults.[3, 24, 26] No congenital deficiencies of α_2-macroglobulin are recognized.

Tissue Factor Pathway Inhibitor

Tissue factor pathway inhibitor is a glycoprotein with three Kunitz domains. It is located on the microvascular endothelium and circulates in plasma in an unbound ("free") form and in a bound form associated with platelets and lipoproteins. It is a major inhibitor of coagulation initiation. Tissue factor pathway inhibitor binds factor Xa, forming a complex. The tissue factor pathway inhibitor/factor Xa complex then binds factor VIIa of the tissue factor/factor VIIa complex, forming a quaternary complex that lacks catalytic activity.[3, 26, 27] No congenital deficiencies of tissue factor pathway inhibitor are recognized.

Thrombomodulin

Thrombomodulin is a glycoprotein that serves as the endothelial cell surface receptor for thrombin. It is present on endothelial surfaces throughout the body, including the brain and the syncytiotrophoblast of the placenta.[28, 29] Thrombomodulin circulates in plasma, and increased concentrations might represent a marker for endothelial damage.[30–32] Thrombin binds thrombomodulin, forming 1:1 complexes. The conformation of thrombin reversibly changes when bound in thrombin/thrombomodulin complexes.[33] Thrombin/thrombomodulin complexes convert protein C to activated protein C by limited proteolysis.[33] Once bound to thrombomodulin, thrombin loses its capacity to cleave fibrinogen and to activate factor IX.[34] Thrombomodulin, fibrinogen, platelets, and factor V compete for the same binding site on thrombin, offering some insight into mechanisms of thrombin inhibition.[35] No congenital deficiencies of thrombomodulin are recognized.

Protein C

Protein C is a vitamin K–dependent zymogen that is produced primarily in the liver.[36] It is activated by the thrombin/thrombomodulin complex. Once activated, protein C proteolytically inactivates factors VIII and VIIIa[37] and factors V and Va by way of cleavage reactions.[38–41] Congenital deficiencies of protein C result in increased risks of thromboses.[42]

Protein S

Protein S is a vitamin K–dependent glycoprotein that is synthesized by hepatocytes,[36] vascular endothelial cells,[43] megakaryocytes,[44] and osteoblasts.[45] It serves as a cofactor for activated protein C, potentiating the inactivation of coagulation factors Va[46] and VIIIa.[47] Protein S is inactivated by factor Xa in the presence of ionized calcium and phospholipid, a reaction that is markedly inhibited by factor Va.[48] Protein S circulates in free and bound forms. The bound form complexes with C4b binding protein, a component of the complement system,[49] and loses its anticoagulant properties, forming a C4b binding protein/protein C/protein S complex that competitively inhibits free protein C/active protein S binding.[50] Congenital deficiencies result in increased risks of thromboses.[50–54]

Fetal and Neonatal Coagulation System

Coagulation proteins are synthesized independently by the fetus and do not cross the fetal-placental barrier. Plasma concentrations of most coagulation proteins are measurable by 5 to 10 weeks of gestational age[55] and increase gradually with advancing gestational age. Plasma concentrations of the coagulation system proteins in premature and healthy term infants differ markedly from those in adults. Reference ranges have been established (Tables 12–1 and 12–2).[1, 2] The pattern of differences is not homogeneous. Plasma concentrations of the vitamin K–dependent coagulant factors (factors II, VII, IX, and X) and the "contact factors" (factors XI and XII, prekallekrein, and high-molecular-weight kininogen) are less than 70% of adult values. Plasma concentrations of fibrinogen, factor V, factor VIII, von Willebrand's factor, and factor XIII are greater than 70% of normal adult values.[56]

Plasma concentrations of inhibitors of coagulation are also markedly different in neonates compared with adults (Table 12–3). Plasma concentrations of antithrombin and heparin cofactor II are decreased in neonates compared with adult values, and are within the concentration range at which spontaneous thromboses could occur in adults. Plasma concentrations of protein C and protein S are reduced at birth to 30% of adult plasma concentrations and remain decreased during the first weeks of life.[1, 2] Protein C circulates in a fetal form that differs from the adult form by a twofold increase in single-chain protein C.[57] Protein S, which circulates as both a free (active) and C4b binding protein bound (inactive) form in adults, circulates primarily in the free (active) form in neonates, because C4b binding protein is absent in neonatal plasma. Because most neonatal protein S is in the free form, protein S activity is approximately 75% of adult activity, even though plasma concentrations of protein S are 25% of adult concentrations.[58, 59]

In contrast to the decreased plasma concentrations of protein C and protein S, plasma concentrations of thrombomodulin are severalfold higher in neonates than in adults and remain increased during early childhood. The influence of age on endothelial cell expression of thrombomodulin has not been determined. Plasma concentrations of antithrombin, heparin cofactor II, and protein S increase to within the adult range by 6 months of age. Protein C plasma concentrations do not reach adult plasma concentrations until early childhood.[60]

Plasma concentrations of α_2-macroglobulin and C1-esterase inhibitor are within the adult range at birth and increase to well above the adult range by 6 months of postnatal life. α_2-Macroglobulin is a more important inhibitor than C1-esterase inhibitor in neonates. Increased plasma concentrations of α_2-macroglobin might compensate in part for decreased plasma concentrations of antithrombin in neonates.[26, 61] Plasma concentrations of tissue factor pathway inhibitor are available from one small series and its plasma activities have been studied in another series. Cord blood concentrations of tissue factor pathway inhibitor are approximately 30% of adult concentrations in fetuses 19 to 38 weeks of gestational age and are 50% in healthy term neonates.[62] Tissue factor pathway inhibitor activities from venipuncture specimens from healthy term neonates are approximately 88% of normal adult activities.[63]

The unique balance of coagulant proteins and inhibitors of coagulation in neonates influences overall generation of thrombin. Thrombin generation in neonates is similar to that in adults receiving therapeutic doses of warfarin or heparin.[64] The quantity of thrombin generated is directly proportional to prothrombin concentrations, whereas the rate of generation reflects concentrations of other procoagulants.

Neonatal thrombin generation is influenced by the presence of fetal anticoagulant. Fetal

Text continued on page 247

Table 12–1. **Reference Values for Coagulation Tests in Healthy Full-Term Infants During the First 6 Months of Life and in Adults**

Coagulation Tests	Day 1 M (B)	Day 5 M (B)	Day 30 M (B)	Day 90 M (B)	Day 180 M (B)	Adult M (B)
PT (s)	13.0 (10.1–15.9)*	12.4 (10.0–15.3)*	11.8 (10.0–14.3)*	11.9 (10.0–14.2)*	12.3 (10.7–13.9)*	12.4 (10.8–13.9)
INR	1.00 (0.53–1.62)	0.89 (0.53–1.48)	0.79 (0.53–1.26)	0.81 (0.53–1.26)	0.88 (0.61–1.17)	0.89 (0.64–1.17)
APTT (s)	42.9 (31.3–54.5)	42.6 (25.4–59.8)	40.4 (32.0–55.2)	37.1 (29.0–50.1)*	35.5 (28.1–42.9)*	33.5 (26.6–40.3)
TCT (s)	23.5 (19.0–28.3)*	23.1 (18.0–29.2)	24.3 (19.4–29.2)	25.1 (20.5–29.7)*	25.5 (19.8–31.2)*	25.0 (19.7–30.3)
Fibrinogen (g/L)	2.83 (1.67–3.99)*	3.12 (1.62–4.62)*	2.70 (1.62–3.78)*	2.43 (1.50–3.79)*	2.51 (1.50–3.87)*	2.78 (1.56–4.00)
Factor II (U/mL)	0.48 (0.26–0.70)	0.63 (0.33–0.93)	0.68 (0.34–1.02)	0.75 (0.45–1.05)	0.88 (0.60–1.16)	1.08 (0.70–1.46)
Factor V (U/mL)	0.72 (0.34–1.08)	0.95 (0.45–1.45)	0.98 (0.62–1.34)	0.90 (0.45–1.32)	0.91 (0.55–1.27)	1.06 (0.62–1.50)
Factor VII (U/mL)	0.66 (0.28–1.04)	0.89 (0.35–1.43)	0.90 (0.42–1.38)	0.91 (0.39–1.43)	0.87 (0.47–1.27)	1.05 (0.67–1.43)
Factor VIII (U/mL)	1.00 (0.50–1.78)*	0.88 (0.50–1.54)*	0.91 (0.50–1.57)	0.79 (0.50–1.25)*	0.73 (0.50–1.09)	0.99 (0.50–1.49)
vWf (U/mL)	1.53 (0.50–2.87)	1.40 (0.50–2.54)	1.28 (0.50–2.46)	1.18 (0.50–2.06)	1.07 (0.50–1.97)	0.92 (0.50–1.58)
Factor IX (U/mL)	0.53 (0.15–0.91)	0.53 (0.15–0.91)	0.51 (0.21–0.81)	0.67 (0.21–1.13)	0.86 (0.36–1.36)	1.09 (0.55–1.63)
Factor X (U/mL)	0.40 (0.12–0.68)	0.49 (0.19–0.79)	0.59 (0.31–0.87)	0.71 (0.35–1.07)	0.78 (0.38–1.18)	1.06 (0.70–1.52)
Factor XI (U/mL)	0.38 (0.10–0.66)	0.55 (0.23–0.87)	0.53 (0.27–0.79)	0.69 (0.41–0.97)	0.86 (0.49–1.34)	0.97 (0.67–1.27)
Factor XII (U/mL)	0.53 (0.13–0.93)	0.47 (0.11–0.83)	0.49 (0.17–0.81)	0.67 (0.25–1.09)	0.77 (0.39–1.15)	1.08 (0.52–1.64)
PK (U/mL)	0.37 (0.18–0.69)	0.48 (0.20–0.76)	0.57 (0.23–0.91)	0.73 (0.41–1.05)	0.86 (0.56–1.16)	1.12 (0.62–1.62)
HMWK (U/mL)	0.54 (0.06–1.02)	0.74 (0.16–1.32)	0.77 (0.33–1.21)	0.82 (0.30–1.46)*	0.82 (0.36–1.28)*	0.92 (0.50–1.36)
Factor XIIIa (U/mL)	0.79 (0.27–1.31)	0.94 (0.44–1.44)*	0.93 (0.39–1.47)*	1.04 (0.36–1.72)*	1.04 (0.46–1.62)*	1.05 (0.55–1.55)
Factor XIIIb (U/mL)	0.76 (0.30–1.22)	1.06 (0.32–1.80)	1.11 (0.39–1.73)*	1.16 (0.48–1.84)*	1.10 (0.50–1.70)	0.97 (0.57–1.37)

All factors except fibrinogen are expressed as units per milliliter (U/mL) where pooled plasma contains 1.0 U/mL. All values are expressed as mean (M) followed by the lower and upper boundary encompassing 95% of the population (B). Between 40 and 77 samples were assayed for each value for the population.

INR = International normalized ratio; TCT = thrombin clotting time; vWf = von Willibrand's factor; HMWK = high molecular weight lininogen.

*Values indistinguishable from those of the adult.

(From Andrew M, Paes B, Johnston M: Development of the hemostatic system in the neonate and young infant. Am J Pediatr Hematol Oncol 1990;12:95.)

Table 12–2. **Reference Values for Coagulation Tests in Healthy Premature Infants (30–36 Weeks' Gestation) During the First 6 Months of Life and Adults**

Coagulation Tests	Day 1 M (B)	Day 5 M (B)	Day 30 M (B)	Day 90 M (B)	Day 180 M (B)	Adult M (B)
PT (s)	13.0 (10.6–16.2)*	12.5 (10.0–15.3)*	11.8 (10.0–13.6)*	12.3 (10.0–14.6)	12.5 (10.0–15.0)*	12.4 (10.8–13.9)
INR	1.0 (0.61–1.70)	0.91 (0.53–1.48)	0.79 (0.53–1.11)	0.88 (0.53–1.32)	0.91 (0.53–1.48)	0.89 (0.64–1.17)
APTT (s)	53.6 (27.5–79.4)†	50.5 (26.9–74.1)	44.7 (26.9–62.5)	39.5 (28.3–50.7)	37.5 (27.2–53.3)	33.5 (26.6–40.3)
TCT (s)	24.8 (19.2–30.4)	24.1 (18.8–29.4)*	24.4 (18.8–29.9)	25.1 (19.4–30.8)	25.2 (18.9–31.5)	25.0 (19.7–30.3)
Fibrinogen (g/L)	2.43 (1.50–3.73)*,†	2.80 (1.60–4.18)*,†	2.54 (1.50–4.14)	2.46 (1.50–3.52)	2.28 (1.50–3.60)	2.78 (1.56–4.00)
Factor II (U/mL)	0.45 (0.20–0.77)	0.57 (0.29–0.85)†	0.57 (0.36–0.95)	0.68 (0.30–1.06)	0.87 (0.51–1.23)	1.08 (0.70–1.46)
Factor V (U/mL)	0.88 (0.41–1.44)*,†	1.00 (0.46–1.54)*	1.02 (0.48–1.56)*	0.99 (0.59–1.39)	1.02 (0.58–1.46)*	1.06 (0.62–1.50)
Factor VII (U/mL)	0.67 (0.21–1.13)	0.84 (0.30–1.38)	0.83 (0.21–1.45)	0.87 (0.31–1.43)	0.99 (0.47–1.51)*	1.05 (0.67–1.43)
Factor VIII (U/mL)	1.11 (0.50–2.13)	1.15 (0.53–2.05)*,†	1.11 (0.50–1.99)	1.06 (0.58–1.88)*,†	0.99 (0.50–1.87)*,†	0.99 (0.50–1.49)
vWf (U/mL)	1.36 (0.78–2.10)	1.33 (0.72–2.19)	1.36 (0.66–2.16)	1.12 (0.75–1.84)*,†	0.98 (0.54–1.58)*	0.92 (0.50–1.58)
Factor IX (U/mL)	0.35 (0.19–0.65)†	0.42 (0.14–0.74)†	0.44 (0.13–0.80)	0.59 (0.25–0.93)	0.81 (0.50–1.20)	1.09 (0.55–1.63)
Factor X (U/mL)	0.41 (0.11–0.71)	0.51 (0.19–0.83)	0.56 (0.20–0.92)	0.67 (0.35–0.99)	0.77 (0.35–1.19)	1.06 (0.70–1.52)
Factor XI (U/mL)	0.30 (0.08–0.52)†	0.41 (0.13–0.69)†	0.43 (0.15–0.71)†	0.59 (0.25–0.93)	0.78 (0.46–1.10)	0.97 (0.67–1.27)
Factor XII (U/mL)	0.38 (0.10–0.66)†	0.39 (0.09–0.69)†	0.43 (0.11–0.75)	0.61 (0.15–1.07)	0.82 (0.22–1.42)	1.08 (0.52–1.64)
PK (U/mL)	0.33 (0.09–0.57)	0.45 (0.25–0.75)	0.59 (0.31–0.87)	0.79 (0.37–1.21)	0.78 (0.40–1.16)	1.12 (0.62–1.62)
HMWK (U/mL)	0.49 (0.09–0.89)	0.62 (0.24–1.00)†	0.64 (0.16–1.12)†	0.78 (0.32–1.24)	0.83 (0.41–1.25)*	0.92 (0.50–1.36)
Factor XIIIa (U/mL)	0.70 (0.32–1.08)	1.01 (0.57–1.45)*	0.99 (0.51–1.47)*	1.13 (0.71–1.55)*	1.13 (0.65–1.61)*	1.05 (0.55–1.55)
Factor XIIIb (U/mL)	0.81 (0.35–1.27)	1.10 (0.68–1.58)*	1.07 (0.57–1.57)*	1.21 (0.75–1.67)	1.15 (0.67–1.63)	0.97 (0.57–1.37)

All factors except fibrinogen are expressed as units per milliliter (U/mL) where pooled plasma contains 1.0 U/mL. All values are given as a mean (M) followed by the lower and upper boundary encompassing 95% of the population (B). Between 40 and 96 samples were assayed for each value for the newborn. Some measurements were skewed owing to a disproportionate number of high values. The lower limits exclude the lower 2.5% of the population.

*Values indistinguishable from those of adults.

†Measurements are skewed owing to a disproportionate number of high values.

(From Andrew M, Paes B, Johnston M: Development of the human coagulation system in the healthy premature infant. Blood 1988;72:1651.)

Table 12–3. **Reference Values for the Inhibitors of Coagulation in Infants During the First 6 Months of Life and Adults**

Inhibitor Levels	Day 1 M (B)	Day 5 M (B)	Day 30 M (B)	Day 90 M (B)	Day 180 M (B)	Adult M (B)
Healthy Full-Term Infants						
AT (U/mL)	0.63 (0.39–0.87)	0.67 (0.41–0.93)	0.78 (0.48–1.08)	0.97 (0.73–1.21)*	1.04 (0.84–1.24)*	1.05 (0.79–1.31)
α_2M (U/mL)	1.39 (0.95–1.83)	1.48 (0.98–1.98)	1.50 (1.06–1.94)	1.76 (1.26–2.26)	1.91 (1.49–2.33)	0.86 (0.52–1.20)
C1E-INH (U/mL)	0.72 (0.36–1.08)	0.90 (0.60–1.20)*	0.89 (0.47–1.31)	1.15 (0.71–1.59)	1.41 (0.89–1.93)	1.01 (0.71–1.31)
α_1AT (U/mL)	0.93 (0.49–1.37)*	0.89 (0.49–1.29)*	0.62 (0.36–0.88)	0.72 (0.42–1.02)	0.77 (0.47–1.07)	0.93 (0.55–1.31)
HCII (U/mL)	0.43 (0.10–0.93)	0.48 (0.00–0.96)	0.47 (0.10–0.87)	0.72 (0.10–1.46)	1.20 (0.50–1.90)	0.96 (0.66–1.26)
Protein C (U/mL)	0.35 (0.17–0.53)	0.42 (0.20–0.64)	0.43 (0.21–0.65)	0.54 (0.28–0.80)	0.59 (0.37–0.81)	0.96 (0.64–1.28)
Protein S (U/mL)	0.36 (0.12–0.60)	0.50 (0.22–0.78)	0.63 (0.33–0.93)	0.86 (0.54–1.18)*	0.87 (0.55–1.19)*	0.92 (0.60–1.24)
TM (AU)	10.55 (4.84–16.25)				7.26 (3.96–10.56)	4.60 (2.9–6.3)
TFPI (U/mL)‡	0.7331*					0.8270
Healthy Premature Infants (30–36 Weeks' Gestation)						
AT (U/mL)	0.38 (0.14–0.62)†	0.56 (0.30–0.82)	0.59 (0.37–0.81)†	0.83 (0.45–1.21)†	0.90 (0.52–1.28)†	1.05 (0.79–1.31)
α_2M (U/mL)	1.10 (0.56–1.82)†	1.25 (0.71–1.77)	1.38 (0.72–2.04)	1.80 (1.20–2.66)	2.09 (1.10–3.21)	0.86 (0.52–1.20)
C1E-INH (U/mL)	0.65 (0.31–0.99)	0.83 (0.45–1.21)	0.74 (0.40–1.24)†	1.14 (0.60–1.68)*	1.40 (0.96–2.04)	1.01 (0.71–1.31)
α_1AT (U/mL)	0.90 (0.36–1.44)*	0.94 (0.42–1.46)*	0.76 (0.38–1.12)†	0.81 (0.49–1.13)*,†	0.82 (0.48–1.16)*	0.93 (0.55–1.31)
HCII (U/mL)	0.32 (0.10–0.60)†	0.34 (0.10–0.69)	0.43 (0.15–0.71)	0.61 (0.20–1.11)	0.89 (0.45–1.40)*,†	0.96 (0.66–1.26)
Protein C (U/mL)	0.28 (0.12–0.44)†	0.31 (0.11–0.51)	0.37 (0.15–0.59)†	0.45 (0.23–0.67)†	0.57 (0.31–0.83)	0.96 (0.64–1.28)
Protein S (U/mL)	0.26 (0.14–0.38)†	0.37 (0.13–0.61)	0.56 (0.22–0.90)	0.76 (0.40–1.12)†	0.82 (0.44–1.20)	0.92 (0.60–1.24)

AT = antithrombin; α_2M = α_2-macroglobulin; C1E-INH = C1 esterase inhibitor; α_1AT = α_1-antitrypsin; TM = thrombomodulin.

All values are expressed in units per milliliter (U/mL) where pooled plasma contains 1.0 U/mL. All values are given as a mean (M) followed by the lower and upper boundary encompassing 95% of the population (B). Between 40 and 75 samples were assayed for each value for the newborn. Some measurements were skewed owing to a disproportionate number of high values. The lower limits exclude the lower 2.5% of the population.

*Values indistinguishable from those of adults.

†Values different from those of full-term infants.

‡Cord blood.

(From Andrew M, Paes B, Johnston M: Development of the hemostatic system in the neonate and young infant. Am J Pediatr Hematol Oncol 1990;12:95.)

anticoagulant has a molecular weight of 150,000 and catalyzes heparin cofactor II inhibition of thrombin.[65, 66] It is present in the plasma of pregnant women and neonates and is produced by the placenta.[67] The length of time fetal anticoagulant persists in neonates is not precisely known, but it is detectable during the first week of life in sick premature infants with hyaline membrane disease.[68]

Plasma concentrations of fibrinogen are similar in neonates and adults. However, fibrinogen in neonates is characterized by an increased sialic acid content compared with adult fibrinogen. If sialic acid is removed, fetal fibrinogen is indistinguishable from adult fibrinogen.[69–72] The physiologic significance of fetal fibrinogen is unknown, and it disappears during early infancy.

The capacity of neonatal fibrin clots to bind thrombin has been assessed by measuring fibrinopeptide A production.[73] Cord plasma clots generate significantly less fibrinopeptide A than clots formed in adult plasma because of the decreased concentrations of prothrombin in cord plasma.[73] In vitro, the addition of prothrombin to cord plasma increases fibrinopeptide A production by cord plasma clots, which suggests that thrombi in neonates might not have the same propensity to propagate as in adults.

Potential mechanisms to explain the physiologic differences in the coagulation system in neonates include (1) decreased synthesis, (2) increased clearance, and (3) increased consumption.

Synthesis of coagulation factors has been assessed for factors VII, VIII, IX, and X and for fibrinogen, antithrombin, and protein C in hepatocytes from 5- to 10-week gestational age embryos, fetuses, and adults. mRNA transcripts are similar in size for adults, embryos, and fetuses, and the nucleotide sequences for mRNA of factors X and IX are identical in adults, embryos, and fetuses. Expression of mRNA in fetal hepatocytes is variable, resulting in concentrations of factor IX that are similar to those of adults but concentrations of factors VII and X that are discordant. Similarly, hepatocyte content of specific coagulation proteins differs and does not necessarily match mRNA expression,[55] suggesting that differences in synthesis of coagulation factors account for some, but not all, of the age-related differences.

Clearance of coagulation proteins is more rapid in neonates than in adults. The half-life of fibrinogen is significantly shorter in healthy neonatal animals and in infants with HMD compared with adults. The half-life of antithrombin is shorter in infants requiring exchange transfusion due to hyperbilirubinemia than it is in healthy adults. Mechanisms for faster clearance of coagulation proteins in neonates are incompletely understood but might reflect an increased basal metabolic rate. Rapid clearance of coagulation proteins in neonates influences factor replacement strategies for sick neonates.[3, 74–76]

Increased consumption of coagulation proteins during the birth process is suggested by detectable cord blood plasma concentrations of fibrinopeptide A and thrombin–antithrombin complexes. However, consumption appears to be well controlled and self-limited, and does not likely contribute to decreased plasma concentrations of coagulation proteins or clinical morbidity.[3, 65, 77–79] Following birth, the coagulation system of premature and term infants gradually becomes similar to the adult system. By 6 months of age, most plasma concentrations of coagulation proteins approximate adult concentrations.[1, 2]

FIBRINOLYSIS

Principles

The fibrinolytic system comprises activators and inhibitors that regulate the conversion of plasminogen to plasmin and thereby control the remodeling and degradation of fibrin clots. Plasminogen, the central zymogen in the fibrinolytic process, is synthesized in the liver as Glu-plasminogen (a single-chain protein) and cleaved by an activator at a single bond to generate plasmin. Plasmin consists of two chains: a heavy chain, containing five structures called *kringles*, four of which participate in fibrin binding, and a light chain, which contains the fibrin catalytic site. Plasmin is a serine protease that hydrolyzes fibrin and fibrinogen at specific sites, resulting in proteolytic degradation. The proteolytic activities of plasmin are nonspecific, resulting in the proteolytic degradation of factor V, factor VIII, growth hormone, corticotropin, and some components of the complement system. Plasmin also cleaves Glu-plasminogen, generating Lys-plasminogen, which accelerates the conversion of plasminogen to plasmin because the Lys form of plasminogen is more readily activated.[80]

The fibrinolytic system is activated by two specific activators: tissue-plasminogen activator (t-PA) and urokinase-plasminogen activator (u-PA). t-PA is located primarily on the vascular endothelium and is released upon stimulation by thrombin.[81, 82] t-PA exists as a single-chain form[81, 82] which is rapidly converted by plasmin or kallikrein to a more active double-chain form.[83] t-PA has high affinity for fibrin and, once bound to fibrin, rapidly converts plasminogen to plasmin.[81] u-PA exists in two forms: single-chain u-PA, with minimal intrinsic fibrinolytic activity, and two-chain u-PA (also known as urokinase), which is formed from single-chain u-PA. u-PA is normally present in urine.[80]

The fibrinolytic system is also activated by the "contact" pathway. Factors XIa and XIIa and kallikrein all cause conversion of plasminogen to plasmin. The physiologic role of "contact" pathway activation of the fibrinolytic system is uncertain, however, because deficiencies of "contact" factors do not to result in increased risks of thrombotic events.[84, 85]

The activation of the fibrinolytic system results in proteolysis of fibrinogen and fibrin. Fibrinogen and non-cross-linked fibrin are proteolyzed into several fragments. The largest and first to appear is the X fragment. Proteolysis of the X fragment yields a Y fragment and one "D piece." The Y fragment is further degraded to a "D piece" and an "E piece." Cross-linked fibrin is proteolyzed into distinct degradation products, the structure of which depends on where in the fibrin polymer proteolysis occurs. The final degradation products from complete proteolysis of cross-linked fibrin are D-dimers and "E pieces."[13] D-dimers are unique to the breakdown of cross-linked fibrin and serve as clinical markers for fibrinolysis.[80]

α_2-Antiplasmin and plasminogen activator inhibitor are important inhibitors of fibrinolysis. α_2-Antiplasmin directly inhibits plasmin by forming catalytic site complexes.[86] It is present in plasma and functions to confine plasmin activity to fibrin, thus preventing systemic fibrinolysis.[87] Factor XIII cross-links α_2-antiplasmin to fibrin, which makes fibrin more resistant to degredation by plasmin.[88, 89] Plasminogen activator inhibitor exists in four forms, of which only plasminogen activator inhibitor-1 is known to have fibrinolytic activity. Plasminogen activator inhibitor is synthesized by endothelial cells and hepatocytes and is present in plasma and on the surface of platelets.[90] Synthesis of plasminogen activator inhibitor is stimulated by endotoxin,[91] thrombin,[92] interleukin-1,[93] tumor necrosis factor-α,[94] and transforming growth factor-β.[95] Plasminogen activator inhibitor activity is inhibited enzymatically by thrombin.[92]

The complex process of fibrinolysis is predominantly a local event. As a clot forms and fibrin polymerizes, plasminogen is incorporated into the clot. The presence of fibrin stimulates t-PA and u-PA, which are located in or on the involved endothelium. Thus, t-PA and u-PA are immediately available to convert plasminogen to plasmin. Plasmin then degrades fibrin and fibrinogen in the clot and stimulates further formation of plasmin. Plasmin released from the clot is rapidly inactivated by ubiquitously circulating inhibitor α_2-antiplasmin. t-PA and u-PA molecules that enter the systemic circulation are rapidly inactivated by plasminogen activator inhibitor-1. Plasminogen activator inhibitor and α_2-antiplasmin are also incorporated into the clot structure, aiding in local control of plasmin generation. Therefore, under physiologic conditions, the balance of fibrinolytic activators and inhibitors prevents systemic fibrinolysis while limiting local thrombosis[80] (Fig. 12–2).

Neonatal Fibrinolysis

Similar to the coagulation system, the fibrinolytic system in neonates is dynamic. Plasma concentrations of plasminogen are decreased at birth (58% of adult concentrations) and increase gradually to approximate adult concentrations by 6 months after birth. Plasma concentrations of t-PA are approximately twice adult concentrations and decrease to normal adult plasma concentrations by day 5 of life. α_2-Antiplasmin plasma concentrations are moderately decreased compared with adult values and reach adult plasma concentrations by day 5 of life. Plasma concentrations of plasminogen activator inhibitor are also approximately twice adult concentrations at birth, decrease to adult plasma concentration values by day 5 of life

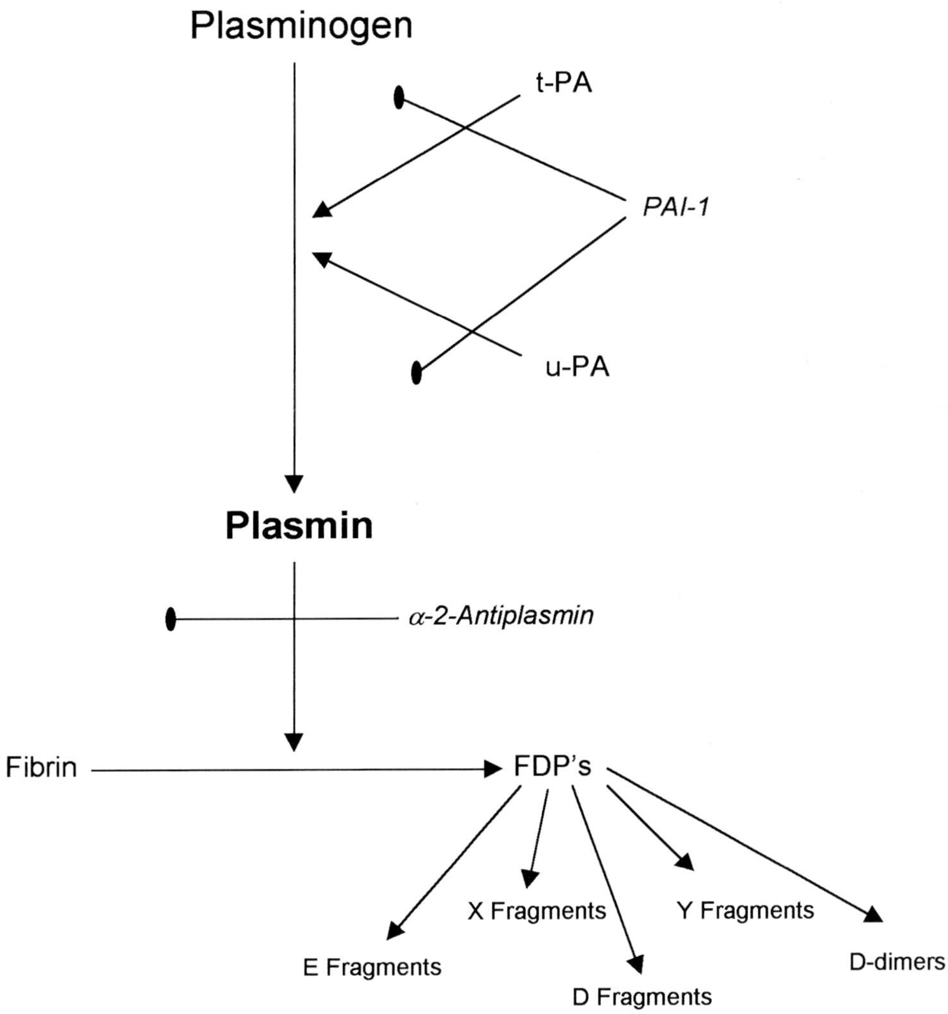

Figure 12–2. The blood fibrinolysis system. t-PA, tissue plasminogen activator; u-PA, urokinase plasminogen activator; PAI-1, plasminogen activator inhibitor-1; FDP, fibrin degradation product; filled oval attached to a line, inhibition.

and then increase throughout the next several months. By 6 months of age, plasma concentrations of plasminogen activator inhibitor are greater than twice the normal adult plasma concentrations[5, 56] (Table 12–4).

GENERAL APPROACH TO NEONATAL BLEEDING DISORDERS

Neonates with clinically significant bleeding should be evaluated for hemostatic deficits. Although acquired bleeding problems are most common in neonates, severe forms of congenital factor deficiencies present in the neonatal period and must be seriously considered, especially in healthy infants with unexplained bleeding.

Clinical Presentation

The clinical presentation of bleeding disorders is different in neonates compared with children or adults. Abnormal bleeding presents with oozing from the umbilicus, bleeding into the scalp, large cephalohematomas, bleeding following circumcision, oozing from peripheral venipuncture sites, and bleeding into the skin. A small but important portion of infants present with an intracranial hemorrhage as the first manifestation of a bleeding problem. Critically ill neonates also have bleeding from mucous membranes, the bladder, and sites of invasive procedures. In contrast to older children, neonates rarely develop hemarthroses.

Clinically significant bleeding in healthy-appearing neonates is most often caused by thrombocytopenia secondary to transplacental passage of maternal antiplatelet antibody, vitamin K deficiency, or, less commonly, severe congenital coagulation factor deficiencies. Sick neonates with clinically significant bleeding most often have acquired disorders such as disseminated intravascular coagulation or liver failure. However, clinically significant bleeding in sick neonates can be the result of underlying congenital coagulation deficiencies.[3]

Laboratory Evaluation

The initial laboratory evaluation of infants with bleeding complications includes a prothrombin time (PT), activated partial thromboplastin time (aPTT), thrombin time, fibrinogen level, platelet count, and, in some patients, a bleeding time. Abnormal results from these tests guide the selection of additional tests such as specific factor assays and paracoagulation tests. For a male child in whom hemophilia A or B is suspected, specific factor assays should be performed regardless of the aPTT value. Deficiencies of factor XIII and α_2-antiplasmin do not prolong screening tests and must be measured directly if suspected. Differentiation of congenital and acquired deficiencies by physiologic values can be difficult for some coagulation proteins because of physiologically decreased plasma concentrations in neonates.[3]

Management

The appropriate management of infants with bleeding disorders depends on the correct identification of the hemostatic defect. Appropriate diagnosis allows for replacement therapy with specific factor concentrates, fresh frozen plasma, stored plasma, platelet concentrates, or cryoprecipitate.

INHERITED BLEEDING DISORDERS

Inheritance Pattern and Clinical Features

Deficiencies of factors II, V, VII, XI, and XII and prekallikrein and high-molecular-weight kininogen are rare, autosomally inherited disorders. Consanguinity is frequently present in families of homozygous patients. Deficiencies of factor XII, prekallikrein, and high-molecular-weight kininogen do not result in bleeding disorders. Deficiencies of factors VIII and IX are X-linked recessive disorders and are the most common inherited causes of bleeding in neonates. Combined deficiencies are rare and do present in the neonatal period.[3]

Most patients with inherited factor deficiencies do not present in the neonatal period unless confronted with a hemostatic challenge. Full-term neonates with intracranial hemorrhage or healthy neonates with hemostatic abnormalities

Table 12–4. **Reference Values for the Components of the Fibrinolytic System During the First 6 Months of Life and Adults**

Fibrinolytic System	Day 1 M (B)	Day 5 M (B)	Day 30 M (B)	Day 90 M (B)	Day 180 M (B)	Adult M (B)
Healthy Full-Term Infants						
Plasminogen (U/mL)	0.58 (0.37–0.79)	0.65 (0.42–0.87)	0.59 (0.38–0.80)	0.74 (0.52–0.96)	0.90 (0.66–1.13)	1.00 (0.74–1.26)
TPA (ng/mL)	9.60 (5.00–18.9)	5.60 (4.00–10.0)*	4.10 (1.00–6.00)*	2.10 (1.00–5.00)*	2.80 (1.00–6.00)	4.90 (1.40–8.40)
α_2AP (U/mL)	0.85 (0.55–1.15)	1.00 (0.70–1.30)*	1.00 (0.76–1.24)*	1.08 (0.76–1.40)*	1.11 (0.83–1.39)*	1.02 (0.68–1.36)
PAI (U/mL)	6.40 (2.00–15.1)	2.30 (0.00–8.10)*	3.4 (0.00–8.80)*	7.20 (1.00–15.3)	8.10 (6.00–13.0)	3.6 (0.00–11.0)
Healthy Premature Infants						
Plasminogen (U/mL)	0.51 (0.33–0.74)†	0.56 (0.36–0.78)†	0.54 (0.32–0.75)	0.71 (0.47–0.95)	0.82 (0.57–1.07)	1.00 (0.74–1.26)
TPA (ng/mL)	8.48 (3.00–16.70)	3.97 (2.00–6.93)*	4.13 (2.00–7.79)*	3.31 (2.00–5.07)*	3.48 (2.00–5.85)*	4.96 (1.46–8.46)
α_2AP (U/mL)	0.78 (0.40–1.16)	0.81 (0.49–1.13)†	0.89 (0.55–1.23)†	1.06 (0.64–1.48)*	1.15 (0.77–1.53)	1.02 (0.68–1.36)
PAI (U/mL)	5.40 (0.00–12.2)*,†	2.50 (0.00–7.10)*	4.30 (0.00–11.8)*	4.80 (1.00–10.2)*,†	4.90 (1.00–10.2)*,†	3.60 (0.00–11.0)
μ-PA (ng/mL)	0.18 (0.08–0.28)‡					0.32 (0.18–0.46)
PAI-2 (ng/mL)	<1.6‡					<1.6

TPA = tissue plasminogen activator; PAI = plasminogen activator inhibitor; μ-PA = urokinase plasminogen activator.

For α_2AP, values are expressed as units per milliliter (U/mL) where pooled plasma contains 1.0 U/mL. Plasminogen units are those recommended by the Committee on Thrombolytic Agents. Values for TPA are given as nanograms per milliliter. Values for PAI are given as units per millliliter where one unit of PAI-1 activity is defined as the amount of PAI-1 that inhibits one international unit of human single chain TPA. All values are given as a mean (M) followed by the lower and upper boundary encompassing 95% of the population (B).

*Values indistinguishable from those of adults.

†Values different from those of full-term infant.

‡Cord blood.

(Data from Andrew M, Paes B, Johnston M: Development of the hemostatic system in the neonate and young infant. Am J Pediatr Hematol Oncol 1990;12:95, and Reverdiau-Moalic P, Gruel Y, et al: Comparative study of the fibrinolytic system in human fetuses and in pregnant women. Thromb Res 1991;61:489.)

require evaluation for inherited bleeding disorders.[96–98] Severe factor VII deficiency is the most common inherited factor deficiency causing intracranial hemorrhage in neonates. However, deficiencies of factors II, V, VII, VIII, IX, X, XI, or XIII can cause neonatal intracranial hemorrhage.[99]

Diagnosis

The diagnosis of inherited coagulation deficiencies is established based on interpretation of abnormal screening tests, followed by evaluation for specific factor deficiencies. Test results for plasma concentrations of coagulation factors should be interpreted in the context of established age-specific and gestational age-specific reference ranges.[1, 2] Homozygous deficiencies of factors V, VII, or XIII result in plasma concentrations of deficient factor that are less than 0.01, 0.03, and 0.01 unit/mL, respectively; these plasma concentrations are significantly decreased compared to physiologic neonatal plasma concentrations. Severe homozygous deficiencies of factors VIII or IX are defined by plasma concentrations of deficient factor that are less than 0.01 unit/mL, which are significantly decreased compared with physiologic neonatal plasma concentrations. In contrast, homozygous deficiencies of factors II, X, and XI are defined by plasma concentrations of deficient factor that are less than 0.20, 0.10, and 0.15 unit/mL, respectively; these plasma concentrations overlap neonatal physiologic ranges. The overlap between physiologic and deficient plasma concentrations makes diagnosis of homozygous deficiencies of factors II, X, and XI difficult, although not impossible, during the neonatal period.[3] Diagnosis of homozygous deficiencies of factors II, X, or XI in neonates can be facilitated by studies of parents, and molecular techniques can be employed when specific factor deficiencies are suspected. Prenatal diagnosis is possible for most coagulation factor deficiencies, and in utero factor replacement has been accomplished for some infants.[100]

Specific Bleeding Disorders

Factor II (Prothrombin) Deficiency

Two neonates with severe factor II deficiency have been identified. One infant experienced mild gastrointestinal bleeding[101] and the second infant presented with intracranial hemorrhage.[102] Adult patients with factor II deficiency present with bleeding following venipuncture or circumcision.[103]

Factor V Deficiency

Five neonates with severe factor V deficiency have been identified. Three of the neonates presented with intracranial hemorrhage. One intracranial hemorrhage occurred prenatally. Two of the neonates with intracranial hemorrhage died during the neonatal period. Besides intracranial hemorrhage, other manifestations of severe factor V deficiency include umbilical bleeding and soft tissue bleeding.[100, 104–106] Replacement therapy for severe factor V deficiency includes whole blood, fresh frozen plasma, and supportive care. Thrombotic complications occur in adults with factor V deficiency, but no thrombotic complications have been reported in affected neonates.[3]

Factor VII Deficiency

Many neonates with severe factor VII deficiency have been identified. Neonates with factor VII plasma concentrations less than 1% generally have severe bleeding complications, and neonates with plasma concentrations greater than 5% have mild bleeding complications.[107] Most neonates with severe factor VII deficiency present with intracranial bleeding and bleeding from other sites,[108–113] and many neonates die as a result of intracranial hemorrhage.[7] Factor VII deficiency has been associated with Dubin-Johnson syndrome and Gilbert syndrome.[114, 115] Factor VII concentrate is the replacement product of choice for treatment of factor VII deficiency bleeding. Replacement of other blood products can be required during a severe hemorrhagic event. Prenatal diagnosis of factor VII deficiency and in utero factor VII replacement are possible.[100]

Factor VIII Deficiency

Factor VIII deficiency (also known as hemophilia A) is an X-linked recessive, relatively common, bleeding disorder that can present during the neonatal period.[116] Severe factor VIII deficiency bleeding occurs in male neonates following circumcision or as intracranial hemorrhage.[97, 98, 117–121] Neonates with factor VIII deficiency rarely develop hemarthroses, in contrast to older children with factor VIII deficiency.[122] Approximately 10% of neonates with severe factor VIII deficiency experience bleeding events during the neonatal period. By 18 months of postnatal age, 70% of children with severe factor VIII deficiency have experienced a bleeding event. The severity of factor VIII deficiency is defined by plasma concentrations: factor VIII plasma concentrations of less than 1% are severe, factor VIII plasma concentrations of 1% to 5% are moderate, and factor VIII plasma concentrations of 5% to 50% are mild deficiencies.[99, 116, 122]

Neonates with factor VIII deficiency may be readily diagnosed during the neonatal period because physiologic neonatal factor VIII plasma concentrations are the same as physiologic adult plasma concentrations. Therefore, decreased plasma concentrations of factor VIII in neonates are pathologic. Neonates with factor VIII deficiency are treated with factor VIII replacement.[3] Prenatal diagnosis of factor VIII deficiency and in utero factor VIII replacement are possible.[100]

Factor IX Deficiency

Factor IX deficiency (also known as hemophilia B) is an X-linked recessive disorder that can present during the neonatal period. Neonates with factor IX deficiency commonly present with bleeding following circumcision or with intracranial hemorrhage. Bleeding from venipuncture sites, hematomas, and umbilical bleeding also occur in neonates with factor IX deficiency.[98, 117, 118, 120, 121] The severity of factor IX deficiency is defined the same as the severity of factor VIII deficiency: factor IX plasma concentrations of less than 1% are severe, factor IX plasma concentrations of 1% to 5% are moderate, and factor IX plasma concentrations of 5% to 50% are mild deficiencies.[99, 116, 122]

Diagnosis of mild forms of factor IX deficiency can be difficult during the neonatal period because in normal neonates physiologic neonatal plasma concentrations of factor IX are decreased compared with adults. The replacement therapy of choice for factor IX deficiency bleeding is factor IX concentrate. Fresh frozen plasma and other blood products may also be required during an acute bleeding episode.[3] Prenatal diagnosis of factor VIII deficiency and in utero factor VIII replacement are possible.[100]

Factor X Deficiency

Five neonates with severe factor X deficiency have been identified. Four of these neonates developed intracranial hemorrhage, and two neonates with intracranial hemorrhage died. Bleeding from umbilical, intra-abdominal, and gastrointestinal sites also occurred in neonates with factor X deficiency. Treatment has included fresh frozen plasma, whole blood, and prothrombin complex concentrate.[123–128]

Factor XI Deficiency

One neonate with severe factor XI deficiency has been identified. This patient bled following circumcision and was successfully treated with fresh frozen plasma.[129, 130] Factor XI deficiency differs from other coagulation factor deficiencies in that the severity of bleeding does not correlate with factor XI plasma concentrations and not all patients with factor XI deficiency have bleeding complications. In adults, bleeding occurs after surgery or trauma.[129, 130]

Factor XIII Deficiency

Several neonates with bleeding as a result of homozygous factor XIII deficiency have been identified. The majority of neonates with factor XIII deficiency present with prolonged bleeding from the umbilicus, and many present with intracranial hemorrhage. In children and adults, intracranial hemorrhage occurs in approximately 25% of reported cases of factor XIII deficiency.[131–135] Factor XIII–deficient individuals can be treated with either cryoprecipitate or factor XIII concentrate. A prophylactic regimen of factor XIII replacement is recommended for neonates with factor XIII deficiency because of the high incidence of intracranial hemorrhage. Plasma concentrations of factor XIII greater than 1% effectively prevent bleeding complications, and once a month therapy is possible due to the long half-life of factor XIII concentrate.[3]

von Willebrand's Disease

Patients with von Willebrand's disease rarely present during the neonatal period because plasma concentrations of von Willebrand's factor and high-molecular-weight multimers are physiologically increased in neonates.[3] von Willebrand's disease is the most common inherited bleeding disorder and has autosomal (dominant or recessive, depending on the specific variant) inheritance. Several variants of von Willebrand's disease have been identified. The variants can be caused by deficiency of von Willebrand's factor or production of von Willebrand's factor with abnormal structure.

Three neonates with bleeding secondary to von Willebrand's disease have been identified. Two neonates presented with bleeding from blood sampling and soft tissue sites.[136, 137] Laboratory investigation for these two neonates revealed prolonged aPTTs, prolonged bleeding times, thrombocytopenia, absence of high-molecular-weight multimers, and platelet aggregation at decreased plasma ristocetin concentrations. The third neonate with von Willebrand's disease presented with intracranial hemorrhage on day 7 of life. The factor VIII concentration for this neonate was significantly decreased (0.03 unit/mL), von Willebrand's antigen and von Willebrand's ristocetin cofactor were undetectable, and the neonate recovered following treatment with factor VIII concentrate twice a day for 10 days, followed by treatment once daily for 10 days.[138]

Familial Multiple Factor Deficiencies

Two neonates with familial multiple factor deficiencies have been identified. One neonate had deficiencies of factors II, VII, IX, and X and presented with spontaneous bruising and umbilical bleeding that persisted until the infant was treated with fresh frozen plasma at 3 months of age. The second neonate had deficiencies of factors V and VIII and presented with "serious bleeding" in the first week of life.[139, 140]

Fibrinogen Disorders

Neonates with inherited fibrinogen disorders (afibrinogenemia, hypofibrinogenemia, dysfibrinogenemia) have been identified. Inherited fibrinogen disorders that present during the neonatal period are usually homozygous.[141] Neonates with inherited fibrinogen disorders present with bleeding from the umbilicus, oozing from venipuncture sites, bleeding after circumcision, gastric bleeding, and epidural bleeding. Neonates with afibrinogenemia can experience severe bleeding that requires transfusion. Older children with afibrinogenemia can present with bleeding into the skin and oral mucosa, subdural bleeding, and splenic rupture.[142] Neonates with inherited fibrinogen disorders have been effectively treated with cryoprecipitate.[141]

ACQUIRED BLEEDING DISORDERS

Vitamin K–Deficiency Bleeding or Hemorrhagic Disease of the Newborn

Hemorrhagic disease of the newborn was first described over 100 years ago by Charles Townsend.[143] Vitamin K was discovered 35 years later by Henrik Dam.[144] In 1952,[145] Dam published a large study demonstrating that hemorrhagic disease of the newborn primarily occurs in breast-fed infants during the first days of life.[145] Vitamin K is an essential cofactor for coagulation factors II (prothrombin), VII, IX, and X and for the inhibitors protein S and protein C. In utero, decreased plasma concentrations of vitamin K are maintained by a placental/fetal vitamin K gradient of 20:1 to 40:1. At birth, vitamin K plasma concentrations are undetectable but rise rapidly and approximate physiologic adult vitamin K plasma concentrations by 4 days of postnatal age.[146] Vitamin K deficiency results in reduced activity of vitamin K–dependent factors and inhibitors. Reduced activity of vitamin K–dependent factors and inhibitors results in bleeding tendencies.[146] The term *vitamin K–deficiency bleeding* is preferable to the term *hemorrhagic disease of the newborn* for bleeding secondary to deficient is required, protamine sulfate can be used to neutralize the activity of heparin.[282] Neonatal doses for heparin and protamine sulfate are extrapolated form pediatric dosages.[286]

Heparin is widely used in neonatal intensive care units for maintenance of indwelling catheter patency. When given as a continuous infusion, heparin prolongs indwelling arterial catheter patency but does not affect the incidence of thrombus formation or of indwelling vascular catheter complications.[287, 288] Heparin is no better than normal saline for maintaining patency of peripheral intravenous catheters.[289–291] Heparin therapy is usually reserved for neonates with serious, symptomatic venous or arterial thromboses who are not at high risk for bleeding complications.

Low-Molecular-Weight Heparin

Low-molecular-weight heparin offers several advantages when compared with standard heparin therapy. In children, (1) the pharmacokinetics are more predictable, which decreases the monitoring required; (2) low-molecular-weight heparin is given every 12 hours, which reduces cost and the need for continuous intravenous access; (3) the frequency of bleeding complications is significantly lower; and (4) low-molecular-weight heparin is at least as effective as standard heparin.[282] The subcutaneous dose for neonates is increased compared with those for adults and children, averaging 1.69 mg/kg/d twice a day (for enoxaparin) to achieve therapeutic levels.[292] Low-molecular-weight heparin has considerably less activity against thrombin than does standard heparin, so anti-factor Xa assays rather than aPTTs are required to monitor low-molecular-weight heparin therapy.[282] At therapeutic doses, low-molecular-weight heparin does not prolong PTs or aPTTs.

Thrombolytic Therapy and Thrombectomy

Available thrombolytic agents are streptokinase, u-PA, and t-PA. Streptokinase is not recommended for neonates and children because of risks of allergic reactions. Streptokinase, u-PA, and t-PA convert endogenous plasminogen to plasmin, thereby increasing activation of the fibrinolytic pathway and increasing degradation of fibrin. Plasminogen plasma concentrations are physiologically decreased in neonates, which makes the efficacy of thrombolytics unpredictable.[293, 294] Thrombolytic therapy is sometimes used in neonates in low doses to restore catheter patency and in higher systemic doses for treatment of serious clinical thromboses. Contraindications for thrombolytic therapy include active bleeding, significant potential for severe local bleeding, general surgery within the past 10 days, or neurosurgery within the past 3 weeks.[286] Case reports suggest that clot resolution occurs in many neonates following thrombolytic therapy, but bleeding complications are common. Intracranial hemorrhage is uncommon following thrombolytic therapy, but it is a significant risk for sick neonates.[282] Optimal dosing and appropriate uses of thrombolytic therapy in neonates are undefined and are extrapolated from pediatric information.

The small size of neonatal blood vessels and the severity of illness in neonates with thromboses preclude the use of surgical thrombectomy in the majority of neonates.

Prevention

Prevention of neonatal thrombotic events is an important goal for neonatologists. Attention to placement of indwelling catheters and removal of catheters that are not clearly needed will benefit sick and recovering neonates. Early detection of developing thromboses requires a high index of suspicion and early investigation of symptoms suggestive of thromboses. Controlled clinical trials are needed to evaluate treatment modalities and to enable development of specific indications and medication dosages for neonates. Continued research into catheter materials is needed.

Treatment Recommendations for Neonates with Thromboses

The use of anticoagulant therapy or thrombolytic agents for neonates with pulmonary emboli, arterial thromboses, or venous thromboses must be individualized. The lack of adequate

bin activity of fibrin clots prepared in cord plasma compared with adult plasma. Pediatr Res 1996;39:826–830.
74. Andrew M, Mitchell L, Berry LR, et al: Fibrinogen has a rapid turnover in the healthy newborn lamb. Pediatr Res 1988;23:249–252.
75. McDonald MM, Hathaway WE: Anticoagulant therapy by continuous heparinization in newborn and older infants. J Pediatr 1982;101:451–457.
76. Schmidt B, Wais U, Pringsheim W, Kunzer W: Plasma elimination of antithrombin III (heparin cofactor activity) is accelerated in term newborn infants. Eur J Pediatr 1984;141:225–227.
77. Yuen PM, Yin JA, Lao TT: Fibrinopeptide A levels in maternal and newborn plasma. Eur J Obstet Gynecol Reprod Biol 1989;30:239–244.
78. Lao TT, Yin JA, Yuen PM: Coagulation and anticoagulation systems in newborns—correlation with their mothers at delivery. Lower levels of anticoagulants and fibrinolytic activity in the newborn. Gynecol Obstet Invest 1990;29:181–184.
79. Suarez CR, Walenga J, Mangogna LC, Fareed J: Neonatal and maternal fibrinolysis: activation at time of birth. Am J Hematol 1985;19:365–372.
80. Francis CW, Marder VJ: Physiologic regulation and pathologic disorders of fibrinolysis. In Colman RW, Hirsh J, Marder VJ (eds): Hemostasis and Thrombosis: Basic Principles and Clinical Practice. Philadelphia: JB Lippincott, 1994, pp 1076–1103.
81. Hoylaerts M, Rijken DC, Lijnen HR, Collen D: Kinetics of the activation of plasminogen by human tissue plasminogen activator. Role of fibrin. J Biol Chem 1982;257:2912–2919.
82. Levin EG, Marzec U, Anderson J, Harker LA: Thrombin stimulates tissue plasminogen activator release from cultured human endothelial cells. J Clin Invest 1984;74:1988–1995.
83. Ichinose A, Kisiel W, Fujikawa K: Proteolytic activation of tissue plasminogen activator by plasma and tissue enzymes. FEBS Lett 1984;175:412–418.
84. Mandle RJJ, Kaplan AP: Hageman-factor-dependent fibrinolysis: generation of fibrinolytic activity by the interaction of human activated factor XI and plasminogen. Blood 1979;54:850–862.
85. Goldsmith GH, Jr., Saito H, Ratnoff OS: The activation of plasminogen by Hageman factor (Factor XII) and Hageman factor fragments. J Clin Invest 1978;62:54–60.
86. Collen D, Wiman B: Fast-acting plasmin inhibitor in human plasma. Blood 1978;51:563–569.
87. Mullertz S, Clemmensen I: The primary inhibitor of plasmin in human plasma. Biochem J 1976;159:545–553.
88. Sakata Y, Aoki N: Cross-linking of alpha 2-plasmin inhibitor to fibrin by fibrin-stabilizing factor. J Clin Invest 1980;65:290–297.
89. Colucci M, Paramo JA, Collen D: Inhibition of one-chain and two-chain forms of human tissue-type plasminogen activator by the fast-acting inhibitor of plasminogen activator in vitro and in vivo. J Lab Clin Med 1986;108:53–59.
90. Erickson LA, Ginsberg MH, Loskutoff DJ: Detection and partial characterization of an inhibitor of plasminogen activator in human platelets. J Clin Invest 1984;74:1465–1472.
91. Colucci M, Paramo JA, Collen D: Generation in plasma of a fast-acting inhibitor of plasminogen activator in response to endotoxin stimulation. J Clin Invest 1985;75:818–824.
92. Madden RM, Levin EG, Marlar RA: Thrombin and the thrombin-thrombomodulin complex interaction with plasminogen activator inhibitor type-1. Blood Coagul Fibrinolysis 1991;2:471–476.
93. Bevilacqua MP, Schleef RR, Gimbrone-MA J, Loskutoff DJ: Regulation of the fibrinolytic system of cultured human vascular endothelium by interleukin 1. J Clin Invest 1986;78:587–591.
94. Schleef RR, Bevilacqua MP, Sawdey M, et al: Cytokine activation of vascular endothelium. Effects on tissue-type plasminogen activator and type 1 plasminogen activator inhibitor. J Biol Chem 1988;263:5797–5803.
95. Saksela O, Moscatelli D, Rifkin DB: The opposing effects of basic fibroblast growth factor and transforming growth factor beta on the regulation of plasminogen activator activity in capillary endothelial cells. J Cell Biol 1987;105:957–963.
96. Rohyans JA, Miser AW, Miser JS: Subgaleal hemorrhage in infants with hemophilia: report of two cases and review of the literature. Pediatrics 1982;70:306–307.
97. Schmidt B, Zipursky A: Disseminated intravascular coagulation masking neonatal hemophilia. J Pediatr 1986;109:886–888.
98. Bray GL, Luban NL: Hemophilia presenting with intracranial hemorrhage. An approach to the infant with intracranial bleeding and coagulopathy. Am J Dis Child 1987;141:1215–1217.
99. Smith PS: Congenital coagulation protein deficiencies in the perinatal period. Semin Perinatol 1990;14:384–392.
100. Daffos F, Forestier F, Kaplan C, Cox W: Prenatal diagnosis and management of bleeding disorders with fetal blood sampling. Am J Obstet Gynecol 1988;158:939–946.
101. Gill FM, Shapiro SS, Schwartz E: Severe congenital hypoprothrombinemia. J Pediatr 1978;93:264–266.
102. Viola L, Chiaretti A, Lazzareschi I, et al: [Intracranial hemorrhage in congenital factor II deficiency]. Pediatr Med Chir 1995;17:593–594.
103. Lewis JH, Spero JA, Ragni MV, Bontempo FA: Transfusion support for congenital clotting deficiencies other than haemophilia. Clin Haematol 1984;13:119–135.
104. Bonvini G, Cotta-Ramusino A, Ricciardi G: [Congenital factor V deficiency and intraventricular hemorrhage of prenatal origin]. Pediatr Med Chir 1994;16:93–94.
105. Whitelaw A, Haines ME, Bolsover W, Harris E: Factor V deficiency and antenatal intraventricular haemorrhage. Arch Dis Child 1984;59:997–999.
106. Seeler RA: Parahemophilia. Factor V deficiency. Med Clin North Am 1972;56:119–125.
107. Triplett DA, Brandt JT, Batard MA, et al: Hereditary factor VII deficiency: heterogeneity defined by combined functional and immunochemical analysis. Blood 1985;66:1284–1287.
108. Chen SC, Chang TK, Chi CS, Shu SG: Factor VII deficiency with intracranial hemorrhage: a case report. Chung Hua I Hsueh Tsa Chih (Taipei) 1993;52:190–193.
109. Ucsel R, Savasan S, Coban A, et al: Fatal intracranial hemorrhage in a newborn with factor VII deficiency. Turk J Pediatr 1996;38:257–260.
110. Ariffin H, Lin HP: Neonatal intracranial hemorrhage secondary to congenital factor VII deficiency: two case reports [letter]. Am J Hematol 1997;54:263.
111. Girolami A, Cattarozzi G, Mengarda G, Lazzarin M: Congenital factor VII deficiency. A case report. Blut 1973;27:236–242.
112. Girolami A, Scorza P, Brunetti A, et al: Congenital

hypoproconvertinemia (factor VII deficiency). A report of two cases belonging to two different kindreds. Acta Haematol 1973;50:228–237.
113. Horng YC, Chou YH, Chen RL, et al: Congenital factor VII deficiency complicated with hemoperitoneum and intracranial hemorrhage: report of a case. J Formos Med Assoc 1993;92:85–87.
114. Seligsohn U, Shani M, Ramot B, et al: Dubin-Johnson syndrome in Israel. II. Association with factor-VII deficiency. Q J Med 1970;39:569–584.
115. Seligsohn U, Shani M, Ramot B: Gilbert syndrome and factor-VII deficiency. Lancet 1970;1:1398.
116. Adcock DM, Brozna J, Marlar RA: Proposed classification and pathologic mechanisms of purpura fulminans and skin necrosis. Semin Thromb Hemost 1990;16:333–340.
117. Yoffe G, Buchanan GR: Intracranial hemorrhage in newborn and young infants with hemophilia. J Pediatr 1988;113:333–336.
118. Ljung R, Petrini P, Nilsson IM: Diagnostic symptoms of severe and moderate haemophilia A and B. A survey of 140 cases. Acta Paediatr Scand 1990;79:196–200.
119. Kletzel M, Miller CH, Becton DL, et al: Postdelivery head bleeding in hemophilic neonates. Causes and management. Am J Dis Child 1989;143:1107–1110.
120. Eyster ME, Gill FM, Blatt PM, et al: Central nervous system bleeding in hemophiliacs. Blood 1978;51:1179–1188.
121. Volpe JJ, Manica JP, Land VJ, Coxe WS: Neonatal subdural hematoma associated with severe hemophilia A. J Pediatr 1976;88:1023–1025.
122. Rosendaal FR, Smit C, Briet E: Hemophilia treatment in historical perspective: a review of medical and social developments. Ann Hematol 1991;62:5–15.
123. Girolami A, Molaro G, Calligaris A, De Luca G: Severe congenital factor X deficiency in 5-month-old child. Thromb Diath Haemorrh 1970;24:175–184.
124. Girolami A, Molaro G, Lazzarin M, et al: A "new" congenital haemorrhagic condition due to the presence of an abnormal factor X (factor X Friuli): study of a large kindred. Br J Haematol 1970;19:179–192.
125. Machin SJ, Winter MR, Davies SC, Mackie IJ: Factor X deficiency in the neonatal period. Arch Dis Child 1980;55:406–408.
126. de Sousa C, Clark T, Bradshaw A: Antenatally diagnosed subdural haemorrhage in congenital factor X deficiency. Arch Dis Child 1988;63:1168–1170.
127. Sandler E, Gross S: Prevention of recurrent intracranial hemorrhage in a factor X-deficient infant. Am J Pediatr Hematol Oncol 1992;14:163–165.
128. Ruane BJ, McCord FB: Factor X deficiency—a rare cause of scrotal haemorrhage [letter]. Ir Med J 1990;83:163.
129. Kitchens CS: Factor XI: a review of its biochemistry and deficiency. Semin Thromb Hemost 1991;17:55–72.
130. Lemaire B, Michaud P, Tescher M: [Retroplacental hematoma and factor XI deficiency]. Rev Fr Gynecol Obstet 1990;85:706–708.
131. Anwar R, Miloszewski KJ, Markham AF: Identification of a large deletion, spanning exons 4 to 11 of the human factor XIIIA gene, in a factor XIII-deficient family. Blood 1998;91:149–153.
132. Ozsoylu S, Altay C, Hi CG: Congenital factor 13 deficiency. Observation of two new cases in the newborn period. Am J Dis Child 1971;122:541–543.
133. Francis J, Todd P: Congenital factor XIII deficiency in a neonate. Br Med J 1978;2:1532.
134. Merchant RH, Agarwal BR, Currimbhoy Z, et al: Congenital factor XIII deficiency. Indian Pediatr 1992;29:831–836.
135. Patel AP, Chandy M, Raghupathy P, et al: Hereditary factor XIII deficiency. Indian J Pediatr 1993;60:441–444.
136. Donner M, Holmberg L, Nilsson IM: Type IIB von Willebrand's disease with probable autosomal recessive inheritance and presenting as thrombocytopenia in infancy. Br J Haematol 1987;66:349–354.
137. Zeitler P, von Stockhausen HB: [Type IIB von Willebrand Jurgens syndrome as the cause of neonatal thrombocytopenia]. Klin Padiatr 1998;210:85–88.
138. Pasi KJ, Williams MD, Enayat MS, Hill FG: Clinical and laboratory evaluation of the treatment of von Willebrand's disease patients with heat-treated factor VIII concentrate (BPL 8Y). Br J Haematol 1990;75:228–233.
139. Mazzone D, Fichera A, Pratico G, Sciacca F: Combined congenital deficiency of factor V and factor VIII. Acta Haematol 1982;68:337–338.
140. McMillan CW, Roberts HR: Congenital combined deficiency of coagulation factors II, VII, IX and X. Report of a case. N Engl J Med 1966;274:1313–1315.
141. Andrew M, Schmidt B: Thrombotic and hemorrhagic complications in children. In Colman RW, Hirsh J, Marder VJ, Salzman EW (eds): Hemostasis and Thrombosis. Philadelphia: JB Lippincott, 1994, pp 989–1022.
142. Fried K, Kaufman S: Congenital afibrinogenemia in 10 offspring of uncle-niece marriages. Clin Genet 1980;17:223–227.
143. Townsend CW: The haemorrhagic disease of the newborn. Arch Pediatr 1894;11:559–565.
144. Dam H, Dyggve H, Larsen H, et al: Cholesterinstoffwechsel in Huhnereiern und Huhnchen. Biochem Z 1929;215:475–492.
145. Dam H, Dyggve H, Larsen H, et al: The relation of vitamin K deficiency to hemorrhagic disease of the newborn. Adv Pediatr 1952;5:129–153.
146. Sutor AH: Vitamin K deficiency bleeding in infants and children. Semin Thromb Hemost 1995;21:317–329.
147. Cornelissen M, Steegers-Theunissen R, Kollee L, et al: Increased incidence of neonatal vitamin K deficiency resulting from maternal anticonvulsant therapy. Am J Obstet Gynecol 1993;168:923–928.
148. von Kries R, Shearer M, McCarthy PT, et al: Vitamin K1 content of maternal milk: influence of the stage of lactation, lipid composition, and vitamin K1 supplements given to the mother. Pediatr Res 1987;22:513–517.
149. von Kries R, Becker A, Gobel U: Vitamin K in the newborn: influence of nutritional factors on acarboxy-prothrombin detectability and factor II and VII clotting activity. Eur J Pediatr 1987;146:123–127.
150. Greer FR, Marshall S, Cherry J, Suttie JW: Vitamin K status of lactating mothers, human milk, and breast-feeding infants. Pediatrics 1991;88:751–756.
151. Sutor AH, Dagres N, Niederhoff H: Late form of vitamin K deficiency bleeding in Germany. Klin Padiatr 1995;207:89–97.
152. Greer FR: Vitamin K deficiency and hemorrhage in infancy. Clin Perinatol 1995;22:759–777.
153. von Kries R, Gobel U: Vitamin K prophylaxis and vitamin K deficiency bleeding (VKDB) in early infancy. Acta Paediatr 1992;81:655–657.
154. McNinch AW, Tripp JH: Haemorrhagic disease of the newborn in the British Isles: two year prospective study. BMJ 1991;303:1105–1109.
155. Hansen KN, Ebbesen F: Neonatal vitamin K prophylaxis in Denmark: three years' experience with oral administration during the first three months of life

compared with one oral administration at birth. Acta Paediatr 1996;85:1137–1139.
156. Golding J, Paterson M, Kinlen LJ: Factors associated with childhood cancer in a national cohort study. Br J Cancer 1990;62:304–308.
157. Golding J, Greenwood R, Birmingham K, Mott M: Childhood cancer, intramuscular vitamin K, and pethidine given during labour. BMJ 1992;305:341–346.
158. Ekelund H, Finnstrom O, Gunnarskog J, et al: Administration of vitamin K to newborn infants and childhood cancer. BMJ 1993;307:89–91.
159. Klebanoff MA, Read JS, Mills JL, Shiono PH: The risk of childhood cancer after neonatal exposure to vitamin K. N Engl J Med 1993;329:905–908.
160. von Kries R, Gobel U, Hachmeister A, et al: Vitamin K and childhood cancer: a population based case-control study in Lower Saxony, Germany. BMJ 1996;313:199–203.
161. American Academy of Pediatrics Vitamin K Ad Hoc Task Force: Controversies concerning vitamin K and the newborn. Pediatrics 1993;91:1001–1003.
162. Rodgers GM: Hemostatic properties of normal and perturbed vascular cells. FASEB J 1988;2:116–123.
163. Okajima K, Uchiba M, Murakami K, et al: Plasma levels of soluble E-selectin in patients with disseminated intravascular coagulation. Am J Hematol 1997;54:219–224.
164. Carey MJ, Rodgers GM: Disseminated intravascular coagulation: clinical and laboratory aspects. Am J Hematol 1998;59:65–73.
165. Schmidt BK, Vegh P, Andrew M, Johnston M: Coagulation screening tests in high risk neonates: a prospective cohort study. Arch Dis Child 1992;67:1196–1197.
166. Gross SJ, Filston HC, Anderson JC: Controlled study of treatment for disseminated intravascular coagulation in the neonate. J Pediatr 1982;100:445–448.
167. von Kries R, Stannigel H, Gobel U: Anticoagulant therapy by continuous heparin-antithrombin III infusion in newborns with disseminated intravascular coagulation. Eur J Pediatr 1985;144:191–194.
168. Gray OP, Ackerman A, Fraser AJ: Intracranial haemorrhage and clotting defects in low-birth-weight infants. Lancet 1968;1:545–548.
169. McDonald MM, Johnson ML, Rumack CM, et al: Role of coagulopathy in newborn intracranial hemorrhage. Pediatrics 1984;74:26–31.
170. Beverley DW, Chance GW, Inwood MJ, et al: Intraventricular haemorrhage and haemostasis defects. Arch Dis Child 1984;59:444–448.
171. Beverley DW, Pitts-Tucker TJ, Congdon PJ, et al: Prevention of intraventricular haemorrhage by fresh frozen plasma. Arch Dis Child 1985;60:710–713.
172. Shirahata A, Nakamura T, Shimono M, et al: Blood coagulation findings and the efficacy of factor XIII concentrate in premature infants with intracranial hemorrhages. Thromb Res 1990;57:755–763.
173. Hensey OJ, Morgan ME, Cooke RW: Tranexamic acid in the prevention of periventricular haemorrhage. Arch Dis Child 1984;59:719–721.
174. Seeger W, Stohr G, Wolf HR, Neuhof H: Alteration of surfactant function due to protein leakage: special interaction with fibrin monomer. J Appl Physiol 1985;58:326–338.
175. Saldeen T: Fibrin-derived peptides and pulmonary injury. Ann NY Acad Sci 1982;384:319–31:319–331.
176. Fukuda Y, Ishizaki M, Masuda Y, et al: The role of intraalveolar fibrosis in the process of pulmonary structural remodeling in patients with diffuse alveolar damage. Am J Pathol 1987;126:171–182.
177. Damiano VV, Cherian PV, Frankel FR, et al: Intraluminal fibrosis induced unilaterally by lobar instillation of CdC12 into the rat lung. Am J Pathol 1990;137:883–894.
178. Ambrus CM, Weintrb DH, Ambrus JL: Studies on hyaline membrane disease. 3. Thrapeutic trial of urokinase-activated human plasmin. Pediatrics 1966; 38:231–243.
179. Ambrus CM, Choi TS, Cunnanan E, et al: Prevention of hyaline membrane disease with plasminogen. A cooperative study. JAMA 1977;237:1837–1841.
180. Markarian M, Lubchenco LO, Rosenblut E, et al: Hypercoagulability in premature infants with special reference to the respiratory distress syndrome and hemorrhage. II. The effect of heparin. Biol Neonate 1971;17:98–111.
181. Schmidt B, Gillie P, Mitchell L, et al: A placebo-controlled randomized trial of antithrombin therapy in neonatal respiratory distress syndrome. Am J Respir Crit Care Med 1998;158:470–476.
182. Zreik H, Bengur AR, Meliones JN, et al: Superior vena cava obstruction after extracorporeal membrane oxygenation. J Pediatr 1995;127:314–316.
183. Truog RD: Randomized controlled trials: lessons from ECMO. Clin Res 1992;40:519–527.
184. Bartlett RH, Roloff DW, Cornell RG, et al: Extracorporeal circulation in neonatal respiratory failure: a prospective randomized study. Pediatrics 1985;76:479–487.
185. Rosenberger WF, Lachin JM: The use of response-adaptive designs in clinical trials. Control Clin Trials 1993;14:471–484.
186. Robinson TM, Kickler TS, Walker LK, et al: Effect of extracorporeal membrane oxygenation on platelets in newborns. Crit Care Med 1993;21:1029–1034.
187. Plotz FB, Van Oeveren W, Bartlett RH, Wildevuur CR: Blood activation during neonatal extracorporeal life support. J Thorac Cardiovasc Surg 1993;105:823–832.
188. Kulhanjian J: Fever, hepatitis and coagulopathy in a newborn infant. Pediatr Infect Dis J 1992;11:1069, 1072.
189. Kelly DA, Summerfield JA: Hemostasis in liver disease. Semin Liver Dis 1987;7:182–191.
190. Rubin MH, Weston MJ, Bullock G, et al: Abnormal platelet function and ultrastructure in fulminant hepatic failure. Q J Med 1977;46:339–352.
191. Blanchard RA, Furie BC, Jorgensen M, et al: Acquired vitamin K-dependent carboxylation deficiency in liver disease. N Engl J Med 1981;305:242–248.
192. Griffin JH, Heeb MJ, Kojima Y, et al: Activated protein C resistance: molecular mechanisms. Thromb Haemost 1995;74:444–448.
193. Kalafatis M, Rand MD, Mann KG: The mechanism of inactivation of human factor Va by activated protein C. J Biol Chem 1994;269:31869–31880.
194. Bertina RM, Koeleman BP, Koster T, et al: Mutation in blood coagulation factor V associated with resistance to activated protein C. Nature 1994;369:64–67.
195. Dahlback B: Resistance to activated protein C caused by the R506Q mutation in the gene for factor V is a common risk factor for venous thrombosis. J Intern Med Suppl 1997;740:1–8.
196. Stenbjerg S: Inherited alpha 2 macroglobulin deficiency. Thromb Res 1981;22:491–495.
197. Nowak-Gottl U, Strater R, Dubbers A, et al: Ischaemic stroke in infancy and childhood: role of the Arg506 to Gln mutation in the factor V gene. Blood Coagul Fibrinolysis 1996;7:684–688.
198. Nowak-Gottl U, Dubbers A, Kececioglu D, et al: Factor V Leiden, protein C, and lipoprotein (a) in

catheter-related thrombosis in childhood: a prospective study. J Pediatr 1997;131:608–612.
199. Poort SR, Rosendaal FR, Reitsma PH, Bertina RM: A common genetic variation in the 3′-untranslated region of the prothrombin gene is associated with elevated plasma prothrombin levels and an increase in venous thrombosis. Blood 1996;88:3698–3703.
200. Rosendaal FR, Doggen CJ, Zivelin A, et al: Geographic distribution of the 20210 G to A prothrombin variant. Thromb Haemost 1998;79:706–708.
201. Arruda VR, Annichino-Bizzacchi JM, Goncalves MS, Costa FF: Prevalence of the prothrombin gene variant (nt20210A) in venous thrombosis and arterial disease. Thromb Haemost 1997;78:1430–1433.
202. Cumming AM, Keeney S, Salden A, et al: The prothrombin gene G20210A variant: prevalence in a U.K. anticoagulant clinic population. Br J Haematol 1997;98:353–355.
203. Biousse V, Conard J, Brouzes C, et al: Frequency of the 20210 G — A mutation in the 3′-untranslated region of the prothrombin gene in 35 cases of cerebral venous thrombosis. Stroke 1998;29:1398–1400.
204. Makris M, Preston FE, Beauchamp NJ, et al: Coinheritance of the 20210A allele of the prothrombin gene increases the risk of thrombosis in subjects with familial thrombophilia. Thromb Haemost 1997; 78:1426–1429.
205. Arruda VR, Siquiera LH, Chiaparini LC, et al: Prevalence of the prothrombin gene variant 20210 G — A among patients with myocardial infarction. Cardiovasc Res 1998;37:42–45.
206. Kyrle PA, Mannhalter C, Beguin S, et al: Clinical studies and thrombin generation in patients homozygous or heterozygous for the G20210A mutation in the prothrombin gene. Arterioscler Thromb Vasc Biol 1998;18:1287–1291.
207. Marlar RA, Neumann A: Neonatal purpura fulminans due to homozygous protein C or protein S deficiencies. Semin Thromb Hemos 1990;16:299–309.
208. Goodwin TM, Gazit G, Gordon EM: Heterozygous protein C deficiency presenting as severe protein C deficiency and peripartum thrombosis: successful treatment with protein C concentrate. Obstet Gynecol 1995;86:662–664.
209. Marlar RA, Montgomery RR, Broekmans AW: Diagnosis and treatment of homozygous protein C deficiency. Report of the Working Party on Homozygous Protein C Deficiency of the Subcommittee on Protein C and Protein S, International Committee on Thrombosis and Haemostasis. J Pediatr 1989;114:528–534.
210. Rogers PC, Silva MP, Carter JE, Wadsworth LD: Renal vein thrombosis and response to therapy in a newborn due to protein C deficiency. Eur J Pediatr 1989;149:124–125.
211. Marlar RA, Sills RH, Groncy PK, et al: Protein C survival during replacement therapy in homozygous protein C deficiency. Am J Hematol 1992;41:24–31.
212. Branson HE, Katz J, Marble R, Griffin JH: Inherited protein C deficiency and coumarin-responsive chronic relapsing purpura fulminans in a newborn infant. Lancet 1983;2:1165–1168.
213. Hartman KR, Manco-Johnson M, Rawlings JS, et al: Homozygous protein C deficiency: early treatment with warfarin. Am J Pediatr Hematol Oncol 1989;11:395–401.
214. Peters C, Casella JF, Marlar RA, et al: Homozygous protein C deficiency: observations on the nature of the molecular abnormality and the effectiveness of warfarin therapy. Pediatrics 1988;81:272–276.
215. Rappaport ES, Speights VO, Helbert B, et al: Protein C deficiency. South Med J 1987;80:240–242.
216. Yuen P, Cheung A, Lin HJ, et al: Purpura fulminans in a Chinese boy with congenital protein C deficiency. Pediatrics 1986;77:670–676.
217. Baliga V, Thwaites R, Tillyer ML, et al: Homozygous protein C deficiency—management with protein C concentrate. Eur J Pediatr 1995;154:534–538.
218. Zoller B: Familial thrombophilia: clinical and molecular analysis of Swedish families with inherited resistance to activated protein C or protein S deficiency. Scand J Clin Lab Invest Suppl 1996;226:19–46.
219. Broekmans AW, Bertina RM, Reinalda PJ, et al: Hereditary protein S deficiency and venous thromboembolism. A study in three Dutch families. Thromb Haemost 1985;53:273–277.
220. Engesser L, Broekmans AW, Briet E, et al: Hereditary protein S deficiency: clinical manifestations. Ann Intern Med 1987;106:677–682.
221. Pegelow CH, Ledford M, Young JN, Zilleruelo G: Severe protein S deficiency in a newborn. Pediatrics 1992;89:674–676.
222. Mahasandana C, Suvatte V, Chuansumrit A, et al: Homozygous protein S deficiency in an infant with purpura fulminans. J Pediatr 1990;117:750–753.
223. Mannucci PM, Tripodi A, Bertina RM: Protein S deficiency associated with "juvenile" arterial and venous thrombosis [letter]. Thromb Haemost 1986;55:440.
224. DeStefano V, Leone G, Ferrelli R, et al: Severe deep vein thrombosis in a 2-year-old child with protein S deficiency [letter]. Thromb Haemost 1987;58:1089.
225. Winter JH, Fenech A, Ridley W, et al: Familial antithrombin III deficiency. Q J Med 1982;51:373–395.
226. Peeters S, Vandenplas Y, Jochmans K, et al: Myocardial infarction in a neonate with hereditary antithrombin III deficiency. Acta Paediatr 1993;82:610–613.
227. Sanchez J, Velasco F, Alvarez R, et al: Aortic thrombosis in a neonate with hereditary antithrombin III deficiency: successful outcome with thrombolytic and replacement treatment. Acta Paediatr 1996;85:245–247.
228. Brenner B, Fishman A, Goldsher D, et al: Cerebral thrombosis in a newborn with a congenital deficiency of antithrombin III. Am J Hematol 1988;27:209–211.
229. Furlan AJ, Lucas FV, Craciun R, Wohl RC: Stroke in a young adult with familial plasminogen disorder. Stroke 1991;22:1598–1602.
230. Liu Y, Lyons RM, McDonagh J: Plasminogen San Antonio: an abnormal plasminogen with a more cathodic migration, decreased activation and associated thrombosis. Thromb Haemost 1988;59:49–53.
231. Nagayama T, Shinohara Y, Nagayama M, et al: Congenitally abnormal plasminogen in juvenile ischemic cerebrovascular disease. Stroke 1993:24:2104–2107.
232. Robbins KC: Dysplasminogenemias. Enzyme 1988;40:70–78.
233. Scharrer IM, Wohl RC, Hach V, et al: Investigation of a congenital abnormal plasminogen, Frankfurt I, and its relationship to thrombosis. Thromb Haemost 1986;55:396–401.
234. Haverkate F, Samama M: Familial dysfibrinogenemia and thrombophilia. Report on a study of the SSC Subcommittee on Fibrinogen. Thromb Haemost 1995;73:151–161.
235. Soria J, Soria C, Collet JP, et al: Dysfibrinogenemia and thrombosis. Nouv Rev Fr Hematol 1991;33:457–459.
236. Engesser L, Brommer EJ, Kluft C, Briet E: Elevated plasminogen activator inhibitor (PAI), a cause of thrombophilia? A study in 203 patients with familial or sporadic venous thrombophilia. Thromb Haemost 1989;62:673–680.

237. Manco-Johnson MJ: Diagnosis and management of thromboses in the perinatal period. Semin Perinatol 1990;14:393–402.
238. Schmidt B, Andrew M: Neonatal thrombosis: report of a prospective Canadian and international registry. Pediatrics 1995;96:939–943.
239. Kavaler E, Hensle TW: Renal artery thrombosis in the newborn infant. Urology 1997;50:282–284.
240. Molteni KH, George J, Messersmith R, et al: Intrathrombic urokinase reverses neonatal renal artery thrombosis. Pediatr Nephrol 1993;7:413–415.
241. Munoz-Arizpe R, Walsh RF, Edge W: Obstructive aortic and renal thrombosis in the newborn—spontaneous recovery. Pediatr Nephrol 1992;6:190–191.
242. Joseph R, Chong A, Teh M, et al: Thrombotic complication of umbilical arterial catheterization and its sequelae. Ann Acad Med Singapore 1985;14:576–582.
243. Tabbutt S, Griswold WR, Ogino MT, et al: Multiple thromboses in a premature infant associated with maternal phospholipid antibody syndrome. J Perinatol 1994;14:66–70.
244. Hibbert J, Howlett DC, Greenwood KL, et al: The ultrasound appearances of neonatal renal vein thrombosis. Br J Radiol 1997;70:1191–1194.
245. Orazi C, Fariello G, Malena S, et al: Renal vein thrombosis and adrenal hemorrhage in the newborn: ultrasound evaluation of 4 cases. J Clin Ultrasound 1993;21:163–169.
246. Brill PW, Jagannath A, Winchester P, et al: Adrenal hemorrhage and renal vein thrombosis in the newborn: MR imaging. Radiology 1989;170:95–98.
247. Lebowitz JM, Belman AB: Simultaneous idiopathic adrenal hemorrhage and renal vein thrombosis in the newborn. J Urol 1983;129:574–576.
248. Laplante S, Patriquin HB, Robitaille P, et al: Renal vein thrombosis in children: evidence of early flow recovery with Doppler US. Radiology 1993;189:37–42.
249. Harms K, Speer CP: [Thrombosis: an underestimated complication of central catheters? Subclavian vein, vena cava and renal vein thrombosis after silastic catheters]. Monatsschr Kinderheilkd 1993;141:21–25.
250. Duncan BW, Adzick NS, Longaker MT, et al: In utero arterial embolism from renal vein thrombosis with successful postnatal thrombolytic therapy. J Pediatr Surg 1991;26:741–743.
251. Lalmand B, Avni EF, Nasr A, et al: Perinatal renal vein thrombosis. Sonographic demonstration. J Ultrasound Med 1990;9:437–442.
252. Levine C: Intestinal obstruction in a neonate with adrenal hemorrhage and renal vein thrombosis. Pediatr Radiol 1989;19:477–478.
253. Sanders LD, Jequier S: Ultrasound demonstration of prenatal renal vein thrombosis. Pediatr Radiol 1989;19:133–135.
254. Al-Samarrai SF, Kato A, Urano Y: Renal vein thrombosis in stillborn infant of diabetic mother. Acta Pathol Jpn 1984;34:1441–1447.
255. Pohl M, Zimmerhackl LB, Heinen F, et al: Bilateral renal vein thrombosis and venous sinus thrombosis in a neonate with factor V mutation (FV Leiden). J Pediatr 1998;132:159–161.
256. Andrew M, Brooker LA: Hemostatic complications in renal disorders of the young. Pediatr Nephrol 1996;10:88–99.
257. Wright NB, Blanch G, Walkinshaw S, Pilling DW: Antenatal and neonatal renal vein thrombosis: new ultrasonic features with high frequency transducers. Pediatr Radiol 1996;26:686–689.
258. Fishman JE, Joseph RC: Renal vein thrombosis in utero: duplex sonography in diagnosis and follow-up. Pediatr Radiol 1994;24:135–136.
259. Nuss R, Hays T, Manco-Johnson M: Efficacy and safety of heparin anticoagulation for neonatal renal vein thrombosis. Am J Pediatr Hematol Oncol 1994;16:127–131.
260. Brun P, Beaufils F, Pillion G, et al: [Thrombosis of the renal veins in the newborn: treatment and long term prognosis]. Ann Pediatr (Paris) 1993;40:75–80.
261. Nuss R, Hays T, Manco-Johnson M: Efficacy and safety of heparin anticoagulation for neonatal renal vein thrombosis. Am J Pediatr Hematol Oncol 1994;16:127–131.
262. Jobin J, O'Regan S, Demay G, et al: Neonatal renal vein thrombosis—long-term follow-up after conservative management. Clin Nephrol 1982;17:36–40.
263. O'Neill JA, Jr, Neblett WW, Born ML: Management of major thromboembolic complications of umbilical artery catheters. J Pediatr Surg 1981;16:972–978.
264. Seibert JJ, Taylor BJ, Williamson SL, et al: Sonographic detection of neonatal umbilical-artery thrombosis: clinical correlation. AJR Am J Roentgenol 1987;148:965–968.
265. Horgan MJ, Bartoletti A, Polansky S, et al: Effect of heparin infusates in umbilical arterial catheters on frequency of thrombotic complications. J Pediatr 1987;111:774–778.
266. Oppenheimer DA, Carroll BA, Garth KE: Ultrasonic detection of complications following umbilical arterial catheterization in the neonate. Radiology 1982; 145:667–672.
267. Olinsky A, Aitken FG, Isdale JM: Thrombus formation after umbilical arterial catheterisation. An angiographic study. S Afr Med J 1975;49:1467–1470.
268. Vailas GN, Brouillette RT, Scott JP, et al: Neonatal aortic thrombosis: recent experience. J Pediatr 1986;109:101–108.
269. Tanke RB, van-Megen R, Daniels O: Thrombus detection on central venous catheters in the neonatal intensive care unit. Angiology 1994;45:477–480.
270. Bjorklund LJ, Malmgren N, Lindroth M: Pulmonary complications of umbilical venous catheters. Pediatr Radiol 1995;25:149–152.
271. Rocha E, Alfaro MJ, Paramo JA, Canadell JM: Preoperative identification of patients at high risk of deep venous thrombosis despite prophylaxis in total hip replacement. Thromb Haemost 1988;59:93–95.
272. Paramo JA, Alfaro MJ, Rocha E: Postoperative changes in the plasmatic levels of tissue-type plasminogen activator and its fast-acting inhibitor—relationship to deep vein thrombosis and influence of prophylaxis. Thromb Haemost 1985;54:713–716.
273. Vincent JG, Lacquet LK, Wal HJ, et al: A denaturated venous homograft as an alternative material for shunts and other reconstructions in congenital cardiac surgery. J Cardiovasc Surg Torino 1990;31:766–770.
274. Nagaraj HS, Mitchell KA, Fallat ME, et al: Surgical complications and procedures in neonates on extracorporeal membrane oxygenation. J Pediatr Surg 1992;27:1106–1109.
275. Riccabona M, Kuttnig-Haim M, Dacar D, et al: Venous thrombosis in and after extracorporeal membrane oxygenation: detection and follow-up by color Doppler sonography. Eur Radiol 1997;7:1383–1386.
276. Bruni B, Gandolfo CM: Arterial thrombosis of the arm in infant of diabetic mother. Acta Diabetol Lat 1979;16:85–87.
277. Hsi AC, Davis DJ, Sherman FC: Neonatal gangrene in the newborn infant of a diabetic mother. J Pediatr Orthop 1985;5:358–360.

278. Nazer H, Abu RA, Qaryouti S, et al: Neonatal limb gangrene and renal vein thrombosis. Case report with review of literature. Eur J Pediatr 1987;146:429–431.
279. Morriss FHJ: Infants of diabetic mothers. Fetal and neonatal pathophysiology. Perspect Pediatr Pathol 1984;8:223–234.
280. de Klerk OL, de Vries TW, Sinnige LGF: An unusual cause of neonatal seizures in a newborn infant. Pediatrics 1997;100:E8.
281. Hage ML, Liu R, Marcheschi DG, et al: Fetal renal vein thrombosis, hydrops fetalis, and maternal lupus anticoagulant. A case report. Prenat Diagn 1994;14:873–877.
282. Andrew M, Michelson AD, Bovill E, et al: Guidelines for antithrombotic therapy in pediatric patients. J Pediatr 1998;132:575–588.
283. Andrew M, Ofosu F, Schmidt B, et al: Heparin clearance and ex vivo recovery in newborn piglets and adult pigs. Thromb Res 1988;52:517–527.
284. Spadone D, Clark F, James E, et al: Heparin-induced thrombocytopenia in the newborn. J Vasc Surg 1992;15:306–311.
285. Andrew M, Marzinotto V, Massicotte P, et al: Heparin therapy in pediatric patients: a prospective cohort study. Pediatr Res 1994;35:78–83.
286. Andrew M, deVeber G: Pediatric Thromboembolism and Stroke Protocols. Hamilton, Ontario: BC Decker, 1997.
287. David RJ, Merten DF, Anderson JC, Gross S: Prevention of umbilical artery catheter clots with heparinized infusates. Dev Pharmacol Ther 1981;2:117–126.
288. Rajani K, Goetzman BW, Wennberg RP, et al: Effect of heparinization of fluids infused through an umbilical artery catheter on catheter patency and frequency of complications. Pediatrics 1979;63:552–556.
289. Kotter RW: Heparin vs saline for intermittent intravenous device maintenance in neonates. Neonatal Netw 1996;15:43–47.
290. Chang GY, Lueder FL, DiMichele DM, et al: Heparin and the risk of intraventricular hemorrhage in premature infants. J Pediatr 1997;131:362–366.
291. Krafte-Jacobs B, Sivit CJ, Mejia R, Pollack MM: Catheter-related thrombosis in critically ill children: comparison of catheters with and without heparin bonding. J Pediatr 1995;126:50–54.
292. Massicotte P, Adams M, Marzinotto V, et al: Low-molecular-weight heparin in pediatric patients with thrombotic disease: a dose finding study. J Pediatr 1996;128:313–318.
293. Leaker MT, Brooker LA, Mitchell LG, et al: Fibrin clot lysis by tissue plasminogen activator (tPA) is impaired in plasma from pediatric patients undergoing orthotopic liver transplantation. Transplantation 1995;60:144–147.
294. Andrew M, Brooker L, Leaker M, et al: Fibrin clot lysis by thrombolytic agents is impaired in newborns due to a low plasminogen concentration. Thromb Haemost 1992;68:325–330.

CHAPTER 13

Developmental Aspects of Platelets and Disorders of Platelets in the Neonatal Period

Martha C. Sola, M.D., and Robert D. Christensen, M.D.

Intracranial bleeding is a common problem among patients in neonatal intensive care units (NICUs) and one that is frequently associated with adverse neurodevelopmental consequences.[1] Hemorrhages, particularly periventricular and intraventricular varieties, are much more common among the smallest and most ill neonates than in any other age group or population, and these hemorrhages can be caused or worsened by thrombocytopenia.[2, 3] Because thrombocytopenia is a problem that affects 20% to 30% of all patients admitted to NICUs,[4, 5] with even higher frequencies among the smallest and most ill neonates, the study of thrombocytopenia and other platelet disorders affecting neonates is essential for neonatologists.

Although thrombocytopenia is by far the most common platelet disorder of neonates, several congenital or acquired conditions affecting platelet function also occur. We briefly review the normal platelet characteristics of preterm and term neonates and then discuss the quantitative and qualitative platelet disorders that manifest in the neonatal period.

PLATELET COUNTS IN NEONATES

Platelets are small, anucleated fragments of megakaryocytes that circulate in the blood as disks with an average volume of about 7.5 fL; they are 14 times smaller than erythrocytes.[6] The characteristics of neonatal megakaryocytes and their progenitors and the mechanisms involved in the regulation of platelet production in neonates are detailed in Chapter 3.

In 1990, van den Hof reported that fetal platelet counts increase linearly with gestation, from a mean concentration of 187,000/μL at 15 weeks to 274,000/μL at 40 weeks.[7] Premature infants, on average, have a slightly lower platelet count than term infants, but it remains within the same range observed in healthy older children and adults (150,000 to 450,000/μL).[8] The definition of thrombocytopenia for preterm and term neonates is the same as for adults: a platelet count of less than 150,000/μL.[9] The significance of platelet counts between 100,000 and 150,000/μL in neonates is unclear, because a higher incidence of counts in this range has been found in otherwise healthy neonates.[10] An approach taken by many neonatologists is to repeat platelet counts that are 100,000 to 150,000/μL and to monitor the infant, with further study depending on the subsequent platelet counts and the infant's clinical condition. Platelet counts less than 100,000/μL should be considered definitely abnormal at any gestational age.

PLATELET FUNCTION IN NEONATES

Under normal circumstances, platelets circulate in a relatively inactive state and do not interact with the intact endothelium lining the blood vessels. When the endothelial lining is damaged, exposure of the blood to the subendothelial layers triggers a series of events that leads to the formation of a platelet-fibrin plug that stops bleeding from the injured vessel. Formation of this hemostatic plug depends on multiple interactions among the vessel wall, platelets, and coagulation proteins. In this chapter, we focus on the role of platelets in the process of thrombus formation, specifically platelet adhesion and platelet aggregation, with an emphasis on the differences between neonates and adults.

Platelet Adhesion

As soon as the endothelial surface is damaged or removed, platelets adhere to the exposed subendothelium, experience a change in shape with the formation of pseudopods, and spread over the surface (Fig. 13–1).[11] The adhesion of the platelets to the subendothelium is mediated by the binding of a plasma protein, von Willebrand's factor, to a specific platelet membrane component, glycoprotein Ib (GPIb). After this binding takes place, von Willebrand's factor acts like a bridge between the subendothelial surface and the platelet membrane. Studies of neonatal platelet adhesiveness have rendered conflicting results,[12, 13] most likely related to the lack of sensitive and reproducible assays. However, it is known that GPIb appears on platelets early in fetal life and is present in fetuses of 18 to 26 weeks' gestation in amounts higher than those found in adults.[14] The plasma of neonates contains higher concentrations of von Willebrand's factor than adult plasma,[15] with an increased proportion of functional high-molecular-weight forms.[16]

Platelet Aggregation

Several factors generated at the interface between the disrupted vessel wall and the blood can activate platelets. These factors include adenosine diphosphate (ADP), thrombin, epinephrine, thromboxane A_2, platelet-activating factor (PAF), and exposed subendothelial collagen. The interactions of these agonists with their specific receptors on the platelet membrane activate different intracellular signaling pathways that ultimately lead to the secretion of platelet granules contents and to platelet aggregation.

Independent of the signaling pathway involved, the aggregation process is mediated by a conformational change experienced by the surface glycoprotein complex GPIIb-IIIa, which converts it into a receptor for fibrinogen. After binding to this receptor, fibrinogen acts as a bridge between adjacent platelets.[11] The thrombin-mediated transformation of fibrinogen to fibrin stabilizes this platelet aggregate and forms a hemostatic plug (Fig. 13–2). Similar to GPIb, platelets express GPIIb-IIIa early in gestation.[14] By 27 weeks' gestation, fibrinogen is also found in concentrations similar to those in adults,[17] and although this fibrinogen is a "fetal" form

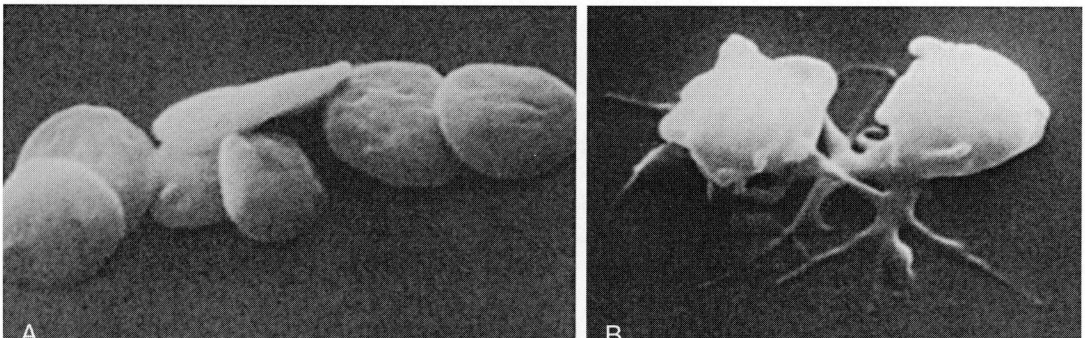

Figure 13–1. *A*, Scanning electron micrograph of a platelet in the resting state. Notice the discoid shape and smooth cell surface. *B*, Scanning electron micrograph taken during platelet adhesion and early shape change. (Photograph courtesy of James G. White, MD, University of Minnesota.) (From Schultz Beardsley D: Platelet abnormalities in infancy and childhood. In Nathan DG, Oski FA [eds]: Hematology of Infancy and Childhood, 4th ed. Philadelphia: WB Saunders, 1992, p 1562.)

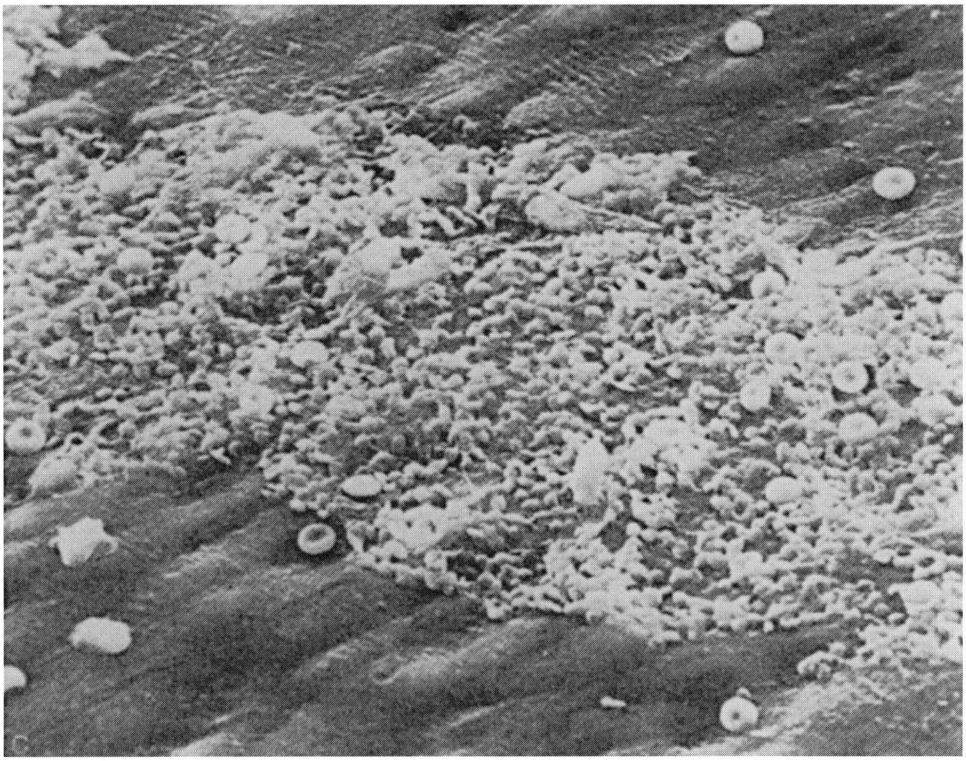

Figure 13–2. Scanning electron micrograph of a platelet plug. (Photograph courtesy of James G. White, MD, University of Minnesota.) (From Schultz Beardsley D: Platelet abnormalities in infancy and childhood. In Nathan DG, Oski FA [eds]: Hematology of Infancy and Childhood, 4th ed. Philadelphia: WB Saunders, 1992, p 1562.)

with a higher phosphorus content than that of adult fibrinogen,[18] it binds normally to newborn platelets.

Unlike the process of platelet adhesion, platelet aggregation in the neonate has several differences from that of adults. The platelet aggregation in response to epinephrine is significantly *decreased* in neonates compared with adults,[19, 20] a finding probably related to a deficiency of α-adrenergic receptors in neonatal platelets.[21, 22] In contrast, the aggregation of neonatal platelets in response to ristocetin is markedly *increased* compared with adult platelets,[23] probably because of the elevated levels of von Willebrand's factor[15] and the increased proportion of high-molecular-weight multimers of this factor found in neonatal plasma.[16] It is important to remember this difference when attempting to diagnose von Willebrand's disease in the neonatal period, because affected infants could falsely be labeled as normal.

Earlier studies evaluating the responses of neonatal platelets to other agonists generated conflicting results.[24–26] Later studies using flow cytometry, however, demonstrated a generalized hyporeactivity of platelets from term and preterm neonates to thrombin, collagen, ADP, and U46619 (a stable thromboxane A_2 analogue).[27–29] Serial evaluations of cord blood and peripheral blood obtained from term infants in the first 10 days of life have shown that, under physiologic conditions, the platelet responses to ADP, collagen, and U46619 reach normal adult levels between the fifth and the ninth day of life.[30] The persistence of platelet dysfunction in neonates after the 10th day of life may therefore be an indicator of a platelet disorder. The mechanisms responsible for this hyporeactivity of neonatal platelets have not been adequately explained. For a long time, it was hypothesized that this transient "dysfunction" resulted from platelet activation during birth, a hypothesis supported by the findings of elevated levels of β-thromboglobulin, thromboxane B_2, and platelet factor 4 in the plasma of neonates and their mothers at the time of birth.[31] However, flow cytometric analysis of cord blood and blood obtained from healthy term and preterm neonates in the first days of life has failed to demonstrate any evidence of circulating activated platelets,[32, 33] regardless of sex, age, or mode of delivery. These data suggest that the decreased reactivity of neonatal platelets represents a developmental phenomenon, perhaps designed to protect the neonate from the possible harmful effects of birth stress on the coagulation system.[33]

In contrast to the decreased reactivity of neonatal platelets, the bleeding time (which is probably the most important in vivo test of platelet interaction with the vessel wall)[34] is slightly shortened in neonates compared with adults.[15] Factors that may explain this discordance include the increased von Willebrand factor concentration and function in neonates,[35] their high hematocrit,[36] and the large size of their erythrocytes.[37] All of these factors enhance the platelet–vessel wall interaction and probably contribute to normalize the bleeding time in presence of platelet hyporeactivity.

In summary, the functional properties of newborn platelets, rather than representing a dysfunction that reflects immaturity, may be elements of an optimally functioning hemostatic system adapted to the physiologic needs of the neonate. Under nonphysiologic circumstances, however, these characteristics can gain considerable pathogenic significance, as occurs in preterm and sick neonates.[38]

QUALITATIVE PLATELET DISORDERS

A disorder of platelet function should be considered in a neonate who manifests platelet-type bleeding (e.g., petechiae, purpura, mucous membrane bleeding) but has a *normal platelet count*. The bleeding time is a useful screening test for this category of disorders,[34] but false-positive and false-negative values are common, perhaps because bleeding times are tested so uncommonly in most NICUs that experience in performing the test is usually minimal (Table 13–1).

Table 13–1. **Instructions for Conducting a Bleeding Time Test in a Neonate**

Equipment Needed

1. Neonatal blood pressure cuff, appropriate size for forearm (if the thumb is to be used), the upper arm (if the volar surface is to be used), or the lower leg (if the toe is to be used)
2. Betadine and alcohol wipes
3. Filter paper
4. Device for producing the standardized incision
   a. Autolet (Tenderfoot) (International Technidyne Corporation, Edison, NJ)
   b. Surgicutt Newborn (International Technidyne Corporation, Edison, NJ)
   c. Simplate Paediatric (Organon Teknika, Sweden)
5. Stopwatch
6. When it is important to keep track of the "blood out," it is useful to have a scale for weighing the filter paper before and after completion of the test to estimate the blood loss.

Procedure

1. Measure blood pressure in the extremity to be tested.
2. Apply a constant "holding pressure" to the blood pressure cuff equal to the diastolic pressure.
3. Clean the site to be tested with Betadine, and then wipe clean with alcohol and air dry. (If the Autolet is to be used, select the thumb or large toe. If the Surgicutt or Simplate devices are to be used, select the volar surface of the forearm.)
4. Produce the standard puncture (Autolet) or incision (Surgicutt or Simplate).
5. Immediately start the stopwatch.
6. Ballot the blood from the incision, using filter paper, every 15 seconds until the bleeding stops, and then stop the stopwatch.
7. The time taken for the bleeding to stop is the *bleeding time.*

Interpretation of Results

1. Normal infants (97%) have bleeding times of less than 3.5 minutes. A prolonged bleeding time in a neonate with a normal platelet count indicates an abnormality in one of four functions:
   a. Platelet adhesion
   b. Platelet activation
   c. Platelet aggregation
   d. Vascular defectiveness (Marfan's or Ehlers-Danlos syndrome)
2. Blood loss from a bleeding time test in a neonate is usually only 0.1 to 0.3 mL, and in cases with very prolonged bleeding times, it rarely exceeds 1.0 mL. When the bleeding time exceeds 10 minutes, we generally stop the test and apply a small bandage.

The process resulting in cessation of bleeding from bleeding time incisions involves platelet adhesion, activation, and aggregation. A prolonged bleeding time does not discriminate among these platelet functions. Prolonged bleeding times can also occur because of defective blood vessels, as are seen in patients with Marfan's syndrome[39] or Ehlers-Danlos syndrome.[40, 41]

Bleeding times from the thumbs of neonates have been reported using standardized microlancet incisions (i.e., Autolet), with a blood pressure cuff on the forearm inflated to a point just above the diastolic blood pressure. The Tenderfoot automated incision device (International Technidyne Corporation, Edison, NJ) makes a standardized incision that is 2.5 mm long and 1.0 mm deep. The blood is then gently balloted from the incision site every few seconds using filter paper, and the time taken for the bleeding to stop (timed with a stopwatch) indicates the *bleeding time*. Testing this method on 82 healthy, term neonates resulted in bleeding times of less than 3.5 seconds for 97% of the subjects.[42]

Specific template devices have been produced for making standardized bleeding time incisions in neonates (including the Surgicutt Newborn device made by International Technidyne Corporation, Edison, NJ), modeled after the instruments used for adults. These devices make a cut 2.5 mm long and 0.5 mm deep and give more reproducible results than the Autolet or template methods.[43] The newest bleeding time device released for use in children is the Simplate Paediatric (Organon Teknika, Sweden), which uses a retractable blade to reduce accidental injury and makes a cut of 3 × 0.5 mm. That device appears to function very well in children, but data have not yet been reported for neonates.[44]

Bleeding times are not particularly useful for neonates who have thrombocytopenia. Their bleeding times usually are prolonged in proportion to the degree of thrombocytopenia. The bleeding time is useful only in evaluating patients who have platelet-type bleeding but have normal platelet counts. In such cases, a prolonged bleeding time suggests the diagnosis of hereditary or acquired disturbances of platelet function.

Hereditary Disorders

Genetic disorders that result in deficient platelet function are rare causes of pathologic bleeding in neonates. Most patients with these rare congenital qualitative platelet disorders do not present during the neonatal period, but rather later in life. Such patients develop platelet-type bleeding, such as petechiae, epistaxis, anemia from occult gastrointestinal hemorrhage, or menorrhagia. At least two cases of neonates with pathologic bleeding from Glanzmann's thrombasthenia have been reported.[45] One neonate had "profuse bleeding" after a circumcision on the 8th day after birth, and at 10 months, he required a transfusion because of bleeding from an abrasion on the lips and tongue that continued to bleed for 4 days. Three years later, he had a female sibling who developed severe purpura immediately after birth. The siblings were evaluated for bleeding problems at the ages of 7 and 4 years, respectively, and were found to have normal platelet counts, prolonged bleeding times, and no in vitro platelet aggregation with the addition of thrombin and collagen. Although uncommon, hereditary platelet dysfunction can present with hemorrhagic problems during the neonatal period, and neonatologists should be aware of this possibility.

Glanzmann's thrombasthenia is an autosomal recessive disorder characterized by failure of platelets to aggregate in response to any of the normal agonists.[46] The platelets look normal microscopically, their blood concentration is normal, and they adhere normally to exposed subendothelial adhesive proteins. The problem is that the platelets lack the fibrinogen receptor glycoproteins (GPIIb-IIIa) that are needed for normal platelet aggregation.[47, 48] The condition is generally classified as type 1 Glanzmann's, which is caused by a total lack of the GPIIb-IIIa complex, or type II Glanzmann's, which is a partial deficiency, usually in the range of 5% to 20% of normal levels. However, more than 20 different genetic defects in the GPIIb or GPIIIa genes have been described, each constituting a different genotype for the Glanzmann's phenotype. Neonatologists should consider this rare set of hereditary disorders of platelet function when platelet-type bleeding is observed in a neonate who has a normal platelet count and normal platelet morphology, and no exposure to agents known to cause acquired platelet dysfunction can be identified. These disorders should be considered if the family history suggests congenital disorders of platelet function. The only treatment for neonates who have Glanzmann's thrombasthenia is platelet transfusion, which should be reserved for instances of serious hemorrhage or the need for surgery.

Most of the other congenital disorders of platelet function have not been recognized as a problem during the neonatal period. For instance, patients with Bernard-Soulier syndrome, an autosomal recessive disorder characterized by very large platelets and defective adhesion resulting from abnormalities in glycoprotein Ib, have not had hemorrhagic problems as neonates.

Acquired Disorders

Platelet function can be impaired by pharmacologic agents administered to or ingested by the mother or used to treat the neonate (Table 13–2). Certain pathologic states, such as uremia and liver disease, also can impair platelet function. The prototype for pharmacologic impairment of platelet function is aspirin (acetylsalicylic acid)—one of the most commonly used drugs during pregnancy in the United States.[49] It results in a potent, irreversible inhibition of the cyclooxygenase enzyme and subsequent increase in the bleeding time. A single dose of aspirin (5 to 10 mg/kg) increases the bleeding time for several days because of its covalent linking to the cyclooxygenase enzyme, which persists for the life span of the platelets (about 10 days).

Salicylates cross the placenta, and after maternal ingestion, they are detected in the fetal circulation. Bleyer and Breckenridge[50] reported three incidents of bleeding (i.e., cephalhematoma, melena, and periorbital edema) among 14 neonates of mothers who had received aspirin. Haslam[51] reported one infant with severe gastrointestinal bleeding with no apparent cause other than maternal aspirin ingestion. Prospectively designed studies, however, have shown no definite link between maternal aspirin ingestion and subsequent hemorrhagic problems in the neonate. Perhaps this link depends on the time between maternal aspirin ingestion and delivery. This correlation is suggested by a study of Stuart and colleagues,[52] in which abnormal bleeding was observed in 9 of 10 neonates whose mothers took aspirin less than 5 days before delivery but in none of 6 whose mothers took aspirin 6 days or more before delivery. The neonate's bleeding time probably will be increased somewhat when aspirin has been ingested within a few days of delivery, but the risk of pathologic hemorrhage in these infants appears to be very low. However, in healthy pregnancies for which alternatives to aspirin can be used to treat headaches and to provide analgesia, it seems prudent to advise against the use of aspirin during the last month of pregnancy.

Like aspirin, indomethacin can interfere with cyclooxygenase function, but unlike aspirin, it does not form a covalent complex with the enzyme, and its antiplatelet effects therefore disappear as soon as the indomethacin serum level falls. Corazza and associates[53] observed that, after indomethacin was administered to 25 preterm infants for closure of a patent ductus arteriosus (PDA), the bleeding time increased from 3.6 to 8.7 minutes and remained elevated for at least 48 hours after completion of therapy. They observed clinical bleeding in only 6 of the 25, and this was generally limited to occult hematuria.[53] Occasionally, surgical ligation of a PDA is performed immediately after several consecutive days of indomethacin administration have failed to close the ductus. These infants on indomethacin who undergo ligation surgery are probably at somewhat higher risk for postoperative hemorrhage than similar infants not on indomethacin. Postoperative hemorrhages in such infants are generally limited to excessive blood in the chest tube or saturating the surgical dressing. Treatment of these patients with platelet transfusions (even though their platelet counts are normal) usually resolves the hemorrhage.

Nitric oxide modulates vessel wall tone, interferes with platelet adhesion and aggregation, and stimulates disaggregation of preformed platelet aggregates. Adults receiving inhaled nitric oxide have a prolonged bleeding time,[54] but it is not clear to what extent nitric oxide administered to neonates results in platelet dysfunction. Although a clinically significant problem has not yet been described, it is prudent to consider nitric oxide–induced platelet dysfunc-

Table 13–2. **Disease States and Medications or Treatments That Can Diminish Platelet Function in Neonates**

- Disease states
  - Uremia
  - Liver disease
  - Hyperbilirubinemia
  - Fatty acid deficiency
  - Intracranial hemorrhage
- Medications or treatments
  - Aspirin (acetylsalicylic acid)
  - Indomethacin
  - Nitric oxide
  - Ampicillin
  - Furosemide
  - Theophylline
  - Phototherapy
  - Extracorporeal membrane oxygenation

tion when platelet-type bleeding is observed in a patient who has a normal platelet count and is being treated with nitric oxide.

Several medications commonly used to treat NICU patients, including ampicillin, furosemide, and theophylline, have been reported to inhibit platelet function in vitro. These medications have not, however, been reported to prolong the bleeding time or to result in clinical hemorrhage in neonates, but this has not been subjected to testing.

In adults and older children, renal failure can induce platelet dysfunction. The exact mechanisms by which this occurs are unknown, but excessive production of nitric oxide by endothelial cells and abnormalities of cyclooxygenase may contribute.[55] Liver disease can result in bleeding problems from a variety of causes, and one such cause is the induction of a state of platelet dysfunction.[56] Clinically significant hemorrhage because of platelet dysfunction caused by renal failure or liver disease does not appear to be prominent in neonates. Perhaps neonatologists should consider the possibility of platelet dysfunction when unexplained platelet-type bleeding problems appear in their patients who have renal or liver disease. However, the lack of descriptions of bleeding problems from platelet dysfunction in such patients probably indicates that these are relatively unimportant in clinical neonatology.

Bilirubin interferes with platelet aggregation in vitro[57] and so does phototherapy.[58] The clinical significance of the platelet dysfunction induced by hyperbilirubinemia and phototherapy is minimal, because platelet-type bleeding is not a frequent finding among otherwise well neonates who develop jaundice or require phototherapy.

Dietary fatty acid deficiency has been reported as a cause of platelet dysfunction. Three varieties have been described, although none of the reported neonates had significant bleeding consequences. The three dietary scenarios are breast-feeding infants of women who are fatty acid deficient, infants receiving a formula deficient in essential fatty acids, and vitamin E–deficient infants. All three conditions result in arachidonic acid depletion and platelet dysfunction.[59] Changes in infant formulas in the mid-1980s, with increased vitamin E to polyunsaturated fat ratios, have almost made the second and third scenarios extinct in the United States. Neonatologists should be aware of these remote possibilities in evaluating a neonate who has a normal platelet count but platelet-type bleeding.[60–65]

Intracranial hemorrhage (intraventricular or subarachnoid) appears capable of inducing platelet dysfunction. This was reported by Setzer and coworkers, who tested the bleeding times of 58 very-low-birth-weight infants[66] using a template device described by Feusner.[67] They observed normal bleeding times (3.3 ± 0.2 minutes) for 16 patients who did not have intraventricular hemorrhages but prolonged times for the group of 7 who had subarachnoid hemorrhages (5.4 ± 0.8 minutes) and in the group of 30 who had intraventricular hemorrhages (5.5 ± 0.4 minutes). At least 13 of the infants in the latter group had normal platelet counts but prolonged bleeding times. It was not clear whether prolongation of the bleeding times in the very-low-birth-weight infants with intracranial hemorrhages preceded their hemorrhage or resulted from the hemorrhage, but this and subsequent studies suggest that the latter is more likely.

Abnormal platelet function has been reported on neonates receiving extracorporeal membrane oxygenation (ECMO). Robinson and colleagues prospectively studied these effects using 10 infants younger than 1 week old who were receiving ECMO for respiratory failure. In addition to the anticipated decrease in platelet number (a 26% fall in blood platelet concentration occurred within 15 minutes of initiation of ECMO), they observed about a 50% decrease in platelet function. Aggregation was reduced in response to collagen, ristocetin, and adenosine 5′-diphosphate. Platelet number, but not platelet function, was restored by periodic platelet transfusions. Normalization of platelet function occurred 8 hours after ECMO was discontinued.[68]

QUANTITATIVE PLATELET DISORDERS

Thrombocytosis

Thrombocytosis (i.e., thrombocythemia), defined by a moderately elevated platelet count in the range of 450,000 to 600,000/μL, is not a rarity in the NICU.[69–70] Preterm infants who spend more than 4 to 6 weeks in the NICU often have an increased platelet count during this period (Table 13–3). For instance, Appleyard and Brinton found that the average platelet count of a preterm infant increased from 203,000/μL at birth to 384,000/μL at 4 weeks of age.[71] Aballi[10] observed that 3% of preterm infants had an elevated platelet count (>400,000/μL) at birth, but 13% did so by 2 weeks of age, and 23% did so by 4 weeks. Effiong reported similar findings from Nigerian neonates.[72] It was rare, however, in any of these reports to have a platelet count peak at greater than 600,000/μL.

In many preterm infants, the peak platelet count is observed just after the nadir of their "anemia of prematurity." When Halperin first reported the administration of recombinant erythropoietin (rEPO) to preterm infants, he found that the treatment, which elevated the reticulocyte and hematocrit levels, was followed by a period of iron deficiency. This iron deficiency, with a fall in ferritin, was accompanied by a significant elevation in platelet count.[73] Iron deficiency can cause thrombocytosis in older children and is seen in experimentally induced iron deficiency in newborn animals,[74] but it was uncommon among patients in the NICU until the advent of rEPO treatment. If rEPO is instituted without adequate iron, iron deficiency can develop, and thrombocytosis can occur in this setting.

A variety of unusual associations with thrombocytosis have been observed in neonates. Turba and associates reported three neonates who had platelet counts of higher than 700,000/μL and who subsequently developed subcutaneous fat necrosis between the 4th and 21st days of life. They postulated that the thrombocytosis might have resulted in a localized subcutaneous thrombosis with subsequent hypoxia and necrosis.[75]

Table 13–3. **Causes of Thrombocytosis in Neonates**

- "Physiologic" (in preterm infants, platelet counts can increase to 600,000/μL by about 4 weeks of age)
- "Reactive" (variety of conditions characterized by infection or inflammation)
- Iron deficiency (especially in preterm receiving recombinant erythropoietin without adequate iron reserves or adequate iron intake)
- Medications (rarely reported for a variety of antibiotics, particularly cephalosporins)
- Asplenia syndrome
- Down syndrome
- Vitamin E deficiency
- Congenital neoplasms
- Congenital adrenal hyperplasia
- Recombinant thrombopoietin administration

Buss and coworkers reported 280 hospitalized adults patients who had extreme thrombocytosis (platelet count >1,000,000/μL). Eighty-two percent of these cases were thought to be "reactive thrombocytosis"; these were patients with acute inflammation or infection, blood loss, or iron deficiency. Fourteen percent of the patients with extreme thrombocytosis had a myeloproliferative disorder, and 4% were idiopathic.[76] Perhaps this larger category of reactive thrombocytosis also accounts for most neonatal cases.

A large study of children with thrombocytosis (platelet count >800,000/μL) was reported by Vora and Lilleyman.[77] Of nearly 8000 children who had platelet counts during a 12-month period in a children's hospital in Sheffield, 36 (0.5%) had a count of more than 800,000/μL. The mean age was 13 months. Twenty seven (75%) of the 36 had an infection, which was bacterial in 18 and viral in 9. The other cases were postoperative, iron deficient, or recovering from antineoplastic chemotherapy. They concluded that secondary reactive thrombocytosis is not rare in very young infants, particularly during infection. No morbidity was recognized as a result of the elevated platelet counts, and no treatments were given.

Another large study of thrombocytosis in children was reported by Chan and colleagues, who in a 12-month period observed 100 episodes of marked thrombocytosis (>900,000/μL). These were all infants, and most had infections. The elevated counts declined after about 3 days, and no hemorrhagic or thrombotic complications were encountered. They interpreted this variety of thrombocytosis in infants to be relatively common and benign.[78]

Thrombocytosis in neonates has regularly been cited as an adverse effect of antimicrobial therapy. Specific reports appear from the use of aztreonam,[79] imipenem-cilastatin,[80] ceftriaxone,[81, 82] and ceftizoxime.[83] Several physicians have cited withdrawal from maternal drug abuse as a cause of neonatal thrombocytosis. Hanssler reviewed 16 neonates with methadone withdrawal who had thrombocytosis after the first week of life. Median counts increased from 566,000/μL in the second week of life to 639,000/μL in the sixth week.[84] The incidence of this variety of thrombocytosis and the responsible mechanism are unknown.

Before the mid-1980s, vitamin E deficiency was not an infrequent cause of thrombocytosis in preterm infants. This condition occurred in the setting of a hemolytic anemia in preterm infants given high amounts of polyunsaturated fatty acids in their formula, was accompanied by thrombocytosis and edema, and was responsive to vitamin E treatment. This disorder has been largely or entirely eliminated in the United States with addition of vitamin E and by reducing the content of linoleic acid.

Many neonates with Down syndrome have a slightly elevated platelet count,[85] but occasionally, they have marked thrombocytosis as part of a congenital myeloproliferative disorder[86] or rarely as a manifestation of acute megakaryoblastic leukemia.[87] Neonates with other malignancies, especially neuroblastoma, sometimes have thrombocytosis.[88] Thrombocytosis has also been reported in neonates with congenital adrenal hyperplasia[89, 90] but the cause and significance are unclear.

Thrombocytopenia

The reported incidence of thrombocytopenia in the neonate is extremely variable, depending on the definition of thrombocytopenia and the patient population studied. Large studies have addressed the incidence of neonatal thrombocytopenia in a nonselected population. Uhrynowska and associates[91] determined platelet counts in the cord blood of 9142 neonates born consecutively in an obstetric unit to mothers without thrombocytopenia. Sixty-four of these had a platelet count less than 100,000/μL, resulting in an overall incidence of neonatal thrombocytopenia of 0.7%. Serologic investigations revealed that approximately 10% of these cases had neonatal alloimmune thrombocytopenia (NAIT), giving an overall incidence of NAIT of 0.06%, or 1 case per 1800 neonates. Dreyfus and coworkers[92] performed a similar study of 5632 neonates and found the incidence of neonatal thrombocytopenia to be approximately 0.9% (48 affected infants). The slightly higher incidence probably results from the fact that they defined thrombocytopenia as a platelet count of less than 150,000/μL and did not exclude children born to women known to have platelet alloantibodies or autoantibodies.

Severe thrombocytopenia, defined as a platelet count <50,000/μL, was present at birth in 9 of the 48 thrombocytopenic neonates and developed after birth in 9 additional cases in which the platelet count continued to decrease. If only the cord blood values are considered for statistical analysis, the incidence of severe neonatal thrombocytopenia is 0.14% in the general population, a value consistent with the incidence of 0.12% found by Burrows and associates in more than 15,000 neonates screened.[93] However, the incidence increases to 0.28% if those infants whose platelet counts drop below that threshold during the first few days of life are included. Of the 4 million births annually in the United States, about 36,000 can be expected to have congenital thrombocytopenia, and about 11,000 of these can be expected to have severe thrombocytopenia.

The relatively low frequency of thrombocytopenia in the general population of neonates is in marked contrast with the very high incidence among sick neonates. In 1980, Mehta and coworkers published the results of a large study evaluating the incidence and causes of neonatal thrombocytopenia in infants admitted to the NICU.[4] They found an incidence of 35% and were unable to establish the cause of the thrombocytopenia in 60% of the affected infants. However, they suggested that decreased platelet production accounted for most cases, based on the lack of changes in the mean platelet volume (MPV) and the finding of decreased bone marrow megakaryocytes on bone marrow aspiration analyses performed for 14 infants at postmortem examinations. In 1986, Castle and colleagues published the results of a 1-year prospective study of 807 consecutive infants admitted to a regional NICU.[5] Twenty-two percent of those infants developed thrombocytopenia, defined as a platelet count of less than 150,000/μL. Among the affected neonates, 38% had platelet counts between 50,000 and 100,000/μL, and 20% had platelet counts less than 50,000/μL. Increased platelet destruction was thought to be the mechanism responsible for most cases of neonatal thrombocytopenia, based on an increased MPV, normal megakaryocytes in the bone marrow, and a poor response to platelet transfusions. Oren and associates conducted a 2-year prospective study of 643 neonates admitted to a NICU; 18.2% of the preterm neonates and 0.8% of the term neonates admitted developed thrombocytopenia.[94]

Of the 400,000 infants admitted annually to NICUs in the United States, 80,000 to 140,000 develop thrombocytopenia. Multiple clinical conditions have been causally associated with neonatal thrombocytopenia, including sepsis, disseminated intravascular coagulation (DIC), necrotizing enterocolitis (NEC), asphyxia, exchange transfusion, intrauterine growth retardation, maternal hypertension, maternal anti-platelet antibodies, Rh hemolytic disease, genetic syndromes, drug effects, and congenital infections. Despite the large number of causes, only four kinetic mechanisms are responsible: decreased platelet production, increased platelet destruction, platelet sequestration, or a combination of these processes. In 40% to 60% of affected infants, the kinetic mechanism leading to thrombocytopenia remains unclear despite extensive evaluation.[4]

The technical difficulties associated with obtaining a bone marrow specimen in small, ill neonates have prompted reliance on indirect measurements of the state of platelet production. MPV,[5, 95] platelet-associated immunoglobulin G (PAIgG),[5, 96] reticulated platelet count,[97, 98] survival of platelets labeled with indium-111–tagged 8-hydroxiquinoline (oxine),[99] and quantification of circulating megakaryocytes and their progenitors in the peripheral blood[100, 101] have all been used to evaluate the kinetic mechanisms responsible for neonatal thrombocytopenia. Although some studies applying these techniques suggest that increased consumption of platelets accounts for most cases,[5, 96, 99] others suggest that reduced platelet production is generally responsible.[4, 101]

CAUSES OF THROMBOCYTOPENIA IN NEONATES

No system that has been proposed for classifying the causes of thrombocytopenia in neonates is entirely acceptable. One such system is the *kinetic classification*, which was described previously. The difficulty with this system is that the assignment to any given category is only as accurate as is the method for determining the kinetics involved, and the methods used for determining the kinetics in neonates have been inaccurate and basically flawed. For example, to categorize a particular adult case as being caused by "decreased platelet production," marrow biopsies or flow cytometric analysis of bone marrow aspirates are generally employed to assess the marrow megakaryocyte mass. Marrow biopsies and marrow megakaryocyte mass calculations, however, have not been reported from thrombocytopenic neonates. Marrow aspirates are instead performed to assess the kinetics, although this is flawed by invariable dilution of the sample with peripheral blood. Moreover, the methods for determining "accelerated platelet destruction" in neonates are all indirect, such as the MPV, the reticulated platelet count, and the PAIgG. These methods have all been criticized as inaccurate and as occasionally misleading.

Better methods for determining the kinetic mechanisms responsible for thrombocytopenia in neonates are being developed. Until such new methods have been sufficiently perfected and adequately tested, we must remain skeptical of a kinetic-based classification system for thrombocytopenic neonates.

The classification system we have chosen for use in this chapter is summarized in Table 13–4. Our classification system is not based on kinetics but on assignment to one of six pathophysiologic categories: immune mediated, infectious, genetic, drug or medication related, DIC, or miscellaneous.

Immune-Mediated Thrombocytopenia

Alloimmune Thrombocytopenia

In 1953, Harrington and coworkers described a variety of thrombocytopenia that affects healthy neonates who have no other evidence of disease.[102] The pathogenesis of this type of thrombocytopenia, now known as NAIT, resembles that of erythroblastosis fetalis

Table 13–4. **Etiologic Categories of Thrombocytopenia in Neonates**

1. Immune mediated
   a. Passive
   b. Active
2. Infections
   a. Bacterial
   b. Nonbacterial
3. Genetic causes
4. Drugs or medications
5. Disseminated intravascular coagulation
6. Miscellaneous

in that it is mediated by maternal antibodies directed against antigens on fetal platelets. When incompatibility between parental platelet antigens exists, the mother can become sensitized to an antigen expressed on the fetal platelets. When a maternal antibody is formed and subsequently crosses the placenta, it can coat the fetal platelets, which are then removed from the circulation by the fetal reticuloendothelial system. Unlike neonatal Rh disease, however, the first pregnancy can produce an affected fetus, and no routine prenatal screening test is available.

The study of NAIT has been complicated by the multiple antigens expressed on platelets, including class I human leukocyte antigens (HLAs), ABO antigens, and five biallelic platelet alloantigen systems that represent polymorphisms of the platelet surface glycoproteins. As an additional complicating feature, the nomenclature for these alloantigens has undergone multiple changes over the last few decades. These platelet antigens have been designated human platelet antigens (HPAs) 1 to 9, and the different allelic forms are distinguished by an a or b suffix, with a indicating the more common and b indicating the uncommon allele.[103] Table 13–5 summarizes the new nomenclature and the names previously assigned to the different antigens. The frequency with which a particular antigen is responsible for cases of NAIT in a specific population depends on the relative frequency of this antigen in that population. For example, the genotype HPA-1a/HPA-1a is prevalent among Caucasians, with a frequency of 68.9%, but only 2.9% of the population is homozygous for the HPA-1b antigen. For that reason, HPA-1a (also known as PLA-1) is the most common antigen responsible for NAIT in white individuals, accounting for 80% to 90% of the cases.[104] Cases mediated by antibodies against HPA-5,[105] HPA-3,[106] HPA-2,[107] and more rarely HPA-6[108] have also been described, although with much smaller frequency.[109] In Asian subjects, the HPA-4 (or Yuk/Pen) system is most frequently implicated in the pathogenesis of NAIT.[103] Rare cases of immunization against "low-frequency" or "private" platelet alloantigens have also been reported.[110]

The incidence of NAIT has been the subject of many studies. Based on the frequency of

Table 13–5. **Platelet Antigen Systems**

Antigen System	Other Names	Antigens	Other Names
HPA-1	Zw, P1A	HPA-1a	Zw^a, $P1^{A1}$
		HPA-1b	Zw^b, $P1^{A2}$
HPA-2	Ko, Sib	HPA-2a	Ko^b
		HPA-2b	Ko^a, Sib^a
HPA-3	Bak, Lek	HPA-3a	Bak^b
		HPA-3b	Bak^a, Lek^a
HPA-4	Pen, Yuk	HPA-4a	Pen^a, Yuk^b
		HPA-4b	Pen^b, Yuk^a
HPA-5	Br, Zav, Hc	HPA-5a	Br^b, Zav^b
		HPA-5b	Br^a, Zav^a, Hc^a
HPA-6	Ca, Tu	HPA-6b	Ca, Tu
HPA-7	Mo	HPA-7b	Mo^a
HPA-8	Sr	HPA-8b	Sr^a
HPA-9W	Max	HPA-9Wb	Max^a

HPA, human platelet antigens; W, workshop (refers to systems that are still under evaluation).

Adapted from Iverson C, Flanagin A, Fontanarosa PB, et al: American Medical Association Manual of Style: A Guide for Authors and Editors, 9th ed. Baltimore: Williams & Wilkins, 1998, p 343. Copyright © 1998, American Medical Association.

HPA-1b in the Caucasian population (2% to 3%), that same percentage of pregnancies in Caucasian women should be at risk for generating anti-HPA-1a antibodies that cross the placenta and induce NAIT in the fetus. However, large studies have shown the incidence of NAIT to be only 1 case per 1000 to 2000 live births,[91, 92] suggesting that HPA-1 incompatibility itself is not sufficient to produce NAIT. An association has been demonstrated between certain maternal HLA antigens and the development of different anti-HPA antibodies,[111–114] probably because the maternal immune response to the HPA antigens is mediated by HLA class II molecules.

Platelet antigens appear in the fetus early in gestation, and the maternal antibodies can cross the placenta early in the second trimester,[115] thereby inducing severe fetal thrombocytopenia. Bussel and coworkers[115] studied 107 fetuses who had siblings with alloimmune thrombocytopenia. The mean (±SD) gestational age of the fetuses was 25 ± 4 weeks, and 50% had an initial platelet count 50,000/μL or less, including 21 fetuses who were evaluated before 24 weeks of gestation. The only good predictive factor for severe thrombocytopenia was a history of antenatal intracranial hemorrhage in the sibling. Of all these fetuses, only one had an intracranial hemorrhage.

After a pregnancy has been affected by NAIT, the proportion of subsequent pregnancies affected mostly depends on the father's genotype. If the father is heterozygous for the alloantigen responsible for the incompatibility (HPA-1a/HPA-1b), the risk is approximately 50%. If the father is homozygous (HPA-1a/HPA-1a), the recurrence risk is close to 100%.[104] As demonstrated by Bussel and colleagues,[115] the severity of the thrombocytopenia in an affected fetus is unpredictable, unless a sibling had a history of intracranial hemorrhage. However, certain clinical features are characteristic of alloimmune thrombocytopenia when compared with nonimmune thrombocytopenia. As shown in Table 13–6, NAIT tends to induce severe thrombocytopenia (<50,000/μL), and it is rarely associated with other disorders or factors that account for the thrombocytopenia.[116]

The platelet count of neonates with NAIT is usually quite low at birth, continues to fall over the first days of life, and then increases over 1 to 4 weeks. The most perilous complication of the thrombocytopenia is intracranial hemorrhage, which occurs in approximately 10% to 15% of all cases.[117] It is likely that at least one half of these occur in utero, and almost all have severe neurodevelopmental sequelae.[118] Because of this, it is recommended that any infant with NAIT and a platelet nadir of less than 50,000/μL have a cranial ultrasonographic examination before hospital discharge.

Although the classic mechanism responsible for the thrombocytopenia in NAIT is antibody-mediated platelet consumption, later studies suggest that reduced platelet production also contributes. Warwick and associates[119] demonstrated that maternal sera from PlA-1–negative mothers (i.e., mothers with the HPA-1b phenotype) whose pregnancies were complicated by anti-PlA-1 (anti-HPA-1a) inhibited the in vitro growth of PlA-1–positive fetal and neonatal colony-forming unit–megakaryocyte (CFU-MK) cultures. In contrast, the anti-PlA-1–containing sera stimulated the growth of CFU-MK from PlA-1–negative individuals, suggesting the pres-

Table 13–6. **Comparison of Neonatal Alloimmune Thrombocytopenia and Other Types of Thrombocytopenia**

Clinical Data	Group I: NAIT (46 cases)	Group II: Other Thrombocytopenias (192 cases)	Significance
Platelet count <50,000/μL	87.0%	39.6%	$P < .001$
Hemorrhagic diathesis	82.6%	65.6%	$P < .05$
Petechiae	80.4%	61.5%	$P < .05$
Gastrointestinal bleeding or other sites	15.2%	5.7%	$P > .05$
Intracranial hemorrhage	10.9%	7.8%	$P > .05$
Associated disorder or factor	6.5%	80.2%	$P < .001$

From Uhrynowska M, Maslanka K, Zupanska: Neonatal thrombocytopenia: incidence, serological, and clinical observations. Am J Perinatol 1997;14:417.

ence of large quantities of cytokines that stimulate CFU-MK growth. Moreover, the degree of inhibition of CFU-MK (unlike platelet antibody titers) correlated well with the clinical severity of the thrombocytopenia.

Cases of immune amegakaryocytic thrombocytopenia in neonates have been associated with maternal anti-HLA-A2 antibodies.[120] Anti-HLA-A2 can cause neonatal thrombocytopenia by directly affecting the megakaryocytes instead of or in addition to any direct effect on the platelets. The cases reported were also associated with transient neonatal leukopenia.

The role of anti-HLA antibodies (found in one third of mothers) in neonatal thrombocytopenia is still controversial. King and coworkers prospectively studied 493 women for the presence of anti-HLA antibodies at delivery and found no significant relationship between maternal HLA alloimmunization or presence of anti-HLA antibodies in the cord blood and neonatal thrombocytopenia.[121]

Autoimmune Thrombocytopenia

As in NAIT, autoimmune neonatal thrombocytopenia is mediated by the transplacental passage of maternal anti-platelet antibodies. In contrast to NAIT, the antibody responsible for these cases binds the maternal and the fetal platelets and therefore causes thrombocytopenia in the mother and the neonate. In most cases, the underlying maternal disease is idiopathic thrombocytopenic purpura (ITP), but other disorders, such as systemic lupus erythematosus, lymphoproliferative disorders, or hyperthyroidism, can also produce this syndrome.[15] Not uncommonly, an otherwise healthy woman without a history of ITP or other autoimmune process presents with a mild decrease in the platelet count that is first detected during pregnancy and resolves after delivery. This condition, which has been called *gestational* or *incidental thrombocytopenia*, is associated with a low risk of fetal or neonatal thrombocytopenia.[103, 122] Of 756 mothers with this disorder, only one gave birth to an infant with severe thrombocytopenia.[123] Unfortunately, ITP can also manifest de novo during the pregnancy, making the differentiation between these types of thrombocytopenia difficult. Severe transient neonatal thrombocytopenia in infants delivered to mothers who have normal platelet counts and no evidence of alloimmunization can be the only sign of mild maternal ITP, characterized by compensated thrombocytolysis in the mother.[124]

Although the association between maternal ITP and neonatal autoimmune thrombocytopenia has long been recognized, consensus about the incidence of neonatal thrombocytopenia in this group is lacking. Earlier reports found an incidence of neonatal thrombocytopenia (platelet count <150,000/μL) as high as 64%, but only 7% had severe thrombocytopenia.[125] Later studies reported a lower incidence of neonatal thrombocytopenia associated with maternal ITP, ranging from 13% to 56%.[126–131] In those series, the incidence of severe neonatal thrombocytopenia (platelet count <50,000/μL) varied from 5% to 20%.[127–129, 132] The disparity between studies can be explained by the differences in the definition of thrombocytopenia (platelet count <100,000 versus <150,000/μL) and by the timing of the neonatal platelet count, because autoimmune thrombocytopenia classically reaches its nadir 2 to 5 days after birth. In one study, the incidence of severe neonatal thrombocytopenia among infants born to mothers with ITP was 14.3% 3 days after delivery, compared with only 3.6% at the time of birth.[132]

In contrast to the controversies regarding the incidence of neonatal thrombocytopenia associated with maternal ITP, later studies coincide in reporting a very low rate of significant bleeding complications in these infants, particularly intracranial hemorrhages. Cook and colleagues,[133] in an analysis of 474 infants born to mothers with ITP reported in the literature until 1991, found an incidence of intracranial hemorrhage of 3% among infants with moderate or severe thrombocytopenia. They did not find a significant association between the delivery mode (cesarean section versus vaginal delivery) and the rate of intracranial hemorrhage. Later studies have confirmed a very low fetal morbidity associated with maternal ITP, and some series have not reported any cases of intracranial hemorrhage.[127, 129, 131–133]

Factors predictive of the severity of neonatal thrombocytopenia have been the subject of significant research. Maternal platelet count, history of splenectomy, titers of PAIgG or serum platelet-bindable IgG, and platelet counts of older siblings have all been investigated with nonconcordant results.[129, 130, 131, 134, 135] Samuels and associates[136] studied 162 women with the presumptive diagnosis of ITP, looking for predictive factors for neonatal thrombocytopenia, and found that the absence of a history of ITP and negative results on circulating-antibody testing were associated with a minimal risk of severe neonatal thrombocytopenia. The lack of uniform predictive factors has complicated the obstetric management of pregnant women with ITP.

Infectious Causes

Thrombocytopenia commonly accompanies systemic infections in neonates. If thrombocytopenia is diagnosed as a platelet count of less than 150,000/μL, perhaps 80% of neonates who have proven infections are thrombocytopenic.[137] If thrombocytopenia is diagnosed as a platelet count of less than 100,000/μL, 55% to 65% of neonates who have proven infections are thrombocytopenic.[138, 139]

Bacterial Infections

Most studies indicate that with the onset of systemic bacterial infection, the first complete blood cell count change is generally a leukocyte "left shift," followed by a fall in platelet count. The studies of Zipursky and Tchernia indicate that, at the time sepsis is diagnosed, about 25% of neonates have thrombocytopenia, but by 36 to 48 hours later, most have developed thrombocytopenia.[137, 138] The duration of thrombocytopenia during an episode of systemic bacterial infection varies. In the series of Modanlou, 6 days was the average duration of such thrombocytopenia.[139]

Some septic neonates develop thrombocytopenia because of DIC, but others have thrombocytopenia without the laboratory findings of DIC. In a study of septic adults by Neame,[140] thrombocytopenia occurred in about 75% of patients, but DIC was only diagnosed in a small minority, and these were the subgroup who had platelet counts of less than 50,000/μL. The principal mechanism responsible for thrombocytopenia in infected neonates is accelerated platelet destruction. This conclusion is drawn from the rapidity of the fall in platelet count,[141] the shortened platelet survival time when platelet transfusions are administered to these patients[142, 143] and the increase in MPV,[144] suggesting the marrow is compensating by releasing platelets. The reason that platelets have a short life span during sepsis probably involves endothelial damage with subsequent platelet adhesion and aggregation and perhaps involves platelet lysis or removal by the reticuloendothelial system.[145, 146]

Decreased platelet production has also been proposed as a contributing mechanism.[101] Our findings of a plasma thrombopoietin (TPO) concentration of more than 1000 pg/mL in some neonates with sepsis suggest that a decrease in marrow megakaryocyte mass may be a contributing factor, because very high plasma TPO concentrations often correlate with very small megakaryocyte masses. The extent to which bone marrow suppression of platelet production occurs in some septic neonates is unclear.

Clinical bleeding abnormalities because of the thrombocytopenia of bacterial infection are rare, perhaps because this variety of thrombocytopenia usually is not severe, with platelet counts typically in the 50,000 to 100,000/μL range. In contrast, when a septic neonate develops thrombocytopenia as a manifestation of DIC, platelet counts are commonly less than 20,000/μL, and bleeding is common. In such cases, platelet transfusions can be helpful.

It appears that virtually any bacterial organism capable of causing sepsis in a neonate is also capable of inducing thrombocytopenia. Thrombocytopenia (in the absence of DIC) has been reported during infections with a wide variety of common and unusual organisms; the latter group include *Acinetobacter*,[147] *Shigella*,[148] *Flavobacterium meningosepticum*,[149, 150] and *Aeromonas*.[151]

Fungal Infections

Fungal organisms are increasingly important as causes of sepsis in very-low-birth-weight neonates. Padovani and coworkers reported 26 neonates who had fungal sepsis and observed that 19 (73%) presented with thrombocytopenia.[152] Fungal sepsis is a particularly common problem among extremely-low-birth-weight neonates. As an example, Melville and colleagues reported seven extremely preterm neonates who developed severe *Candida* infection during a 1-month period in the Regional Neonatal Intensive Care Unit in Whitechapel.[153] All seven were less than 26 weeks' gestation, and all weighed less than 750 g at birth. The median age of onset of *Candida* sepsis was 7 days, and thrombocytopenia was the most consistent early laboratory finding. The problem of *Candida* sepsis in extremely-low-birth-weight infants prompted McDonnell and Isaacs to recommend empirical antifungal treatment while awaiting culture results when thrombocytopenia is seen in an extremely-low-birth-weight infant who is clinically septic with a nosocomial infection.[154]

Infection with *Malassezia furfur* has also emerged as a problem among extremely-low-birth-weight infants, particularly among those receiving intravenous lipid emulsions. Since the first report in a neonate in 1981, many cases and series have been published. Surmont and associates described six such neonates, all of whom presented with thrombocytopenia.[155] Richet and coworkers reported three similar neonates (all with birth weights of less than 1000 g), two of whom died, in whom thrombocytopenia developed along with respiratory failure and bronchopneumonia.[156] Kim reported the cases of two preterm infants in whom the Silastic catheter used for hyperalimentation (including lipid infusions) became adherent to the vessel wall and difficult to remove in association with *M. furfur* fungemia.[157] In contrast to the thrombocytopenia that accompanies bacterial infection, the variety seen with fungal sepsis is generally severe, with most counts falling below 50,000/μL unless periodic transfusions are employed.[158]

Viral Infections

Thrombocytopenia is fairly common in women with human immunodeficiency virus (HIV) infection because of disease progression or antiviral treatment.[159] In contrast, thrombocytopenia seems to be rare in the HIV-infected neonates of these women.[160] Other congenital viral infections, however, typically cause thrombocytopenia. All of the organisms that cause TORCH (i.e., toxoplasmosis, other infections, rubella, cytomegalovirus [CMV], and herpes simplex) can cause thrombocytopenia, and CMV is a classic cause of congenital thrombocytopenia. Results of a phase II study of ganciclovir treatment of symptomatic, congenitally CMV-infected neonates showed that most of the study patients had severe thrombocytopenia (platelet count <50,000/μL).[161]

Coxsackievirus B can cause a fulminant hepatitis and thrombocytopenia that is evident at birth. Sometimes, myocarditis and central nervous system involvement are minimal, and liver failure, respiratory failure, and profound thrombocytopenia are the principal findings.[162] A similar syndrome can be seen in congenital echovirus 11 infection.[163, 164] Congenital parvovirus (B19) is most commonly associated with hydrops and anemia, but thrombocytopenia can be part of the pathology.[165] Congenital Epstein-Barr virus,[166] mumps,[167] and adenovirus infections have caused thrombocytopenia.[168]

The kinetic mechanism resulting in thrombocytopenia of congenital viral infections is most likely a mixture of diminished production and accelerated destruction. The few cases for which marrow aspirates have been reported generally indicate reduced marrow megakaryocytes, but the accuracy of aspirates for this purpose is suspect. Vacuolization of megakaryocytes has been reported, suggesting virus-induced megakaryocyte dysfunction.[169] The splenomegaly and reticuloendothelial hyperactivity that accompany most of these congenital viral infections may lead to platelet removal from the circulation, and endothelial damage from the virus or its sequela could lead to platelet activation, aggregation, and removal.

Genetic Associations

A variety of syndromes and congenital disorders have historically been associated with neonatal thrombocytopenia (Table 13–7). In most cases, the mechanism responsible for the thrombocytopenia is decreased platelet production as a consequence of reduced megakaryocytes or impaired platelet production from megakaryocytes. Although cases of congenital amegakaryocytic thrombocytopenia without associated anomalies have been described, they are unusual. Most of these patients present with obvi-

Table 13–7. Genetic Causes of Thrombocytopenia in Neonates

Thrombocytopenia with absent radii (TAR) syndrome
Fanconi's anemia
Congenital amegakaryocytic thrombocytopenia
Congenital hypoplastic thrombocytopenia with microcephaly
Congenital thrombocytopenia, Robin sequence, agenesis of the corpus callosum, distinctive facies, and developmental delay
Familial macrothrombocytopenias
- Bernard-Soulier syndrome
- May-Hegglin anomaly
- Paris-Trousseau thrombocytopenia
- X-linked recessive thrombocytopenia

Chromosomal abnormalities
- Trisomy 13
- Trisomy 18
- Trisomy 21 (Down syndrome)
- Turner's syndrome

Neonatal thrombocytopenia associated with other genetic disorders
- Wiskott-Aldrich syndrome (WAS)
- Noonan syndrome
- Alport's syndrome
- Inherited metabolic disorders
  - Methyl malonic acidemia
  - Ketotic glycinemia
  - Isovaleric acidemia
  - Holocarboxylase synthetase deficiency

ous anomalies that are detected on physical examination.

Thrombocytopenia with Absent Radii Syndrome

Thrombocytopenia with absent radii (TAR) syndrome is a congenital syndrome transmitted in an autosomal recessive fashion and characterized by severe thrombocytopenia and bilateral absent radii.[170] In 1988, Hedberg and Lipton published a review of 100 cases of TAR syndrome and summarized the characteristics of the disorder.[171] All affected individuals have bilateral absence of the radius and abnormalities of the ulna. Other skeletal abnormalities are frequently observed, most commonly involving the upper extremities, but the thumbs and digits are almost always present, a feature that distinguishes TAR from Fanconi's anemia. Approximately one third of the patients have associated heart defects, primarily tetralogy of Fallot and atrial septal defect.[170]

The most striking hematologic feature of the syndrome is severe thrombocytopenia (platelet count <10,000 to 30,000/μL) in 59% of the cases at birth or before 1 week of age and in 90% of the patients by 4 months of age. Approximately 25% of affected individuals die,[172] usually of intracranial hemorrhage. Most deaths occur during the first year of life, particularly in the first 4 months. The natural history of the disorder during infancy is complicated by exacerbations of the thrombocytopenia by viral illnesses (particularly gastrointestinal) and cow's milk allergy or intolerance. If the affected individuals survive through this period, the thrombocytopenia generally resolves over a variable period, with normal platelet counts usually present by school age.[103]

Affected infants can have other hematologic abnormalities. Leukemoid reactions occur in 63%, usually in association with exacerbations of the thrombocytopenia.[173] Eosinophilia and anemia also occur frequently. Bone marrow examination reveals absent or reduced megakaryocytes, and the remaining megakaryocytes are hypoplastic or immature.[174] Bone marrow cellularity is normal, and myeloid and erythroid cell lines are normal or increased.[172]

Until recently, the pathophysiology of the thrombocytopenia in TAR syndrome was the subject of multiple hypotheses. After the cloning of TPO, however, it was demonstrated that these patients had elevated serum concentrations of TPO and that they expressed the TPO receptor on the surface of their platelets. However, the TPO-induced tyrosine phosphorylation of platelet proteins was completely absent or markedly decreased, suggesting that the underlying mechanism is a lack of response to TPO in the signal transduction pathway of its receptor (MPL).[175] Sekine and colleagues[176] subsequently cultured bone marrow cells from a patient with TAR syndrome in the presence of TPO, and demonstrated the presence of megakaryocyte colonies in greater numbers than in age-matched control marrow cells. However, the colonies grown from the patient's progenitor cells appeared to be smaller, suggesting a decreased proliferative response to TPO.

Whether pharmacologic dosages or recombinant TPO (rTPO) will result in improved platelet production in these patients is unknown. The only treatment available is vigorous support with platelet transfusions to maintain the platelet counts above 10,000 to 15,000/μL until spontaneous resolution of the thrombocytopenia occurs. This support is rarely necessary beyond the first year of life.

Fanconi's Anemia

Since Fanconi's first description of three brothers with pancytopenia and physical anomalies, in 1927,[177] more than 700 cases have been reported.[178] Fanconi's anemia is an autosomal recessive disorder with marked variability in the clinical phenotype. Classic features include radial ray defects in 49% of cases, including hypoplasia to aplasia of the thumb or supernumerary thumbs (a feature that distinguishes it from TAR syndrome), short stature (frequently of prenatal onset), microcephaly (25%), eye anomalies (41%), renal and urinary tract anomalies (34%), brownish pigmentation of the skin (64%), and pancytopenia that usually does not manifest until childhood (median age, 7 years).[179] Occasionally, Fanconi's anemia can present with isolated thrombocytopenia and absent or hypoplastic radii, resembling TAR syndrome. The aplasia or hypoplasia of the thumbs seen in Fanconi's anemia is then an important characteristic for differentiating the two syndromes.

These patients rarely experience any hematologic problems in the neonatal period.[180, 181] The problems usually manifest later in childhood with isolated thrombocytopenia or leukopenia that eventually progresses to pancytopenia.[182] Classically, their erythrocytes have fetal characteristics even in the pre-anemic state, including macrocytosis, increased hemoglobin F, and I antigen.[183, 184] The diagnosis is usually based on the clinical presentation and the presence of a high proportion of chromosomal breaks, gaps, and rearrangements in baseline cultures and more so when clastogenic agents such as diepoxybutane are used.[185] A new molecular diagnostic test has also been described.[186]

When making the diagnosis, it is important to consider that 25% of the affected individuals are structurally normal. For this reason, the diagnosis should be considered whenever a child presents with thrombocytopenia, anemia, leukopenia, or pancytopenia accompanied by chromosome breaks, even in the absence of dysmorphic features. Conversely, because the median age of onset of hematologic problems is 7 years, the diagnosis should be entertained for every neonate with clinical features suggestive of Fanconi's anemia, even in the absence of hematologic manifestations.[179]

Butturini and associates[182] published data analyzed from 388 patients with Fanconi's anemia. Thirty-five percent of the patients died at a median age of 13 years, mostly as a consequence of hematologic problems. Twenty-eight percent of these hematologic-related deaths were caused by development of myeloid leukemias or myelodysplastic syndromes. Current treatment modalities for patients with Fanconi's anemia include supportive care, androgen therapy, and bone marrow transplantation. Several reports of successful umbilical cord blood-derived progenitor cell transplantation from histocompatible siblings[187–189] offer a new therapeutic alternative to these patients. The use of recombinant hematopoietic growth factors has not been adequately tested.

Congenital Amegakaryocytic Thrombocytopenia

Congenital amegakaryocytic thrombocytopenia is a rare disorder characterized by isolated, moderate to severe thrombocytopenia in the first year of life in the absence of other physical abnormalities. These infants are frequently diagnosed initially with NAIT, but no maternal alloantibodies can be demonstrated. The bone marrow examination reveals absent or extremely scarce and small megakaryocytes with normal marrow cellularity.[190] Of the 21 cases reported, 12 presented in the first week of life and the remainder in the first 9 years.[190] The male to female ratio is 2:3, suggesting X-linked transmission in some cases.[191]

The platelet count at the time of diagnosis ranges from 0 to 80,000/μL. Approximately one half of the patients initially diagnosed with amegakaryocytic thrombocytopenia eventually develop aplastic anemia; the median age is 3.5 years.[190] Some patients also develop leukemia or preleukemia.[190] Mortality from this disorder is extremely high, usually because of hemorrhagic problems or infections related to the pancytopenia. Bone marrow transplantation has been curative in some patients.[192]

The pathophysiology of congenital amegakaryocytic thrombocytopenia has begun to be disclosed. Muraoka and coworkers[193] studied the expression of TPO and its receptor (MPL) in a patient with congenital amegakaryocytic thrombocytopenia. They found that the serum TPO level in this patient was significantly higher than in normal controls but that the response of bone marrow progenitors to rTPO in vitro was defective. They did not detect expression of the TPO receptor mRNA in the marrow mononuclear cells from the patient, suggesting that the defect responsible for the thrombocytopenia and subsequent aplastic anemia might be an impaired expression of the TPO receptor. The response of bone marrow cells to other cytokines has also been investigated.[194] In vitro studies demonstrated that the megakaryocyte progenitors responded to the addition of interleukin-3 (IL-3), granulocyte-macrophage colony-stimulating factor (GM-CSF), or the combination of both with increased numbers of CFU-MK derived colonies. In a phase I/II trial, both cytokines were administered to five patients with this disorder. IL-3 administration resulted in improved platelet counts in two patients and decreased bleeding and transfusion requirements in the remaining three. No clinical benefit was demonstrated from GM-CSF administration.

Congenital Hypoplastic Thrombocytopenia with Microcephaly

A few cases of congenital amegakaryocytic thrombocytopenia associated with microcephaly have been reported.[195–197] The absence of other associated anomalies and the persistence of the thrombocytopenia beyond the first year of life suggests that a viral infection is not the etiologic factor responsible for this association.

Congenital Thrombocytopenia, Robin Sequence, Agenesis of the Corpus Callosum, Distinctive Facies, and Developmental Delay

Braddock and Carey[198] described two children with a distinctive pattern of malformations, thought to constitute a previously undescribed syndrome. Both patients presented with Robin sequence, agenesis of the corpus callosum, and persistent thrombocytopenia with onset in the newborn period. Both progressed to growth delay, microcephaly, mental retardation, and enamel hypoplasia. Bone marrow aspiration showed adequate megakaryocytes in the first patient and decreased megakaryocytes in the second. This discrepancy may reflect difficulties in the interpretation of bone marrow aspirates rather than differences in the disease processes.

Familial Macrothrombocytopenias

Certain forms of congenital thrombocytopenia are associated with an increased platelet volume (i.e., macrothrombocytopenia), with or without any other hematologic abnormalities. Bernard-Soulier syndrome is an autosomal recessive disorder characterized by mild thrombocytopenia, giant platelets seen on the blood smear, and easy bruising and severe bleeding associated with injuries or surgery.[199] The primary defect responsible for this disorder is the absence of glycoprotein Ib from the platelet membrane,[200] accompanied by a deficiency of glycoproteins V and IX.[201, 202] In normal subjects, these proteins associate on the platelet surface to form a receptor called the GPIb-IX-V complex, which serves two important functions. It mediates platelet adhesion to the blood vessel wall at sites of injury by binding von Willebrand's factor, and it facilitates thrombin-mediated platelet activation.[203]

May-Hegglin anomaly is a rare autosomal dominant disorder also characterized by thrombocytopenia and giant platelets, accompanied by blue-staining inclusions in the cytoplasm of neutrophils, eosinophils, basophils, and monocytes.[204] Ultrastructural and functional platelet defects have been described in patients with May-Hegglin anomaly.[205] A novel congenital macrothrombocytopenia associated with giant platelet α-granules in a subpopulation of platelets (Paris-Trousseau thrombocytopenia) has been described in a woman and her 1-month old son. This disorder, characterized by mild hemorrhagic manifestations, unusual facial features, and mental retardation, is associated with a chromosome 11 deletion at 11q23. The bone marrow examination disclosed an increased number of megakaryocytes, including micromegakaryocytes, and evidence of massive cell lysis at the end of the maturation in bone marrow cultures.[206]

A form of X-linked thrombocytopenia associated with large platelets and a hypermegakaryocytic bone marrow has also been described in three brothers from Saudi Arabia.[207] DNA analysis in the affected boys indicated that the locus of the relevant gene lies close to or is identical to the locus of the gene for the Wiskott-Aldrich syndrome.

Chromosomal Abnormalities

Infants with trisomies of chromosomes 13, 18, or 21 and infants with Turner's syndrome can present with neonatal thrombocytopenia in addition to the characteristic physical features.[208] Hohlfeld and colleagues[209] examined platelet counts in 5194 fetal blood samples (17 to 41 weeks), and 247 fetuses had platelet counts less than 150,000/μL, 43 (17%) because of chromosomal abnormalities, including trisomy 13 (6), trisomy 18 (26), trisomy 21 (3), Turner's syndrome (5), and triploidy (3). In that study, 87% of all fetuses diagnosed with trisomy 18, 54% of those with trisomy 13, 31% of those with Turner's syndrome, and 7% of those with Down syndrome had thrombocytopenia. In all cases, the thrombocytopenia was mild to moderate (50,000 to 150,000/μL). Although historically, trisomy 21 has been mostly associated with other hematologic disorders, such as polycythemia, transient myeloproliferative disorder, and acute leukemia,[210] isolated neonatal thrombocytopenia is a frequent finding.

In a study of 25 neonates with Down syndrome, Hord and associates[211] found an incidence of isolated thrombocytopenia, defined as a platelet count of less than 100,000/μL, of 28%. In all cases, the thrombocytopenia was mild to moderate (platelet count >40,000/μL) and transient, with resolution at 2 to 3 weeks of life. Based on these findings, they suggested not performing an extensive evaluation of mild to moderate thrombocytopenia in neonates with Down syndrome.

Neonatal Thrombocytopenia Associated with Other Genetic Disorders

The Wiskott-Aldrich syndrome (WAS) is classically described as an X-linked immunodeficiency disease associated with thrombocytopenia, severe bleeding tendency, and eczema.[212] The responsible gene has been mapped to the short arm of the X chromosome, at Xp11.2.[213] The first symptoms usually occur early in infancy, when the infants present with gastrointestinal bleeding or excessive bleeding after circumcision. The eczematous skin also tends to become infected, mostly with *Staphylococcus* organisms. On laboratory evaluation, these patients invariably have low levels of platelets that are also very small and have impaired aggregation in response to ADP, epinephrine, ristocetin, and collagen.[214] The megakaryocytes are normal, but the production of viable platelets is decreased.[212] The immunodeficiency results from impairment of cellular and humoral immunity. Although splenectomy usually improves the platelet counts, it increases the risk of overwhelming infections with encapsulated organisms. For that reason, bone marrow transplantation is considered the treatment of choice.[212]

Thrombocytopenia has also been observed in infants with Noonan syndrome, a rare autosomal dominant disorder characterized by facial anomalies, congenital heart disease, skeletal abnormalities, genital malformations, and mild mental retardation. In these patients, the thrombocytopenia has been associated with a myeloproliferative disorder[215] or with a wide variety of hemostatic abnormalities.[216] A case of congenital cutaneous lymphangioma and amegakaryocytic thrombocytopenia in an infant with Noonan syndrome has been reported.[217] Patients with Alport's syndrome, characterized by hereditary nephritis and nerve deafness, can also present with thrombocytopenia and large platelets (macrothrombocytopenia), sometimes in association with defects of platelet function.[218, 219] Neonatal thrombocytopenia has been associated with certain inherited metabolic disorders, including methyl malonic acidemia, ketotic glycinemia, isovaleric acidemia, and holocarboxylase synthetase deficiency.[173]

The mechanism responsible for the thrombocytopenia in these disorders is unclear. Other hereditary disorders that are associated with thrombocytopenia or pancytopenia, such as dyskeratosis congenita, are not discussed here because they almost never have hematologic manifestations in the neonatal period.

Drugs That Produce Thrombocytopenia in the Mother and Fetus

Numerous chemical agents have been reported to cause thrombocytopenia.[220] Only a few drugs, however, have been implicated beyond the statistical probability of coincidence. For medications that are taken by a significant portion of the population, an apparent association between drug ingestion and development of thrombocytopenia in any given case report can be entirely coincidental.

Certain drugs administered to pregnant women have been reported to cause thrombocytopenia in the women and in their fetuses or neonates.[221] Generally, only a very small minority of the mothers who receive the particular drug in question have this reaction. In any given case, it is not possible to know whether this is coincidental to the medication or a drug-induced dyscrasia. When statistical probability suggests that the drug is likely to be responsible, the rarity of the occurrence indicates that the reaction is "idiosyncratic." The mechanism by which drugs produce idiosyncratic thrombocytopenia in the mother and fetus is unclear but may involve an immune reaction in which antibody is formed against a drug-haptene complex that cross-reacts with a platelet antigen. When such an antibody is of the IgG subclass, not only can it attach to maternal platelets, but it can also cross the placenta and simultaneously attach to the fetal platelets. An early example of this was reported by Mauer.[222] A mother who took quinine developed thrombocytopenia, and at delivery, her neonate also had thrombocytopenia, and platelet agglutinins were demonstrated in both. The drugs, besides quinine, that have been implicated in this condition include thiazide diuretics, hydralazine, and tolbutamide.[223]

Thiazide diuretics are noteworthy because two different mechanisms have been proposed, each causing a kinetically different variety of neonatal thrombocytopenia. One mechanism is reduced platelet production in the fetus, with reduced megakaryocytes in the fetal marrow, and without affecting the mother's platelet count. The second is a hapten-antibody–mediated destruction of platelets, as was proposed for quinine. The former mechanism has been suggested as the more common of the two.[224, 225] Rodriguez reported seven purpuric neonates of mothers taking thiazides, but the mothers themselves were not thrombocytopenic. One of these infants died at 40 hours of life of subdural and pulmonary hemorrhages. In the others, bleeding was not abnormal or was very mild, and all recovered spontaneously after 2 to 12 weeks. Bone marrow aspirates revealed decreased megakaryocytes in four of five studied. This should be interpreted with some skepticism, however, because quantification of megakaryocytes in marrow aspirates of neonates is very difficult, and no studies employing marrow biopsy techniques to quantify megakaryocytes of these infants have been reported. It is possible that both varieties of chlorothiazide-induced thrombocytopenia are antibody mediated. The apparent hyporegenerative variety could be the result of antibodies directed against megakaryocyte antigens, thereby suppressing platelet production, whereas the hyperregenerative variety could be the result of antibodies directed against antigens on platelets, with marrow megakaryocytes increased in an attempt to compensate. In prospective studies following mothers and neonates when the women were taking or not taking thiazides, no statistical differences have been seen in the platelet counts of mothers or neonates. There is a general impression that thiazide administration to pregnant women rarely or never causes neonatal thrombocytopenia.

Kumar and Yu reported thrombocytopenia to be a minor and transient complication of indomethacin treatment of very-low-birth-weight infants.[226] In a larger study (n = 90), Couser and coworkers did not observe a higher incidence of thrombocytopenia among neonates who were treated with indomethacin than among those treated with placebo.[227]

Disseminated Intravascular Coagulation (DIC)

It is impossible to make a diagnosis of DIC in a neonate unless thrombocytopenia, or at least a falling platelet count, is detected. Thrombocytopenia is a consistent finding and usually a very early finding in neonates with DIC. Although the thrombocytopenia is sometimes severe, it is more often in the 50,000 to 100,000/μL range.

The rapidity with which the platelet count often falls in neonates who develop DIC suggests that accelerated platelet destruction is the responsible kinetic mechanism. Decreased platelet production, however, may be an accompanying feature, but the studies to determine this are incomplete. The exact mechanisms by which the platelets are damaged and removed from the circulation in neonates with DIC have not been elucidated. Presumably, some platelets are removed because of attachment to damaged endothelium or thrombi. Perhaps some are removed because of sequestration or uptake by reticuloendothelial cells. Other issues of DIC diagnosis and management are provided in Chapter 12.

Miscellaneous Causes of Neonatal Thrombocytopenia

In the miscellaneous category (Table 13–8), we include thrombocytopenias caused by thrombosis (renal vein, intracardiac, vascular), NEC, intrauterine growth retardation, pregnancy-induced hypertension, asphyxia, and idiopathic conditions.

Thrombosis

Thrombocytopenia sometimes occurs in neonates who have none of the other etiologic factors discussed elsewhere in this chapter but who have localized thrombi. These thrombi may be located in the renal vein, attached to an indwelling catheter, or in the ECMO circuit. In such cases, it is not always clear whether the thrombocytopenia is caused by platelet attachment to a developing thrombus or by platelet destruction through interactions between the circulating platelets and whatever pathologic surfaces in the vascular system caused the thrombosis in the first place. Pathologic alterations of vessels that can damage platelets include indwelling catheters,[228] stenotic heart valves,[229] and ECMO circuits.[68]

Table 13–8. **Miscellaneous Causes of Thrombocytopenia in Neonates**

Thrombosis
Renal vein
Intracardiac
Vascular
Necrotizing enterocolitis
Small for gestational age or delivered to hypertensive women
Asphyxia
Idiopathic

When platelets interact with foreign surfaces, a sequence of events is initiated that is similar to that which occurs when platelets are activated normally. For instance, when platelets contact the ECMO circuits, a preferential release of α-granule constituents occurs.[230] As more extensive platelet activation occurs in the circulation, the damaged platelets are removed from the circulation by the reticuloendothelial system. When this process occurs more rapidly than platelets can be produced, thrombocytopenia occurs. In such cases, the thrombocytopenia can be treated by platelet transfusions, but until the underlying cause of the platelet destruction has been removed, the need for platelet transfusions can be expected to continue.

Infected right atrial thrombosis is a rare complication of neonatal intensive care. The thrombus generally develops around a right atrial catheter. De Schepper and colleagues reported two infants with such thrombi who presented with protracted thrombocytopenia after episodes of catheter-related sepsis and were treated by administering antibiotics through the catheters.[231] Cardiotomies were performed for removal of the infected thrombi in both cases.

Sometimes, ill neonates develop thrombocytopenia associated with platelet thrombi on the cardiac valves.[232] The absence of the other coagulation defects distinguishes this variety of thrombocytopenia from DIC. Favara postulated that injury to the endothelium initiated local platelet adhesion and aggregation. Morrow[233] observed thrombocytopenia in neonates with pulmonary hypertension and persistent fetal circulation and postulated that the hypertension was caused by vasoconstriction from substances released by the platelets aggregated in the pulmonary capillaries.

Necrotizing Enterocolitis

Thrombocytopenia occurs frequently in neonates who have necrotizing enterocolitis (NEC).[234, 235] Probably 80% to 90% of patients with NEC develop thrombocytopenia (platelet count <150,000/μL) as part of the presentation, and many have platelet counts in the range of 30,000 to 60,000/μL. A minority of these patients have DIC, but like patients with DIC, platelet destruction seems to be the operative mechanism, because platelet transfusions do not generally maintain a normal blood platelet concentration for more than 1 or 2 days.

The inflammatory mediator, PAF, appears to play a role in the pathogenesis of NEC. Administration of a PAF-receptor antagonist can largely prevent NEC in an neonatal rat model.[236] Similarly, administration of an enzyme that degrades PAF reduces or eliminates NEC in this model.[237] The intestinal tissue of neonates appears to have a greater capacity for synthesizing PAF on a gram for gram basis than the intestinal tissue of adults.[238] The extent to which PAF is involved in the genesis of the thrombocytopenia that so commonly accompanies NEC is unknown.

Intrauterine Growth Retardation

Thrombocytopenia was first recognized as a problem among small for gestational age (SGA) preterm infants in 1982, when Meberg and associates contrasted the hematologic findings of 14 appropriately grown (AGA) infants with 16 who were SGA.[239] The SGA infants had significantly higher hematocrits but significantly lower platelet counts. Subsequently, Philip studied 374 preterm infants during their first day of life, and observed that the SGA infants had significantly higher circulating nucleated red cells but lower levels of neutrophils and platelets than AGA infants.[240] Thrombocytopenia is particularly common in preterm SGA infants but is relatively uncommon in term SGA infants.[241]

The cause of the thrombocytopenia and the neutropenia so commonly seen in preterm SGA infants is unknown. Peters suggested that the pathogenesis involved accelerated platelet removal from the blood. Specifically, it was postulated that the development of polycythemia, from reduced oxygen delivery in utero, led to increased fetal blood viscosity and reduced blood flow on the fetal side of the placenta, increasing the risk of placental infarction with thrombus formation and platelet removal.[242] Koyama also postulated accelerated platelet removal but thought it was the result of maternal anti-HLA antibodies, which were detected in the sera of 10 of 11 mothers who gave birth to an SGA thrombocytopenic infant.[243]

Another theory to explain the kinetic mechanism of thrombocytopenia among preterm SGA infants was proposed by Murray and Roberts,[101] who cultured megakaryocyte progenitors from the peripheral blood of 26 thrombocytopenic and 37 normal neonates. Twenty-one of the 26 with thrombocytopenia were SGA or born after pregnancy-induced hypertension (PIH), and all had low circulating levels of megakaryocyte progenitors. The thrombocytopenia generally resolved by 10 days and was preceded by an increase in circulating megakaryocyte progenitors. Subsequently, they studied 13 thrombocytopenic neonates, 11 of whom were SGA or were born after PIH. Circulating TPO concentrations were no different in the thrombocytopenic than in the control infants.[244] The researchers postulated that these two common forms of thrombocytopenia are the kinetic result of reduced platelet production associated with low quantities of megakaryocyte progenitors and a failure to compensate by increasing TPO production. Additional studies are needed to determine the kinetic mechanism responsible for these common varieties of thrombocytopenia and to test treatment alternatives to repeated platelet transfusions.

Pregnancy-Induced Hypertension

Thrombocytopenia is common among neonates delivered to women with PIH,[245] but the pathogenesis of the condition and best method of treatment are unclear. Neutropenia is also common in these neonates, and our group and others have evaluated the pathogenesis, natural history, and treatment of that variety of neutropenia.[246] The neutropenia is the kinetic result of decreased neutrophil production.[246, 247] An as yet unidentified inhibitor of neutrophil production, elaborated by the placenta, is likely to be involved, because placental extracts from these pregnancies (but not from matched nonhypertensive pregnancies) cause a diminution in neutrophil production when cocultured with hematopoietic progenitors from normal adults.[247]

Some overlap probably exists between the varieties of thrombocytopenia among preterm SGA infants and infants born to women with PIH. Many thrombocytopenic neonates are SGA and born after PIH. Most thrombocytopenic SGA infants, however, are not born after PIH.[239] It is likely that the thrombocytopenia observed in neonates delivered to women with PIH, like the neutropenia also seen in these neonates, is the kinetic result of decreased production. In support of this theory is our observation that the MPV in 10 thrombocytopenic neonates born after PIH was normal, not increased, as often occurs when neonatal thrombocytopenia is the result of accelerated platelet destruction.[246] We found that thrombocytopenia almost exclusively occurs in the subset of neonates whose mothers had severe hypertension. We observed that essentially all such thrombocytopenic neonates had severe neutropenia also and that these patients had the longest duration of cytopenia of any identified subset.[246]

Because PIH is common, this variety of neonatal thrombocytopenia is also common. PIH occurs in up to 12% of pregnancies, and severe hypertension occurs in up to 3%.[248] Neonates delivered to women with severe hypertension have a 75% to 90% incidence of neutropenia, and one third to one half of these have severe thrombocytopenia lasting up to 21 days or sometimes longer.[245–247] Based on these statistics, we can expect an incidence of PIH-related neonatal thrombocytopenia of 1 case per 100 live births. Among all infants born to women with PIH, preterm babies are at higher risk of developing thrombocytopenia; term infants of hypertensive mothers are not more likely to be thrombocytopenic than are control infants.[249]

Other than platelet transfusions, no treatment is available for these patients, and until the responsible kinetic mechanism is understood, advances in treating this common variety of thrombocytopenia are probably unlikely.

Asphyxia

Castle and coworkers performed a 1-year prospective study of 807 infants admitted to an NICU and observed that thrombocytopenia developed in 22%. Birth asphyxia appeared to be a significant risk factor, because it was seen significantly more often in those who developed thrombocytopenia than in those who did not.[5] Ropert and colleagues described 64 cases of severe neonatal thrombocytopenia (platelet count <50,000/μL) for whom they attempted to determine the cause. Classic causes were found for 33%, but in the remaining 67% (idiopathic), hypoxia was significantly more common than in the group with thrombocytopenia of a determined cause. They concluded that hypoxia plays a role in the pathogenesis of idiopathic thrombocytopenia in neonates.[250]

Similarly, Oren and associates reported a 2-year prospective study of 643 neonates admitted to their NICU, where 18.2% developed thrombocytopenia. As in the studies of Castle and Ropert, hypoxia was more common among the thrombocytopenic than the nonthrombocytopenic patients.[94]

The effect of hypoxia on platelet survival was studied in newborn and adults rabbits. Inhalation of 5% oxygen for 15 minutes did not produce acidemia or thrombocytopenia but did shorten the ^{111}In-oxine–labeled platelet survival because of platelet sequestration in the liver and spleen.[251]

Idiopathic Conditions

Many cases of thrombocytopenia remain idiopathic after extensive evaluation. In two large studies, up to 60% of all cases of neonatal thrombocytopenia fell into this category.[4, 252] In these two studies, thrombocytopenia associated with SGA infants or maternal hypertension was listed as idiopathic, but other neonates fell into this idiopathic category, because not all were SGA or delivered to hypertensive women. Neonates with idiopathic thrombocytopenia usually have platelet counts in the 50,000 to 100,000/μL range and are not severely thrombocytopenic, although the thrombocytopenia can be problematic and persist for many weeks.

Some of these neonates with idiopathic thrombocytopenia may have heparin-induced conditions. In adults, as many as 10% of patients receiving heparin develop a mild form of heparin-induced thrombocytopenia,[253] and bovine heparin seems to produce a higher incidence of such than porcine heparin. Bleeding problems usually do not occur. Patients recover rapidly when the heparin is stopped, and the disorder is not associated with thrombosis. The new low-molecular-weight heparin products have a much lower incidence of this complication.

A severe form of heparin-induced thrombocytopenia (i.e., “white clot” syndrome) is associated with thrombocytopenia and widespread thrombosis (often arterial). The cause is an antibody that damages the platelets and the endothelium.[254] Treatment involves discontinuation of heparin and perhaps switching to low-molecular-weight heparin, which is usually effective without producing heparin-induced thrombocytopenia.

Spadone and coworkers[255] attempted to determine whether heparin-induced thrombocytopenia occurs in neonates and evaluated 34 neonates who had thrombocytopenia (<70,000/μL) of unknown origin while receiving heparin. Heparin-associated anti-platelet antibodies were demonstrated in 14 infants by platelet aggregation testing. An umbilical artery catheter was present in all except one, and aortic thrombosis was documented by abdominal ultrasonography in 12 (85%). Abnormal bleeding was not observed in these patients. In one, the thrombocytopenia remitted when the heparin was removed but returned with its reintroduction. The researchers concluded that heparin-induced thrombocytopenia does occur in preterm infants receiving heparin and that it is associated with arterial thromboses. In neonates who have idiopathic thrombocytopenia and are receiving heparin, this variety should be considered.

Some patients receiving phototherapy for hyperbilirubinemia develop a diminution of their platelet counts. We consider this form to be in the category of idiopathic thrombocytopenia, because the mechanism is not clear. Platelet destruction is likely, perhaps occurring in the phototherapy-exposed skin vasculature, because the counts fall faster than would be expected if decreased production were responsible.[256] This variety does not appear to cause severe thrombocytopenia or bleeding risks, and the platelet counts increase to normal within 2 days of stopping the phototherapy.

EVALUATION OF THE KINETIC MECHANISMS OF THROMBOCYTOPENIA IN NEONATES

The state of platelet production can be assessed by direct measurements of the marrow or indirect methods that examine elements in the peripheral blood (Table 13–9).

Table 13–9. **Methods for Evaluating the Kinetic Mechanism Responsible for Thrombocytopenia in Neonates**

Direct methods
Bone marrow biopsy
Megakaryocyte mass
Megakaryocyte ploidy
Indirect methods
Mean platelet volume
Reticulated platelet count
Platelet-associated immunoglobulin G
^{111}In-labeled platelet survival and scintography
Plasma thrombopoietin concentrations

Direct Methods

Bone Marrow Biopsy

Direct aspiration of cells from a neonate's bone marrow can sometimes provide a neonatologist with important information about the state of platelet production that is not otherwise available.[257, 258] Unfortunately, bone marrow aspirates of neonates can be so diluted with peripheral blood that the interpretation is limited. Marrow biopsies avoid this problem, because biopsies preserve the basic in situ architecture of the marrow.[259] Biopsies are generally more useful than aspirates in evaluating patients for thrombocytopenia when an estimate of the marrow megakaryocyte mass is needed. Unfortunately, the smallest Jamshidi-type needles, which are the most frequently used variety for bone marrow biopsies of adults and older children, are 14-gauge needles, and instructions call for their introduction 2 to 2.5 cm into the bone.[260] This approach is impractical for neonates.

We have developed a biopsy method for the tibial bone marrow of thrombocytopenic neonates using an Osgood (New Hyde Park, NY) 0.5-inch, 19-gauge needle. The procedure is identical to the marrow aspirate illustrated in Chapter 7. However, after the operator feels the needle penetrating the cortex of the tibia, the stylet (trocar) is completely withdrawn from the needle. The (hollow) needle is then advanced into the marrow space an additional 3 to 5 mm. The hollow needle "cores" a small segment of marrow into the needle, and this is pushed out of the needle by reintroducing the stylet directly into fixative for subsequent sectioning and staining to appreciate the cellularity and number of megakaryocytes.

Megakaryocyte Mass

Conceptually, the *megakaryocyte mass* is the sum of the marrow concentration of megakaryocytes multiplied by the total body marrow space. In this way, the entire thrombopoietic capacity is evaluated. Detailed methods for this measurement have been made in adult animals and adult humans, as described by Harker and colleagues.[261, 262] Determination of the megakaryocyte mass requires a marrow biopsy or flow cytometric analysis. No such measurements have been reported for neonates. It is not clear whether neonates have a megakaryocyte mass, on a per kilogram of body weight basis, that is less than, equal to, or greater than the megakaryocyte mass of adults. Similarly, megakaryocyte mass measurements have not been reported for thrombocytopenic neonates as a direct means of determining the kinetic contribution of production to the overall cause of the thrombocytopenia.

Megakaryocyte Ploidy

Analysis of megakaryocyte size and ploidy has emerged as a useful tool for the study of the mechanisms that regulate megakaryocytopoiesis. In 1988, Tomer and associates[263] described a method to analyze megakaryocytes from routine human bone marrow aspirates for size, granularity, and ploidy using flow cytometry. These investigators reported that megakaryocytes of adults have a mean diameter of 28.1 μm, and a modal ploidy of 16 N. One year later, the same group applied the newly described technique to the study of 40 patients with quantitative platelet disorders.[264] They found that thrombocytopenic patients with decreased bone marrow megakaryocytes seen on biopsy had an increase in low ploidy cells (53.2% had ≤8N), and thrombocytopenic patients with platelet destruction and normal or increased megakaryocytes on biopsy showed an increased proportion of high ploidy cells (39.2% had ≥32N).

Although flow cytometric studies of bone marrow megakaryocytes have not been published for neonates, studies of fetal bone marrow biopsies or cord blood cultured megakaryocytes have shown that fetal megakaryocytes are smaller, less mature, and of lower ploidy than adult megakaryocytes.[265–267] The reported size and mean ploidy of fetal megakaryocytes varied depending of whether the determination was done on fetal bone marrow biopsy specimens (8N)[266] or by flow cytometry of cultured cord blood or fetal liver megakaryocytes (4N),[265] probably because cultured megakaryocytes tend to be smaller and less polyploid that those seen in vivo.

Indirect Measurements

Mean Platelet Volume

The MPV is a measure of the average size of circulating platelets. Because younger platelets usually are larger, a high MPV suggests increased platelet production, presumably as a compensation for accelerated platelet destruction. In a thrombocytopenic neonate, an elevated MPV is sometimes taken as evidence that the kinetic mechanism causing the thrombocytopenia is accelerated platelet destruction. In NICU patients who develop sepsis with coagulase-negative staphylococci, the MPV increases whether or not thrombocytopenia occurs during the infection, and this suggests that an increase in platelet production accompanies the infection.

Patrick and Lazarchick[268] reported that high MPVs occur during bacterial infections in neonates. In a sample of 156 infants, they observed a high specificity (95%) for an MPV of greater than 10.8 fL in detecting bacteremia. The tenet that the MPV reflects accelerated platelet production has been challenged by several observations. After treatment of newborn rhesus monkeys with recombinant thrombopoietin (which significantly increased their platelet production and their blood platelet concentrations), their MPVs consistently diminished. A falling MPV after rTPO treatment has also been observed in adult subjects. It is unclear how useful an MPV is in establishing the kinetic mechanism responsible for thrombocytopenia in neonates.

Reticulated Platelet Count

Newly produced platelets have a higher ribonucleic acid content than do platelets that have been circulating for days. These new platelets, which can be recognized by flow cytometry, are called *reticulated platelets*.[97–98] In term neonates, 3% to 5% of the circulating platelets are reticulated platelets. Increased production of platelets is expected to increase the reticulated platelet count. Although this tenet seems true in general, it has not been particularly helpful in classifying thrombocytopenic states of neonates, perhaps because of the lack of a reliable standard for neonates for determining whether platelet production is decreased, normal, or increased. Without such a standard, the indirect, surrogate methods that putatively assess the state of platelet production are unverifiable.

Platelet-Associated Immunoglobulin G

Assays have been developed to assess the presence of IgG on platelets. In a thrombocytopenic neonate, the presence of IgG on platelets presumably signifies that the thrombocytopenia is the result of platelet destruction. About 85% of children with ITP have elevated PAIgG levels.[269] Most tests for PAIgG are performed on intact platelets, but perhaps higher positivity rates are observed on lysed platelets.[270] Although initially developed as a test for ITP, it was seen that thrombocytopenic patients with bacterial sepsis had falsely positive PAIgG results.[271] As a result of this finding, it was suggested that part or all of the IgG detected on the platelets by the PAIgG assays is nonspecifically bound to the platelet.[272]

Yamamoto suggested that, in infants and children with ITP, the presence of PAIgG corresponded with prolonged time to recovery.[273] Ware and coworkers suggested that a high PAIgG level in a child with ITP suggests an acute course, and a modestly elevated level suggests a chronic course.[274] Winiarski and colleagues reported that high-dose IgG treatment reduced PAIgG levels in four children with ITP.[275]

The exact interpretation of finding PAIgG in a thrombocytopenic neonate is still uncertain, because Stilliman and associates found that platelets from healthy neonates have increased levels of IgG compared with adults controls.[276] Castle and coworkers performed PAIgG, MPV, and coagulation tests on 177 thrombocytopenic neonates over a 1-year period,[5] and they observed elevated PAIgG levels in 52% of cases. Elevated PAIgG levels were also found in 15% of control, nonthrombocytopenic neonates.

In another report, Castle observed that elevated PAIgG levels in thrombocytopenic neonates corresponded with reduced platelet survival.[99] She suggested that accelerated platelet destruction is involved in the pathogenesis of many cases of thrombocytopenia in the NICU.

Indium-111–Labeled Platelet Survival

Labeling of platelets with ^{111}In-oxine has been encouraging as a means of determining platelet survival and, in cases of accelerated platelet destruction, of identifying the anatomic site of the platelet destruction.[277] The high photon yield of ^{111}In results in clear images of the sites of in vivo distribution of the labeled platelets, and the function of In-labeled platelets appears to be normal.[278] The technique has been useful in localizing the anatomic sites of platelet consumption, particularly when the differential diagnosis has included platelet consumption in intracardiac or arterial thrombi.[279–281] The use of ^{111}In platelet scans has been useful in the detection of and as a means of following the treatment of Kasabach-Merritt syndrome.[282–284]

Castle and colleagues observed that survival of ^{111}In-oxine–labeled platelets in neonates and adults is similar, indicating that platelet life span in the circulation in neonates is 7 to 10 days, as is the case in adults.[99] In 31 thrombocytopenic neonates, she measured ^{111}In-oxine–labeled platelet life spans, and in every patient, the platelet life span was significantly shortened (65 ± 6 hours, compared with 212 ± 8 hours in adults). She observed that the group of patients who had the lowest platelet counts were the ones with the shortest platelet survival. Many of these had immune-mediated thrombocytopenia or DIC.[99] Castle also reported scintigraphic studies and platelet survival times of 10 thrombocytopenic children after infusing heterologous (donor) platelets that were labeled with ^{111}In.[285] The studies were generally helpful in determining whether the thrombocytopenia was the result of decreased platelet production or accelerated destruction, and for the latter, identified whether the anatomic site of the platelet destruction was within a hemangioma, the spleen, or diffuse. In thrombocytopenic neonates, ^{111}In-oxine–labeled platelet survival and scintigraphy can sometimes be useful tests to document platelet survival time and, when shortened, to determine the anatomic site of the platelet destruction.

Thrombopoietin Concentrations

TPO is a physiologic regulator of platelet production. Shortly after TPO was isolated and purified,[286–289] several laboratories developed enzyme immunoassays that allowed accurate measurement of TPO concentrations in plasma. In 1996, Emmons published TPO concentrations of 48 adult patients with thrombocytopenia. He reported that patients with abnormally low concentrations of megakaryocytes in their bone marrow had elevated plasma TPO concentrations and that patients with a high marrow megakaryocyte mass had low blood TPO levels.[290] Several subsequent studies confirmed this inverse relationship between plasma TPO concentration and marrow megakaryocyte mass.[291–293] Measurement of plasma TPO levels may constitute an indirect assessment of the megakaryocyte mass and be a useful method of assessing the kinetic mechanism causing thrombocytopenia.

Murray and associates[244] measured plasma TPO levels by enzyme-linked immunosorbent assay at birth in healthy term (n = 17) and preterm babies (n = 16) and in preterm babies with early thrombocytopenia (n = 13). They showed that the median TPO levels were similar in term (145 pg/mL) and preterm infants (132 pg/mL) and that thrombocytopenic preterm infants did not have a significant increase in TPO (median, 185 pg/mL). Among their thrombocytopenic neonates, 24% were SGA, and 45% were born to women with PIH. The TPO levels, however, were measured at birth and not at the time of the thrombocytopenia, raising the question of whether these thrombocytopenic neonates would have had higher TPO concentrations at the time of their platelet nadir.

As is the case in thrombocytopenic adults, elevated TPO levels in thrombocytopenic neonates suggest a small marrow megakaryocyte mass and decreased platelet production. Based on our findings, a reduced number of megakaryocytes is a contributing factor in many cases of neonatal thrombocytopenia, such as the variety affecting SGA preterm infants and certain cases of NAIT and sepsis.

THERAPEUTIC OPTIONS

The decision about whether to provide specific treatment for a thrombocytopenic neonate in an attempt to elevate the platelet count is sometimes complex and inexplicit. In part, the decision should be based on the platelet count, but the platelet count selected as a "trigger" (i.e., below which treatment is to be instituted) should vary with knowledge of the underlying cause of the thrombocytopenia, the likelihood of bleeding consequences if untreated, and the risks and benefits of the treatment options selected.

If there is no evidence of active bleeding in adults and older children, a platelet count as low as 20,000/μL, and perhaps as low as 10,000/μL, may be sufficient to prevent spontaneous serious hemorrhage.[294–295] Most neonatologists are reluctant to let their thrombocytopenic NICU patients' platelet counts fall to this level—and with good justification. For instance, Feusner observed a much greater prolongation of the bleeding time of thrombocytopenic neonates than adults as the platelet count fell below 50,000/μL.[296] Depending on the individual case, many sick, thrombocytopenic neonates have significant platelet dysfunction accompanying their thrombocytopenia. Many such patients, particularly those with birth weights less than 1000 g, are at risk for intraventricular hemorrhage. Others, such as thrombocytopenic patients with NEC, may require prompt surgery and require platelet counts above 50,000/μL to reduce intraoperative and postoperative hemorrhage. Because of these concerns, neonatologists generally consider treatment at a level of 50,000/μL, but they lower this threshold, perhaps to as low as 20,000/μL, for a stable term or near-term infant when the count has been stable or increasing.

Treatment of Alloimmune and Autoimmune Thrombocytopenia in Neonates with Intravenous Immunoglobulin and Corticosteroids

The principal means by which neonatologists manage their patients who have alloimmune thrombocytopenia is with the transfusion of washed maternal platelets (Chapter 18), but the administration of intravenous immunoglobulin (IVIG) is also useful.[297–299] Corticosteroids were typically used for these neonates before the availability of IVIG but seem to be less frequently employed now (Table 13–10).[300] The antenatal administration of IVIG or steroids has been attempted for PlA1-negative women carrying PlA1-positive fetuses, and these approaches are being evaluated.[301–303] The combination of IVIG and steroids given antenatally to the mother, coupled with transfusions of platelets to the fetus, using ultrasound-guided intraumbilical cord infusion techniques, were reported in the successful management of one woman who previously had a severely affected child.[304]

Neonates delivered to women who have autoimmune disease generally have a milder depression of platelet count than neonates with alloimmune thrombocytopenia. Typically, neonates with autoimmune thrombocytopenia have platelet counts in the 50,000 to 70,000/μL range and rarely require platelet transfusions. IVIG has been administered to these neonates, resulting in an 80% to 90% response rate. Published dosing schedules for IVIG have included 400 mg/kg/d for 3 to 5 consecutive days or a single dose of 1000 mg/kg on day 1.[305, 306]

It is not known whether the addition of corticosteroids to the IVIG infusion regimen is beneficial. In children with ITP, IVIG produces a more rapid resolution in platelet count than does steroid treatment, but this effect is not clear in neonates. We suggest starting treatment with IVIG when the diagnosis is made and then adding steroids only if the count falls significantly. For these neonates, platelet transfusions usually are not needed because of the only moderately depressed platelet counts. Platelet transfusions usually do not effect a significant increase in these neonates' platelet counts. Transfusions should be administered, however, along with IVIG and steroids, for those unusual cases of autoimmune neonatal thrombocytopenia in which clinical bleeding is a problem.

Table 13–10. **Options for Treating Thrombocytopenic Neonates**

Intravenous immunoglobulin and corticosteroids (for alloimmune thrombocytopenia)
Platelet transfusions
Recombinant thrombopoietin administration

Platelet Transfusions

An extensive discussion of platelet transfusions for NICU patients is provided in Chapter 18, and they are only briefly mentioned here. Treatment of patients who have severe nonimmune neonatal thrombocytopenia (platelet count <50,000/μL) with platelet transfusions is generally provided in an attempt to diminish the occurrence or severity of hemorrhage. Intracranial hemorrhage, particularly periventricular and intraventricular hemorrhage, can be caused or worsened by thrombocytopenia,[2, 3] and a significant intracranial hemorrhage almost invariably indicates adverse neurodevelopmental consequences.[1] Platelet transfusions are the only treatment available for NICU patients with nonimmune thrombocytopenia.

Although platelet donors are screened extensively, contamination with bacterial or viral pathogens such as CMV can occur, placing susceptible neonates at risk of iatrogenic disease. At many medical centers, each time a platelet transfusion is given, the recipient neonate is exposed to three different donors, because three packed and pooled units are used for each transfusion. It is not uncommon for thrombocytopenic neonates to be exposed to more than 20 donors during the course of treatment, and this can increase the potential for transfusion reactions and platelet refractoriness.

Recombinant Thrombopoietin

The rTPO and a recombinant human polypeptide that contains the receptor-binding N-terminal domain of TPO (rhMGDF) have been the subject of multiple animal studies. When injected into normal animals,[307–311] rTPO and rhMGDF induced significant thrombocytosis, with peak mean platelet counts up to 670% of baseline. When administered to animals that were previously exposed to myelosuppressive chemotherapy, rhMGDF was able to ameliorate or completely prevent the anticipated thrombocytopenia,[307] and it also accelerated the red blood cell and neutrophil recovery.[312] Later studies using myelosuppressed mice and primates have shown a synergistic effect of rTPO and recombinant granulocyte colony-stimulating factor (G-CSF) or recombinant GM-CSF in the prevention of the thrombocytopenia and neutropenia associated with marrow suppressive chemotherapy.[313–315] The pegylated form of recombinant human MGDF (PEG-rhMGDF) is 5 to 10 times more potent in vivo than the unconjugated polypeptide, as demonstrated in normal nonhuman primates,[310] and this has been the formulation chosen for most of the human studies published.

Phase I and II human trials, although in early stages, have demonstrated the efficacy of rTPO and PEG-rhMGDF as potent simulators of platelet production in nonthrombocytopenic adults[316–318] and in patients with chemotherapy-induced thrombocytopenia.[318, 319] Only mild side effects have been reported, including isolated thromboembolic events in treated patients at times when the platelet count was not abnormally elevated. Although rTPO has not been tested yet in cases of thrombocytopenia unassociated with the administration of myelosuppressive agents, it is reasonable to speculate that it will be beneficial in treating many diseases and syndromes.

Little is known about the role of TPO or the theoretical benefits of rTPO administration in the neonatal population. In 1996, Nishihira and coworkers[320] reported the effects of rTPO on megakaryocyte progenitors isolated from nonthrombocytopenic human cord blood at different gestational ages. Their results indicated that rTPO alone supports the growth of megakaryocyte colonies and that progenitors from preterm infants tend to be more sensitive to rTPO than do those from term infants. Murray and colleagues[244] cultured megakaryocyte progenitors from the blood of neonates with different concentrations of rTPO and showed a greater response in preterm infants. Nishihira and Murray performed their studies using megakaryocyte progenitors isolated from cord blood or peripheral blood of the neonates. However, it is not clear whether the number of circulating megakaryocyte progenitors truly reflects megakaryocytopoiesis in general, and the responsiveness of neonatal bone marrow progenitors to rTPO has never been tested. Studies by our group and others suggest that certain thrombocytopenic infants fail to generate TPO adequately. If that is so, we speculate that treatment with rTPO may be particularly beneficial for these neonates.

Van de Ven and associates demonstrated that treatment of neonatal rats with rTPO enhanced thrombopoiesis and that no additive effect was observed when rmIL-3 or rhIL-11 were included.[321] It is unknown whether there are any age-related differences in the dose-response relationship, pharmacokinetics, thrombopoietic effects, or potential toxicity of PEG-rhMGDF. In 1990, a study comparing the erythropoietic responses to recombinant human erythropoietin (which has significant homology with TPO) in adult and infant rhesus monkeys showed that rEPO had very different pharmacokinetic properties in infants.[322] The infants had a much larger volume of distribution and more rapid clearance, and higher doses per kilogram of body weight were needed to produce an effect comparable to that in adults. This study was the first step toward the current successful use of much higher doses of rEPO to treat the anemia of prematurity.

We have observed that TPO pharmacokinetics and pharmacodynamics do not differ significantly between neonatal and adult rhesus monkeys. Unlike the case with rEPO, in which neonatal animals require larger doses per kilogram of body weight than do adults to achieve a similar erythropoietic effect, the neonatal monkeys seem to require a slightly lower dose of rTPO than the adults to achieve a quadrupling of platelet counts. Adult and neonatal animals require about 4 days of dosing before any change in circulating platelet count occurs. It is not clear whether rTPO will have the desired biologic effects in thrombocytopenic human neonates, what its risk-benefit profile will be, or whether it will become an important therapeutic agent in the NICU.

References

1. Papile LA, Burstein J, Bursetin R: Incidence and evolution of subependymal and intraventricular hemorrhage: a study of infants with birth weights less than 1,500 gm. Pediatrics 1978;92:529.
2. Andrew M, Castle, Saigal S, et al: Clinical impact of neonatal thrombocytopenia. J Pediatr 1987;110:457.
3. Setzer ES, Webb IB, Wassenaar JW, et al: Platelet dysfunction and coagulopathy in intraventricular hemorrhages in the premature infant. J Pediatr 1982;100:599.

4. Mehta P, Vasa R, Neumann L, et al: Thrombocytopenia in the high-risk infant. J Pediatr 1980;97:791.
5. Castle V, Andrew M, Kelton J, et al: Frequency and mechanism of neonatal thrombocytopenia. J Pediatr 1986;108:749.
6. Radley JM, Scurfield G: The mechanism of platelet release. Blood 1980;56:996.
7. Van den Hof MC, Nicolaides KH: Platelet count in normal, small, and anemic fetuses. Am J Obstet Gynecol 1990;162:735.
8. Hathaway WE, Bonnar J: Perinatal Coagulation. New York: Grune & Stratton, 1978.
9. Andrew M: Neonatal thrombocytopenia. Clin Perinatol 1984;11:359.
10. Aballi A, Puapondh Y, Desposito F: Platelet counts in thriving premature infants. Pediatrics 1968;42:685.
11. Blanchette VS, Rand ML: Platelet disorders in newborn infants: diagnosis and management. Semin Perinatol 1997;21:53.
12. Hrodek O: Blood platelets in the newborn: platelet adhesiveness in vitro. Acta Univ Carol Med Monogr 1966;22:26.
13. Mull MM, Hathaway WE: Altered platelet function in newborns. Pediatr Res 1970;4:229.
14. Boizard GY, Daffos F, Forester F, et al: Determination of platelet antigens and glycoproteins in the human fetus. Blood 1986;68:488.
15. Andrew M: The hemostatic system in the infant. In Nathan DG, Oski FA (eds): Hematology of Infancy and Childhood. Philadelphia: WB Saunders, 1992, p 119.
16. Weinstein JM, Blanchard R, et al: Fetal and neonatal von Willebrand factor (vWF) is unusually large and similar to the vWF in patients with thrombotic thrombocytopenic purpura. Br J Haematol 1989;72:68.
17. Sell EJ, Corrigan JJ: Platelet counts, fibrinogen concentrations, and factor V and factor VIII levels in healthy infants according to gestational age. J Pediatr 1973;82:1028.
18. Hamulyak K, Nieuwenhuizen W, Devilee PP, Hemker HC: Reevaluation of some properties of fibrinogen, purified from cord blood of normal newborns. Thromb Res 1983;32:301.
19. Stuart MJ, Dusse J, Clary DA, Walenga RW: Differences in thromboxane production between neonatal and adult platelets in response to arachidonic acid and epinephrine. Pediatr Res 1984;18:823.
20. Stuart MJ: Platelet function in the neonate. Am J Pediatr Hematol Oncol 1979;1:227.
21. Jones CR, McCabe R, Hamilton CA, Reid JL: Maternal and fetal platelet responses and adrenoceptor binding characteristics. Thromb Haemost 1985;53:95.
22. Corby DG, O'Barr TP: Decreased alpha-adrenergic receptors in newborn platelets: cause of abnormal response to epinephrine. Dev Pharmacol Ther 1981;2:215.
23. Ts'ao CH, Green D, Schultz K: Function and ultrastructure of platelets of neonates: enhanced ristocetin aggregation of neonatal platelets. Br J Haematol 1976;32:225.
24. Gader AM, Bahkim H, Jabbar FA, et al: Dose-response aggregometry in maternal/neonatal platelets. Thromb Haemost 1988;60:314.
25. Barradas MA, Mikhailidis DP, Imoedemhe DA, et al: An investigation of maternal and neonatal platelet function. Biol Res Pregnancy Perinatol 1986;7:60.
26. Corby DG, Zuck TF: Newborn platelet dysfunction: a storage pool and release defect. Thromb Haemost 1976;36:200.
27. Israels SJ, Odaibo FS, Robertson C, et al: Deficient thromboxane synthesis and response in platelets from premature infants. Pediatr Res 1997;41:218.
28. Rajasekhar D, Kestin AS, Bednarek FJ, et al: Neonatal platelets are less reactive than adult platelets to physiological agonists in whole blood. Thromb Haemost 1994;72:957.
29. Israels SJ, Daniels M, McMillan EM: Deficient collagen-induced activation in the newborn platelet. Pediatr Res 1990;27:337.
30. Tanindi S, Kurekci AE, Koseogly V, et al: The normalization period of platelet aggregation in newborns. Thromb Res 1995;80:57.
31. Suarez CR, Gonzalez J, Mendendez C, et al: Neonatal and maternal platelets: activation at time of birth. Am J Hematol 1988;29:18.
32. Irken G, Mutafoglu Uysal K, Olgun, et al: Platelet activation during the early neonatal period. Biol Neonate 1998;73:166.
33. Grosshaupt B, Muntean W, Sedlmayr P: Hyporeactivity of neonatal platelets is not caused by preactivation during birth. Eur J Pediatr 1997;156:944.
34. Harker LA, Slichter SJ: The bleeding time as a screening test for evaluation of platelet function. N Engl J Med 1972;287:155.
35. Andrew M, Paes B, Johnston M: Development of the hemostatic system in the neonate and young infant. Am J Pediatr Hematol Oncol 1990;12:95.
36. Fernandez F, Goudable C, Sie P, et al: Low hematocrit and prolonged bleeding time in uraemic patients: effects of red cell transfusions. Br J Haematol 1985;59:139.
37. Aarts PA, Bolhuis PA, Sakariassen KS, et al: Red blood cell size is important for adherence of blood platelets to artery subendothelium. Blood 1983;62:214.
38. Niederhoff H, Kunzer W: Physiology of hemostasis in newborn infants, I. Monatsschr Kinderheilk 1985;133:130.
39. Estes JW, Carey RJ, et al: Marfan's syndrome: hematological abnormalities in a family. Arch Intern Med 1965;116:889.
40. Estes S: Platelet abnormalities in heritable disorders of connective tissue. Ann N Y Acad Sci 1972;201:445.
41. Hathaway WE: Bleeding disorders due to platelet dysfunction. Am J Dis Child 1971;121:127.
42. Rennie JM, Gibson T, Cooke RW: Micromethod for bleeding time in the newborn. Arch Dis Child 1985;60:51.
43. Andrew M, Paes B, Bowker J, Begh P: Evaluation of an automated bleeding time device in the newborn. Am J Hematol 1990;35:275.
44. Lethagen S, Kling S: New bleeding time devices with retractable blades evaluated in children, healthy volunteers and patients with prolonged bleeding time. Thromb Haemost 1993;70:595.
45. Zaizov R, Cohen I, and Matoth Y: Thrombasthenia: 1968 study of two siblings. Acta Paediatr Scand 1968;57:522.
46. Glanzmann E: Hereditare haemorrhagische Thromboasthenie, ein Beitrag zur Pathologie der Blut Plattchen. Jahrb Kinderheilk 1918;88:1.
47. Phillips DR, Agin PP: Platelet membrane defects in Glanzmann's thrombasthenia: evidence for decreased amounts of two major glycoproteins. J Clin Invest 1977;60:535.
48. Tomiyama Y, Kashiwagi H, Kosugi S, et al: Demonstration of a marked reduction in the amount of GPIIb in most type II patients with Glanzmann's thrombasthenia. Br J Haematol 1994;87:119.
49. Bleyer WA, Au WY, Lange WA, et al: Studies on the detection of adverse drug reactions in the newborn. I.

Fetal exposure to maternal medication. JAMA 1970;213:2046.
50. Bleyer WA, Breckenridge RT: Studies in the detection of adverse drug reactions in the newborn. II. The effects of prenatal aspirin on newborn hemostasis. JAMA 1970;213:2049.
51. Haslam RR, Ekert H, Gilliam GL: Hemorrhage in a neonate possibly due to maternal ingestion of salicylate. J Pediatr 1974;84:556.
52. Stuart MJ, Gross SJ, Graeber JE, et al: The effect of prenatal acetyl salicylic acid (ASA) ingestion on maternal and neonatal hemostasis. Pediatr Res 1978;12:475.
53. Corazza MS, Davis RF, Merritt TA, et al: Prolonged bleeding time in preterm infant receiving indomethacin for patent ductus arteriosus. J Pediatr 1984;105:292.
54. Cheung PY, Salas E, Schultz R, Radomski MW: Nitric oxide and platelet function: implication for neonatology. Semin Perinatol 1997;21:409.
55. Remuzzi G, Benigni A, Dodesini P, et al: Reduced platelet thromboxane formation in uremia: evidence for a functional cyclooxygenase defect. J Clin Invest 1983;71:762.
56. Russ JS Johan MH: Platelet dysfunction in extrahepatic biliary obstruction. South Med J 1982;75:506.
57. Maurer HM, Caul J: Influence of bilirubin on human platelets. Pediatr Res 1972;6:84.
58. Maurer HM, Haggins JC, Still WJS: Platelet injury during phototherapy. Am J Hematol 1976;1:89.
59. Kaapa P, Uhari M, Nikkari T, et al: Dietary fatty acids and platelet thromboxane production in puerperal women and their offspring. Am J Obstet Gynecol 1986;155:146.
60. Khurshid M, Lee TJ, Peake IR, et al: Vitamin E deficiency and platelet functional defect in a jaundiced infant. BMJ 1975;4:19.
61. Lake AM, Stuart MJ, Oski FA: Vitamin E deficiency and enhanced platelet function: reversal following E supplementation. J Pediatr 1977;90:722.
62. Friedman Z, Lamberth ELJ, Stahlman MT: Platelet dysfunction in the neonate with essential fatty acid deficiency. J Pediatr 90:439. 1977.
63. Friedman Z, Danon A, Stahlman MT, et al: Rapid onset of essential fatty acid deficiency in the newborn. Pediatrics 1976;58:640.
64. Friedman Z, Seyberth H, Lamberth EL, et al: Decreased prostaglandin E turnover in infants with essential fatty acid deficiency. Pediatr Res 1978;12:711.
65. Stuart MJ: Vitamin E deficiency: its effect on platelet-vascular interaction in various pathologic states. Ann N Y Acad Sci 1982;393:277.
66. Setzer ES, Webb IB, Wassenaar JW, et al: Platelet dysfunction and coagulopathy in intraventricular hemorrhages in the premature infant. J Pediatr 1982;100:599.
67. Feusner JH: Normal and abnormal bleeding times in neonates and young children using a fully standardized template technique. Am J Clin Pathol 1980;74:73.
68. Robinson TM, Kickler TS, Walker LK, et al: Effect of extracorporeal membrane oxygenation on platelets in newborns. Crit Care Med 1993;21:1029.
69. Sirota L, Bessler H, Weissman Z, et al: Thrombopoietic activity in preterm newborns and infants. Arch Dis Child 1986;67:585.
70. Sutor AH: Thrombocytosis in childhood. Semin Thromb Hemost 1995;21:330.
71. Appleyard WJ, Brinton A: Venous platelet counts in low birth weight infants. Biol Neonate 1971;17:340.
72. Effiong CE, Usanga EA, Mellits ED: Platelet counts in healthy full term Nigerian neonates. Trop Geogr Med 1976;28:329.
73. Halperin DS, Washer P, Lacourt G, et al: Effects of recombinant human erythropoietin in infants with the anemia of prematurity: a pilot study. J Pediatr 1990;116:779.
74. Holter PH, Refusm HE: Postnatal anemia and thrombocytosis in suckling rabbits: influence of delayed weaning and iron supplies. Pediatr Hematol Oncol 1988;5:157.
75. Turba R, Bianchi C, Cella D, et al: Thrombocytosis and neonatal subcutaneous adiponecrosis. Minerva Pediatr 1994;46:343.
76. Buss CH, Cashell AW, O'Connor ML, et al: Occurrence, etiology, and clinical significance of extreme thrombocytosis: as study of 280 cases. Am J Med 1994;96:247.
77. Vora AJ, Lilleyman JS: Secondary thrombocytosis. Arch Dis Child 1993;68:88.
78. Chan KW, Kailov Y, Wadsworth LD: Thrombocytosis in childhood: a survey of 94 patients. Pediatrics 1989;84:1064.
79. Azagami S, Isohata E, Oikawa T, et al: Pharmacokinetics and clinical safety of aztreonam in neonates. Jpn J Antibiot 1990;43:405.
80. Ahonkhai IV, Cyhan GM, Wilson SE, et al: Imipenem-cilastatin in pediatric patients: an overview of safety and efficacy in studies conducted in the United States. Pediatr Infect Dis J 1989;8:740.
81. Fujii R, Hashira S, Sakata H, et al: Pharmacokinetics and clinical evaluation of ceftriaxone in neonates. Jpn J Antibiot 1988;41:1237.
82. Van-Reempts PJ, Van-Overmeire B, Mahieu LM, et al: Clinical experience with ceftriaxone treatment in the neonate. Chemotherapy 1995;41:316.
83. Fujii R, Yoshioka H, Osano M, et al: Pharmacokinetic and clinical studies on the use of ceftizoxime in premature and newborn infants. Jpn J Antibiot 1988;41:1030.
84. Hanssler L, Roll C: Increased thrombocyte count in newborn infants of drug-dependent mothers. Klin Padiatr 1994;206:55.
85. Kivivuori SM, Rajantie J, Siimes MA: Peripheral blood cell counts in infants with Down's syndrome. Clin Genet 1996;49:15.
86. Suda J, Eguchi M, Akiyamna Y, et al: Differentiation of blast cells from a Down's syndrome patient with transient myeloproliferative disorder. Blood 1987;69:508.
87. Yokoyama S, Nito T, Irimada K: Acute megakaryoblastic leukemia preceded by refractory anemia with an excess of blast cells: leukemic transformation in an infant of Down syndrome recovering from transient abnormal myelopoiesis. Nippon Ketsueki Gakkai Zasshi 1984;47:62.
88. Rao SP, Falter ML, Brown AK: Thrombocytosis in neuroblastoma. J Pediatr 1976;89:682.
89. Gasparini N, Franzese A, Argenziano A, et al: Thrombocytosis in congenital adrenal hyperplasia at diagnosis. Clin Pediatr (Phila) 1996;35:267.
90. Yohannan MD, Santhosh-Kumar CR: Thrombocytosis in congenital adrenal hyperplasia at diagnosis. Clin Pediatr (Phila) 1997;36:186.
91. Uhrynowska M, Maslanka K, Zupanska B: Neonatal thrombocytopenia: incidence, serological and clinical observations. Am J Perinatol 1997;14:415.
92. Dreyfus M, Kaplan C, Verdy E, et al: Frequency of immune thrombocytopenia in newborns: a prospective study. Blood 1997;89:4402.
93. Burrows RF, Kelton JG: Fetal thrombocytopenia and its relation to maternal thrombocytopenia. N Engl J Med 1993;329:1463.
94. Oren H, Irken G, Oren B, et al: Assessment of clinical

impact and predisposing factors for neonatal thrombocytopenia. Indian J Pediatr 1994;61:551.

95. Corash L, Chen HY, Levin J, et al: Regulation of thrombopoiesis: effects of the degree of thrombocytopenia on megakaryocyte ploidy and platelet volume. Blood 1987;70:177.
96. Tate DY, Carlton GT, Johnson D, et al: Immune thrombocytopenia in severe neonatal infections. J Pediatr 1981;98:449.
97. Joseph MA, Adams D, Maragos J, Saving KL: Flow cytometry of neonatal platelet RNA. J Pediatr Hematol Oncol 1996;18:277.
98. Peterec SM, Brennan SA, Rinder HM, et al: Reticulated platelet values in normal and thrombocytopenic neonates. J Pediatr 1996;129:269.
99. Castle V, Coates G, Kelton JG, Andrew M: ^{111}In-oxine platelet survivals in thrombocytopenic infants. Blood 1987;70:652.
100. Murray NA, Roberts IAG: Circulating megakaryocytes and their progenitors (BFU-MK and CFU-MK) in term and pre-term neonates. Br J Haematol 1995;89:41.
101. Murray NA, Roberts IAG: Circulating megakaryocytes and their progenitors in early thrombocytopenia in preterm neonates. Pediatr Res 1996;40:112.
102. Harrington W, Sprague C, Minnich V, et al: Immunologic mechanisms in idiopathic and neonatal thrombocytopenic purpura. Ann Intern Med 1953;38:433.
103. George D, Bussel J: Neonatal thrombocytopenia. Semin Thromb Hemost 1995;21:278.
104. Homans A: Thrombocytopenia in the neonate. Pediatr Clin North Am 1996;43:737.
105. Kaplan C, Morel-Kopp MC, Kroll H, et al: HPA-5b (Br[a]) neonatal alloimmune thrombocytopenia: clinical and immunological analysis of 39 cases. Br J Haematol 1991;78:425.
106. Von dem Borne AEGK, von Riesz E, Verheugt FWA, et al: Bak[a], a new platelet-specific antigen involved in neonatal allo-immune thrombocytopenia. Vox Sang 1980;39:113.
107. Kroll H, Muntean W, Kiefel V, et al: Anti Ko(a) as a cause of neonatal alloimmune thrombocytopenia. Beitr Infusionsther Transfusionsmed 1994;32:244.
108. Westman P, Hashemi-Tavoularis S, Blanchette V, et al: Maternal DRB1*1501, DQA1*0102, DQB1*0602 haplotype in fetomaternal alloimmunization against human platelet alloantigen HPA-6b (GPIIIa-Gln489). Tissue Antigens 1997;50:113.
109. Mueller-Eckhardt C, Kiefel V, Grubert A, et al: 348 Cases of suspected neonatal alloimmune thrombocytopenia. Lancet 1989;1:363.
110. Kiefel V, Vicariot M, Breitfeld C, et al: Immunization against a new, infrequent alloantigen (Iy) on the platelet glycoprotein Ib/IX as a cause of a serious case of neonatal alloimmune thrombocytopenia. Beitr Infusionsther Transfusionsmed 1994;32:247.
111. L'Abbe D, Tremblay L, Filion M, et al: Alloimmunization to platelet antigen HPA-1a (PLA1) is strongly associated with both HLA-DRB3*0101 and HLA-DQB1*0201. Hum Immunol 1992;34:107.
112. De Waal LP, Van Dalen CM, et al: Alloimmunization against the platelet-specific Zw[a] antigen, resulting in neonatal thrombocytopenia or posttransfusion purpura, is associated with the supertypic Drw52 antigen including DR3 and DRw6. Hum Immunol 1986;17:45.
113. Reznikoff-Etievant MF, Dangu C, et al: HLA-B8 antigens and anti-PL[a1] allo-immunization. Tissue Antigens 1981;18:66.
114. Semana G, Zazoun T, Alizadeh M, et al: Genetic susceptibility and anti-human platelet antigen 5b alloimmunization role of HLA class II and TAP genes. Hum Immunol 1996;46:114.
115. Bussel JB, Zabusky M, Berkowitz RL, et al: Fetal alloimmune thrombocytopenia. N Engl J Med 1997;337:22.
116. Cohen DL, Baglin TP: Assessment and management of immune thrombocytopenia in pregnancy and in neonates. Arch Dis Child 1995;72:71.
117. Blanchette VS: Neonatal alloimmune thrombocytopenia: a clinical perspective. Curr Stud Hematol Blood Transfus 1988;54:112.
118. Bonacossa IA, Jocelyn LJ: Alloimmune thrombocytopenia of the newborn: neurodevelopmental sequelae. Am J Perinatol 1996;13:211.
119. Warwick RM, Vaughan J, Murray N, et al: In Vitro culture of colony forming unit-megakaryocyte (CFU-MK) in fetal alloimmune thrombocytopenia. Br J Haematol 1994;88:874.
120. Evans D: Immune amegakaryocytic thrombocytopenia of the newborn: association with anti-HLA-A2. J Clin Pathol 1987;40:258.
121. King KE, Kao KJ, Bray PF, et al: The role of HLA antibodies in neonatal thrombocytopenia: a prospective study. Tissue Antigens 1996;47:206.
122. Anteby E, Shalev O: Clinical relevance of gestational thrombocytopenia of $<100,000/\mu L$. Am J Hematol 1994;47:118.
123. Burrows RF, Kelton JG: Fetal thrombocytopenia and its relation to maternal thrombocytopenia. N Engl J Med 1993;329:1463.
124. Tchernia G, Morel-Kopp MC, Yvart J, et al: Neonatal thrombocytopenia and hidden maternal autoimmunity. Br J Haematol 1993;84:457.
125. Christiaens GCML, Nieuwenhuis HK, von Dem AEGK, et al: Idiopathic thrombocytopenic purpura in pregnancy: a randomized trial on the effect of antenatal low dose corticosteroids on neonatal platelet count. Br J Obstet Gynecol 1990;97:893.
126. Moutet A, Fromont P, Farcet JP, et al: Pregnancy in women with immune thrombocytopenic purpura. Arch Intern Med 1990;150:2141.
127. Burrows RF, Kelton JG: Low fetal risks in pregnancies associated with idiopathic thrombocytopenic purpura. Am J Obstet Gynecol 1990;163:1147.
128. Sharon R, Tatarsky I: Low fetal morbidity in pregnancy associated with acute and chronic idiopathic thrombocytopenic purpura. Am J Hematol 1994;46:87.
129. Al Mofada SM, Osman ME, Kides E, et al: Risk of thrombocytopenia in the infants of mothers with idiopathic thrombocytopenia. Am J Perinatol 11:423,1994.
130. Hwa HL, Chen RJ, Chen YC, et al: Maternal and fetal outcome of pregnant women with idiopathic thrombocytopenic purpura: retrospective analysis of 25 pregnancies. J Formos Med Assoc 1993;92:957.
131. Wanachiwanawin W, Chansung K, Visudhiphan, Piankijagum A: Outcomes of pregnancy in adult idiopathic thrombocytopenic purpura. J Med Assoc Thai 1992;75:584.
132. Sainio S, Joutsi L, Jarvenpaa AL, et al: Idiopathic thrombocytopenic purpura in pregnancy. Acta Obstet Gynecol Scand 1998;77:272.
133. Cook RL, Miller RC, Katz VL, Cefalo RC: Immune thrombocytopenic purpura in pregnancy: a reappraisal of management. Obstet Gynecol 1991;78:578.
134. Mazzucconi MG, Petrelli V, Gandolfo GM, et al: Autoimmune thrombocytopenic purpura in pregnancy: maternal risk factors predictive of neonatal thrombocytopenia. Autoimmunity 1993;16:209.

135. Christiaens GC, Nieuwenhuis HK, Bussel JB: Comparison of platelet counts in first and second newborns of mothers with immune thrombocytopenic purpura. Obstet Gynecol 1997;90:546.
136. Samuels P, Bussel JB, Braitman LE, et al: Estimation of the risk of thrombocytopenia in the offspring of pregnant women with presumed immune thrombocytopenia purpura. N Engl J Med 1990;323:229.
137. Tchernia G, Subtil E, Dehan M, et al: Thrombocytopenia with bacterial infections in neonates. Nouv Rev Fr Hematol 1975;15:484.
138. Zipursky A, Jaber HM: The haematology of bacterial infection. Clin Haematol 1978;7:175.
139. Modanlou HD, Ortiz OB: Thrombocytopenia in neonatal infection. Clin Pediatr 1981;20:402.
140. Neame PB, Kelton JG, Walker IR, et al: Thrombocytopenia in septicemia: the role of disseminated intravascular coagulation. Blood 1980;56:88.
141. Reidler GF, Straub PW, Frick PG: Thrombocytopenia in septicemia. Helv Med Acta 1971;36:23.
142. Zipursky A, Jaber HM: The haematology of bacterial infection in newborn infants. Clin Haematol 1978;7:175.
143. Harker LA, Slichter SJ: Platelet and fibrinogen consumption in man. N Engl J Med 1972;287:999.
144. Patrick CH, Lazarchick J: The effect of bacteremia on automated platelet measurements in the neonate. Am J Clin Pathol 1990;93:391.
145. Corrigan JJ: Thrombocytopenia: a laboratory sign of septicemia in infants and children. J Pediatr 1974;85:219.
146. Tate DY, Carlton GT, Johnson D, et al: Immune thrombocytopenia in severe neonatal infections. J Pediatr 1981;98:449.
147. Ng PC, Herrington RA, Beane CA, et al: An outbreak of *Acinetobacter* septicaemia in a neonatal intensive care unit. J Hosp Infect 1989;14:363.
148. Struelens MJ, Patte D, Kabir I, et al: *Shigella* septicemia: prevalence, presentation, risk factors, and outcome. J Infect Dis 1985;152:784.
149. Linder N, Korman SH, Cyal F, et al: Trimethoprim-sulfamethoxazole in neonatal *Flavobacterium meningosepticum* infection. Arch Dis Child 1984;59:582.
150. Amit Y, Peleg O, Singer R, et al: Intravenous immunoglobulin for *Flavobacterium*-induced thrombocytopenia in a premature infant. Am J Perinatol 1991;8:161.
151. Sirinavin S, Likitnukul S, Lolekha S: Aeromonas sepsis in infants and children. Pediatr Infect Dis 1984;3:122.
152. Padovani EM, Michielutte F, Dall'Agnola A, et al: Sepsis caused by *Candida* in the neonatal period. Pediatr Med Chir 1997;19:83.
153. Melville C, Kempley S, Graham J, et al: Early onset systemic *Candida* infection in extremely preterm neonates. Eur J Pediatr 1966;155:904.
154. McDonnell M, Isaacs D: Neonatal systemic candidiasis. J Paediatr Child Health 1995;31:490.
155. Surmont I, Gavilanes A, Vandepitte J, et al: *Malassezia furfur* fungaemia in infants receiving intravenous lipid emulsions: a rarity or just underestimated? Eur J Pediatr 1989;148:435.
156. Richet HM, McNeil MM, Edwards MC, et al: Cluster of *Malassezia furfur* pulmonary infections in infants in a neonatal intensive-care unit. J Clin Microbiol 1989;27:1197.
157. Kim EH, Cohen RS, Ramachandran P, et al: Adhesion of percutaneously inserted Silastic central venous lines to the vein wall associated with *Malassezia furfur* infection. J Parenter Enteral Nutr 1993;17:458.
158. Dyke MP, Ott K: Severe thrombocytopenia in extremely low birth weight infants with systemic candidiasis. J Paediatr Child Health 1993;29:298.
159. Mandelbrot L, Schlienger I, Bongain A, et al: Thrombocytopenia in pregnant women infected with human immunodeficiency virus: maternal and neonatal outcome. Am J Obstet Gynecol 1994;171:252.
160. Joshi VV: Pathology of acquired immunodeficiency syndrome (AIDS) in children. Keio J Med 1996;45:306.
161. Whitley RJ, Cloud G, Gruber W, et al: Gancyclovir treatment of symptomatic congenital cytomegalovirus infection: results of a phase II study. J Infect Dis 1997;175:1080.
162. Chou LL, Chang CP, Wu LC: Neonatal coxsackievirus B1 infection associated with severe hepatitis: report of three cases. Chung Hua Min Kuo Hsiao Erh Ko I Hsueh Hui Tsa Chih 1995;36:296.
163. Pruekprasert P, Stout C, Patamasucon P: Neonatal enterovirus infection. J Assoc Acad Minor Phys 1995;6:134.
164. Abzug MJ, Levin MJ, Rotbart HA: Profile of enterovirus disease in the first two weeks of life. Pediatr Infect Dis J 1993;12:820.
165. Vogel H, Kornman M, Ledet SC, et al: Congenital parvovirus infection. Pediat Pathol Lab Med 1997;17:903.
166. Schuster V, Janssen W, Seidenspinner S, et al: Congenital Epstein-Barr virus infection. Monatsschr Kinderheilk 1993;141:401.
167. Lacour M, Maherzi M, Vienny H, et al: Thrombocytopenia in a case of neonatal mumps infection: evidence for further clinical presentations. Eur J Pediatr 1993;152:739.
168. Abzug MJ, Levin MJ: Neonatal adenovirus infection: four patients and review of the literature. Pediatrics 1991;87:890.
169. Chesney PJ, Taher A, Gilbert EMG, et al: Intranuclear inclusions in megakaryocytes in congenital cytomegalovirus infection. J Pediatr 1978;92:957.
170. Jones KL: Smith's recognizable patterns of human malformation, 5th ed. Philadelphia: WB Saunders, 1997, p 322.
171. Hedberg VA, Lipton JM: Thrombocytopenia with absent radii. A review of 100 cases. Am J Pediatr Hematol Oncol 1988;10:51.
172. Alter BP, Young NS: The bone marrow failure syndromes. In Nathan DG, Oski FA (eds): Hematology of Infancy and Childhood. Philadelphia: WB Saunders, 1992, p 278.
173. Andrew M, Kelton J: Neonatal thrombocytopenia. Clin Perinatol 1984;11:359.
174. Gounder DS, Pullon HW, Ockelford PA, Nicol RO: Clinical manifestations of the thrombocytopenia and absent radii (TAR) syndrome. Aust N Z J Med 1989;19:479.
175. Ballmaier M, Schulze H, Strauss G, et al: Thrombopoietin in patients with congenital thrombocytopenia and absent radii: elevated serum levels, normal receptor expression, but defective reactivity to thrombopoietin. Blood 1997;90:612.
176. Sekine I, Hagiwara T, Miyazaki H, et al: Thrombocytopenia with absent radii syndrome: studies on serum thrombopoietin levels and megakaryopoiesis in vitro. J Pediatr Hematol Oncol 1998;20:74.
177. Fanconi G: Familiare infantile perniziosaartige Anamie (pernizioses Blutbild und Konstitution). Jahrb Kinderheilk 1927;117:257.
178. Alter BP, Young NS: The bone marrow failure syndromes. In Nathan DG, Oski FA (eds): Hematology of Infancy and Childhood. Philadelphia: WB Saunders, 1992, p 237.
179. Jones KL: Smith's Recognizable Patterns of Human

Malformation, 5th ed. Philadelphia: WB Saunders, 1997, p 320.
180. Gershanik JJ, Morgan SK, Akers R: Fanconi's anemia in a neonate. Acta Paediatr Scand 1972;61:623.
181. O'Neill EM, Varadi S: Neonatal aplastic anemia and Fanconi's anemia. Arch Dis Child 1963;38:92.
182. Butturini A, Gale RP, Verlander PC, et al: Hematologic abnormalities in Fanconi anemia: an International Fanconi Anemia Registry study. Blood 1994;84:1650.
183. Jones JH: Foetal haemoglobin in Fanconi type anaemia. Nature 1961;192:982.
184. Shahidi NT, Gerald PS, Diamond LK: Alkali-resistant hemoglobin in aplastic anemia of both acquired and congenital types. N Engl J Med 1962;266:117.
185. Swift MR, Hirschhorn K: Fanconi's anemia. Inherited susceptibility to chromosome breakage in various tissues. Ann Intern Med 1966;65:496.
186. Auerbach AD, Verlander PC, Brown KE, et al: New molecular diagnostic tests for two congenital forms of anemia. J Clin Lab Anal 1997;11:17.
187. Honig GR, Vida LN, Hoganson GE: Fetal hemoglobin expression in transplant recipients of placental blood hematopoietic progenitor cells. Pediatr Res 1995;37:432.
188. Auerbach AD: Umbilical cord transplants for genetic diseases: diagnostic and ethical issues in fetal studies. Blood Cells 1994;20:303.
189. Gluckman E, Devergie A, Thierry D, et al: Clinical applications of stem cell transfusion from cord blood and rationale for cord blood banking. Bone marrow Transplant 1992;9:114.
190. Alter BP, Young NS: The bone marrow failure syndromes. In Nathan DG, Oski FA (eds): Hematology of Infancy and Childhood. Philadelphia: WB Saunders, 1992, p 255.
191. Alter BP, Potter NU, Li FP: Classification and aetiology of the aplastic anemias. Clin Haematol 1978;7:431.
192. Henter JI, Winiarski J, Ljungman P, et al: Bone marrow transplantation in two children with congenital amegakaryocytic thrombocytopenia. Bone Marrow Transplant 1995;15:799.
193. Muraoka K, Ishii E, Tsuji K, et al: Defective response to thrombopoietin and impaired expression of c-mpl mRNA of bone marrow cells in congenital amegakaryocytic thrombocytopenia. Br J Haematol 1997;96:287.
194. Guinan EC, Lee YS, Lopez KD, et al: Effects of interleukin-3 and granulocyte-macrophage colony-stimulating factor on thrombopoiesis in congenital amegakaryocytic thrombocytopenia. Blood 1993;81:1691.
195. Eisenstein EM: Congenital amegakaryocytic thrombocytopenic purpura. Clin Pediatr 1966;5:143.
196. Hoyeraal HM, Lamvik J, Moe PJ: Congenital hypoplastic thrombocytopenia and cerebral malformations in two brothers. Acta Paediatr Scand 1970;59:185.
197. Hreidarsson S, Kristjansson K, Johannesson G, et al: A syndrome of progressive pancytopenia with microcephaly, cerebellar hypoplasia and growth failure. Acta Paediatr Scand 1988;77:773.
198. Braddock SR, Carey JC: A new syndrome: congenital thrombocytopenia, Robin sequence, agenesis of the corpus callosum, distinctive facies, and developmental delay. Clin Dysmorphol 1994;3:75.
199. Bernard J, Soulier J: Sur une nouvelle variete de dystrophie thrombocytaire hemmorragipare congenitale. Semin Hop Paris 1948;24:3217.
200. Nurden AT, Caen JP: Specific roles for platelet surface glycoproteins in platelet function. Nature 1975;255:720.
201. Clemetson KJ, McGregor JL, James E, et al: Characterization of the platelet membrane glycoprotein abnormalities in Bernard-Soulier syndrome and comparison with normal by surface-labeling techniques and high-resolution two-dimensional gel electrophoresis. J Clin Invest 1982;70:304.
202. Berndt MC, Gregory C, Chong BH, et al: Additional glycoprotein defects in Bernard-soulier's syndrome: confirmation of genetic basis by parental analysis. Blood 1983;62:800.
203. Lopez JA, Andrews RK, Afshar-Kharghan V, Berndt MC: Bernard-Soulier syndrome. Blood 1998;91:4397.
204. Davidson WM: Inherited variations in leukocytes. Br Med Bull 1960;17:190.
205. Hamilton RW, Shaikh BS, Ottie JN, et al: Platelet function, ultrastructure and survival in the May-Hegglin anomaly. Am J Clin Pathol 1980;74:663.
206. Breton-Gorius J, Favier R, Guichard J, et al: A new congenital dysmegakaryopoietic thrombocytopenia (Paris-Trousseau) associated with giant platelet α-granules and chromosome 11 deletion at 11Q23. Blood 1995;85:1805.
207. Knox-Macaulay HH, Bashawri L, Davies KE: X-linked recessive thrombocytopenia. J Med Genet 1993;30:968.
208. Markenson AL, Hilgartner MW, Miller DR: Transient thrombocytopenia in 18-trisomy. J Pediatr 1975;87:834.
209. Hohlfeld P, Forestier F, Kaplan C, et al: Fetal thrombocytopenia: a retrospective survey of 5,194 fetal blood samplings. Blood 1994;84:1851.
210. Miller M, Cosgriff JM: Hematological abnormalities in newborn infants with Down syndrome. Am J Med Genet 1983;16:173.
211. Hord JD, Gay JC, Whitlock JA: Thrombocytopenia in neonates with trisomy 21. Arch Pediatr Adolesc Med 1995;149:824.
212. Geha RS, Rosen FS, Chatila T: Primary immunodeficiency diseases. In Nathan DG, Oski FA (eds): Hematology of Infancy and Childhood. Philadelphia: WB Saunders, 1992, p 1040.
213. Kwan SP, Sandkuyl LA, Blaese M, et al: Genetic mapping of the Wiskott-Aldrich syndrome with two highly linked polymorphic DNA markers. Genomics 1988;3:39.
214. Parkman R, Remold-O'Donnell E, Kenney DM, et al: Surface protein abnormalities in lymphocytes and platelets from patients with Wiskott-Aldrich syndrome. Lancet 1981;2:1387.
215. Bader-Meunier B, Tchernia G, Mielot F, et al: Occurrence of myeloproliferative disorder in patients with Noonan syndrome. J Pediatr 1997;130:885.
216. Singer ST, Hurst D, Addiego JE: Bleeding disorders in Noonan syndrome: three case reports and review of the literature. J Pediatr Hematol Oncol 1997;19:130.
217. Evans DG, Lonsdale RN, Patron MA: Cutaneous lymphangioma and amegakaryocytic thrombocytopenia in Noonan syndrome. Clin Genet 1991;39:228.
218. Epstein DJ, Sahud MA, et al: Hereditary macrothrombocytopathia, nephritis and deafness. Am J Med 1972;52:299.
219. Eckstein JD, Filip DJ, Watts JC: Hereditary thrombocytopenia, deafness and renal disease. Ann Intern Med 1975;82:639.
220. Bithell TC: Thrombocytopenia caused by immunologic platelet destruction: idiopathic thrombocytopenic purpura, drug-induced thrombocytopenia, and miscellaneous forms. In Lee GR, Bithell TC, Foerster J, et al (eds): Wintrobe's Clinical Hematology, 9th ed. Philadelphia: Lea & Febiger, 1993, pp 1345–1347.

221. Whaun JM, Smith GR, Sochor V: Effect of prenatal drug administration on maternal and neonatal platelet aggregation and PF4 release. Haemostasis 1980;9:226.
222. Mauer AM, De Vauz LO, Lahey ME: Neonatal and maternal thrombocytopenic purpura due to quinine. Pediatrics 1957;19:84.
223. Corby DG, Schulman I: The effects of antenatal drug administration on aggregation of platelets of newborn infants. J Pediatr 1971;79:307.
224. Merenstein GB, O'Loughlin EP, Plunket DC: Effect of maternal thiazides on platelet counts of newborn infants. J Pediatr 1970;76:766.
225. Rodriguez SU, Leikin SL, Hiller MC: Neonatal thrombocytopenia associated with antepartum administration of thiazide drugs. N Engl J Med 1964;270:881.
226. Kumar RK, Yu VY: Prolonged low-dose indomethacin therapy for patent ductus arteriosus in very low birth weight infants. J Paediatr Child Health 1997;33:38.
227. Couser RJ, Ferrara TB, Wright GB: Prophylactic indomethacin therapy in the first twenty-four hours of life for the prevention of patent ductus arteriosus in preterm infants treated prophylactically with surfactant in the delivery room. J Pediatr 1996;128:631.
228. Mokrohisky ST, et al: Low positioning of umbilical-artery catheters increases associated complications in newborn infants. N Engl J Med 1978;299:561.
229. Jacobson RJ, Rath CE, Perloff JK: Intravascular hemolysis and thrombocytopenia in left ventricular outflow obstruction. Br Heart J 1973;35:849.
230. Harker LA, Malpass TW, Branson HE, et al: Mechanism of normal bleeding in patients undergoing cardiopulmonary bypass: Acquired transient dysfunction associated with selective α-granule release. Blood 1980;56:824.
231. De Schepper J, Hachimi-Idrisse S, Cham B: Diagnosis and management of catheter-related infected intracardiac thrombosis in premature infants. Am J Perinatol 1993;10:39.
232. Favara BE, Francisoe RA, Butterfield LJ: Disseminated intravascular and cardiac thrombosis of the neonate. Am J Dis Child 1974;127:197.
233. Morrow WR, Haas JE, Benjamin DR: Nonbacterial endocardial thrombosis in neonates: relationship to persistent fetal circulation. J Pediatr 1982;100:117.
234. Hutter JJ, Hathaway WE, Wayne ER: Hematologic abnormalities in severe neonatal necrotizing enterocolitis. J Pediatr 1976;88:1026.
235. Patel CC: Hematologic abnormalities in acute necrotizing enterocolitis. Pediatr Clin North Am 1977;24:579.
236. Caplan MS, Hedlund E, Adler L, et al: The platelet-activating factor receptor antagonist WEB 2170 prevents neonatal necrotizing enterocolitis in rats. J Pediatr Gastroenterol Nutr 1977;24:296.
237. Caplan MS, Lickerman, Adler L, et al: The role of recombinant platelet-activating factor acetylhydrolase in a neonatal rat model of necrotizing enterocolitis. Pediatr Res 1997;42:7798.
238. Muguruma K, Gray PW, Tjoelker LW, et al: The central role of PAF in necrotizing enterocolitis development. Adv Exp Med Biol 1977;407:379.
239. Meberg A, Jakobsen E, Halvorsen K: Humoral regulation of erythropoiesis and thrombopoiesis in appropriate and small for gestational age infants. Acta Paediatr Scand 1982;71:769.
240. Philip AG, Tito AM: Increased nucleated red blood cell counts in small for gestational age infants with very low birth weight. Am J Dis Child 1989;143:164.
241. Christensen RD, Sola MC: Unpublished observations, 1998.
242. Peters M, ten-Cate JW, Koo LH, et al: Persistent antithrombin III deficiency: risk factor for thromboembolic complications in neonates small for gestational age. J Pediatr 1984;105:310.
243. Koyama N, Ohama Y, Kaneko K, et al: Association of neonatal thrombocytopenia and maternal anti-HLA antibodies. Acta Paediatr Jpn 1991;33:71.
244. Murray NA, Watts TL, Roberts IAG: Endogenous thrombopoietin levels and effect of recombinant human thrombopoietin on megakaryocyte precursors in term and preterm babies. Pediatr Res 1998;43:148.
245. Brazy JE, Grimm JK, Little VA: Neonatal manifestations of severe maternal hypertension occurring before the thirty-sixth week of pregnancy. J Pediatr 1982;100:265.
246. Koenig JM, Christensen RD: Incidence, neutrophil kinetics, and natural history of neonatal neutropenia associated with maternal hypertension. N Engl J Med 1989;321:557.
247. Koenig JM, Christensen RD: The mechanism responsible for diminished neutrophil production in neonates delivered to women with pregnancy-induced hypertension. Am J Obstet Gynecol 1991;165:467.
248. Zuspan FP: New concepts in the understanding of hypertensive disease during pregnancy: an overview. Clin Perinatol 1991;18:653.
249. Burrows RF, Andrew M: Neonatal thrombocytopenia in the hypertensive disorders of pregnancy. Obstet Gynecol 1990;76:234.
250. Ropert JC, Dreyfus M, Dehan M, et al: Severe neonatal thrombocytopenia: analysis of the etiologic data on 64 cases. Arch Fr Pediatr 1984;41:85.
251. Castle V, Coates G, Mitchell LG, et al: The effect of hypoxia on platelet survival and site of sequestration in the newborn rabbit. Thromb Haemost 1988;59:45.
252. Hathaway WE, Bonnar J: Perinatal Coagulation. New York: Grune & Stratton, 1978, p 124.
253. Ansell J, Slepchuk N Jr, Kumar R, et al: Heparin-induced thrombocytopenia: a prospective study. Thromb Haemost 1980;43:61.
254. Kelton JG, Sheridan D, Santos A, et al: Heparin-induced thrombocytopenia: laboratory studies. Blood 1988;72:925.
255. Spadone D, Clark F, James E, et al: Heparin-induced thrombocytopenia in the newborn. J Vasc Surg 1992;15:306.
256. Maurer HM, Haggins JC, Still WJS: Platelet injury during phototherapy. Am J Hematol 1976;1:89.
257. Christensen RD, Rothstein G: Exhaustion of mature marrow neutrophils in neonates with sepsis. J Pediatr 1980;96:316.
258. Al-Mulla ZS, Christensen RD: Neutropenia in the neonate. Clin Perinatol 1995;22:711.
259. Rothstein G: Origin and development of the blood and blood-forming tissues. In Lee GR, Bithell TC, Foerster J, et al (eds): Wintrobe's Clinical Hematology, 9th ed. Philadelphia: Lea & Febiger, 1993, p 74.
260. Weber M, Johannisson R, Bolte M, et al: Fine needle tissue aspiration for accurate localization of histological specimens from complex structures. Biotech Histochem 1997;72:243.
261. Harker LA: Kinetics of thrombopoiesis. J Clin Invest 1968;47:458.
262. Harker LA, Finch CA: Thrombokinetics in man. J Clin Invest 1969;48:963.
263. Tomer A, Harker LA, Burstein SA: Flow cytometric analysis of normal human megakaryocytes. Blood 1988;71:1244.
264. Tomer A, Friese P, Conklin R, et al: Flow cytometric analysis of megakaryocytes from patients with abnormal platelet counts. Blood 1989;74:594.

265. Hegyi E, Nakazawa M, Debili N, et al: Developmental changes in human megakaryocyte ploidy. Exp Hematol 1991;19:87.
266. De Alarcon PA, Graeve JLA: Analysis of megakaryocyte ploidy in fetal bone marrow biopsies using a new adaptation of the Feulgen technique to measure DNA content and estimate megakaryocyte ploidy from biopsy specimens. Pediatr Res 1996;39:166.
267. Olson TA, Levine RF, Mazur EM, et al: Megakaryocytes and megakaryocyte progenitors in human cord blood. Am J Pediatr Hematol Oncol 1992;14:241.
268. Patrick CH, Lazarchick J: The effect of bacteremia on automated platelet measurements in neonates. Am J Clin Pathol 1990;93:391.
269. Cheugh NK, Hilgartner MW, Schulman I, et al: Platelet-associated immunoglobulin G in childhood idiopathic thrombocytopenic purpura. J Pediatr 1983;102:366.
270. Kelton JG, Denomme G, Lucarelli A, et al: Comparison of the measurement of surface or total platelet-associated IgG in the diagnosis of immune thrombocytopenia. Am J Hematol 1985;18:1.
271. Kelton JG: Elevated platelet-associated IgG in the thrombocytopenia of septicemia. N Engl J Med 1979;300:760.
272. Shulman NR, Leissinger CA, Hotchkiss AJ, et al: The nonspecific nature of platelet-associated IgG. Trans Assoc Am Physians 1982;95:213.
273. Yamamoto T, Kinoshita T, Miyata H: Idiopathic thrombocytopenic purpura in childhood: Retrospective analysis of the clinical prognosis. Rinsho Ketsueki 1993;34:1445.
274. Ware R, Kjinney TR, Friedman HS, et al: Prognostic implications for direct platelet-associated IgG in childhood idiopathic thrombocytopenic purpura. Am J Pediatr Hematol Oncol 1986;8:32.
275. Winiarski J, Kreuger A, Ejderhamn J, et al: High dose IgG reduces platelet associated immunoglobulins and complement in idiopathic thrombocytopenic purpura. Scand J Haematol 1983;31:342.
276. Stilliman CC, Cusack NA, Swanson NJ, et al: Platelets and neutrophils from healthy term neonates exhibit increased levels of immunoglobulins. Pediatr Res 1995;38:993.
277. Heyns AD, Lotter MG, Badenhorst PN, et al: Kinetics, distribution and sites of destruction of ^{111}indium-labeled human platelets. Br J Haematol 1980;44:269.
278. Hill-Zobel RL, Scheffel U, McIntyre PA, et al: ^{111}In-oxine–labeled rabbit platelets: in vivo distribution and sites of destruction. Blood 1983;61:149.
279. Ikeoka K, Todo Y, Konishiike A, et al: Scintigraphic detection of thrombi using indium-111–labeled autologous platelets. J Cardiol 1985;15:67.
280. Najean Y, Rain JD, Billotey C: The site of destruction of autologous ^{111}In-labeled platelets and the efficiency of splenectomy in children and adults with idiopathic thrombocytopenic purpura: a study of 578 patients with 268 splenectomies. Br J Haematol 1997;97:547.
281. Ezekowitz MD, Wilson DA, Smith EO, et al: Comparison of indium-111 platelet scintigraphy and two-dimensional echocardiography in the diagnosis of left ventricular thrombi. N Engl J Med 1982;306:1509.
282. Sondel PM, Ritter MW, Wilson DG, et al: Use of ^{111}In platelet scans in the detection and treatment of Kasabach-Merritt syndrome. J Pediatr 1984;104:87.
283. Hanada T, Nakahara S, Takita H, et al: ^{111}In-labeled platelet scintigraphy in Kasabach- Merritt syndrome. Nippon Ketsueki Gakkai Zasshi 1984;47:1359.
284. Shulkin BL, Argenta LC, Chio KJ, et al: Kasabach-Merritt syndrome: treatment with epsilon-aminocaproic acid and assessment by indium 111 platelet scintigraphy. J Pediatr 1990;117:746.
285. Castle VP, Shulkin BL, Coats G, et al: The use of indium-111 oxine platelet scintigraphy and survival studies in pediatric patients with thrombocytopenia. J Nucl Med 1989;30:1819.
286. de Sauvage FJ, Hass PE, Spencer SD, et al: Stimulation of megakaryocytopoiesis and thrombopoiesis by the c-Mpl ligand. Nature 1994;369:533.
287. Lok S, Kaushansky K, Holly RD, et al: Cloning and expression of murine thrombopoietin cDNA and stimulation of platelet production in vivo. Nature 1994;369:565.
288. Bartley TD, Bogenberger J, Hunt P, et al: Identification and cloning of a megakaryocyte growth and development factor that is a ligand for the cytokine receptor Mpl. Cell 1994;77:1117.
289. Kuter DJ, Beeler DL, Rosenberg RD: The purification of megapoietin: a physiological regulator of megakaryocyte growth and platelet production. Proc Natl Acad Sci USA 1994;91:11104.
290. Emmons RVB, Reid DM, Cohen RL, et al: Human thrombopoietin levels are high when thrombocytopenia is due to megakaryocyte deficiency and low when due to increased platelet destruction. Blood 1996;87:4068.
291. Chang M, Suen Y, Meng G, et al: Differential mechanisms in the regulation of endogenous levels of thrombopoietin and interleukin-11 during thrombocytopenia: insight into the regulation of platelet production. Blood 1996;88:3354.
292. Ichikawa N, Ishido F, Shimodaira S, et al: Regulation of serum thrombopoietin levels by platelets and megakaryocytes in patients with aplastic anaemia and idiopathic thrombocytopenic purpura. Thromb Haemost 1996;76:156.
293. Kunishima S, Tahara T, Kato T, et al: Serum thrombopoietin and plasma glycocalicin concentrations as useful diagnostic markers in thrombocytopenic disorders. Eur J Haematol 1996;57:68.
294. Consensus Development Conference. Platelet transfusion. JAMA 1987;257:1777.
295. Beutler E: Platelet transfusions: the 20,000/μL trigger. Blood 1993;81:1411.
296. Feusner JH, Slichter SJ, Harker LA: Acquired haemostatic defects in the ill newborn. Br J Haematol 1983;53:73.
297. Mueller-Eckhardt C, Kiefel V, Grubert A, et al: 348 Cases of suspected neonatal alloimmune thrombocytopenia. Lancet 1989;1:363.
298. Blanchette VS, Chen L, de Friedberg ZS, et al: Alloimmunization to the PlA1 platelet antigen: results of a prospective study. Br J Haematol 1990;74:209.
299. Sidiropulous D, Straume B: The treatment of neonatal isoimmune thrombocytopenia with intravenous immunoglobulin. Blut 1984;48:383.
300. Pearson HA, Shulman R, Marder VJ, et al: Isoimmune neonatal thrombocytopenic purpura: clinical and therapeutic considerations. Blood 1964;23:154.
301. Kaplan C, Murphy MF, Kroll H, et al: Feto-maternal alloimmune thrombocytopenia: antenatal therapy with IVIG and steoids—more questions than answers. European Working Group of FMAIT. Br J Haematol 1998;100:62.
302. Kroll H, Kiefel V, Giers G, et al: Prenatal management of fetuses with alloimmune thrombocytopenia. Beitr Infusionsther Transfusionsmed 1996;33:150.
303. Lynch L, Bussel JB, McFarland JG, et al: Antenatal treatment of alloimmune thrombocytopenia. Obstet Gynecol 1992;80:67.

304. Schechter Y, Zeides I, Shalev E, et al: Neonatal alloimmune thrombocytopenia. Harefuah 1994;127:505.
305. Chirico G, Duse M, Ugazio AG, et al: High-dose intravenous gamma-globulin therapy for passive immune thrombocytopenia in the neonate. J Pediatr 1983;103:654.
306. Ballin A, Andrew M, Ling E, et al: High dose intravenous gamma-globulin therapy for neonatal autoimmune thrombocytopenia. J Pediatr 1988;112:789.
307. Ulich TR, del Castillo J, Yin S, et al: Megakaryocyte growth and development factor ameliorates carboplatin-induced thrombocytopenia in mice. Blood 1995;86:971.
308. Farese AM, Hunt P, Boone T, MacVittie T: Recombinant human megakaryocyte growth and development factor stimulates thrombocytopoiesis in normal nonhuman primates. Blood 1996;86:54.
309. Harker LA, Hunt P, Marzec UM, et al: Regulation of platelet production and function by megakaryocyte growth and development factor in nonhuman primates. Blood 1996;87:1833.
310. Harker LA, Marzec UM, Hunt P, et al: Dose-response effects of pegylated human megakaryocyte growth and development factor on platelet production and function in nonhuman primates. Blood 1996;88:511.
311. Daw NC, Arnold JT, Abushullaih BA, et al: A single intravenous dose of murine megakaryocyte growth and development factor potently stimulates platelet production, challenging the necessity for daily administration. Blood 1988;91:466.
312. Grossmann A, Lenox J, Ren HP, et al: Thrombopoietin accelerates platelet, red blood cell, and neutrophil recovery in myelosuppressed mice. Exp Hematol 1996;24:1238.
313. Grossmann A, Lenox J, Deisher TA, et al: Synergistic effects of thrombopoietin and granulocyte colony-stimulating factor on neutrophil recovery in myelosuppressed mice. Blood 1996;88:3363.
314. Harker LA, Marzec UM, Kelly AB, et al: Prevention of thrombocytopenia and neutropenia in a nonhuman primate model of marrow suppressive chemotherapy by combining pegylated recombinant human megakaryocyte growth and development factor and recombinant human granulocyte colony-stimulating factor. Blood 1997;89:155.
315. Neelis KJ, Hartong SCC, Egeland T, et al: The efficacy of single-dose administration of thrombopoietin with coadministration of either granulocyte/macrophage of granulocyte colony-stimulating factor in myelosuppressed rhesus monkeys. Blood 1997;90:2565.
316. Basser RL, Rasko JEJ, Clarke K, et al: Thrombopoietic effects of pegylated recombinant human megakaryocyte growth and development factor (PEG-rHuMGDF) in patients with advanced cancer. Lancet 1996;348:1279.
317. Vadhan-Raj S, Murray LJ, Bueso-Ramos C, et al: Stimulation of megakaryocyte and platelet production by a single dose of recombinant human thrombopoietin in patients with cancer. Ann Intern Med 1997;126:673.
318. Fanucchi M, Glaspy J, Crawford J, et al: Effects of polyethylene glycol-conjugated recombinant human megakaryocyte growth and development factor on platelet counts after chemotherapy for lung cancer. N Engl J Med 1997;336:404.
319. Basser RL, Rasko JEJ, Clarke K, et al: Randomized, blinded, placebo-controlled phase I trial of pegylated recombinant human megakaryocyte growth and development factor with filgrastim after dose-intensive chemotherapy in patients with advanced cancer. Blood 1997;89:3118.
320. Nishihira H, Toyoda Y, Miyazaki H, et al: Growth of macroscopic human megakaryocyte colonies from cord blood in culture with recombinant human thrombopoietin (c-mpl ligand) and the effects of gestational age on frequency of colonies. Br J Haematol 1996;92:23.
321. van de Ven C, Fernandez GW, Herbst T, et al: Sequential treatment with rmIL-3 or simultaneous treatment with rmIL-3 or rhIL-11 with thrombopoietin (TPO) fails to enhance in vivo neonatal rat thrombocytopoiesis. Exp Hematol 1997;25:1005.
322. George JW, Bracco CA, Shannon KM, et al: Age-related differences in erythropoietic response to recombinant human erythropoietin: comparison in adult and infant rhesus monkeys. Pediatr Res 1990;28:567.

CHAPTER 14

Leukocyte Development and Disorders During the Neonatal Period

Kurt Schibler, M.D.

The chief disorders of leukocytes observed in the newborn period include quantitative abnormalities such as neutropenia, lymphopenia, and leukemoid reactions and qualitative defects in multiple lineages of leukocytes, including neutrophils, monocytes, and T lymphocytes.

GRANULOPOIESIS AND LYMPHOPOIESIS

The conventional view of hematopoiesis holds that all varieties of blood cells are derived from a population of hematopoietic stem cells and that these pluripotent stem cells progress through a series of commitment steps toward single-lineage progenitor cells that ultimately mature into various fully differentiated formed elements in the blood, as shown in Figure 14–1. The existence of such a hematopoietic hierarchy was initially postulated by Maximow in 1924,[1] and this concept was further refined years later by Downey.[2] Experiments demonstrating that bone marrow cells administered to lethally irradiated mice were capable of reconstituting the entire hematopoietic system confirmed these theories.[3]

The development of techniques to culture hematopoietic cells during the past 3 decades has added considerably to our understanding of hematopoietic commitment and differentiation. The ability to culture hematopoietic progenitor cells has enabled categorization, functional analysis, and definition of growth factor requirements for various committed progenitors.[4–6] Culture systems have been developed to selectively support progenitor cell maintenance of myeloid development, B lymphocyte development, or T lymphocyte development.[7–9] These systems have enabled investigators to define many of the growth factors required for regulation of survival, proliferation, and differentiation of hematopoietic progenitor cells and committed hematopoietic cells.

Some of these factors act on stem cells and primitive progenitors capable of giving rise to multiple blood cell lineages. Among these are stem cell factor, interleukin (IL)-3, IL-6, and IL-11.[10–12] Other factors support lineage-committed multipotential hematopoietic progenitors at intermediate stages of differentiation. Such factors include IL-3, IL-4, and granulocyte-macrophage colony-stimulating factor (GM-CSF).[13–15]

A group of lineage-specific factors support proliferation and maturation of committed progenitor cells and regulate effector functions of mature blood cells. Examples of these factors include granulocyte colony-stimulating factor (G-CSF), IL-5, and monocyte colony-stimulating factor (M-CSF). G-CSF is a physiologic regulator of neutrophil maturation and function.[16] It also acts on primitive progenitors.[10] IL-5 and M-CSF are believed to be specific for eosinophil and monocyte-macrophage progenitors.[17, 18]

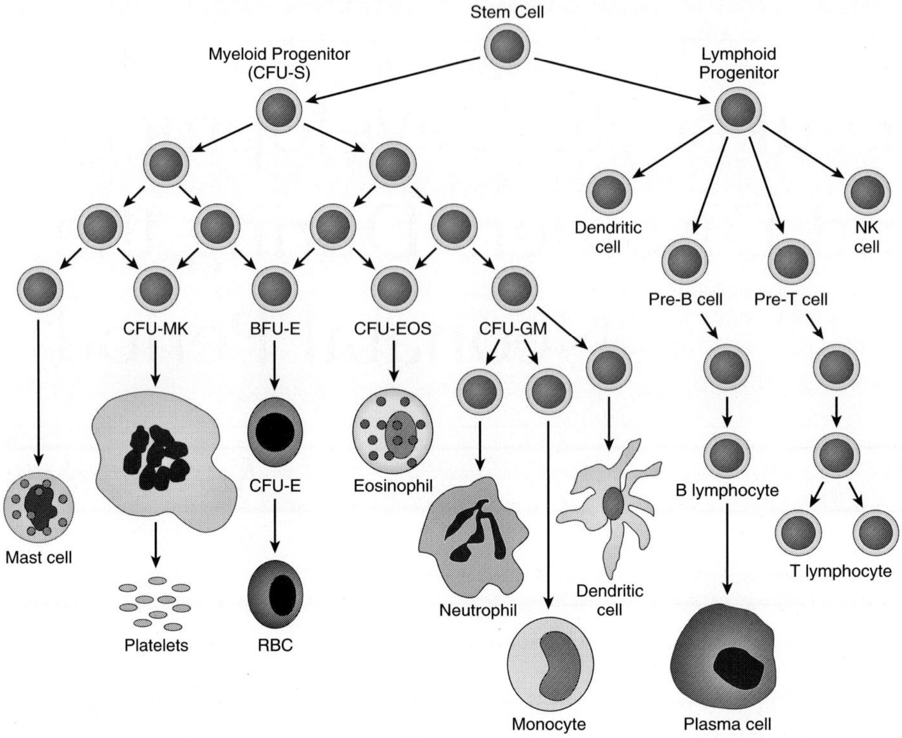

Figure 14–1. Hematopoietic progenitors. (BFU, burst-forming unit; CFU, colony-forming unit; E, erythroid; EOS, eosinophil; GM, granulocyte-macrophage; RBC, red blood cell; S, spleen.)

NEUTROPHILS

Function

Bacterial and fungal sepsis are major causes of morbidity and mortality in neonates. Infection rates are high among infants hospitalized in intensive care units and particularly among extremely-low-birth-weight infants, for whom infection rates are approximately 40%.[19] An ongoing survey of neonatal infections at Yale University has documented a decline in neonatal deaths due to sepsis commensurate with the liberal use of antibiotics and the improvement in supportive care in neonatal intensive care units.[20] Mortality from sepsis declined steadily until the early 1980s, but it has remained relatively constant since that time. Significant developmental defects in host immunity among preterm and term neonates and survival of increasing numbers of extremely-low-birth-weight infants probably are responsible for this plateau in mortality.

Neutrophils are central to the defense against bacterial infection, and neutrophil production and function are immature processes in neonates. The functional defects are largely involved in the phagocytic process (Table 14–1). This process involves motility, recognition, ingestion, and intracellular killing.

Cell Movement

After neutrophils have emigrated from the circulation, migration occurs in two ways: by random movement and by directed movement toward a chemoattractant. This movement is not related to a stimulus and occurs in any direction with equal probability. The ability of neutrophils to undergo directed migration de-

Table 14–1. **Normal and Deficient Functions of Neutrophils from Neonates**

Normal Functions	Deficient Functions
Random movement	Directed migration
Mobilization of intracellular granules	Phagocytosis
Myeloperoxidase content	Lactoferrin content
Lysozyme content	Gelatinase content
Ingestion of microorganisms*	Antiviral activity
Intracellular killing of bacteria*	

*May be deficient in preterm and "stressed" neonates.

pends on sensory mechanisms capable of detecting differences in concentration of chemotactic molecules and linking this information to the locomotory apparatus within the cell.[21]

Random movement of neonatal neutrophils is normal compared with that observed in adult cells.[22, 23] On the contrary, the consensus derived from a number of studies is that directed migration of neutrophils from preterm and term neonates to defined chemotactic stimuli is impaired.[24–27] The mechanism underlying this defect has not been defined. Neonatal neutrophils express receptors involved in the chemotactic factor-receptor interaction at the cell surface. Receptors on the plasma membrane for formyl-peptides (e.g., N-formyl-L-methionyl-L-leucyl-L-phenylalanine [FMLP]) and for complement components such as C3bi and C5a have been characterized.[28–30] The binding kinetics and concentrations of FMLP required to saturate receptors are comparable on neonatal and adult neutrophils.[13, 27] In contrast, C3bi receptors on activated neutrophils are only 75% of adult values and may limit chemotaxis.[29] Other mechanisms that have been postulated include signal transduction abnormalities related to low levels of free intracellular calcium,[31, 32] impaired generation of new plasma membrane during the migratory process,[33, 34] and impaired energy metabolism resulting from the inability to increase hexose uptake adequately during migration toward chemotactic stimuli.[35]

Phagocytosis

Neutrophils establish contact with invading microorganisms through opsonins, including complement and IgG antibody. The phagocyte envelops the microorganism completely by sequential and circumferential interactions between opsonins and receptors. Once engulfed, the newly formed phagocytic vacuole is internalized, and products of intracellular granules are mobilized and discharged into the vacuole.[36, 37] Mobilization of granules appears to be normal in neutrophils from newborns compared with adults.[38] Neutrophils from newborn infants are equivalent to those of adults in the content of myeloperoxidase and lysozyme,[39] but they possess diminished quantities of lactoferrin and gelatinase.[38–40]

In several experiments, neutrophils from healthy term infants were suspended in pooled adult serum. Results demonstrated that the phagocytic capacity of newborn cells was similar to that of cells from adult controls in the ingestion of a variety of microorganisms and foreign particles. Microorganisms evaluated included *Escherichia coli*,[41, 42] group B streptococci,[41, 43] *Pseudomonas aeruginosa*,[42] *Serratia marcescens*,[44] *Staphylococcus aureus*,[41, 42] and *Candida albicans*.[45]

Phagocytosis by neutrophils from preterm infants is less well characterized. In the studies available, neutrophils from healthy preterm infants exhibited normal ingestion capabilities for bacteria and foreign particles.[42, 44] Ingestion of *Candida albicans* by neutrophils from preterm infants was reported as normal in one study[45] and decreased in others.[46, 47]

Intracellular Killing

Bactericidal activity of neutrophils against a variety of microorganisms appears to be normal in healthy newborns. The microorganisms evaluated in these studies include *E. coli*,[41, 42, 48] group B streptococci,[41 48] *P. aeruginosa*,[42] *S. marcescens*,[44] and *Staphylococcus pyogenes*.[48] Among infants stressed by conditions such as respiratory distress or sepsis, diminished bactericidal activity was documented against *E. coli* and *S. aureus*.[49] Neonatal neutrophils are less effective in killing group B streptococci when concomitant pathologic conditions are present.[50] Microbicidal activity against *C. albicans* was reported to be low in one study[47] but normal compared with adults in another study.[45] Antiviral activity of newborn neutrophils is also diminished compared with that of adults.[51]

Changes with Infection

Myeloblasts, promyelocytes, and myelocytes are collectively called the neutrophil proliferative pool, because these cells have the capacity for cell division. As committed neutrophil precursors mature, their capacity to undergo cell division is lost. This population of postmitotic cells that includes metamyelocytes, band neutrophils, and mature segmented neutrophils is called the neutrophil storage pool (NSP). Neutrophils are released from the NSP to maintain the circulating and marginated neutrophil pools in equilibrium with approximately equal numbers of cells in each pool. About 0.3×10^9 neutrophils per 1 kg of body weight are present in the circulating pool of healthy human adults.[52]

Adults have a large NSP and can increase circulating neutrophils rapidly in response to infection.[52] Unlike adults, newborn infants have a relatively small NSP per 1 kg of body weight.[53] These differences in the available reserve of postmitotic neutrophils limit the ability of newborn infants to respond to bacterial challenge. The circulating neutrophil concentration is relatively low in humans during gestation but rises progressively to term.[53] A fourfold increase in the circulating neutrophil count occurs between 14 and 32 weeks' gestation.[54] Postnatally, the circulating neutrophil counts are much higher. A study by Manroe and associates[55] delineated neutrophil ranges in normal term newborns during the first 28 days of life. This study demonstrated a rise in neutrophil concentrations to a peak occurring between 12 and 24 hours. The range of normal neutrophil concentrations at that time is between 7800 and 14,500 cells/μL. The neutrophil count subsequently decreases and stabilizes, with a lower value of 1750 cells/μL by 72 hours. Mouzihno and coworkers[56] established reference ranges for blood neutrophil concentrations in very-low-birth-weight infants. The upper range for normal neutrophil concentrations was similar to those observed in term infants, but the very-low-birth-weight infants exhibited a substantially wider range of values. The lower levels defining neutropenia were about 2000 cells/μL at 12 hours postpartum, falling and stabilizing at 1000 cells/μL by 48 hours of life.

The proportion of band neutrophils to segmented neutrophils in the bone marrow is much higher than in the circulation. On that basis, selective release of cells from the NSP occurs in response to infection.

NEUTROPENIA

Causes and Associated Disorders

Infants of Mothers with Hypertension

A high proportion of neonates delivered of women with hypertension have reduced circulating blood neutrophil concentrations (Table 14–2).[57–60] The neutrophil kinetic abnormality is decreased neutrophil production.[61] This idea is supported by studies delineating a decrease in neutrophil progenitor cells, decreased cycling of these cells, a relatively normal neutrophil proliferative pool and NSP, and the absence of a "left shift." This variety of neutropenia is particularly common in severe maternal hypertension accompanied by fetal growth restriction.[61] The cause of the reduced neutrophil production is uncertain, but it does not appear to be related to maternal medications.[60, 61] Extracts of placental tissue and from neutropenic neonates contain substances that inhibit neutrophil production.[62] This substance also occurs in umbilical cord blood of neutropenic neonates.

The significance of neutropenia associated with maternal hypertension is that nonspecific host defenses are impaired in these infants. Moreover, several investigators have documented a higher incidence of nosocomial infection in infants who were neutropenic compared with infants with normal neutrophil counts delivered of hypertensive mothers.[61, 63, 64] One

Table 14–2. **Causes of Neonatal Neutropenia**

Increased Neutrophil Destruction	Diminished Neutrophil Production
Infection	Infants of hypertensive mothers
Isoimmunization (alloimmune) neonatal neutropenia	Donor in twin-to-twin transfusion
Autoimmune neonatal neutropenia	Rh hemolytic disease
Chronic benign neutropenia	Severe congenital neutropenia (Kostmann's syndrome)
	Cyclic neutropenia
	Schwachman syndrome
	Reticular dysgenesis
	Drug or toxin induced

group reviewed records of 301 low-birth-weight infants delivered of hypertensive mothers and reported an incidence of neutropenia of 48% and a significant difference in the incidence of sepsis in neutropenic (6%) and non-neutropenic infants (0%) in this cohort.[63] Another group reported a significant increase in the incidence of nosocomial infection in 101 consecutive infants with this variety of neutropenia (29%) compared with infants with normal neutrophil counts (5%).[64]

Multiple Gestation

A transient, hyporegenerative neutropenia has been reported among donors in twin-to-twin transfusion. This neutrophil abnormality can manifest at delivery and persist for up to 8 days.[65] Accelerated erythropoiesis is evidenced by elevated concentrations of erythroid precursors in the circulation and rapid cycling rates among these progenitor cells. The accelerated erythropoiesis is probably a compensatory response to intrauterine anemia caused by transfusion of the recipient twin. As has been observed with other states of accelerated erythropoiesis, reduced neutrophil production can occur. Concentrations of circulating myeloid precursors are low in these infants, and no left shift is observed. The cycling status in circulating myeloid precursor cells also is reduced.

Rh Hemolytic Disease

A well-documented complication of severe Rh erythroblastosis fetalis is a reduction in the concentration of other formed elements in the blood, particularly platelets and neutrophils.[66, 67] In one series of 20 patients delivered of mothers with Rh sensitization, 11 had severe disease requiring multiple transfusions.[66] Before exchange transfusion, all infants with severe disease had neutropenia that persisted for 3 to 5 days, whereas none with mild disease exhibited neutrophil depletion. Marrow studies revealed markedly accelerated erythropoiesis and decreased myelopoiesis.

Cyclic Neutropenia

Cyclic neutropenia is a rare disorder characterized by neutropenic episodes occurring in cycles of 21 ± 3 days.[68–70] The duration of neutropenic episodes is typically 3 to 10 days. In most cases, other formed elements in the blood such as reticulocytes and platelets also cycle. Bone marrow aspiration during neutropenia demonstrates cellular hypoplasia or maturational arrest.[68, 70] Patients have histories of repetitive infections occurring in tandem with the cyclic oscillations in circulating neutrophil concentrations. The severity of the infections tends to correlate with the degree of neutropenia. Between neutropenic nadirs, patients remain free of infections, but during neutropenic episodes, fever of unknown source, oral ulceration, gingivitis, stomatitis, pharyngitis, cellulitis, perirectal abscess, and lymphadenopathy are observed. Although the disorder is usually benign, death from overwhelming sepsis occurs in as many as 10% of affected individuals. Although some patients experience clinical improvement as they grow older, the disease persists throughout the patients' lifetimes. Cyclic neutropenia does not progress to leukemia or aplastic anemia.[71] The disorder may occur sporadically, but in approximately one third of patients, a pattern of autosomal inheritance is likely.[72]

Treatment with splenectomy, steroids, and lithium have been ineffective.[69, 70] Trials of recombinant G-CSF have reported promising results, with significant decreases in severity and duration of neutropenia and in the incidence of infection.[69, 73]

Severe Congenital Neutropenia

Severe congenital neutropenia, or Kostmann syndrome, is an autosomal recessive disorder of myelopoiesis characterized by severe neutropenia with absolute blood neutrophil counts generally less than 200 cells/μL.[74, 75] Bone marrow smears usually demonstrate normal cellularity with impaired myeloid differentiation at the promyelocyte-myelocyte stage.[76] Daily administration of G-CSF to these patients results in circulating neutrophil counts in the range of 1000 cells/μL and is associated with a dramatic clinical improvement.[76, 77] The hematopoietic defect is believed to reside in the G-CSF receptor molecule or the G-CSF–mediated signal transduction cascade. In patients with severe congenital neutropenia who subsequently develop myeloid leukemia, point mutations are present in the cytoplasmic portion of the G-CSF receptor gene.[78–80] Most individuals with this disorder do not have mutations in the G-CSF receptor.

Neonatal Isoimmune Neutropenia

Isoimmune neonatal neutropenia results from maternal production of IgG directed against antigens on fetal neutrophils.[81] This disorder is analogous to Rh hemolytic anemia in that maternal sensitization to fetal neutrophil antigens results in IgG antibodies that cross the placenta and destroy the infant's neutrophils.[82, 83] Maternal sensitization against antigens on the fetal neutrophil can occur at any time during gestation and can occur in the fetus of a primagravida.[83, 84] Isoimmune neutropenia should be considered in any infant with neutropenia persisting for several days. The incidence of this disorder is estimated to be 0.5 to 2 per 1000 live births.[85]

Affected infants frequently develop fever in the first days of life and are particularly susceptible to cutaneous infections caused by *S. aureus*. Less commonly, β-hemolytic streptococci and *E. coli* are causative. The onset of symptoms is concurrent with severe neutropenia. Other myeloid lineages, particularly monocytes and eosinophils, are often increased in the circulation. Bone marrow evaluation characteristically shows myeloid hyperplasia with depletion of mature neutrophils. Marrow erythropoiesis and megakaryopoiesis are normal.

Neutrophil antibodies are detected in the sera of mother and infant. The antibodies react against neutrophils of the patient, the father, and some siblings, but they do not react against neutrophils from the mother. The infant's neutrophil count typically normalizes over the first 1 to 5 weeks of life, as would be anticipated with the half-life of maternal IgG. Several neutrophil-specific antibodies have been implicated, including most commonly NA1, NA2, NB1, and NC1. NA1 and NA2 have been identified as isotypes of the FcγIII receptor.[86]

Appropriate treatment of infections with antibiotics and close clinical follow-up are recommended for these patients. The use of prophylactic antibiotics is controversial. In the event of life-threatening infections that are poorly responsive to antibiotics and supportive care, transfusion with maternal or compatible donor neutrophils can be considered.[83, 84] Intravenous immunoglobulin (IVIG) administration has not produced consistent effects on circulating neutrophil counts.[84]

Neonatal Autoimmune Neutropenia

Transplacental transfer of maternal IgG autoantibodies reacting against neutrophil antigens can rarely cause transient neonatal neutropenia. Mothers of these infants can be asymptomatic or have autoimmune neutropenia from systemic lupus erythematosus or idiopathic thrombocytopenic purpura.[87, 88] The diagnosis of neonatal autoimmune neutropenia is established by demonstrating neutrophil autoantibodies in the sera of mother and infant. Administration of IVIG can transiently increase neutrophil concentrations in these infants.

Autoimmune Neutropenia

Autoimmune neutropenia (AIN) is a disorder caused by increased destruction of neutrophils as a result of antibodies in the patient's blood directed against his or her own neutrophils. The incidence is approximately 1 case per 100,000 live births.[89] Primary AIN is not associated with other autoimmune disease such as lupus erythematosus. Although AIN was convincingly demonstrated in 1975, the cause of this disorder is still unknown.[90, 91] Patients with this disorder present within the first 3 years of life with a variety of infections and neutropenia. In most patients, approximately 80%, infections are mild, consisting of upper respiratory infections, otitis media, gastroenteritis, pyoderma, abscesses, conjunctivitis, and lymphadenitis coli, but in the remaining patients, AIN predisposes to severe infections such as sepsis, pneumonia, and meningitis.[92]

The laboratory study in these infants consists of blood counts and bone marrow evaluation. At diagnosis, the concentration of blood neutrophils is below 1500 cells/μL and remains low for several months.[92] The bone marrow evaluation shows normal to increased cellularity in more than 95% of patients. The numbers of metamyelocytes, bands, and mature neutrophils vary. Although in a few cases a maturational arrest appears to occur, maturation at least reaches the myelocyte-metamyelocyte stage in all cases. This profile contrasts with that of severe congenital neutropenia, in which a maturational arrest in myelopoiesis occurs at the promyelocyte-myelocyte stage. Antibody-mediated destruction of mature neutrophils and band forms can mimic maturational arrest in the myelocyte-metamyelocyte stage.

The key to diagnosis of AIN is detection of granulocyte-specific antibodies in the patient's serum. Granulocyte-specific antibodies are directed most commonly against FcγIIIb. This neutrophil-restricted glycoprotein appears to be very immunogenic, because the most clinically significant granulocyte-specific antigens—NA1, NA2, and SH antigen—are located on this molecule.[93, 94] Antibodies to the leukocyte adhesion molecule, CD11/CD18, have been detected to a lesser extent.[92, 95]

Patients with AIN usually do not require specific treatment for the neutropenia. Infections are treated symptomatically with antibiotics. Infants with recurrent infections are treated with prophylactic antibiotics. To increase circulating neutrophil concentrations in cases of severe infection or before elective surgery, patients have been treated with corticosteroids, high-dose IVIG, or recombinant human G-CSF. Corticosteroids and IVIG were effective in approximately 50% of cases, whereas G-CSF increased the neutrophil count in all patients treated.

The natural course of this disease in most cases is resolution of the neutropenia after spontaneous disappearance of autoantibodies.[91, 92] Because AIN shows a self-limited course, G-CSF treatment is typically reserved for patients with severe infections or before surgical intervention. No evidence of predisposition to other autoimmune diseases has been observed in patients with AIN.

Exocrine Pancreatic Insufficiency

The Schwachman syndrome is a rare multiorgan disease of unknown origin characterized by metaphyseal chondrodysplasia, dwarfism, pancreatic exocrine insufficiency, and neutropenia.[96, 97] In the neonatal period, clinical manifestations include diarrhea, weight loss, failure to thrive, eczema, otitis media, and pneumonia.[98–101] Growth failure and dwarfism usually are identified in the first 2 years of life. Later, gait disturbances result from the metaphyseal chondrodysplasia. The steatorrhea tends to diminish with time, but the pancreatic insufficiency persists. Treatment of malabsorption does not improve the neutropenia. In approximately 25% of cases, aplastic anemia develops. Leukemic transformation has also occurred.[99]

The circulating neutrophil counts vary, with the average between 200 and 400 cells per 1 μL. Although this syndrome can resemble cystic fibrosis in infancy, the sweat chloride test result is negative in this disorder. Patients suffer from recurrent infections resulting from the neutropenia and occasionally from a concomitant neutrophil motility defect. The pathophysiology underlying the hematopoietic defect has not been identified. Normal numbers of granulocytic progenitor cells have been observed in this disorder, and they respond normally to G-CSF and GM-CSF but not to IL-3 in clonal culture.[102] In vivo administration of G-CSF has been reported to increase the neutrophil count to normal levels.[103]

Hair-Cartilage Hypoplasia Syndrome

Cartilage-hair hypoplasia is an autosomal recessive disorder characterized by short-limbed dwarfism, fine hair, and moderate neutropenia.[104] This disorder is common among the Amish population. Affected individuals have an increased susceptibility to infections, particularly varicella zoster viral infections. Immunologic defects are variable, but cellular immune functions are frequently impaired.[105]

Reticular Dysgenesis

Reticular dysgenesis, also called congenital aleukocytosis, is distinguished by severe neutropenia associated with leukopenia; rudimentary thymic, lymphoid, and splenic tissue; and agammaglobulinemia.[106] Histologic examination of the bone marrow, spleen, and lymphoid compartments shows normal reticular structure with normal erythroid and megakaryocyte elements but absent or sparse myeloid cells. The mechanism underlying this disorder is unknown, but it is postulated that a defect in maturation of a lymphohematopoietic progenitor cell is responsible.[107] Bacterial and viral infections occur early in life and are severe. Aggressive antibiotic and supportive treatment are necessary for survival. Use of the hematopoietic growth factors G-CSF and GM-CSF has been ineffective.[108, 109] Bone marrow transplantation remains the only long-term treatment option available for infants with reticular dysgenesis.[110]

Approach and Therapeutic Options

Evaluation

The evaluation of infants with neutropenia relies heavily on a thorough history and physical examination. Inquiries into family and obstetric history should emphasize detection of infection, elucidation of obstetric causes of neutropenia, identification of associated phenotypic abnormalities, and evaluation for signs of underlying chronic illness such as hepatosplenomegaly and lymphadenopathy. The history should gather pertinent details about the duration of symptoms, exposure to drugs or toxins capable of inducing neutropenia, and the family history of other individuals with recurrent infections.

The timing, duration, and severity of neutropenia should guide the laboratory evaluation. For infants presenting with neutropenia early in the neonatal period, obstetric causes should be sought, including evidence for peripartum infection (i.e., clinical symptoms of chorioamnionitis, prolonged rupture of membranes, and premature rupture of membranes, maternal fever, maternal bacteruria), maternal hypertension, antepartum fetal distress, and birth depression. Multiple births, particularly monozygotic infants with twin-to-twin transfusion,[65] and birth asphyxia have also been associated with neutropenia.[111]

The duration and severity of the neutropenia influence the extent of laboratory evaluation (Table 14–3). Patients with persistent neutropenia should have complete blood cell counts with differential cell counts twice weekly for 5 to 6 weeks to evaluate the periodicity of neutropenia suggestive of a cyclic process. Antineutrophil antibody assays may assist in identification of infants with immune-mediated neutrophil destruction.

Hematopoietic Colony-Stimulating Factors

G-CSF and GM-CSF are naturally occurring proteins that regulate the proliferation and differentiation of myeloid precursors into mature neutrophils.[112] The genes for these factors have been cloned and are commercially available in pharmacologic quantities.[113] These factors have been widely used in adult and general pediatric medicine primarily to treat iatrogenic neutropenia and bone marrow failure syndromes.[114] Both have been used routinely to shorten the duration of neutropenia after chemotherapy for leukemia and solid tumors and after bone marrow transplantation. G-CSF is effective in correcting the neutropenia associated with congenital neutropenia, Kostmann's syndrome, and cyclic neutropenia.[115]

Target cells for these hematopoietic factors differ. For instance, G-CSF is lineage specific for the committed progenitors of the neutrophilic granulocyte pathway. It stimulates proliferation and differentiation, expanding the available pool of neutrophil precursors and shortening their transit time through the bone marrow. It has been reported that G-CSF enhances several functions of mature neutrophils, but this has been questioned.[116] GM-CSF acts on multilineage progenitors and on those of monocyte and neutrophil lineage. GM-CSF also enhances bactericidal activities of mature phagocytes.[116]

Results of several human and animal studies provide a rational basis for the administration of G-CSF and GM-CSF to preterm infants to reduce the incidence and severity of infections. Explanted blood monocytes and mononuclear cells from human neonates produce G-CSF and GM-CSF poorly compared with adults in response to inflammatory agents in vitro, and cells from preterm infants produce these proteins more poorly than do cells from term infants.[117, 118] Plasma concentrations of G-CSF are low in

Table 14–3. **Evaluation of Neutropenia in Neonates**

Laboratory Analysis	Parameter Assessed	Associated Diagnosis
Culture and serologic screening for infection	Active infection	Bacterial, fungal, or viral infection
Complete blood count and differential	Neutrophil and band count	Infection
Serial absolute granulocyte counts	Cycling of myelopoiesis Severity and persistence of neutropenia	Cyclic neutropenia Chronic neutropenia
Bone marrow aspiration	Bone marrow cellularity and morphology; presence or absence of mature neutrophils and their precursors	Agranulocytosis Myeloid maturational arrest Megaloblastic or ineffective myelopoiesis Storage pool depletion
Antineutrophil antibody assay	Presence of neutrophil-specific antibodies	Autoimmune and isoimmune neutropenia
Immunologic evaluation	T and B cell numbers Chemotactic assay Suppressor T cell assay	Reticular dysgenesis Hair-cartilage hypoplasia Chemotactic defect with neutropenia
Serum copper	Nutritional copper status	Copper deficiency with neutropenia
Serum folate	Nutritional folate status	Folate deficiency with megaloblastic marrow
Serum vitamin B_{12}	Nutritional vitamin B_{12} status	Vitamin B_{12} deficiency with megaloblastic marrow
Colony-forming units assay	Adequacy of myeloid committed progenitor cell compartment	Deficiency in colony-forming units Defective response to CSF
Colony-stimulating factor (CSF) assay	Adequacy of CSF production	Defective CSF production Inhibition of CSF effect
Radiographic bone survey	Bony abnormalities	Cartilage-hair hypoplasia Dyskeratosis congenita Schwachman syndrome Preleukemia
Plasma and urine amino acid screening	Amino acid abnormalities	Orotic aciduria Hyperglycinemia
Exocrine pancreatic function	Adequacy of pancreatic enzymes from duodenal fluid	Schwachman syndrome

newborn infants with neutropenia and in infants with presumed sepsis.[117–119] Neonatal hematopoietic progenitor cells are equally as responsive as adult bone marrow progenitors to the actions of G-CSF and GM-CSF in culture.[118] The rapid, "emergency" neutrophil response to infection is impaired in the murine model of G-CSF gene disruption.[120] Animal studies have demonstrated diminished production of G-CSF by neonates compared with adults during bacterial sepsis.[121] G-CSF and GM-CSF administration in animal models of neonatal sepsis have documented improved survival.[122, 123]

A limited number of reports in the literature document administration of the myeloid growth factors, G-CSF and GM-CSF, to infants.[124–129] Three controlled studies of G-CSF administration to infants with clinical signs of infection have been reported. The largest of these studies was a dose-escalation, randomized, placebo-controlled trial of recombinant G-CSF administration to 42 infants with presumed bacterial infection within the first 3 days of life.[124] Gillan and colleagues[124] sought to define safety, pharmacokinetics, and biologic effects of G-CSF in neonates with presumed infection defined as having blood cultures obtained and antibiotics initiated. Bacterial infection was documented in 17%, and neutropenia was observed in 5% of patients enrolled. This trial demonstrated a dose-dependent induction of neutrophilia in the peripheral circulation and bone marrow. Neutrophil function also was enhanced by G-CSF, as indicated by increased C3bi expression on the neutrophil surface membrane. There were no deaths among study participants.

A second study, by Kocherlakota and coworkers,[125] used a concurrently treated, retrospective, case-matched control design to examine G-CSF administration in neonates with sepsis complicated by neutropenia. The study population included 14 G-CSF recipients and 11 case-matched controls, and researchers evaluated cases of early-onset and late-onset infection. These investigators reported a significant increase in the absolute neutrophil count in G-CSF recipients by 24 hours that persisted through day 7 to 10 of the study. Differences between G-CSF recipients and controls in circulating neutrophils were not significant. The mortality rate was lower among G-CSF recipients, but the study did not include sufficient numbers of subjects to attain statistical significance.

In another study, 20 infants with clinical signs of early-onset sepsis and neutropenia were enrolled in a randomized, placebo-controlled trial of G-CSF administration.[126] This trial showed no difference between the G-CSF and placebo recipients in the circulating absolute neutrophil counts, immature to total neutrophil ratios, and bone marrow storage and proliferative pools. Moreover, no differences were observed in the severity of illness or in morbidity or mortality between G-CSF and placebo recipients. Infants who exhibited profound neutropenia and bone marrow storage pool depletion succumbed to sepsis.

Taken together, these studies indicate that G-CSF administration is capable of increasing circulating neutrophil concentrations when target cells are present in the bone marrow, but in many cases, endogenous G-CSF production is sufficient to mediate recovery of normal circulating neutrophil concentrations. In the absence of sufficient numbers of target cells in the bone marrow and in the blood, it does not appear that G-CSF administration can be effective. The studies have not enrolled sufficient numbers of patients to evaluate clinical efficacy.

The risk of developing nosocomial infection in preterm neonates with neutropenia due to maternal hypertension is controversial. Some studies have demonstrated an increased incidence of nosocomial infections in these neonates, but others have not.[61, 130–132] Studies evaluating G-CSF administration to correct the neutropenia caused by maternal hypertension have demonstrated a significant increase in circulating neutrophils compared with study entry.[127, 128] Additional studies are required to determine the efficacy of G-CSF administration to these infants.

GM-CSF has been studied in neonates using slightly different strategies than used in trials of G-CSF administration. In a phase I/II randomized, placebo-controlled trial, GM-CSF or placebo was administered to 20 preterm infants within 72 hours of birth and continued for 7 days.[129] GM-CSF increased the circulating absolute neutrophil count and bone marrow neutrophil storage pool. Neutrophil function was enhanced as defined by up-regulation of surface C3bi expression. Circulating monocytes and platelet counts were increased among GM-CSF recipients.

The results of human and animal studies provide a basis for evaluating the use of myeloid growth factors in newborns with neutropenia caused by a variety of pathologic processes and infection. Studies have demonstrated that target cells in the bone marrow and circulation of newborn infants are responsive to G-CSF and GM-CSF, and in the limited numbers of patients studied, no serious adverse effects have been reported. None of the studies has had the power to establish clinical efficacy or to delineate the most effective strategies for using these hematopoietic growth factors. Strategies probably will be more effective when they promote early administration of myeloid factors, before depletion of target cells, because such designs were more effective in animal models of infection.[122] Strategies to prevent infections in neutropenic infants at increased risk for developing nosocomial infections are also warranted. Multicenter trials are in progress to evaluate the safety and efficacy of G-CSF administration for late-onset neonatal sepsis and for neutropenia caused by early- and late-onset infection, necrotizing enterocolitis, and pregnancy-induced hypertension. A multicenter study of GM-CSF administration to preterm neonates to prevent hospital acquired infections is in progress. These and other clinical trials are needed to define the efficacy and safety of these myeloid factors before they can be used routinely in human newborns.

Clinical applications for other cytokines is progressing in several areas. One cytokine that may find clinical application in the neonate because of its unique effects on hematopoietic and gastrointestinal mucosal stem cells is IL-11. IL-11 is a cytokine that exhibits pleiotropic effects on multiple tissues.[133] Although it was initially characterized as a hematopoietic cytokine with thrombopoietic activity, it is expressed in other tissues, including the central nervous system, gut, and testis.[134] The hematopoietic actions of IL-11 include stimulation of proliferation of primitive stem cells and multipotential and committed progenitor cells.[135] It acts in synergy with other cytokines to support proliferation and differentiation of all lineages of hematopoietic cells.[135, 136]

Efforts to determine clinical applications of IL-11 initially focused on its effects on megakaryocytopoiesis and myelopoiesis.[137] In preclinical studies, including those of murine bone marrow transplantation, and in combined chemotherapy and radiation therapy models, accelerated neutrophil and platelet recovery and enhanced survival were achieved, particularly after bacterial invasion by inoculation with exogenous organisms (e.g., *P. aeruginosa*) or sepsis from endogenous gut organisms.[138] Models of toxic shock syndrome and experimental group B streptococcal sepsis in neonatal rats in which mice were pretreated with IL-11 demonstrated a significant reduction in mortality.[139, 140] In the rabbit endotoxemia model, IL-11 prevented hypotension and decreased gastrointestinal damage.[141] These effects appear to be mediated by inhibition of proinflammatory cytokine synthesis by macrophages.[142]

The gastrointestinal protective effects of IL-11 are significant and have led to studies of IL-11 administration in animal models of chemical-induced acute colitis, chronic inflammatory bowel disease, ischemic bowel necrosis, burn injury, and short bowel syndrome.[143–146] In all of these models, significantly increased survival was observed in IL-11–treated animals. Translocation of enteric bacteria was decreased in the burn injury and bowel necrosis models.

Clinical trials in humans have demonstrated that IL-11 accelerates hematopoietic recovery from multiple cancer therapies.[147–149] Based on the observation of potent effects of IL-11 in models of gut damage, IL-11 may be effective against the bone marrow and gastrointestinal toxicities associated with chemotherapy and irradiation. Phase I/II trials of IL-11 in patients with Crohn's disease have been completed.[150] Additional studies are anticipated for Crohn's disease and chemotherapy-induced mucositis. Studies of IL-11 administration for prevention or treatment of necrotizing enterocolitis in newborns are also under consideration.

CHRONIC GRANULOMATOUS DISEASE

Chronic granulomatous disease (CGD) is an inherited immunodeficiency syndrome in which the generation of superoxide by the respiratory burst oxidase of phagocytic leukocytes (i.e., neutrophils, monocytes-macrophages, and eosinophils) is absent or markedly diminished.[151] The disorder, which has an approximate incidence of 1 case per 500,000 individuals, results from mutations in any one of four essential subunits of the respiratory burst complex.[151, 152]

Approximately two thirds of cases of CGD are caused by defects in the X-linked gene encoding gp91-phox (i.e., phagocyte oxidase), the larger subunit of the flavocytochrome b_{588}, a plasma membrane heterodimer that is the redox center of the oxidase. A rare autosomal recessive form of CGD is caused by mutations in the gene encoding the p22-phox, a small subunit of the flavocytochrome b_{588}. The remaining cases of autosomal recessive CGD involve defects in the genes encoding p47-phox or p67-phox, two soluble proteins that interact with flavocytochrome b_{588} to form the enzymatically active respiratory burst oxidase.

The manifestations of CGD typically develop in infancy or early childhood.[153–155] Superoxide generated during the phagocytic respiratory burst is the precursor for a variety of potent oxidants that are important in killing many microbial pathogens. Patients with CGD lack this pathway and have recurrent purulent bacterial and fungal infections that are difficult to treat and often life threatening. Common sites of infection are the skin, lymph nodes, lungs, bone, liver, and gastrointestinal tract. Individuals with CGD are particularly susceptible to infections with *S. aureus*, *Aspergillus* species, and a variety of gram-negative bacilli, including *Pseudomonas*, *Salmonella*, and *Serratia* species. Many of these organisms express catalase, which prevents phagocytes of CGD patients from scavenging microbe-generated hydrogen peroxide to promote killing within the phagosome. The other hallmark of CGD is the propensity to develop chronic inflammatory granulomas with widespread tissue distribution.[154, 156]

The prognosis for CGD patients has improved continually since the disorder was first described in the 1950s, at which time almost all patients died in childhood. Current management includes aggressive treatment of acute infections with combined use of prophylactic antibiotics and prophylactic interferon-γ (IFN-γ).[157, 158] Although allogenic bone marrow transplantation for CGD has been curative, even in a case in which mixed chimerism resulted in production of about 30% of circulating neutrophils being of donor origin,[159–161] it is used infrequently because of its associated complications and the difficulties in finding a suitable donor. Morbidity and mortality caused by infections and complications of granulomas remain significant for many patients, particularly those with X-linked CGD.[162] The overall mortality has been estimated at 2% per year.[163]

Because the genetic defects of CGD affect primarily cells of the hematopoietic system, this disorder has been considered to be a candidate disease for gene therapy targeted at hematopoietic stem cells.[164, 165] Insertion of a functional copy of the involved gene into hematopoietic stem cells should reconstitute the respiratory burst oxidase activity in circulating and tissue phagocytes and could provide lifelong cure of the disease. Mouse models have been developed for the X-linked (gp91-phox −/−) and the p47-phox–deficient forms of CGD.[166, 167] In murine CGD, retroviral-mediated gene transfer into bone marrow cells can correct the respiratory burst oxidase activity and the defect in host defense against bacterial and fungal pathogens. The ability of gene transfer technology to reconstitute the respiratory burst oxidase activity in human CGD leukocytes cultured in vitro has been established.[168, 169]

Phase I clinical trials of gene therapy have been initiated for the p47-phox–deficient form of CGD. This protocol involved retroviral transduction of p47-phox cDNA into autologous peripheral CD34-positive ($CD34^+$) cells in ex vivo culture and then infusion of these cells back into the patients.[170] Although the respiratory burst activity was corrected in 10% to 20% of neutrophils and monocytes in vitro, a much lower percentage of corrected circulating peripheral blood neutrophils was observed in vivo. Ongoing research in human hematopoietic stem cell biology, alternative vector systems, and alternative transplantation regimens are being explored to provide alternative strategies for making gene therapy an option for the treatment of CGD.

MONOCYTES AND MACROPHAGES

Ontogeny

The development of the mononuclear phagocyte system has been described morphologically at various stages of embryonic and fetal life. Embryonic macrophages are found among hematopoietic cells in the yolk sac at 3 to 4 weeks' gestation.[171, 172] In murine models, macrophages develop in vitro from primitive yolk sac progenitor cells.[173] Later in gestation, when the yolk sac is open to the fetal circulation, monocytes and macrophages are readily identifiable. During the second month of gestation, as hematopoiesis is established in the fetal liver, monocytes are present in high proportions. Approximately 70% of hematopoietic cells at 4.5 weeks' gestation are morphologically identifiable as monocytes.[174] This proportion decreases to 1% to 2% over the next 6 weeks as erythroid cells become predominant. Although monoblasts and promonocytes are present in the fetal liver during this period of fetal liver hematopoiesis, intravascular monocytes are not observed until about the fifth month of gestation.[175] Circulating monocytes remain rare until bone marrow hematopoiesis becomes predominant after the tenth week of gestation.[176] Monocytes comprise 3% to 7% of hematopoietic cells by 30 weeks' gestation.[177]

Study of the development of the mononuclear phagocyte system in the neonatal period has been limited by poor access to sample tissues. The number of circulating granulocyte-monocyte progenitor cells (CFU-GM) is high in cord blood before 32 weeks but falls shortly after birth.[178] Total bone marrow cellularity of the term neonate at birth is approximately 1.36×10^{11} cells/L. Total cell numbers decline over the first 1 to 2 weeks to about 3.5×10^{10}/L.[179] The relative monocytosis at birth persists throughout the neonatal period. Although normal values for circulating monocyte counts vary among studies, they usually are highest in the first week of life, ranging from 1340 to 2200/μL in the first week of life to about 700 cells/μL by 3 weeks, and decline thereafter to about 450/μL at 6 years of age.[180–182] The reason for discrepancies in the numbers of circulating monocytes is that these cells are heterogeneous and appear morphologically similar to other circulating immature cells, such as myeloid precursors and granular lymphocytes.

Analysis of the kinetics of tissue macrophage turnover in the neonatal period has relied on information garnered from pathologic specimens from fetal and neonatal mortality cases. Histologic examination of lung tissue derived from stillborn infants and from infants who died within the early neonatal period demonstrated that few alveolar macrophages were present in lungs of stillborn infants. Alveolar macrophages were identified in specimens from 33 of 46 infants who died within 48 hours and in all specimens from infants surviving longer than 48 hours.[183] Macrophages were detectable in infants of all gestational ages who survived for more than 48 hours. Studies using rodents and primates confirm that few alveolar macrophages are present in fetal life but that they increase rapidly early during postnatal life.[184–186] The increase appears to be caused by an influx of monocytes from the circulation and from local proliferation of macrophages.

Characterization of Monocytes

The morphology of human monocytes and macrophages has been extensively studied at the light and electron microscopic levels.[187] The ultrastructure of monocytes is notable for a well-developed Golgi apparatus with a small endoplasmic reticulum containing ribosomes and polysomes. Mitochondria are abundant. Numerous granules containing a number of lysosomal enzymes are distributed throughout the cytoplasm. The surface membrane of the monocyte includes an extensive system of microvilli.

Compared with monocytes, macrophages are larger, have a larger Golgi apparatus, and have more mitochondria and lysosomal granules. The most prominent feature of macrophages are electron-dense lysosomes along the cell surface.[188] Granules and vacuoles are observed along the periphery of the cell, indicating their enhanced pinocytic function. Phagosomes are seen containing ingested material at various stages of degradation.

Monocytes and macrophages can be delineated by cytochemical techniques that detect cellular constituents and biochemical processes. One of the most reliable of these markers is nonspecific esterase, which can be demonstrated by using α-naphthyl butyrate as a substrate.[189] Many cell types contain nonspecific esterase, but the isozyme present in monocytes can be discerned by its property of being inhibited by sodium fluoride.[190] Nonspecific esterase is expressed on the surface of peripheral blood monocytes, and as monocytes differentiate into macrophages, additional isozymes of nonspecific esterase are expressed, leading to more intense cytoplasmic staining.[191] Although cord blood monocytes stain positively for nonspecific esterase, the proportion of esterase-positive cells is lower than in adult peripheral blood monocytes.[192–194] Peroxidase activity is also prominent in monocytes and diminishes with their maturation into macrophages.[195] No differences are discernible between monocyte peroxidase activity in neonates and adults.

Morphologic and cytochemical characteristics have traditionally been used to identify monocytes. Monoclonal antibodies provide a more precise means of identifying the monocyte lineage differentiation.[196] During ontogeny, macrophages in the fetal liver express CD11b as early as 12 weeks' gestation.[197] CD14 does not appear until about 15 to 21 weeks' gestation and is a mature differentiation antigen. CD14 expression is equivalent in cord blood and adult peripheral blood. In contrast, CD11a, CD11b, and CD11c are expressed at lower densities on cord blood monocytes than on cells from adults. Several investigators have reported that HLA-DR, HLA-DP, and HLA-DQ are expressed in lower proportions on neonatal monocytes than on adult monocytes.[194, 198–200] The density of these class II major histocompatibility complex (MHC) antigens has been correlated with antigen-presenting capacity in vitro.[201] It remains to be determined whether developmental differences in expression of these antigens accounts for the deficient antibody responses to certain foreign antigens in the newborn period.

Properties of monocytes related to phagocytic functions include movement, adherence, endocytosis, and microbicidal activity. Monocytes, like other granulocytes, are capable of moving in random and directed fashion.[202] Chemotaxis, or directed movement, is mediated by receptors to chemotactic substances produced by bacteria or generated through the complement, fibrinolytic, and kinin systems.[203] Comparisons of chemotactic capabilities of neonatal and adult peripheral blood monocytes suggest that chemotactic activity is significantly less pronounced in neonatal cells than adult cells.[204, 205]

Adherence requires interaction between monocytes and vascular endothelium. Emigration of cells from the systemic circulation into tissue occurs by three steps. Monocytes roll along the vascular endothelium using low-affinity interactions between a family of molecules called selectins. L-selectin is constitutively expressed on the surface of monocytes, whereas E- and P-selectins are expressed on activated endothelium.[206–209] The second step in emigration from the circulation is firm adhesion to the endothelial surface, which is mediated by integrins (CD11a–c and CD18) on the surface of activated monocytes and intercellular adhesion molecule-1 (ICAM-1) or ICAM-2 on the endothelial surface or by vascular cell adhesion molecule-1 (VCAM-1).[210] The final step in extravasation involves movement through the endothelium to a site of inflammation or infection.

Individuals with congenital deficiency in the expression of selectins or integrins are susceptible to recurrent bacterial infections, because of the inability of their phagocytic cells to move to sites of infection.[211] Preliminary studies to assess properties of fetal and newborn monocyte adhesion demonstrate levels of adhesion comparable to that of adult blood cells.[212]

Monocytes use several different antimicrobial mechanisms.[213] Oxygen-dependent mechanisms include the respiratory burst, which elaborates reactive oxygen radicals. The initial product of the respiratory burst is superoxide anion. This molecule is capable of breaking down certain proteins and membrane components. Superoxide is also converted to hydrogen peroxide by superoxide dismutase. Hydrogen peroxide is highly toxic to a number of microbes. Its toxicity can be further enhanced by action of the enzyme myeloperoxidase to convert hydrogen peroxide to hypohalous acid.[214] Monocytes exhibit considerably less respiratory burst production of hydrogen peroxide and other toxic reactive molecules than do neutrophils.[215] Oxygen-independent antimicrobial mechanisms include acidification of the phagosome and synthesis of defensins, hydrolases, proteases, and nucleases.[216]

Nitric oxide (NO) also provides antimicrobial activity.[217] NO is synthesized through oxidation of L-arginine by nitric oxide synthases. The antimicrobial effects of NO are mediated through inhibition of enzymes containing nonheme iron complexed to sulfur and through reaction with superoxide to form peroxynitrites.[218] These species undergo decomposition to form highly reactive hydroxyl radicals,[219] molecules that can damage host and microbial cell membranes. The ability of fetal and neonatal monocytes to kill a variety of pathogens including *S. aureus*, *S. epidermidis*, *E. coli*, and *C. albicans* appears to be equivalent to that of adults.[220, 221]

Monocytes and macrophages synthesize and secrete numerous products involved in the inflammatory process. These diverse products include polypeptide hormones, complement components, cytokines, coagulation factors, enzymes, extracellular matrix proteins, bioactive oligopeptides, bioactive lipids, and sterol hormones.[222] Certain products, such as the polypeptides IL-1, IFN-α, and tumor necrosis factor-α, are synthesized in similar concentrations by newborn and adult blood monocytes.[223–225] Other molecules are produced in markedly lower concentrations by fetal and neonatal monocytes and macrophages compared with adult cells. These include polypeptides such as IFN-γ, IL-8, IL-10, and G-CSF; extracellular matrix proteins such as fibronectin; and bioreactive lipids such as leukotriene B_4.[192, 226–230] The relative differences in production of these molecules in neonatal host defenses remains to be determined. Development of techniques that can identify cellular expression of secretory products from small numbers of cells and techniques enabling isolation of pure populations of monocytes from peripheral blood of adults and from cord blood and peripheral blood of newborns may facilitate our ability to define the roles of these products in the human fetus and neonate.

DENDRITIC CELLS

Dendritic cells are a discrete leukocyte population with highly developed antigen-presenting capabilities for initiating primary and secondary T cell responses.[231, 232] Dendritic cells originating from myeloid precursors are associated with T cells within lymphoid tissue and provide critical antigen-presenting activity for initiating specific T cell activation and proliferation. Follicular dendritic cells within B cell follicles probably do not originate from the bone marrow and exhibit a different phenotype than the myeloid-derived dendritic cells. They retain antigen for prolonged periods and are capable of re-stimulating B lymphocytes. The cardinal properties of myeloid lineage-derived dendritic cells include the ability to take up, process, and present antigen; the ability to migrate selectively through tissues; and the ability to interact with, stimulate, and direct T cell responses.[233]

Dendritic cells initially received their name because of their distinctive morphology. They are notable for their irregular shape, with numerous membrane processes, including spiny dendrites, bulbous pseudopods, and lamellipodiae or veils.[234] Distinctive electron microscopic features with a paucity of intracellular organelles and prominent mitochondria are also described. Endosomes and lysosomes essential for antigen processing are prominent in the cytoplasm of dendritic cells.

Morphology alone is insufficient to define dendritic cells, because this cell lineage encompasses populations of leukocytes with very different properties characteristic of their state of activation or differentiation.[235] A working definition has been proposed. First, these cells have the ability to stimulate primary T cell response. Second, they have the ability to migrate through tissues and home to T cell–dependent areas of the lymph nodes. Third, they possess active fluid-phase endocytosis of extracellular material. Fourth, the cell-surface antigen phenotype must distinguish these cells from other leukocytes, particularly monocytes, macrophages, and B cells. Fifth, they express certain dendritic cell–associated antigens according to their state of activation or differentiation. They exhibit certain cytochemical reactions that are distinct from those of monocytes and macrophages.

Cell-Surface and Associated Molecules

Dendritic cells express a variety of surface molecules commonly found on other leukocytes, including MHC molecules, CD45 (leukocyte common) isoforms, adhesion molecules, Fc receptors, and costimulatory molecules. Most dendritic cells express CD33, an early marker of myeloid differentiation, but this surface antigen appears to be down-regulated in dendritic cells within dermal and tonsillar tissue, suggesting a reduction in this molecule with differentiation.[236, 237] Human blood and perivascular skin dendritic cells are CD36$^+$ (thrombospondin receptor). Certain subsets of monocytes and macrophages also express this surface antigen.[238, 239] Blood, dermal, and tonsillar dendritic cells also express CD4.[236, 240, 241]

Dendritic cells express a repertoire of relatively specific antigens that vary with the activation and differentiation status. These include adhesion molecules, antigen uptake receptors, and costimulatory molecules. Adhesion molecules expressed by dendritic cells include members of the immunoglobulin superfamily, including ICAM-1 (CD54), ICAM-2 (CD50), ICAM-3 (CD102), VCAM (CD106), and platelet–endotheial cell adhesion molecule-1 (PECAM-1, CD31).[233] ICAM-3 appears to be the most important lymphocyte function antigen-1 (LFA-1) ligand for the dendritic cell–T cell adhesion.[242] VCAM, although not present on resting cells, is induced on gut dendritic cells.[243] Several members of the integrin and selectin families are expressed. For example, the very-late activation antigen-5 (VLA-5, fibronectin receptor) and VLA-6 (laminin receptor) are thought to be involved in interstitial actions. The β2-integrin, LFA-1 (CD11a), is densely expressed on human dendritic cells.[244] CD11b and CD11c are also expressed on human Langerhans cells.[238] The CD15a on dendritic cells is related to ligands for E and P selectin. Other groups of adhesion molecules, including CD44 (hyaluronidase ligand) and CD138 (syndecan) are involved with connective tissue and interstitial matrix interactions.[245]

Antigen uptake receptors, including CD32 (FcγII) and CD64 (FcγI), are present on dendritic cells early in their differentiation. Nonspecific pattern recognition receptors with binding specificities for structural patterns displayed by microorganisms but not by host cells are also used by dendritic cells. Such receptors include mannose receptor and lectin-like molecules.[246–248]

Costimulatory molecules are expressed predominantly in activated dendritic cells. CD40 can be up-regulated in vitro after cytokine exposure.[249] CD80 and CD86 are not expressed on resting cells but are rapidly up-regulated on activation.[250]

Functional Properties

Dendritic cells exhibit relatively limited phagocytic and proteolytic functions, unlike those observed in other leukocytes such as macrophages and neutrophils.[251] They instead are adapted to ingesting sufficient antigen to be processed into peptide fragments for presentation to T cells. After antigen uptake, the dendritic cell migrates to lymphoid tissues and initiates membrane interactions with T cells and costimulates specific T cell responses.

Dendritic cells are capable of stimulating T cell responses to alloantigens, autoantigens, and exogenous antigens.[236, 252–254] They are considerably more effective than blood B cells or monocytes as stimulators of these reactions. During these interactions, dendritic cells must first receive environmental danger signals such as tissue damage, infection, or inflammation (Fig. 14–2). These signals initiate antigen uptake and processing, MHC expression, and antigen presentation. The dendritic cells then migrate from peripheral tissue to lymphoid organs. Expression of the costimulatory molecules CD40, CD80, and CD86 is up-regulated. T cells contact the dendritic cell through adhesive interactions and MHC-antigen:T cell receptor recognition, followed by increased costimulatory molecule interaction, cytokine production, and T cell activation.

Dendritic Cells in Infectious Diseases

Dendritic cells can present antigens from a variety of organisms, including *Chlamydia*,[255] *Leishmania*,[256] and *Candida*.[257] There is good evidence that viral antigens for influenza and herpes simplex are presented by dendritic cells to generate T cell immune responses.[258, 259] Although major changes in number, localization, and function of dendritic cells can be predicted to occur during infections, no data are available

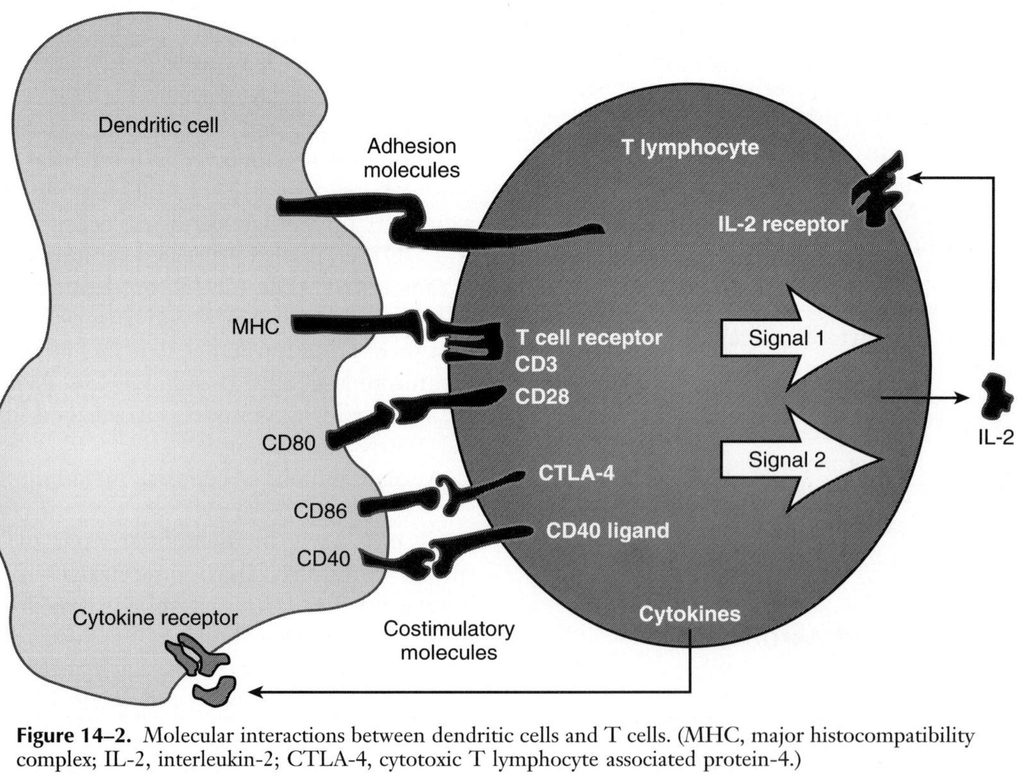

Figure 14–2. Molecular interactions between dendritic cells and T cells. (MHC, major histocompatibility complex; IL-2, interleukin-2; CTLA-4, cytotoxic T lymphocyte associated protein-4.)

on dendritic cell numbers, viability, and trafficking in different clinical infections because of the difficulty of monitoring these cells effectively in vivo.

Dendritic Cell Vaccination and Immunotherapy

Dendritic cells are being studied for use in several forms of immunotherapy. Investigations are in progress using dendritic cells as cellular therapy; these cells may be ideal vehicles for immunization against infectious agents, malignant tissue, and autoimmune lymphocytes. These cells can present bacterial and viral antigens to T cells in vitro.[259–261] Peptide derived from herpes simplex virus (HSV), influenza virus, and human immunodeficiency virus are capable of eliciting strong virus-specific cytotoxic responses in vitro.[259, 262, 263] Animal studies are encouraging; antigen-pulsed dendritic cells are efficacious in providing protective immunity at a level equal to or greater than that established by conventional adjuvant vaccines.[251, 264] No formal clinical comparisons have been undertaken.

LYMPHOCYTES

T Lymphocytes

Ontogeny

In mammals, hematopoietic precursor cells are present in the yolk sac early in embryonic life. These precursors are subsequently found in the fetal liver and ultimately migrate to the bone marrow, where they reside during adult life. A portion of these hematopoietic progenitor cells seed the thymus, which is the principal site of T cell development.[265] A functional thymic epithelium is essential for development of mature T cells.[266] Examples of defective thymic microenvironment include mice with a gene defect causing thymic epithelial development abnormality (i.e., nude mice). These mice have few T cells and exhibit impaired ability to reject grafts.[267] Humans with deletion of certain genes on chromosome 22 have abnormal pharyngeal pouch development and a condition called DiGeorge syndrome. These individuals have various degrees of T cell dysfunction.[268]

T cell development in the human starts about 7 weeks' gestation with the migration of lymphoid progenitor cells to the thymus.[269] These cells express CD7 and CD45 on their surface. By 8.5 weeks' gestation, CD2 and CD3 are expressed, and by 9.5 weeks' gestation, T cell receptor (TCR) β-chains are present in the cytoplasm of a subset of $CD3^+$ cells.[270] TCR α-chains are apparent in the cytoplasm of maturing T cells by 10 weeks. CD1, CD4, and CD8 appear on the cell surface of thymic lymphocytes by 10 weeks. CD3 expression increases by 12 weeks of gestation. T cell migration from the thymus to the spleen and peripheral lymphoid tissue occurs after 12 weeks of gestation. Fetal T cells resemble adult cells in expressing CD4 or CD8 but not both. Their appearance in the blood parallels that in the liver and spleen between 25 and 30 weeks' gestation.

T cells accumulate in the blood and lymphoid organs during second half of gestation. At the time of delivery, 99% of the T cells circulating in cord blood express the CD45 isoforms, CD45RA and CD45RB, associated with naive T cells.[271, 272] On stimulation, T cells of neonates switch to expression of CD45RO, which is present on memory T cells. The low numbers of CD45RO cells in term newborns suggests that little antigen-induced expansion occurs before birth.

Functional Responses of Fetal and Neonatal T Cells

At 12 weeks' gestation, fetal T cells are capable of generating several components of a normal T cell response, including proliferation and IL-2 production in response to alloantigen or phytohemagglutinin antigen stimulation in mixed lymphocyte cultures. T cells of neonates are capable of generating antigen-specific responses, as determined in vitro by proliferation in mixed lymphocyte culture, and of generating cytotoxic T cells. In response to antigens such as staphylococcal enterotoxins and anti-TCR antibodies, responses are diminished compared with those observed in adult cells.[273, 274] This difference is attributable in part to a high proportion of T cells with a naive phenotype,

CD45RA+ or CD45RB+, in the neonate compared with the adult.

The maturation of naive T cells into memory T cells follows an encounter with antigen presented to the T cell by antigen-presenting cells such as dendritic cells, B cells, and monocytes. Encounter with antigen in the absence of proper costimulatory signals by these cells results in a state of unresponsiveness to that antigen, called *anergy*, which may be temporary or permanent.[275] T cells synthesize a host of cytokines in response to antigen stimulation. Naive and memory T cells produce similar quantities of IL-2, but other cytokines, including IFN-γ, IL-4, IL-10, and IL-12, are produced largely by memory T cells. Moreover, newborn T cells produce little IFN-γ or IL-4 unless they undergo further proliferation and maturation.[276]

Differences in cytokine production between newborns and adults probably lead to significant differences in T cell functions. Cells making IFN-γ and IL-12 are called type 1 helper T cells (TH1), and those producing IL-4 and IL-10 are referred to as type 2 helper T cells (TH2) cells. TH1 cells promote local inflammatory responses such as cytotoxic T cell functions and prompt B cells to synthesize IgG. TH2 cells promote B cell replication and IgE antibody isotype production.[277]

Development of naive T cells into memory T cells occurs when surface receptors are cross-linked by antigen appropriately presented with self-MHC and costimulation. This interaction leads to production of IL-2 and surface expression of IL-2 receptor. As long as antigenic stimulation persists, the autocrine IL-2 loop supports expansion of this T cell clone.[278] Development of a useful repertoire of memory T cells depends on antigen experience and T cell proliferation. Response of the naive T cell population to antigenic exposure results in an increase in the population of CD45RO+ cells from less than 5% at birth to between 35% and 45% by 16 years of age. The preponderance of this increase occurs in the first year of life.[279]

On encountering antigen, B cells enter one of two pathways, depending on the presence of signals from T cells. If no signal is received from a helper T cell, the B cell enters an apoptosis pathway. However, when a T cell signal is received, the B cell undergoes proliferation and differentiation.[280] The B cell help function provided by T cells is predominantly supplied by secretion of IL-4. Naive T cells are capable of secreting IL-4 in response to IL-1 stimulation and CD28 signaling.

In addition to proliferation, T cells control the isotype switching of IgM to IgG production. The signal through which this change is mediated appears to be the interaction between CD40 on the B cell surface and the CD40 ligand on memory T cells.[281] The CD40 ligand is not constitutively expressed on T cells but is up-regulated on antigenic exposure. Naive T cells require a significantly longer period to become CD40 ligand positive. In vitro studies suggest that this delay may limit the ability of human newborns to mount a prompt and effective antibody response.[282]

T Cells and Neonatal Host Defense

T cells are important in the control of a variety of microbes encountered by the human neonate. T cells play a limited protective role against pyogenic bacteria such as group B streptococci. The principal line of defense against these organisms resides in the opsonization by antibody and the actions of phagocytic cells and complement. Under normal circumstances, the neonate derives antibody by transplacental transfer of IgG from the mother. Infants delivered before 34 weeks' gestation have markedly reduced circulating antibody titers compared with maternal antibody titers.[283] Among preterm infants, even those with protective antibodies, titers may be insufficient to provide protection.

The absence of passively derived maternal antibodies is the major determinant of risk for neonatal group B streptococcal infection.[284–286] Infected neonates exhibit poor capacity to produce specific antibody to the group B streptococcal capsular polysaccharide. This incapacity probably is caused by B cell and T cell immaturity. The amount and isotype of the antibodies produced is influenced by T cells. For instance, the production of antibody to capsular polypeptide may be enhanced by secretion of cytokines, including IFN-γ by activated T cells. The preponderance of naive T cells and diminished IFN-γ secretion may contribute to ineffective production of specific antibodies.[287]

Antiviral immunity is characterized by an early (nonspecific) phase and a late phase. HSV is a prototype infection in the neonate that illustrates the importance of each of these phases of the immune response. The early phase is critical, because infection may be successfully contained or may be disseminated. This early phase is mediated predominantly by actions of mononuclear phagocytes and natural killer (NK) cells. The late phase uses specific-antibody production by T cells and B cells. T cells are essential components in this phase of antiviral immunity because they up-regulate the actions of mononuclear phagocytes and NK cells through secretion of cytokines and because they directly mediate antigen-specific destruction of cells infected with the invading virus.

Neonates exhibit deficits in both phases of host defense. The early phase probably reflects developmental immaturity of NK cell function. This deficit appears to be the function of poor cell-mediated lysis, rather than a deficiency in the number of NK cells. The cytolytic function of NK cells increases during fetal life to approximately 50% of adult activity by term.[288, 289] This cytolytic deficit parallels the presence of a significant subpopulation of CD56⁻ NK cells in neonates.[290] Neonatal CD56⁺ NK cells exhibit similar cytolytic function to that seen in adult NK cells. The reduced cytolytic activity appears to be caused by decreased recognition and binding of virally infected cells by CD56⁻ NK cells and to defective postbinding cytotoxic activity. Age-related maturation in NK function parallels resistance to certain viruses such as HSV.[291]

In a mouse model of neonatal HSV infection, neonatal mice are protected against HSV by infusion of adult blood mononuclear cells but not by neonatal cells. The failure of neonatal cells to correct the immune deficit can be corrected by infusion of IFN-γ, a cytokine poorly produced by neonatal T cells.[292]

To compound the inability to contain the viral infection with nonspecific early immune surveillance, the T cell–mediated, antigen-specific phase is frequently diminished or delayed in neonates compared with adults.[293] This deficit may be intrinsic to the T cell, such as decreased expression of CD40 ligand or limitations in the production of certain cytokines required to develop antigen-specific T cell responses.[294, 295] Alternatively, diminished numbers or function of dendritic cells may contribute to diminished T cell effectiveness against viral pathogens.[296]

Fungal infections present a particular challenge to human infants, especially those delivered prematurely or requiring hospitalization in neonatal intensive care units. Many of the same cellular and humoral deficits contributing to increased susceptibility to bacterial and viral infections may be implicated in the ineffective neonatal defense against fungal infections. The T cell plays an important role in mucocutaneous and systemic fungal infections with organisms such as *C. albicans*. Mucosal fungal infections are prevalent among humans with inherited (i.e., severe combined immunodeficiency and DiGeorge syndrome) or acquired (i.e., advanced human immunodeficiency virus infection) T cell immunodeficiency.[297] Resistance to mucocutaneous candidiasis correlates with the presence of delayed-type hypersensitivity to *Candida* skin antigens, which depends on antigen-specific TH1 cytokine production by CD4 T cells.[298]

Murine studies, taking advantage of genetic variability between different strains of animals, suggest that T cell immunity, particularly that offered by CD4 T cell subsets, is important in defense against fungal infections. Naive T cells from C57BL/6 mice differentiate into predominantly TH1 effector cells that secrete IL-2 and IFN-γ. However, in BALB/c mice, TH2 CD4 cells predominate, leading to secretion of IL-4 and IL-10.[299] The outcome of fungal infections depends on which cytokine profile is generated by infected animals. C57BL/6 mice in which the TH1 phenotype predominates clear a systemic fungal infection, whereas BALB/c mice depending on TH2 effector T cells succumb to persistent infection.

The finding of a protective role for IFN-γ–producing TH1 cells in experimental invasive candidal infections may provide insight into T cell–mediated deficits in neonatal immunity.[300] IFN-γ production by neonatal cells in vitro is diminished. In other types of infection, such as HSV, infants exhibit a delay in IFN-γ production and T cell proliferation in response to a primary infection compared with adults.[301] It is unknown whether IFN-γ production is delayed or reduced in the premature infant with disseminated *Candida* infection.

Although anecdotal cases of IFN-γ administration to patients with CGD and infection with *Aspergillus* have shown some benefits, it is not clear whether administration of this cytokine to premature infants would be safe or beneficial in preventing or treating systemic *Candida* infections. Certain studies raised the possibility that IFN-γ could be ineffective in mediating antifungal effects in neonatal mononuclear phagocytes.[302]

B Lymphocytes

Ontogeny

Pluripotent stem cells in the fetal liver and bone marrow give rise to pre-B cells, identified by intracytoplasmic expression of the μ chain of IgM. These B cell precursors appear first in the fetal liver between 7 and 8 weeks' gestation. By 9 to 10 weeks' gestation, B cells bearing surface IgM are detectable. B cells expressing membrane-bound IgA, IgD, and IgG appear in low numbers between 10 and 12 weeks' gestation. The proportion of B cells rises sharply between 12 and 16 weeks' gestation, and by 16 weeks, B cell proportions in blood, spleen, and bone marrow are similar to those in adult tissues.[303–305]

The most primitive B cells in fetal mice and humans express only membrane-associated IgM and no other membrane immunoglobulins. Exposure of cells at this stage of development to ligands that cross-link IgM receptors renders these cells nonfunctional.[306, 307] Administration of anti-μ antibodies to neonatal mice blocks development of the entire B cell system.[308] Neonatal B cells exposed to specific antigen in the absence of activated T cells develop tolerance to that particular antigen, whereas B cells of adult mice are unaffected by this treatment.[309] Each B cell clone passes through this period of tolerance susceptibility. B cells are tolerance-susceptible in newborn mice, but they become similar to those of adults by 7 days of age. A subpopulation of B cells remains tolerance-susceptible throughout adulthood.

Immunoglobulin Structure

Immunoglobulins are heterodimeric glycoproteins composed of pairs of identical heavy and light chains connected by disulfide bonds. Monomers (i.e., IgD, IgE, and IgG) contain heavy (H) and light (L) chain pairs, and polymeric (i.e., IgA and IgM) immunoglobulins consist of two secretory (IgA) or five monomeric units (IgM). These polypeptides are encoded by genes on separate chromosomes. The heavy chain locus is on chromosome 14, the light κ chain is on chromosome 2, and the light λ chain is on chromosome 22.

The heavy chain family is composed of tandem arrays of several hundred variable (V_H) genes, a smaller number of diversity (D_H) genes, and six joining (J_H) genes. The J genes are linked to a group of constant (C_H) genes that encode different heavy chain classes. The light chain families are arranged in a similar manner; however, they lack D genes. There are several constant λ chain genes but only one constant κ light chain gene.[310]

A complex series of genetic rearrangements results in production of immunoglobulin peptides unique for each B cell clone.[311] Intact immunoglobulin genes are created during the initial stages of B cell development through rearrangement of gene segments composing each family. For example, a μ gene is composed of a V_H sequence, a D_H segment, a J_H gene, and a C_μ gene. The combined VDJ segment encodes the specificity-determining variable region of the immunoglobulin molecule. The C_μ segment gene encodes the constant region, which confers biologic activity of the IgM class. Light-chain gene rearrangement and assembly occur in a similar manner, resulting in the formation of VJ_λ or VJ_κ genes.

Diversity

Generation of diversity in antibody specificity occurs through several mechanisms. First, diversity of antibody variable regions is expanded from several hundred inherited genes to several million distinct antibody specificities through combinatorial joining of heavy chain V, D, and J regions and light chain V and J regions. Second, during assembly of V, D, and J genes, the splice sites for recombination are not rigidly controlled. This gives rise to generation of nucleotide triplets that encode different amino acids or encode deletions. Third, during gene splicing, extra nucleotides may be added in random fashion by the action of an enzyme called terminal deoxynucleotidyl transferase. Fourth, the repertoire of antibody diversity is enhanced during the clonal selection because V region genes encoding heavy and light chains undergo point mutations at a high frequency during the antigen-driven proliferation stage. The mechanism leading to this high rate of mutation is not operative in the genes encoding constant regions.

B Cell Differentiation

Stages of B cell differentiation are depicted in Figure 14–1. B cell differentiation is initiated in a population of rapidly cycling lymphoblasts in which immunoglobulin gene rearrangement occurs: first, D to J, and subsequently, V to DJ.[312] Cells undergoing these rearrangements are called pro-B cells.

A functional rearrangement on chromosome 14 is followed by transcription of the μ chain of IgM, which identifies the pre-B stage of B cell differentiation. Pre-B cells generate clonal diversity through rearrangement of heavy and light chain genes. The sequence of these rearrangements from heavy to κ light to λ light allows for all combinations of V_H and V_L to be expressed, because pre-B cells may give rise to progeny producing different V_L chains.[313] Rapid proliferation facilitates generation of combinatorial diversity and compensates for nonproductive rearrangements. Because these cells lack surface immunoglobulin, they are not yet subject to clonal deletion by incidental antigen exposure.

After functional heavy and light chain rearrangement has occurred, the cells exit from cell cycle and become immature B cells, which express surface immunoglobulin of the same isotype that is to be secreted. These membrane-associated molecules act as receptors for antigens.[314] These cells have sparse polysomes and small cytoplasmic pools of immunoglobulins. In children and adults, 10% to 20% of circulating blood mononuclear cells are B cells. Of these, approximately 80% express membrane-bound (m) IgM and IgD. The remainder express mIgA or mIgG.

Plasma cells are derived by proliferation and terminal differentiation of B cells. These cells are characterized by abundant rough endoplasmic reticulum and rapid synthesis of immunoglobulin molecules, usually thousands of molecules per second. Plasma cells contain significant intracytoplasmic stores of immunoglobulin, but they lack surface immunoglobulin as they shift to synthesis of a heavy chain lacking the C-terminal membrane anchor.

Immunoglobulin Isotype Heterogeneity

All immature B cell–derived lymphocyte progenitors express mIgM. During ontogeny, interruption of mIgM expression and function at critical times hinders or ablates clonal B cell development.[308, 315, 316] Based on the results of many studies, B cells expressing IgM are thought to generate daughter cells with the same antigen specificity, but expressing a different immunoglobulin isotype.[317] Human and murine studies have led to a model of isotype switching:

1. Primitive B cell progenitors express only mIgM.
2. Cells expressing isotypes other than IgM appear at other times during gestation, but cells expressing new isotypes are found on mIgM-positive cells.
3. Cells later in development that express mIgA or mIgG also express mIgM and mIgD.
4. Most mIgA- or mIgG-expressing cells in adults express only one isotype.

Experimental evidence indicates that isotype switching is antigen driven, is T cell dependent, and requires action of certain cytokines.[318] B cells appear to require a signal between surface CD40 and CD40 ligand on CD4 T cells to initiate cytokine-dependent proliferation, differentiation, and isotype switching.[319] Isotypes produced are regulated by cytokines in the local environment, including IL-4, which promotes IgE synthesis and IL-10 and transforming growth factor-β, which stimulates switching to IgA synthesis.[320]

Neonatal Antibody Response

The newborn infant's capacity to produce antibodies differs quantitatively and qualitatively from that of the adult. During ontogeny,

IgM is detectable by 8 to 10 weeks' gestation, and IgG and IgA synthesis occurs by about 30 weeks' gestation.[321] Serum IgM concentrations in the blood of term infants are about 10% of concentrations in normal adults. IgG concentrations are near normal compared with adults, but most IgG is maternally derived by transplacental transport.[322] Little or no IgA is present in neonatal serum. IgM synthesis increases rapidly and reaches adult levels by 1 to 2 years of life. IgG levels fall, reaching a nadir at 3 to 4 months of life, as maternal IgG is catabolized. IgG reaches adult levels by 4 to 6 years of age and IgA by the onset of puberty.[314, 323]

Intrauterine infection can elicit a significant antibody response, with IgM concentrations occasionally being comparable to those seen in adults. IgA and IgG have been observed at birth in response to congenital infection, but the predominant response is IgM production.[324]

The newborn's response to carbohydrate vaccines is extremely limited,[324] but the reason for this deficit is unknown. The predominant immunoglobulin subclass for carbohydrate antigens is IgG2 in adults. This isotype subclass is delayed in newborns relative to production of IgG1, although this is not thought to be the cause of the poor response to carbohydrate antigens. This deficit limits the efficacy of current vaccines to significant bacterial pathogens afflicting infants.

Interactions between neonatal B cells and T cells appear to be responsible in part for developmental deficits in antibody synthesis. For instance, plasma cells are induced from mononuclear cells in vitro using pokeweed mitogen (PWM). This differentiation does not occur when purified B cells are cultured with PWM.[325] When fetal or neonatal mononuclear cells are stimulated with PMW, plasma cells are induced, but the immunoglobulin is produced in lower quantities and is predominantly IgM.[326] Coculture of PWM-stimulated neonatal cells with adult T cells results in augmented immunoglobulin production and in production of IgG and IgA in addition to IgM.[327] To the contrary, when neonatal T cells are cultured with adult B cells, immunoglobulin production is lower than when the same cells are cultured with adult T cells.[328] Addition of certain cytokines, including IL-2, IL4, or IL-6, to cultures of neonatal cells results in production of immunoglobulin of all isotypes.[329] Activated neonatal T cells have been shown to produce adequate quantities of IL-2 compared with adult cells, but production of other cytokines, including IL-4, IL-6, and IL-10, is diminished compared with adult cells.[330–332]

Studies demonstrate that, in addition to immature cytokine production profiles, neonatal T cells express lower quantities of costimulatory molecules required for B cell activation through cell-cell interaction. One such molecule is the CD40 ligand, a molecule expressed on the membrane of activated CD4 T cells. Binding of this protein to CD40 on the surface of B cells is important in B cell differentiation and isotype switching.[319] Neonatal B cells express lower concentrations of this costimulatory molecule than adult cells.

The importance of CD40 ligand in B cell differentiation is demonstrated in vitro by studies in which neonatal B cells cultured with soluble CD40 ligand and IL-4 produce IgE.[294] The role of this molecule in B cell differentiation is elucidated in individuals with a CD40 signaling defect that results in an X-linked immunodeficiency with increased IgM production.[333, 334] B cells from these individuals produce only IgM when stimulated with activated T cells in vitro. Production of IgG, IgA, and IgE is restored by treatment with CD40 antibody or recombinant CD40 ligand.[333] Moreover, neonatal T cells provide ineffective signals to B cells as a result of developmental deficits in local cytokine production and cell-cell interaction.

CONGENITAL AND NEONATAL LEUKEMIA

Incidence

Leukemia manifesting in infancy represents a small fraction of childhood leukemia cases. Acute lymphoblastic leukemia (ALL) is diagnosed in approximately 2000 children in the United States each year, whereas acute myeloid leukemia (AML) is diagnosed in about 500 children, and chronic myeloid leukemia (CML) in fewer than 100 children.[335] Although current chemotherapeutic regimens cure as many as 70% of children with ALL, AML is less amenable to treatment, with only 30% to 40% cured. Chemotherapy is ineffective against CML without allogeneic bone marrow transplantation. The variety of ALL occurring in 70% of infants has chromosome 11q23 rearrangements (primarily the t(4;11)(q21; q23) translocation) and is far less responsive to chemotherapy than other forms. This rearrangement creates a fusion *MLL-AF4* gene associated with hyperleukocytosis and a poor prognosis.[336] This extremely poor prognosis for infant ALL is limited to those with the t(4;11) translocation or other 11q23 abnormalities.[335]

Rearrangements of 11q23 are also the most common cytogenetic abnormalities in acute monocytic leukemia (M5 subtype). Coagulation disorders and central nervous system involvement are characteristic of 11q23 translocations in AML. The 11q23 breakpoint is identical in lymphoblastic and myeloid leukemia, suggesting that the *MLL* gene plays an important regulatory role in myelopoiesis and lymphopoiesis.

Congenital Leukemia and Down Syndrome

The predisposition of individuals with Down syndrome has been established. The incidence is approximately 10 to 20 times that observed in the general population. On morphologic and cytologic evaluation, three types of leukemia can be determined for children with Down syndrome.[337] Group I leukemias are morphologically and immunologically ALLs, but these malignancies are distinct from those of non-Down syndrome patients in that they lack the translocations and hyperdiploidy often seen in childhood ALL.

Group II leukemias are clearly AML with positive myeloperoxidase and nonspecific esterase cells. These leukemias are readily classified by FAB criteria. The leukemias diagnosed in these groups are similar to the ALL and AML of non-Down syndrome individuals.

Group III leukemias, with the largest group of patients, have prominent megakaryocytic, erythroid, or megakaryocytic-erythroid differentiation patterns. Although most blasts have no differentiating features by cytochemical and ultrastructural evaluation, they are classified as myeloid based on dysmegakaryopoiesis and dyserythropoiesis. Expression of CD36 is consistent with megakaryocytic, monocytic, or erythroid lineage. Although the major population of blasts lacks the platelet antigen CD61, morphologically identifiable megakaryocytes and micromegakaryocytes are present. Dysgranulopoiesis is notably absent. The leukemic process observed in these patients is distinct from that of acute megakaryocytic leukemia in non-Down syndrome patients. Based on changes in megakaryocytic and erythroid cell lines, it is possible that the major cell type found in these leukemias is a common progenitor of the megakaryocyte and erythroblast.

The spontaneous remission of Down syndrome–associated acute leukemia manifesting in the newborn period is a well-known phenomenon. All patients in whom this occurs exhibit the megakaryocytic-erythrocytic variety of leukemia. No specific hematologic or morphologic markers distinguish which infants will experience spontaneous remission and which will develop persistent leukemia requiring intervention. Some studies have suggested that cell culture and cytogenetics can predict the biologic course, but there are insufficient data to substantiate these hypotheses.[338]

References

1. Maximow AA: Relation of blood cells to connective tissues and endothelium. Physiol Rev 1924;4:533.
2. Downey H: Handbook of Hematology. New York: PB Hoeber, 1938.
3. Till JE, McCulloch EA: A direct measurement of the radiation sensitivity of normal mouse bone marrow. Radiat Res 1961;14:213.
4. Pluznik DH, Sachs L: The cloning of normal mast cells in tissue culture. J Cell Comp Physiol 1965;66:319.
5. Bradley TR, Metcalf D: The growth of mouse marrow cells in vitro. Aust J Exp Biol Med Sci 1966;44:287.
6. Metcalf D: Detection and analysis of human granulocyte-monocyte precursors using semi-solid cultures. Clin Haematol 1979;8:263.
7. Whitlock CA, Witte ON: Long term culture of B lymphocytes and their precursors from murine bone marrow. Proc Natl Acad Sci U S A 1982;79:3608.
8. Dexter TM, Lajtha LG: Proliferation of haematopoietic stem cells in vitro. Br J Haematol 1974;28:525.
9. Anderson G, Jenkinson EJ, Moore MC, et al: MHC-class I-positive epithelium and mesenchyme cells are both required for T-cell development in the thymus. Nature 1993;362:70.
10. Bodine DM, Crosier PS, Clark SC: Effects of hematopoietic growth factors on the survival of primitive stem cells in liquid suspension culture. Blood 1991;78:914.
11. Itoh Y, Ikebuchi K, Hirashima K: Interleukin-3 and granulocyte colony-stimulating factor as survival factors in murine hematopoietic stem cells in vitro. Int J Hematol 1992;55:139.

12. Katayama N, Clark SC, Ogawa M: Growth factor requirements for survival in cell cycle dormancy of primitive lymphohematopoietic progenitors. Blood 1993;81:610.
13. Suda T, Suda J, Ogawa M, et al: Permissive role of interleukin-3 in proliferation and differentiation of multipotential hematopoietic progenitors in culture. J Cell Physiol 1985;124:182.
14. Sieff CA, Emerson SG, Donahue RE, et al: Human recombinant granulocyte macrophage colony-stimulating factor: a multilineage hematopoietin. Science 1985;230:1171.
15. Broxmeyer HE, Lu L, Cooper S, et al: Synergistic effects of a purified recombinant human and murine B cell growth factor/IL-4 on colony formation in vitro by hematopoietic progenitor cells. J Immunol 1988;141:3852.
16. Demetri GD, Griffin JD: Granulocyte colony-stimulating factor and its receptor. Blood 1991;78:2791.
17. Sanderson CJ: Interleukin-5, eosinophils, and disease. Blood 1989;79:3101.
18. Ralph P, Warren MK, Nakoinz I, et al: Biological properties and molecular biology of the human macrophage growth factor, CSF-1. Immunobiology 1986;172:194.
19. Baker CJ, Melish ME, Hall RT, et al: Intravenous immune globulin for the prevention of nosocomial infection in low-birth-weight neonates. N Engl J Med 1992;327:213.
20. Freedman RM, Ingram DL, Gross I, et al: A half century of neonatal sepsis at Yale. Am J Dis Child 1981;135:140.
21. Wilkinson PC: Chemotaxis and Inflammation, 2nd ed. New York: Churchill Livingstone, 1982, pp 107–129.
22. Pahwa SC, Pahwa R, Grimes E, et al: Cellular and humoral components of monocyte and neutrophil chemotaxis in cord blood. Pediatr Res 1977;11:677.
23. Tono-Oka T, Nakayama M, Uehara H, et al: Characteristics of impaired chemotactic function in cord blood leukocytes. Pediatr Res 1979;13:148.
24. Krause PJ, Herson VC, Boutin-Lebowitz J, et al: Polymorphonuclear leukocyte adherence and chemotaxis in stressed and healthy neonates. Pediatr Res 1986;20:296.
25. Carr R, Pumford D, Davies JM: Neutrophil chemotaxis and adhesion in preterm babies. Arch Dis Child 1992;67:813.
26. Dos Santros C, Davidson D: Neutrophil chemotaxis to leukotriene B_4 in vitro is decreased for the human neonate. Pediatr Res 1993;33:242.
27. Bokoch GM: Chemoattractant signaling and leukocyte activation. Blood 1995;86:1649.
28. Williams LT, Snyderman R, Pike ML, et al: Specific receptor sites for chemotactic peptides on human polymorphonuclear leukocytes. Proc Natl Acad Sci U S A 1977;74:1204.
29. Bruce MC, Baley JE, Medvik KA, et al: Impaired surface membrane expression of C3bi but not C3b receptors on neonatal neutrophils. Pediatr Res 1987;21:306.
30. Chenoweth DE, Hughi TE: Demonstration of specific C5a receptor on intact human polymorphonuclear leukocytes. Proc Natl Acad Sci U S A 1978;75:3943.
31. Sacchi F, Hill HR: Defective membrane potential changes in neutrophils from human neonates. J Exp Med 1984;160:1247.
32. Santoro P, Agosti V, Viggiano D, et al: Impaired D-myo-inositol 1,4,5-triphosphate generation from cord blood polymorphonuclear leukocytes. Pediatr Res 1995;38:564.
33. Gallin JI, Fletcher MP, Seligmann BE, et al: Human neutrophil specific granule deficiency. Blood 1982;59:1317.
34. Gahr M, Schulze M, Scheffczyk D, et al: Diminished release of lactoferrin for polymorphonuclear leukocytes of human neonates. Acta Haematol 1987;77:90.
35. Abughali N, Dubyak G, Tosi MF: Impaired chemoattractant-stimulated hexose uptake in neonatal neutrophils. Blood 1993;82:2182.
36. Griffin FM, Griffin JA, Silverstein SC: Studies on the mechanism of phagocytosis. II. The interaction of macrophages with anti-immunoglobulin IgG-coated bone marrow-derived lymphocytes. J Exp Med 1976;144:788.
37. Bainton DF: Selective abnormalities of azurophil and specific granules of human neutrophil leukocytes. Fed Proc 1981;40:1443.
38. Kjeldsen L, Sengelov H, Lollike K, et al: Granules and secretory vesicles in human neonatal neutrophils. Pediatr Res 1996;40:120.
39. Ambruso DR, Brentwood B, Henson PM, et al: Oxidative metabolism of cord blood neutrophils: relationship to content and degranulation of cytoplasmic granules. Pediatr Res 1984;18:1148.
40. Ambruso DR, Stark LC, Gibson BE, et al: Increased activity of the respiratory burst in cord blood neutrophils: kinetics of the NAPDH oxidase enzyme system in subcellular fractions. Pediatr Res 1987;21:205.
41. Dossett JH, Williams RC, Quie PG: Studies on the interaction of bacteria, serum factors, and polymorphonuclear leukocytes in mothers and newborns. Pediatrics 1969;44:49.
42. McCracken GH Jr, Eichenwald HOF: Leukocyte function and the development of opsonic and complement activity in the neonate. Am J Dis Child 1971;121:120.
43. Harris MC, Stroobant J, Cody CS, et al: Phagocytosis of group B streptococcus by neutrophils from newborn infants. Pediatr Res 1983;17:358.
44. Forman ML, Stiehm ER: Impaired opsonic activity but normal phagocytosis in low-birth-weight infants. N Engl J Med 1969;281:926.
45. Xanthou M, Valassi-Adam E, Kintsonidou E, et al: Phagocytosis and killing ability of Candida albicans by blood leukocytes of healthy term and preterm babies. Arch Dis Child 1975;50:72.
46. Bektas S, Goetze B, Speer CP: Decreased adherence, chemotaxis, and phagocytic activity of neutrophils from preterm neonates. Acta Paediatr Scand 1990;79:1031.
47. Al-Hadithy H, Addison IE, Goldstone AH, et al: Defective neutrophil function in low-birth-weight, premature infants. J Clin Pathol 1981;34:366.
48. Marodi L, Leijh PCS, Van Furth R: Characteristics and functional capacities of human cord blood granulocytes and monocytes. Pediatr Res 18L1127, 1984.
49. Wright WC, Ank BJ, Herbert J, et al: Decreased bactericidal activity of leukocytes of stressed newborn infants. Pediatrics 1975;56:579.
50. Shigeoka AO, Santos JI, Hill HR: Functional analysis of neutrophil granulocytes from healthy, infected, and stressed neonates. J Pediatr 1979;95:454.
51. Roberts RL, Ank BJ, Stiehm ER: Antiviral properties of neonatal and adult human neutrophils. Pediatr Res 1994;36:792.
52. Athens JW: Granulocytes-neutrophils. In Lee GR, Bithell TC, Foerster J, et al (eds): Wintrobe's Clinical Hematology, 9th ed. Philadelphia: Lea & Febiger, 1993.
53. Christensen RD: Developmental granulopoiesis. In

Polin RA, Fox WW (eds): Fetal and Neonatal Physiology 2nd ed. Philadelphia: WB Saunders, pp 1753–1761.
54. Thomas DB, Yoffey JM: Human foetal hematopoiesis. I. The cellular composition of foetal blood. Br J Haematol 1962;8:290.
55. Manroe BL, Rosenfeld CR, Weinberg AG, et al: The neonatal blood count in health and disease. I. Reference values for neutrophilic cells. J Pediatr 1979;95:89.
56. Mouzihno A, Rosenfeld CR, Sanchez PJ, et al: Revised reference ranges for circulating neutrophils in very-low-birth-weight neonates. Pediatrics 1994;94:76.
57. Manroe BL, Weinberg AG, Rosenfeld CR, et al: The neonatal blood count in health and disease. I. Reference values for neutrophilic cells. J Pediatr 1979;95:89.
58. Brazy JE, Grimm JK, Little VA: Neonatal manifestations of severe maternal hypertension occurring before the thirty-sixth week of pregnancy. J Pediatr 1982;100:265.
59. Engle WD, Rosenfeld CR: Neutropenia in high risk neonates. J Pediatr 1984;105:982.
60. Mouzinho A, Rosenfeld CR, Sanchez PJ, et al: Effects of maternal hypertension on neonatal neutropenia and risk of nosocomial infection. Pediatrics 1992;90:430.
61. Koenig JM, Christensen RD: Incidence, neutrophil kinetics, and natural history of neonatal neutropenia associated with maternal hypertension. N Engl J Med 1989;321:557.
62. Koenig JM, Christensen RD: The mechanism responsible for diminished neutrophil production in neonates delivered of women with pregnancy-induced hypertension. Am J Obstet Gynecol 1991;165:467.
63. Doron MW, Makhlouf RA, Katz VL, et al: Increased incidence of sepsis at birth in neutropenic infants of mothers with preeclampsia. J Pediatr 1994;125:452.
64. Cadnapaphornchai M, Faix RG: Increased nosocomial infection in neutropenic low birth weight (2000 grams or less) infants of hypertensive mothers J Pediatr 1992;121:956.
65. Koenig JM, Hunter DD, Christensen RD: Neutropenia in donor (anemic) twins involved in twin-twin transfusion syndrome. J Perinatol 1991;11:355.
66. Koenig JM, Christensen RD: Neutropenia and thrombocytopenia in infants with Rh hemolytic disease. J Perinatol 1989;9:126.
67. Zipursky A, Bowman JM: Isoimmune hemolytic disease. In Nathan DG, Oski FA (eds): Hematology of Infancy and Childhood. WB Saunders, 1993, p 65.
68. Dale D, Hammond W: Cyclic neutropenia: a clinical review. Blood Rev 1988;2:178.
69. Dale D, Bolyard A, Hammond W: Cyclic neutropenia: Natural history and effects of long-term treatment with recombinant human granulocyte colony-stimulating factor. Cancer Invest 1993;11:219.
70. Lange R: Cyclic hematopoiesis: Human cyclic neutropenia. Exp Hematol 1983;11:4435.
71. Boesen P: Cyclic neutropenia terminating in permanent agranulocytosis. Acta Med Scand 1988;223:91.
72. Jonsson OG, Buchanan GR: Chronic neutropenia during childhood. Am J Dis Child 1991;145:232.
73. Hammond W, Price T, Souza L, Dale D: Treatment of cyclic neutropenia with granulocyte colony-stimulating factor. N Engl J Med 1989;320:306.
74. Kostmann R: Infantile genetic agranulocytosis (agranulocytosis infantilis hereditaria): a new recessive lethal disease in man. Acta Paediatr Scand 1956;45(Suppl 105):1.
75. Kostmann R: Infantile genetic agranulocytosis. A review with presentation of ten cases. Acta Paediatr Scand 1975;64:362.
76. Welte K, Dale D: Pathophysiology and treatment of severe chronic neutropenia. Ann Hematol 1996;72:158.
77. Bonilla MA, Gillio AP, Auggeiro M, et al: Effects of recombinant granulocyte colony-stimulating factor on neutropenia in patients with congenital agranulocytosis. N Engl J Med 1989;320:1574.
78. Tidow N, Pilz C, Teichmann B, et al: Clinical relevance of point mutations in the cytoplasmic domain of the granulocyte colony-stimulating factor receptor gene in patients with severe congenital neutropenia. Blood 1997;89:2369.
79. Dong F, Hoefsloot LH, Schelen AM, et al: Identification of a non-sense mutation in the G-CSF receptor in severe congenital neutropenia. Proc Natl Acad Sci U S A 1994;91:4480.
80. Dong F, Brynes RK, Tidow N, et al: Mutations in the gene for the granulocyte colony-stimulating factor receptor in patients with acute myelogenous leukemia preceded by severe congenital neutropenia. N Engl J Med 1995;333:487.
81. Boxer L, Yokoyama M, Lalezari P: Isoimmune neonatal neutropenia. J Pediatr 1972;80:783.
82. Lalezari P, Radel E: Neutrophil specific antigens: Immunology and clinical significance. Semin Hematol 1974;11:231.
83. Minchinton RM, McGrath KM: Alloimmune neonatal neutropenia—a neglected diagnosis. Med J Aust 1987;147:139.
84. Cartron J, Tchernia G, Celton J, et al: Alloimmune neonatal neutropenia. Am J Pediatr Hematol Oncol 1991;13:21.
85. Levine D, Prema R, Madyastha R: Isoimmune neonatal neutropenia. Am J Perinatol 1986;3:231.
86. Huizinga TWJ, Kleijer M, Tetteroo PA, et al: Biallelic neutrophil NA-antigen system is associated with a polymorphism on the phosphoinositol-induced Fc-gamma receptor III (CD16). Blood 1990;75:213.
87. Conway L, Clay ME, Kline WE, et al: Natural history of primary autoimmune neutropenia of infancy. Pediatrics 1987;79:728.
88. Lalezari P: Autoimmune neutropenia of infancy. J Pediatr 1986;109:764.
89. Boxer LA, Greenberg MS, Boxer GJ, Stossel TP: Autoimmune neutropenia. N Engl J Med 1975; 293:748.
90. Lalezari P, Jiang AF, Yegen L, Santorineou M: Chronic autoimmune neutropenia due to anti-N2 antibody. N Engl J Med 1975;293:744.
91. Lyall EGH, Lucas GF, Eden OB: Autoimmune neutropenia of infancy. J Clin Pathol 1992;45:431.
92. Bux J, Behrens G, Jaeger G, Welte K: Diagnosis and clinical course of autoimmune neutropenia in infancy: analysis of 240 cases. Blood 1998;91:181.
93. Werner G, von dem Borne AEGKR, Bos MJE, et al: Localization of the human NA1 alloantigen on neutrophil Fcγ receptor. In Reinherz EL, Haynes BF, Nadler LM, Bernstein ID (eds): Leukocyte Typing II, White Cell Differentiation Antigens. Vol. 3. New York: Springer-Verlag, 1986, p 109.
94. Bux J, Stein EL, Bierling P, et al: Characterization of a new alloantigen (SH) on the human neutrophil Fcγ receptor IIIb. Blood 1997;89:1027.
95. Hartman KR, Wright DG: Identification of autoantibodies specific for neutrophil adhesion glycoprotein CD11b/CD18 in patients with autoimmune neutropenia. Blood 1991;78:1096.
96. Schwachman H, Diamond LK, Oski FA, et al: The syndrome of pancreatic insufficiency and bone marrow dysfunction. J Pediatr 1964;65:645.

97. Shmerling DH, Prader A, Hitzig WH, et al: The syndrome of exocrine pancreatic insufficiency, neutropenia, metaphyseal dysostosis, and dwarfism. Helv Paediatr Acta 1969;24:547.
98. Saunders EF, Gall G, Freedman MH: Granulopoiesis in Schwachman's syndrome (pancreatic insufficiency and bone marrow dysfunction). Pediatrics 1979; 64:515.
99. Huijgens PC, van der Veen EA, Meijer S, et al: Syndrome of Schwachman and leukemia. Scand J Haematol 1977;18:20.
100. Aggett PJ, Cavanaugh NPC, Matthew DJ, et al: Schwachman's syndrome. Arch Dis Child 1980;55:331.
101. Hill RE, Durie PR, Gaskin KJ, et al: Steatorrhea and pancreatic insufficiency in Schwachman's syndrome. Gastroenterology 1982;83:22.
102. Moore MAS: Clinical implications of positive and negative hematopoietic stem cell regulators. Blood 1991;78:1.
103. Paley C, Murphy S, Karayalcin G, et al: Treatment of neutropenia in Schwachman-Diamond syndrome (SDS) with recombinant human granulocyte colony stimulating factor (RH-G-CSF) (Abstract). Blood 1991;78:3a.
104. McKusick VA, Roswell E, Hostetler JA, et al: Dwarfism in the Amish. II. Cartilage hair hypoplasia. Bull Johns Hopkins Hosp 1965;116:285.
105. Lux SE, Johnston RB Jr, August CS, et al: Chronic neutropenia and abnormal cellular immunity in cartilage-hair hypoplasia. N Engl J Med 1970;282:231.
106. De Vaal O, Seynhaeve V: Reticular dysgenesis. Lancet 1959;2:1123.
107. Roper M, Parmley R, Crist W, et al: Severe congenital leukopenia (reticular dysgenesis). Am J Dis Child 1985;139:832.
108. Bujan W, Ferster A, Azzi N, et al: Use of recombinant human granulocyte colony stimulating factor in reticular dysgenesis. Br J Haematol 1992;81:128.
109. Azcona C, Alzina V, Barona P, et al: Use of recombinant human granulocyte-macrophage colony stimulating factor in an infant with reticular dysgenesis. Eur J Pediatr 1994;153:164.
110. Fischer A, Landais P, Fredrich W, et al: European experience of bone marrow transplantation for severe combined immunodeficiency. Lancet 1990;336:850.
111. Rodwell RL, Taylor KM, Tudehope DI, et al: Hematopoietic scoring system in early diagnosis of sepsis in neutropenic newborns. Pediatr Infect Dis J 1993;12:372.
112. Cannistra SA, Griffin JD: Regulation of the production and action of granulocytes and monocytes. Semin Hematol 1988;25:173.
113. Golde DW, Gasson JC: Hormones that stimulate the growth of blood cells. Sci Am 1988;259:34.
114. Davis I, Morstyn G: Clinical uses of growth factors. Baillieres Clin Haematol 1992;5:753.
115. Dale DC, Bonilla MA, Davis MW, et al: A randomized, controlled phase III trial of recombinant human granulocyte colony-stimulating factor (filgrastim) for treatment of severe chronic neutropenia. Blood 1993;81:2496.
116. Sullivan GW, Carper HT, Mandell GL: The effects of three human recombinant hematopoietic growth factors (granulocyte-macrophage colony-stimulating factor, granulocyte colony-stimulating factor, and interleukin-3) on phagocyte oxidative activity. Blood 1993;81:1963.
117. Cairo M, Suen Y, Knoppel E, et al: Decreased G-CSF and IL-3 production and gene expression from mononuclear cells of newborn infants. Pediatr Res 1992;31:574.
118. Schibler K, Leichty K, White W, Christensen R: Production of granulocyte colony-stimulating factor in vitro by monocytes from preterm and term neonates. Blood 1993;82:2478.
119. Gessler P, Kirchmann N, Kientsch-Engel R, et al: Serum concentrations of granulocyte colony-stimulating factor in healthy term and preterm neonates and in those with various diseases including bacterial infections. Blood 1993;82:3177.
120. Lieschke G, Grail D, Hodgson G, et al: Mice lacking granulocyte colony-stimulating factor have chronic neutropenia, granulocyte and macrophage progenitor deficiency, and impaired neutrophil mobilization. Blood 1994;84:1737.
121. Leichty K, Schibler K, Ohls R, et al: The failure of newborn mice infected with *Escherichia coli* to accelerate neutrophil production correlates with their failure to increase transcripts for granulocyte colony-stimulating factor and interleukin-6. Biol Neonate 1993;64:331.
122. Cairo M, Plunkett J, Mauss D, van de Ven C: Seven-day administration of recombinant granulocyte colony-stimulating factor to newborn rats: modulation of neonatal neutrophilia, myelopoiesis, and group B streptococcal sepsis. Blood 1990;76:1788.
123. Cairo M, Plunkett J, Nguyen A, van de Ven C: Effects of stem cell factor with and without granulocyte colony-stimulating factor on neonatal hematopoiesis: in vivo induction of newborn myelopoiesis and reduction in mortality during experimental group B streptococcal sepsis. Blood 1992;80:96.
124. Gillan E, Christensen R, Suen Y, et al: A randomized, placebo-controlled trial of recombinant human granulocyte colony-stimulating factor administration in newborn infants with presumed sepsis: significant induction of peripheral and bone marrow neutrophilia. Blood 1994;84:1427.
125. Kocherlakota P, La Gamma EF: Human granulocyte colony-stimulating factor may improve outcome attributable to neonatal sepsis complicated by neutropenia. Pediatrics 1997;100:E6.
126. Schibler KR, Osborne KA, Leung LY, et al: A randomized, placebo-controlled trial of granulocyte colony-stimulating factor administration to newborn infants with neutropenia and clinical signs of early-onset sepsis. Pediatrics 1998;102:6.
127. La Gamma EF, Alpan O, Kocherlakota P: Effects of granulocyte colony-stimulating factor on preeclampsia-associated neonatal neutropenia. J Pediatr 1995;126:457.
128. Makhlouf RA, Doron MW, Bose CL, et al: Administration of granulocyte colony-stimulating factor to neutropenic low birth weight infants of mothers with preeclampsia. J Pediatr 1995;126:454.
129. Cairo MS, Christensen R, Sender LS, et al: Results of a phase I/II trial of recombinant human granulocyte-macrophage colony-stimulating factor in very low birth weight neonates: significant induction of circulatory neutrophils, monocytes, platelets, and bone marrow neutrophils. Blood 1995;86:2509.
130. Mouzinho A, Rosenfeld CR, Sanchez PJ, et al: Effects of maternal hypertension on neonatal neutropenia and risk of nosocomial infection. Pediatrics 1992;90:430.
131. Doron MW, Makhlouf RA, Katz VL, et al: Increased incidence of sepsis at birth in neutropenic infants of mothers with preeclampsia. J Pediatr 1994;125:452.
132. Cadnapaphornchai M, Faix RG: Increased nosocomial infection in neutropenic low birth weight (2000 grams or less) infants of hypertensive mothers. J Pediatr 1992;121:956.

133. Du X, Williams DA: Interleukin-11: review of molecular, cell biology, and clinical use. Blood 1997;89:3897.
134. Du XX, Everett ET, Wang G, et al: Murine interleukin-11 (IL-11) is expressed at high levels in the hippocampus and expression is developmentally regulated in the testis. J Cell Physiol 1996;168:362.
135. van de Ven C, Ishizawa L, Law P, et al: IL-11 in combination with SLF and G-CSF or GM-CSF significantly increases expansion of isolated CD34+ cell populations from cord blood versus adult bone marrow. Exp Hematol 1995;23:1289.
136. Lemoli RM, Fogli M, Fortuna A, et al: Interleukin-11 stimulates proliferation of human hematopoietic CD34+ and CD34+CD33−DR− cells and synergizes with stem cell factor, interleukin-3, and granulocyte-macrophage colony-stimulating factor. Exp Hematol 1993;21:1668.
137. Du XX, Neben T, Goldman S, et al: Effects of recombinant human interleukin-11 on hematopoietic reconstitution in transplant mice: acceleration of recovery of peripheral blood neutrophils and platelets. Blood 1993;81:27.
138. Du XX, Keller D, Goldman S, et al: Functional effects of interleukin-11 treatment in vivo following bone marrow transplantation (BMT) and combined modality therapy in mice (Abstract). Exp Hematol 1992; 20:768.
139. Barton BE, Shortall J, Jackson JV: Interleukin-6 and interleukin-11 protect mice from mortality in a staphylococcal enterotoxin-induced toxic shock model. Infect Immun 1996;64:714.
140. Chang M, Williams A, Ishizawa L, et al: Role of interleukin-11 (IL-11) during experimental group B streptococcal (GBS) sepsis in rats: prophylactic use of IL-11 improves survival and enhances platelet recovery (Abstract). Blood 1994;84(Suppl 1):477a.
141. Misra BR, Ferranti TJ, Keith JC, et al: Recombinant human interleukin-11 prevents hypotension in LPS-treated anesthetized rabbits. J Endotox Res 1996; 3:297.
142. Trepicchio WL, Bozza M, Pedneault G, et al: Recombinant human interleukin-11 attenuates the proinflammatory response through regulation of cytokine gene expression. Exp Hematol 1996;24:1009.
143. Keith JCJ, Albert L, Sonis ST, et al: IL-11, a pleiotropic cytokine: exciting new effects of IL-11 on gastrointestinal mucosal biology. Stem Cells 1994;12:79.
144. Du XX, Liu Q, Yang Z, et al: The protective effects of interleukin-11 (IL-11) in a murine model of ischemic bowel necrosis. Am J Physiol 1997;272:545.
145. Schindel D, Maze R, Liu Q, et al: Interleukin-11 improves survival and reduces bacterial translocation and bone marrow suppression in burned mice. J Pediatr Surg 1997;32:312.
146. Liu Q, Du XX, Schindel DT, et al: Tropic effects of interleukin-11 in rats with experimental short bowel syndrome. J Pediatr Surg 1996;31:1047.
147. Gordon MS, McCaskill-Stevens WJ, Battiato LA, et al: A phase I trial of recombinant human interleukin-11 (Neumega rhIL-11 growth factor) in women with breast cancer receiving chemotherapy. Blood 1996; 87:3615.
148. Cairo MS, Davenport V, Reaman G, et al: Accelerated hematopoietic recovery with rhIL-11 following ifosfamide, carboplatin, and etoposide administration in children with solid tumors or lymphoma: preliminary results of a phase I/II trial. Exp Hematol 1996; 24:1104.
149. Tepler I, Elias L, Smith JW 2nd, et al: A randomized placebo-controlled trial of recombinant human interleukin-11 in cancer patients with thrombocytopenia due to chemotherapy. Blood 1996;87:3607.
150. Bank S, Sninsky C, Robinson M, et al: Safety and activity evaluation of rhIL-11 in subjects with active Crohn's disease. Shock 1997;7:520.
151. Curnutte J, Orkin S, Dinauer M: Genetic disorders of phagocyte function. In Stamoyannopoulos G (ed): The Molecular Basis of Blood Diseases. Philadelphia: WB Saunders, 1994, pp 493–522.
152. Roos D, de Boer M, Kuribayashi F, et al: Mutations in the X-linked and autosomal recessive forms of chronic granulomatous disease. Blood 1996;87:1663.
153. Curnutte JT: Molecular basis for the autosomal recessive forms of chronic granulomatous disease. Immunol Rev 1992;4:149.
154. Gallin JI, Buescher ES, Seligmann BE, et al: NIH Conference: recent advances in chronic granulomatous disease. Ann Intern Med 1983;99:657.
155. Finn A, Hadzic N, Morgan G, et al: Prognosis of chronic granulomatous disease. Arch Dis Child 1990;65:942.
156. Segal AW: The NADPH oxidase and chronic granulomatous disease. Mol Med Today 1996;2:129.
157. The International Study Group: A controlled trial of interferon gamma to prevent infection in chronic granulomatous disease. N Engl J Med 1991;3234:509.
158. Weening RS, Kabel P, Pijman P, Roos D: Continuous therapy with sulfamethoxazole-trimethoprim in patients with chronic granulomatous disease. J Pediatr 1983;103:127.
159. Calvino MC, Maldonado MS, Otheo E, et al: Bone marrow transplantation in chronic granulomatous disease. Eur J Pediatr 1996;155:877.
160. Ho CM, Vowels MA, Lockwood L, Ziegler JB: Successful bone marrow transplantation in a child with X-linked chronic granulomatous disease. Bone Marrow Transplant 1996;18:213.
161. Kamani N, August CS, Campbell DE, et al: Marrow transplantation in chronic granulomatous disease: an update, with 6-year follow-up. J Pediatr 1988;113:697.
162. Weening R, Adriaansz L, Weemaes C, et al: Clinical differences in chronic granulomatous disease in patients with cytochrome *b*-negative or cytochrome *b*-positive neutrophils. J Pediatr 1985;107:102.
163. Mardiney M 3rd, Jackson SH, Spratt SK, et al: Enhanced host defense after gene transfer in the murine p47phox-deficient model of chronic granulomatous disease. Blood 1997;89:2268.
164. Karlsson S: Treatment of genetic defects in hematopoietic cell function by gene transfer. Blood 1991;78:2481.
165. Weinberg KI, Kohn DB: Gene therapy for congenital immunodeficiency diseases. Immunol Allergy Clin North Am 1996;16:453.
166. Pollock JD, Williams DA, Gifford MA, et al: Mouse model of X-linked chronic granulomatous disease, an inherited defect in phagocyte superoxide production. Nat Genet 1995;9:202.
167. Jackson SH, Gallin JI, Holland SM: The p47phox mouse knock-out model of chronic granulomatous disease. J Exp Med 1995;182:751.
168. Sekhsaria S, Gallin JI, Linton GF, et al: Peripheral blood progenitors as a target for genetic correction of p47phox-deficient chronic granulomatous disease. Proc Natl Acad Sci U S A 1993;90:7446.
169. Kume A, Dinauer MC: Retrovirus-mediated reconstitution of respiratory burst activity in X-linked chronic granulomatous disease cells. Blood 1994;84:3311.
170. Malech H, Sekhsaria S, Whiting-Theobald N, et al: Development of a phase I clinical trial of gene therapy

for chronic granulomatous disease (Abstract). Blood 1995;86:295a.
171. Jordan HE: The histology of the yolk sac of a 9.2 mm human embryo. Anat Anz 1907;31:291.
172. Takashina T: Hematopoiesis in the human yolk sac. J Anat 1987;151:125.
173. Cline MJ, Moore MAS: Embryonic origin of the mouse macrophage. Blood 1972;87:67.
174. Kelemen E, Janossa M: Macrophages are the first differentiated blood cells formed in human embryonic liver. Exp Hematol 1980;8:996.
175. Kelemen E, Calvo W: Prenatal hematopoiesis in the human bone marrow and its developmental antecedents. In Trubowitz S, Davis S (eds): The Human Bone Marrow: Anatomy, Physiology and Pathophysiology. Boca Raton: CRC Press, 1982, pp 3–41.
176. Porcellini A, Manna A, Manna M, et al: Ontogeny of granulocyte:macrophage progenitor cells in the human fetus. Int J Cell Cloning 1983;1:92.
177. Linch DC, Knott LJ, Rodeck CH, et al: Studies of circulating hematopoietic progenitor cells in human fetal blood. Blood 1982;59:967.
178. Christensen DR: Circulating pluripotent hematopoietic progenitor cells in neonates. J Pediatr 1987; 110:622.
179. Miller DR: Normal values and examination of the blood: Perinatal period, infancy, childhood, and adolescence. In Miller DR (ed): Blood Diseases of Infancy and Childhood. St. Louis: CV Mosby, 1984, pp 21–45.
180. Kato K: Leukocytes in infancy and childhood. J Pediatr 1935;7:7.
181. Xanthou M: Leukocyte blood picture in healthy full term and premature babies during the neonatal period. Arch Dis Child 1970;45:242.
182. Weinberg AG, Rosenfeld CR, Manroe BL, et al: Neonatal blood cell counts in health and disease: II. Values for lymphocytes, monocytes and eosinophils. J Pediatr 1985;106:462.
183. Alenghat E, Esterly JR: Alveolar macrophages in perinatal infants. Pediatrics 1984;74:221.
184. Jacobs RF, Wilson CB, Palmer S, et al: Factors related to the appearance of alveolar macrophages in the developing lung. Am J Respir Dis 1985;131:548.
185. Kurland G, Cheung AT, Miller ME, et al: The ontogeny of pulmonary defenses: alveolar macrophage function in neonatal and juvenile rhesus monkeys. Pediatr Res 1988;23:293.
186. Sherman M, Goldstein E, Lippert W, et al: Neonatal lung defense mechanisms: a study of the alveolar macrophage system in neonatal rabbits. Am Rev Respir Dis 1977;116:433.
187. Johnston RB Jr, Zucker-Franklin D: Monocytes and macrophages. In Zucker-Franklin D (ed): Atlas of Blood Cells: Function and Pathology. Philadelphia: Lea & Febiger, 1988, pp 323–357.
188. Zuckerman SH, Douglas SD: Mononuclear phagocytes: Plasma membrane receptors and dynamics. Annu Rev Microbiol 1979;33:267.
189. Johnston RB Jr: Monocytes and macrophages. N Engl J Med 1988;318:747.
190. Yourno J, Burkart P, Mastro Paolo W, et al: Monocyte nonspecific esterase. J Histochem Cytochem 1986; 34:727.
191. Kreipe H, Radzun HJ, Parwaresch MR: Phenotypic differentiation patterns of the human monocyte/macrophage system. Histochem J 1986;18:441.
192. Yoder MC, Lanker TA, Engle WA: Culture medium oxygen tension affects fibronectin production in human adult blood and cord blood macrophages. Immunol Lett 1988;19:1.
193. Santiago-Schwartz F, Fleit HB: Identification of nonadherent mononuclear cells in human cord blood that differentiate into macrophages. J Leukoc Biol 1988;45:51.
194. Stiehm ER, Sztein MB, Steeg PS, et al: Deficient DR antigen expression on human cord blood monocytes: reversal with lymphokines. Clin Immunol Immunopathol 1984;30:430.
195. Morris RB, Nichols BA, Bainton DF: Ultrastructure and peroxidase cytochemistry of normal human leukocytes at birth. Dev Biol 1975;44:223.
196. Johnston RB Jr, Zucker-Franklin D: Monocytes and macrophages. In Zucker-Franklin D (ed): Atlas of Blood Cells: Function and Pathology. Philadelphia: Lea & Febiger, 1988, pp 323–357.
197. Bhoopat L, Taylor CR, Hofman FM: The differentiation antigens of macrophages in human fetal liver. Clin Immunol Immunopathol 1986;41:184.
198. Edward JA, Jones DB, Evans PR, et al: Differential expression of HLA class II antigens on human fetal and adult lymphocytes and macrophages. Immunology 1985;55:489.
199. Bulmer JN, Morrison L, Smith JC: Expression of class II MHC gene products by macrophages in human uteroplacental tissue. Immunology 1988;63:707.
200. Glover DM, Brownstein D, Burchett S, et al: Expression of HLA class II antigens and secretion of interleukin-1 by monocytes and macrophages from adults and neonates. Immunology 1987;61:195.
201. Gonwa TA, Picker LJ, Raff HV, et al: Antigen-presenting capabilities of human monocytes correlate with their expression of HLA-DS, an Ia determinant distinct from HLA-DR. J Immunol 1983;130:706.
202. Miller ME: Phagocytic cells. In Miller ME (ed): Host Defenses in the Human Neonate. New York: Grune & Stratton, 1978, pp 59–71.
203. Kozin F, Cochrane CG: The contact activation system of plasma: biochemistry and pathophysiology. In Gallin JI, Goldstein IM, Snyderman R (eds): Inflammation: Basic Principles and Clinical Correlates. New York: Raven Press, 1992, pp 103–122.
204. Marodi L, Csorba S, Nagh B: Chemotactic and random movement of human newborn monocytes. Eur J Pediatr 1980;135:73.
205. Klein RB, Fischer TJ, Gard SE, et al: Decreased mononuclear and polymorphonuclear chemotaxis I human newborns, infants, and young children. Pediatrics 1977;60:467.
206. Lasky LA: Selectins: Interpreters of cell-specific carbohydrate information during inflammation. Science 1992;258:964.
207. Bevilacqua MP, Nelson RM: Selectins. J Clin Invest 1993;91:379.
208. Hogg N, Landis RC: Adhesion molecules in cell interactions. Curr Opin Immunol 1993;5:383.
209. Weller A, Isenmann S, Vestweber D: Cloning of the mouse endothelial selectins; expression of both E- and P-selectin is inducible by tumor necrosis factor. J Biol Chem 1992;267:15176.
210. Carlos TM, Harlan JM: Leukocyte-endothelial adhesion molecules. Blood 1994;84:2068.
211. Anderson DC, Springer TA: Leukocyte adhesion deficiency: an inherited defect in Mac-1, LFA-1, p150, 95 glycoproteins. Annu Rev Med 1987;38:175.
212. Roth P, Polin RA: Adherence of human newborn infants' monocytes to matrix-bound fibronectin. J Pediatr 1992;121:285.
213. Nathan CF: Mechanisms of macrophage antimicrobial activity. Trans R Soc Trop Med Hyg 1983;77:620.
214. Nathan CF, Tsunawaki S: Secretion of toxic oxygen

products by macrophages: regulatory cytokines and their effects on the oxidase. Ciba Found Symp 1986;118:211.
215. Reiss M, Roos D: Differences in oxygen metabolism of phagocytosing monocytes and neutrophils. J Clin Invest 1978;61:480.
216. Elsbach P, Weiss J: Oxygen-independent antimicrobial systems of phagocytes. In Gallin JI, Goldstein IM, Snyderman R (eds): Inflammation: Basic Principles and Clinical Concepts. New York: Raven Press, 1992, pp 603–636.
217. Hibbs JB Jr, Taintor RR, Vavrin Z, et al: Nitric oxide: a cytotoxic activated macrophage effector molecule. Biochem Biophys Res Commun 1988;157:87.
218. Drapier JC, Pellat C, Henry Y: Generation of ERR-detectable nitrosyl-iron complexes in tumor target cells cocultured with activated macrophages. J Biol Chem 1991;266:10162.
219. Hogg N, Darley-Usmar VM, Wilson MT, et al: Production of hydroxyl radicals from the simultaneous generation of superoxide and nitric oxide. Biochem J 1992;281:419.
220. Speer CP, Johnston RB Jr: Phagocyte function. In Ogra PL (ed): Neonatal Infections: Nutritional and Immunological Interactions. Orlando: Grune & Stratton, 1984, pp 21–36.
221. D'Ambola JB, Sherman MP, Tashkin DP, et al: Human and rabbit newborn lung macrophages have reduced anti-*Candida* activity. Pediatr Res 1988;24:285.
222. Nathan CF: Secretory products of macrophages. J Clin Invest 1987;79:319.
223. Bessler H, Sirota L, Dulitzky F, et al: Production of interleukin-1 by mononuclear cells of newborns and their mothers. Clin Exp Immunol 1987;68:655.
224. Wilson CB: Immunologic basis for increased susceptibility of the neonate to infection. J Pediatr 1986;108:1.
225. Weatherstone KB, Rich EA: Tumor necrosis factor/cachetin and interleukin-1 expression in cord blood monocytes from term and preterm neonates. Pediatr Res 1989;25:342.
226. Bryson YJ, Winter HS, Gard SE, et al: Deficiency of immune interferon production by leukocytes of normal newborns. Cell Immunol 1980;55:191.
227. Rowen JL, Smith CW, Edwards MS: Group B streptococci elicit leukotriene B_4 and interleukin-8 from human monocytes: neonates exhibit a diminished response. J Infect Dis 1995;172:420.
228. Schibler KR, Trautman MS, Liechty KW, et al: Diminished transcription of interleukin-8 by monocytes from preterm neonates. J Leukoc Biol 1993;53:399.
229. Le TV, Leung L, Carroll WL, et al: Regulation of interleukin-10 gene expression: possible mechanisms accounting for its up-regulation and for maturational differences in its expression by blood mononuclear cells. Blood 1997;89:4112.
230. Schibler KR, Liechty KW, White WL, et al: Production of granulocyte colony-stimulating factor by monocytes from preterm and term neonates. Blood 1993;82:2478.
231. Steinman RM: The dendritic cell system and its role in immunogenicity. Annu Rev Immunol 1991;9:271.
232. Williams L, Egner W, Hart DN: Isolation and function of human dendritic cells. Int Rev Cytol 1994;153:41.
233. Hart D: Dendritic cells: Unique leukocyte populations which control the immune system. Blood 1997;90:3245.
234. Steinman RM, Cohn ZA: Identification of a novel cell type I peripheral lymphoid organs of mice. I. Morphology, quantitation, and tissue distribution. J Exp Med 1973;137:1142.
235. Hart DNJ, Fabre JW: Demonstration and characterization of Ia-positive dendritic cells in the interstitial connective tissue of rat heart and other tissues but not brain. J Exp Med 1981;153:347.
236. Hart DNJ, McKenzie JL: Isolation and characterization of human tonsil dendritic cells. J Exp Med 1988;168:57.
237. Grouard G, Rissoan MC, Filgueira L, et al: The enigmatic plasmacytoid T cells develop into dendritic cells with interleukin-(IL)-3 and CD40 ligand. J Exp Med 1997;185:1101.
238. Weber-Matthiese K, Sterry W: Organization of the monocyte/macrophage system of skin. J Invest Dermatol 1990;95:83.
239. Shen HH, Talle MA, Goldstein G, et al: Functional subset of human monocytes defined by monoclonal antibodies: a distinct subset of monocytes containing the cells capable of inducing the autologous mixed lymphocyte culture. J Immunol 1983;130:698.
240. Davis AL, McKenzie JL, Hart DN: HLA-DR positive leukocyte subpopulations in human skin include dendritic cells, macrophages, and CD7-negative T cells Immunology 1988;65:573.
241. O'Doherty U, Steinman RM, Peng M, et al: Dendritic cells freshly isolated from human blood express CD4 and mature into typical immunostimulatory dendritic cells after culture in monocyte-conditioned medium. J Exp Med 1993;178:1067.
242. Starling GC, McLellan AD, Egner W, et al: Intercellular adhesion molecule-3 is a costimulatory ligand for LFA-1 expressed on human blood dendritic cells. Eur J Immunol 1995;25:2528.
243. Norton J, Sloane JP, Al-Saffar N, et al: Expression of adhesion molecules in human intestinal graft-versus-host disease. Clin Exp Immunol 1992;87:231.
244. Inaba K, Steinman RM: Monoclonal antibodies to LFA-1 and to CD4 inhibit the mixed lymphocyte reaction after the antigen dependent clustering of dendritic cells and T lymphocytes. J Exp Med 1987; 165:1403.
245. Sallusto F, Lanzavecchia A: Efficient presentation of soluble antigen by cultured human dendritic cells is maintained by granulocyte/macrophage colony-stimulating factor plus interleukin-4 and down-regulated by tumor necrosis factor α. J Exp Med 1994;179:1109.
246. Pearson AM: Scavenger receptor in innate immunity. Curr Opin Immunol 1996;8:20.
247. Stahl PD: The mannose receptor and other macrophage lectins. Curr Opin Immunol 1992;4:49.
248. Wu K, Yuan J, Lasky LA: Characterization of novel members of the macrophage mannose receptor type C lectin family. J Biol Chem 1995;271:21323.
249. McLellan AD, Sorg RV, Williams LA, et al: Human dendritic cells activate T lymphocytes via a CD40:CD40 ligand-dependent pathway. Eur J Immunol 1996;26:1204.
250. Hart DNJ, Starling GC, Calder VL, et al: B7/BB-1 is a leukocyte differentiation antigen on dendritic cells induced by activation. Immunology 1993;79:616.
251. Steinman RM: The dendritic cell system and its role in immunogenicity. Annu Rev Immunol 1991;9:271.
252. Egner W, Andreesen R, Hart DN: Allostimulatory cells in fresh human blood: heterogeneity in antigen presenting cell populations. Transplantation 1993; 56:945.
253. Kuntz-Crow M, Kunkel HG: Human dendritic cells: major stimulators of autologous and allogenic MLR. Clin Exp Immunol 1982;49:338.
254. Inaba K, Metlay JP, Crowley MT, et al: Dendritic cells pulsed with protein antigens in vitro can prime

antigen-specific MHC-restricted T cells in situ. J Exp Med 1990;172:1459.
255. Waalen K, Forre O, Teigland J, et al: Human rheumatoid synovial and normal blood dendritic cells as antigen presenting cells—comparison with autologous monocytes. Clin Exp Immunol 1987;70:1.
256. Will A, Blank C, Rollinghoff M, et al: Murine epidermal Langerhans cells are potent stimulators of an antigen-specific T cell response to Leishmania major, the cause of cutaneous leishmaniasis.
257. Van Voorhis WC, Valinsky J, Hoffman E, et al: Relative efficacy of human monocytes and dendritic cells as accessory cells for T cell replication. J Exp Med 1983;158:174.
258. Bender A, Bui LK, Feldman MA, et al: Inactivated influenza virus when presented on dendritic cells elicits human $CD8^+$ cytolytic T cell responses. J Exp Med 1995;182:1663.
259. Nair S, Babu JS, Dunham RG, et al: Induction of primary, antiviral cytotoxic and proliferative responses with antigens administered via dendritic cells. J Virol 1993;67:4062.
260. Corr M, Lee DJ, Carson DA, et al: Gene vaccination with naked plasmid DNA: mechanism of CTL priming. J Exp Med 1996;184:1555.
261. Svensson M, Stockinger B, Wick MJ: Bone marrow-derived dendritic cells can process bacteria for MHC-I and MHC-II presentation to T cells. J Immunol 1997;158:4229.
262. Bhardwaj N, Bender A, Gonzalez N, et al: Influenza virus-infected dendritic cells stimulate strong proliferative and cytolytic responses from human $CD8^+$ T cells. J Clin Invest 1994;94:797.
263. Manca F, Li Pira G, Fenoglio D, et al: Dendritic cells are potent antigen-presenting cells for in vitro induction of primary $CD4^+$ T-cell lines specific for HIV gp120. J Acquir Immune Defic Syndr 1994;7:15.
264. Nonacs R, Humborg C, Tam JP, et al: Mechanisms of mouse spleen dendritic cell function in generation of influenza-specific, cytolytic T lymphocytes. J Exp Med 1992;176:519.
265. Goldstein G, Mackay IR: The Human Thymus. London: William Heinemann, 1969, pp 26–27.
266. Anderson G, Owen JJ, Moore NC, et al: Thymic epithelial cells provide unique signals for positive selection of $CD4^+CD8^+$ thymocytes in vitro. J Exp Med 1994;179:2027.
267. Shultz LD, Sidman CL: Genetically determined murine models of immunodeficiency. Annu Rev Immunol 1987;5:367.
268. Carey AH, Roach S, Williamson R, et al: Localization of 27 markers in the region of human chromosome 22q11-pter deleted in patients with DiGeorge syndrome and duplicated in der22 syndrome. Genomics 1990;27:299.
269. Royo C, Touraine JL, De Bouteiller O: Ontogeny of T lymphocyte differentiation in the human fetus: acquisition of phenotype and function. Thymus 1987;10:57.
270. Hayes BF, Martin ME, Kay HH, et al: Early events in human T cell ontogeny: phenotypic characterization and immunohistologic localization of T cell precursors in early human fetal tissue. J Exp Med 1988;168:1061.
271. Janossy G, Bofill M, Rowe D, et al: Tissue distribution of T lymphocytes expressing different CD45 polypeptides. Immunology 1989;66:517.
272. Bofill M, Akbar AN, Salmon M, et al: Immature CD45RA low RO low T cells in the human cord blood. I. Antecedents of $CD45RA^+$ unprimed T cells. J Immunol 1994;152:5613.
273. Rayfield LS, Brent L, Rodeck CH: Development of cell mediated lympholysis in human foetal blood lymphocytes. Clin Exp Immunol 1980;42:561.
274. Horgan KJ, van Seventer GA, Shimizu Y, et al: Hyporesponsiveness of naive (CD45RA) human T cells to multiple receptor-mediated stimuli but augmentation of responses by co-stimulation. Eur J Immunol 1990;20:1111.
275. Durie FH, Foy TM, Masters SR, et al: The role of CD40 in regulation of humoral and cell mediated immunity. Immunol Today 1994;15:406.
276. Ehlers S, Smith KA: Differentiation of T cell lymphokine expression: the in vitro acquisition of T cell memory. J Exp Med 1991;173:25.
277. Mosmann TR, Coffman RL: TH1 and TH2 cells: different patterns of lymphokine secretion lead to different functional properties. Annu Rev Immunol 1989;7:145.
278. Linsley PS, Brady W, Grosmaire L, et al: Binding of the B cell activation antigen B7 to CD28 costimulates T cell proliferation and interleukin-2 mRNA accumulation. J Exp Med 1991;173:721.
279. Hayward AR, Lee J, Beverley PC: Ontogeny of expression of UCHL1 on TCD1 and TCR-delta positive cells. Eur J Immunol 1989;19:771.
280. Krammer PH, Dhen J, Walczak H, et al: The role of APO-1 mediated apoptosis in the immune system. Immunol Rev 1994;142:175.
281. Spriggs MK, Armitage RJ, Strockbine L, et al: Recombinant human CD40 ligand stimulates B cell proliferation and immunoglobulin E secretion. J Exp Med 1992;176:1543.
282. Durandy A, De Saint Basile G, Lisowska-Grospierre B, et al: Undetectable CD40 ligand expression on T cells and low B cell responses to CD40 binding agonists in human newborns. J Immunol 1995;154:1560.
283. Christensen KK, Christensen P, Duc G, et al: Correlation between serum antibody levels against group B streptococci and gestational age in newborns. Eur J Pediatr 1984;142:86.
284. Baker CJ, Edwards MS, Kasper DL: Role of antibody to native type III polysaccharide of group B streptococcus in infant infection. Pediatrics 1981;68:544.
285. Klegerman ME, Boyer KM, Papierniak CK, et al: Estimation of the protective level of human IgG antibody to the type-specific polysaccharide of group B streptococcus type Ia. J Infect Dis 1983;148:648.
286. Gotoff SP, Papierniak CK, Klegerman ME, et al: Quantitation of IgG antibody to the type specific polysaccharide of group B streptococcus type Ib in pregnant women and infected infants. J Pediatr 1984;105:628.
287. Mond JJ, Vos Q, Lees A, et al: T cell independent antigens. Curr Opin Immunol 1995;7:349.
288. Sancho L, de la Hera A, Gasas J, et al: Two different maturational states of natural killer lymphocytes in human newborns. J Pediatr 1991;119:446.
289. Yabuhara A, Kawai H, Kamiyama A: Development of the natural killer cytotoxicity during childhood: marked increase in the number of natural killer cells with adequate cytotoxic abilities during infancy to early childhood. Pediatr Res 1990;28:316.
290. Gaddy J, Risdon G, Broxmeyer HE: Cord blood natural killer cells are functionally and phenotypically immature but readily respond to interleukin-2 and interleukin-12. J Interferon Cytokine Res 1995;15:527.
291. Kohl S: The neonatal human's immune response to herpes simplex virus infection: a critical review. Pediatr Infect Dis J 1989;8:67.
292. Kohl S: Protection against murine neonatal herpes

simplex virus infection by lymphokine-treated human leukocytes. J Immunol 1990;144:307.
293. Sullender WM, Miller JL, Yasvkawa LL, et al: Humoral and cell-mediated immunity in neonates with herpes simplex virus infections. J Infect Dis 1987;155:28.
294. Nonoyama S, Penix LA, Edwards CP, et al: Diminished expression of CD40 ligand by activated neonatal T cells. J Clin Invest 1995;95:66.
295. Brugnoni D, Airo P, Graf D, et al: Ineffective expression of CD40 ligand on cord blood T cells may contribute to poor immunoglobulin production in newborns. Eur J Immunol 1994;24:1919.
296. Hunt DW, Huppertz HI, Jiang HJ, et al: Studies of human cord blood dendritic cells: evidence for functional immaturity. Blood 1994;84:4333.
297. Hong R: Disorders of the T-cell system. In Stiehm ER (ed): Immunologic Disorders in Infants and Children, 4th ed. Philadelphia: WB Saunders, 1996, pp 339–408.
298. Kirkpatrick CH, Rich RR, Bennett JE: Chronic mucocutaneous candidiasis: model-building in cellular immunity. Ann Intern Med 1971;74:955.
299. Reiner SL, Locksley RM: The regulation of immunity to *Leishmania major*. Annu Rev Immunol 13: 151, 1995.
300. Romani L, Cenci E, Mencacci A, et al: Gamma interferon modifies $CD4^+$ subset expression in murine candidiasis. Infect Immun 1992;60:4950.
301. Burchett SK, Carey L, Mohan KM, et al: Diminished interferon-gamma and lymphocyte proliferation in neonatal and postpartum primary herpes simplex virus infection. J Infect Dis 1992;165:813.
302. Mar'odi L, Kaposzta R, Campbell DE, et al: Candidacidal mechanisms in the human neonate: impaired IFN-gamma activation of macrophages in newborn infants. J Immunol 1994;153:5643.
303. Gathings WE, Mage RG, Cooper MD, et al: Immunofluorescent studies on the development of pre-B cells, B lymphocytes, and immunoglobulin isotype diversity in humans. Eur J Immunol 1977;7:804.
304. Gupta S, Pahwa R, O'Reilly R, et al: Ontogeny of lymphocyte subpopulations in human fetal liver. Proc Natl Acad Sci U S A 1976;73:919.
305. Hayward AR, Ezer G: Development of lymphocyte populations in human thymus and spleen. Clin Exp Immunol 1974;17:169.
306. Nossal GJV: Cellular mechanisms of immunologic tolerance. Annu Rev Immunol 1983;1:33.
307. Raff MC, Owen JJ, Cooper MD, et al: Differences in susceptibility of mature and immature mouse B lymphocytes to anti-immunoglobulin–induced immunoglobulin suppression in vitro. Possible implications for B cell tolerance of self. J Exp Med 142:1975.
308. Manning DD, Jutila JW: Immunosuppression in mice injected with heterologous anti-immunoglobulin antisera. J Immunol 1972;108:282.
309. Metcalf ES, Klinman NR: In vitro tolerance induction of neonatal murine B cells. J Exp Med 1976;143:1327.
310. Lawton AR: B cell development. In Polin RA, Fox WW (eds): Fetal and Neonatal Physiology, 2nd ed. Philadelphia: WB Saunders.
311. Korsmeyer SJ, Hieter PA, Ravetch JV, et al: Developmental hierarchy of immunoglobulin rearrangement in human leukemic pre-B cells. Proc Natl Acad Sci U S A 1981;78:7096–7100.
312. Alt FW, Oltz EM, Young F, et al: VDJ recombination. Immunology Today 1992;13:306.
313. Riley SC, Brock EJ, Kuehl WM: Induction of light chain expression in a pre-B cell line by fusion to myeloma cells. Nature 1981;289:804.
314. Allansmith M, McClellan BH, Butterworth M, et al: The development of immunoglobulin levels in man. J Pediatr 1968;72:276.
315. Kincade PW, Lawton AR, Bockman DE, et al: Suppression of immunoglobulin G synthesis as a result of antibody-mediated suppression of immunoglobulin M synthesis in chickens. Proc Natl Acad Sci U S A 1970;67:1918.
316. Lawton AR, Asofsky R, Hylton MB, et al: Suppression of immunoglobulin class synthesis in mice. I. Effects of treatment with antibody to μ chain. J Exp Med 1972;135:277.
317. Cooper MD, Lawton AR: The development of the immune system. Sci Am 1974;231:58.
318. Purkerson J, Isakson P: A two signal-model for regulation of immunoglobulin isotype switching. FASEB J 1992;6:3245.
319. Noelle RJ, Roy M, Shepherd DM, et al: A 39-kDa protein on activated T helper cells binds CD40 and transduces the signal for cognate activation of B cells. Proc Natl Acad Sci U S A 1992;89:6550.
320. Defrance T, Van Bervliet B, Briere F, et al: Interleukin-10 and transforming growth factor β cooperate to induce anti-CD40-activated naive human B cells to secrete immunoglobulin A. J Exp Med 1992;175:671.
321. Van Furth R, Schuit HR, Hijmans W: The immunologic development of the human fetus. J Exp Med 1965;122:1173.
322. Cates KL, Rowe JC, Ballow M: The premature infant as a compromised host. Curr Prob Pediatr 1983;13:1.
323. Buckley RH, Dees SC, O'Fallon WM: Serum immunoglobulins. I. Levels in normal children and in uncomplicated childhood allergy. Pediatrics 1968;41: 600.
324. Adderson EE, Johnston JM, Shackelford PG, et al: Development of the human antibody repertoire. Pediatr Res 1992;32:257.
325. Keightley RK, Cooper MD, Lawton AR: The T cell dependence of B cell differentiation induced by pokeweed mitogen. J Immunol 1976;117:1538.
326. Wu LYF, Bianco A, Cooper MD, et al: Ontogeny of B lymphocyte differentiation induced by pokeweed mitogen. Clin Immunol Immunopathol 1976;5:208.
327. Hayward AR, Lawton AR: Induction of plasma cell differentiation of human fetal lymphocytes: evidence for functional immaturity of T and B cells. J Immunol 1977;119:1213.
328. Splawski JB, Jelinek DF, Lipsky PE: Delineation of the functional capacity of human neonatal lymphocytes. J Clin Invest 1991;87:545.
329. Splawski JB, Lipsky PE: Cytokine regulation of immunoglobulin secretion by neonatal lymphocytes. J Clin Invest 1991;88:967.
330. Lewis DB, Yu CC, Meyer J, et al: Cellular and molecular mechanisms for reduced interleukin-4 and interferon-gamma production by neonatal T cells. J Clin Invest 1991;87:194.
331. Schibler KR, Liechty KW, White WL, et al: Defective production of interleukin-6 by monocytes: a possible mechanism underlying several host defense deficiencies of neonates. Pediatr Res 1992;31:18.
332. Chheda S, Palkowetz KH, Garofalo R, et al: Decreased interleukin-10 production by neonatal monocytes and T cells: relationship to decreased production and expression of tumor necrosis factor-alpha and its receptors. Pediatr Res 1996;40:475.

333. Allen RL, Armitage RJ, Conley ME, et al: CD40 ligand gene defects responsible for X-linked hyper-IgM syndrome. Science 1993;259:990.
334. Aruffo A, Farrington M, Hollenbaugh D, et al: The CD40 ligand GP39 is defective in activated T cells from patients with X-linked hyper-IgM syndrome. Cell 1993;72:291.
335. Pui CH, Kane JR, Crist WM: Biology and treatment of infant leukemias. Leukemia 1995;9:762.
336. Sorensen PH, Chen CS, Smith FO, et al: Molecular rearrangements of the MLL gene are present in most cases of infant acute myeloid leukemia and are strongly correlated with monocytic or myelomonocytic phenotypes. J Clin Invest 1994;93:429.
337. Lange BJ, Kabrinsky N, Barnard DR, et al: Distinctive demography, biology, and outcome of acute myeloid leukemia and myelodysplastic syndrome in children with Down syndrome: Children's Cancer Group studies 2861 and 2891. Blood 1998;91:608.
338. Zipursky A, Brown E, Christensen H, et al: Leukemia and/or myeloproliferative syndrome in neonates with Down syndrome. Semin Perinatol 1997;21:97.

CHAPTER 15

Complement System Development and Disorders During the Neonatal Period

Herbert A. Lassiter, M.D., Erzsebet Jung, M.D., and Karen M. Cost, Ph.D.

The complement system participates in essential physiologic and pathophysiologic events, including opsonization, cellular adherence, chemotaxis, cytolysis, platelet aggregation, and anticoagulant and procoagulant activity. This chapter summarizes the findings of basic and clinical research on these topics, suggests potential clinical applications of the information, and indicates unexplored areas to direct future research. An exhaustive discussion of the complement system is not attempted because excellent reviews are available.[1–6] Instead, the focus is on the aspects of complement that are most relevant to the hematologic problems observed in newborn infants.

HISTORICAL BACKGROUND

The complement system has been recognized as an important component of host immunity for more than 100 years. Between 1960 and 1980, the chemical nature of complement was demonstrated, the mechanisms of complement-mediated actions were investigated, and functional assessment of the complement system in newborn infants was initiated.[7–11] By 1980, the various proteins that compose the complement system in plasma had been described. Subsequently, intense research efforts were directed toward understanding the molecular mechanisms responsible for the development, expression, activation, regulation, and functions of complement.[12]

During the past 2 decades, investigators have studied the role of complement activation and complement deficiency in the pathogenesis of a variety of conditions relevant to newborn infants. Examples include immune cytopenias,[13–18] blood transfusion reactions,[19] disseminated intravascular coagulation,[20] advanced bacterial sepsis and septic shock,[21, 22] postischemic reperfusion injury,[23, 24] multiorgan failure,[25] intraoperative cardiopulmonary bypass,[26] deleterious complications of extracorporeal membrane oxygenation,[27] and rejection of transplanted organs.[28–32] In these and other conditions, the role of complement is inextricably linked to the roles of leukocytes, platelets, erythrocytes, and the plasma proteins that compose the coagulation system.

The pathogenic role of complement has become increasingly relevant with the discovery of inhibitors of complement activity such as C1 inhibitor, humanized monoclonal anti-C5 antibody, and soluble complement receptor type 1 (sCR1).[33–35] For instance, clinical trials have been initiated to assess the effect of sCR1 in the treatment of adult respiratory distress syndrome, pulmonary transplantation, and myocardial infarction.[36] As new strategies are developed to modulate complement activity for the prevention and treatment of human disease, an understanding of the complement system and its regulation will undoubtedly become increasingly pertinent to health professionals who provide care to newborn infants.

OVERVIEW OF COMPLEMENT ACTIVATION

The complement system, broadly defined, comprises at least 20 circulating plasma proteins, five membrane-bound proteins that regulate the binding or degradation of complement components, and seven membrane-bound protein receptors that bind complement components or cleavage fragments of components (Table 15–1). Functional overlap occurs, as exemplified by CR1, which serves as regulator and receptor.

The complement cascade (Fig. 15–1) may be activated by either of two pathways. The classic pathway of complement is characteristically activated after the binding of plasma C1q by antigen-antibody complexes. For example, after specific IgG antibodies bind to the surface of a bacterium, the Fc (crystalline fraction) portion of the antibody undergoes a conformational change that permits binding of C1q, thereby initiating activation of the complement cascade through the classic pathway. Ultimately, as seen in Figure 15–1, the classic pathway C3/C5 convertase is assembled, and complement component C3 is enzymatically cleaved. C3a is released into the surrounding medium, and C3b binds to the target membrane.[37]

Activation of the alternative pathway characteristically occurs in the absence of specific antibody. Instead, certain biologic surfaces have the capacity to directly activate the alternative pathway by binding C3b, which under normal conditions is spontaneously formed in plasma at a low concentration.[38, 39] Examples of surfaces that activate the alternative pathway include hemodialysis and oxygenator membranes,[40–42] endotoxin, many strains of gram-positive and gram-negative bacteria, and some fungi, viruses, and tumor cells.[43] Surfaces that activate the alternative pathway provide an environment that protects C3b from degradation by the circulating regulatory proteins factors H and I. Consequently, membrane-bound C3b may participate in the formation of the alternative pathway C3/C5 convertase, an enzyme that accelerates cleavage of C3, resulting in amplification of C3b deposition on the activating surface.[44] The two activation pathways are not mutually exclusive. For instance, C3b derived from classic pathway activation may initiate activation of the alternative pathway.

Many of the bacteria that invade neonates

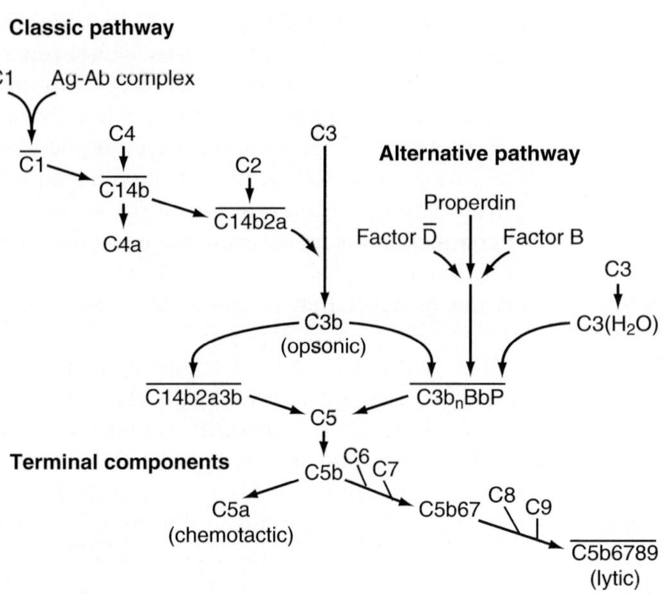

Figure 15–1. Complement activation. The classic and alternative pathways intersect at C3, followed by incorporation of the terminal components to assemble the membrane attack complex $C5b678(9)_n$. Enzymatically active proteases that cleave and activate subsequent components are shown with an overbar. (Adapted from Lewis DB, Wilson CB: Developmental immunology and role of host defenses in neonatal susceptibility to infection. In Remington JS, Klein JO [eds]: Infectious Diseases of the Fetus and Newborn Infant, 4th ed. Philadelphia: WB Saunders, 1995, p 64.)

Table 15–1. **The Proteins of the Human Complement System**

	Component	Molecular Weight (kd)	Subunit Structure	Plasma Concentration mg/L	Plasma Concentration (μM)	Role
Classic pathway	C1q	460	6A chains (26 kd), 6B chains (26 kd), 6C chains (24 kd)	80	(0.15)	Binds Ig; initiates classic pathway activation
	C1r	83	Single, complex with C1q	50	(0.30)	Cleaves/activates C1s
	C1s	83	In plasma ($C1qC1r_2C1s_2$)	50	(0.30)	Cleaves/activates C4 and C2
	C4	205	1 α-chain (97 kd), 1 β-chain (75 kd), 1 γ-chain (33 kd)	600	(3.0)	Binds C2 during activation
	C2	102	Single chain	20	(0.20)	Cleaves/activates C3 and C5
Alternative pathway	Factor B	93	Single chain	210	(2.0)	Cleaves/activates C3 and C5
	Factor D	24	Single chain	2	(0.05)	Cleaves/activates Factor B
	Properdin	220	4 Identical subunits (55 kd)	26	(0.10)	Stabilizes activation pathway convertases
Common	C3	185	1 α-chain (110 kd); 1 β-chain (75 kd)	1300	(7.0)	Binds C5 in convertases; opsonization/chemotaxis, etc.
Membrane attack pathway	C5	190	1 α-chain (115 kd); 1 β-chain (75 kd)	70	(0.4)	Initiates membrane attack; C5a major chemotactic/anaphylactic peptide
	C6	120	Single chain	65	(0.5)	
	C7	110	Single chain	55	(0.5)	Self-associate with cleaved C5 to form membrane sites to which C9 can bind
	C8	150	1 α-chain (64 kg), 1 β-chain	55	(0.4)	
	C9	69	Single chain	60	(0.8)	Major component of MAC
Soluble control	C1-INH	110	Single chain	200	(1.8)	Binds C1r + C1s, dissociates C1
	C4bp	500	8 Identical subunits (70 kd)	250	(0.5)	Accelerates decay of C4b2a cofactor for C4b cleavage by I
	Factor H	150	Single chain	450	(3.0)	Accelerates decay of C3bBb, cofactor for C3b cleavage by I; cleaves/inactivates C4b + C3b
	Factor I	80	1 α-chain (50 kd), 1 β-chain (38 k)	35	(0.4)	
	S-protein	83	Single chain	500	(6.0)	Binds fluid-phase C5b-7
	Sp—40,40	70	2 Subunits (35 kd)	50		Binds fluid-phase C5b-7
Membrane control	CR1	160–250	Single chain			Accelerate decay of C3/C5 convertases; cofactor in C3b cleavage
	DAF	70	Single chain			
	MCP	45–70	Single chain			
	HRF/MIP	65	Single chain			Control of MAC formation/activity
	CD59 antigen	20	Single chain			

CR1, complement receptor-1; DAF, decay accelerating factor; HRF, homologous restriction factor; MAC, membrane attack complex; MCP, membrane cofactor protein; MIP, membrane attack complex inhibitory protein.

Adapted from Morgan BP: The complement system. In Morgan BP (ed): Complement: Clinical Aspects and Relevance to Disease. London: Academic Press, 1990, pp 10–11. Copyright 1990, by permission of the publisher Academic Press Limited.

express capsules that inhibit activation of the alternative pathway. Antibody-mediated activation of complement is consequently required to efficiently prepare (opsonize) these bacteria for recognition, ingestion, and killing by phagocytes. Examples include type III group B streptococci, *Escherichia coli* that express the K1 antigen, and blood isolates of coagulase-negative staphylococci.[45–50]

Activation of the classic or alternative pathway results in the formation of a C3/C5 convertase, which cleaves circulating C5. Biologically active C5a is released into the surrounding fluid medium, and C5b binds to the targeted membrane. The sequential binding of C6, C7, C8, and several molecules of C9 results in assembly of the membrane attack complex, a pore-forming tubular structure that may penetrate the lipid bilayer of cells, resulting in cell activation, injury, or lysis.[51, 52]

ONTOGENY OF COMPLEMENT COMPONENT SYNTHESIS

The appearance in serum of complement components, complement-mediated hemolytic activity, and complement regulatory proteins occurs early in gestation (e.g., between 8 and 14 weeks in the human fetus). The preponderance of evidence suggests that serum concentrations of complement components depend on fetal synthesis and that maternal components are not transferred across the placenta.[53, 54] In the mature subject, the major site of complement component synthesis is the liver, with the notable exception of C7.[55] In the embryo and early fetus, the major sites of synthesis have not been well defined, but extrahepatic sites may possibly predominate. For instance, in the quail embryo, the major site of C3 synthesis is the reticuloendothelial system.[56]

In the various species studied, serum concentrations of complement and complement-mediated hemolytic activity gradually increase during gestation but do not achieve adult levels until several weeks after delivery.[57–59] In human infants, deficiencies of complement components are more pronounced in prematurely born subjects, and the serum concentrations of most complement proteins are within the adult range of normal by 6 to 18 months of age.[60, 61]

The molecular mechanisms that regulate the synthesis of complement components, regulatory proteins, and receptors during development are poorly understood. Although the structures and chromosomal locations of the various genes that code for human complement proteins have in most cases been determined,[62] the mechanisms that control the expression of these genes during development have not been defined. Some information is available. For instance, interleukin (IL)-1α, IL-6, and tumor necrosis factor enhance the synthesis and expression of alternative pathway and terminal complement components by endothelial cells isolated from the umbilical cord veins of human newborn infants.[63, 64] Whether cytokines participate in the gradual maturation of the complement system during gestation and the first few weeks of life is unknown.

PHYSIOLOGIC AND PATHOPHYSIOLOGIC CONSEQUENCES OF COMPLEMENT ACTIVATION

Activation of the complement system is a prerequisite for effective host resistance to invasion by infectious agents, including bacteria, fungi, and viruses. However, focal and systemic complement activation may also participate in the pathogenesis of a wide variety of disease states. Table 15–2 indicates neonatal hematologic disorders in which complement activation occurs and may participate in the pathogenesis. The following discussion addresses the physiologic and pathophysiologic consequences of complement activation on opsonization, cellular adherence, chemotaxis, cytolysis, platelet aggregation, and anticoagulant or procoagulant activity.

Opsonization

Opsonization is the process by which particulate antigens are prepared for recognition and ingestion by phagocytes such as polymorphonuclear neutrophils, circulating monocytes, and tissue macrophages. For instance, most pathogenic bacteria are neither recognized nor ingested by phagocytes unless specific antibody or

Table 15–2. **Neonatal Hematologic Disorders with Complement Activation**

- Anemia and/or hyperbilirubinemia
  - Alloimmune hemolytic anemia (ABO or Rh incompatibility)
  - Autoimmune hemolytic anemia
    - Maternal autoimmune hemolytic anemia
- Thrombocytopenia
  - Alloimmune thrombocytopenia
  - Autoimmune thrombocytopenia
    - Maternal ITP
    - Maternal SLE
  - Bacterial, fungal, viral sepsis
  - Cardiopulmonary bypass, ECMO
- Neutropenia
  - Alloimmune neutropenia
  - Autoimmune neutropenia
    - Maternal autoimmune neutropenia (SLE)
  - Sepsis
  - Cardiopulmonary bypass, ECMO
- Coagulopathy
  - Disseminated intravascular coagulation

ECMO, extracorporeal membrane oxygenation; ITP, idiopathic thrombocytopenic purpura; SLE, systemic lupus erythematosus.

complement components are deposited onto the bacterial surface. Neutrophils, monocytes, and macrophages express surface receptors for the Fc portion of IgG antibodies and for the opsonic cleavage fragments of C3, particularly C3b and iC3b.

Opsonization of bacteria in newborn infants, compared with adults, is relatively inefficient, particularly in prematurely born infants. Consequently, the capacity of neonates to restrict the dissemination of bacteria that colonize mucosal or cutaneous surfaces and become focally invasive is compromised. Much of this opsonic inefficiency can be ascribed to a deficiency of specific antibody.[47, 65–68] However, diminished serum concentrations of complement components (Table 15–3) and functional limitations of the complement system may also restrict the capacity of neutrophils to kill bacteria in the neonatal host. C3 is the major opsonic component of the complement system. In healthy neonatal animals, the deposition of C3 onto bacteria does not appear to be significantly restricted if supplemental opsonic antibody is provided.[49] However, C3 deposition by serum from human neonates with suspected or proven sepsis is reduced even after the administration of intravenous immunoglobulin (IVIG),[69, 70] a phenomenon that may possibly restrict the rate of bacterial clearance and limit the therapeutic efficacy of IVIG in neonatal sepsis.

Compared with C3 from adults, C3 from newborn infants demonstrates reduced reactivity of the internal thiolester bond. After complement activation, the internal thiolester bond of circulating C3 is disrupted, exposing a reactive glutamyl residue that binds covalently to hydroxyl or amino groups on the bacterial surface. Consequently, the expression of opsonic activity by surface-bound cleavage products of C3 (i.e., C3b and iC3b) is facilitated. The developmental restriction of C3 internal thiolester bond reactivity observed in neonates is directly related to the degree of prematurity.[71]

Impairment of opsonization may be exacerbated by the restricted capacity of neutrophils from newborn infants to express and up-regulate complement receptor type 3 (CR3),[72–74] which serves as a ligand for iC3b bound to the surface of opsonized bacteria and also as an adhesion molecule that mediates binding of leukocytes to activated endothelial cells. Although most studies indicate that the capacity of neutrophils from healthy term neonates to ingest and kill bacteria is normal, it is possible that limited expression of CR3 may contribute to the restricted bactericidal capacity observed in neutrophils obtained from ill or premature neonates.[10, 75–80] The administration of human recombinant granulocyte colony-stimulating factor to uninfected, but not to septic, neutropenic neonates enhances the surface expression of the neutrophil complement receptors CR1 and CR3. This observation supports the theory that down-regulation or consumption of neutrophil complement receptors may contribute to the opsonic defect and high mortality of septic neonates.[81]

Adherence

To migrate from the bloodstream to parenchymal sites of infection or tissue injury, leukocytes must first adhere to endothelial cells. The capacity of circulating cells to adhere to microvascular endothelial cells is modulated in part by the complement system. After a variety of focal or systemic insults such as ischemia, hypoxia, bacterial invasion, or cardiopulmonary bypass, adherence molecules may be up-regulated on the surfaces of phagocytes and endothelial cells. Intense investigation is under way to determine the complex mechanisms that control

Table 15–3. **Complement Systems of Preterm and Term Infants Compared with Adult Controls**

	Preterm Newborn (GA 28–33 weeks) (Mean ± 1 SD)	Preterm Newborn (GA 34–36 weeks) (Mean ± 1 SD)	Term Newborn (GA 37–42 weeks) (Mean ± 1 SD)	Adult (Mean ± 1 SD)	*P* Value* 1	*P* Value 2	*P* Value 3	*P* Value 4
AP50	49.2 ± 15.9 (n: 12)	53.3 ± 16.6 (n: 20)	59.9 ± 21.3 (n: 33)	93.1 ± 8.8 (n: 59)	NS	NS	<0.001	<0.001
CH50	57.5 ± 25 (n: 12)	75.1 ± 30.7 (n: 20)	68.9 ± 25.8 (n: 34)	96.1 ± 10.3 (n: 59)	NS	NS	<0.001	<0.001
P	38.8 ± 15.1 (n: 21)	39.4 ± 16 (n: 18)	57.4 ± 15.2 (n: 32)	99.3 ± 11 (n: 59)	NS	<0.001	<0.001	<0.001
B	52.8 ± 17.1 (n: 25)	47.7 ± 19.1 (n: 35)	63.8 ± 25.7 (n: 47)	99.3 ± 13.1 (n: 59)	NS	0.01	<0.001	<0.001
C1q	36.8 ± 16 (n: 16)	35.1 ± 19 (n: 16)	52.6 ± 16.7 (n: 30)	103 ± 10.2 (n: 59)	NS	0.014	<0.001	<0.001
C1r	45.7 ± 18.1 (n: 16)	60.6 ± 21.2 (n: 16)	70.1 ± 20.6 (n: 35)	93.9 ± 8.9 (n: 59)	0.03	0.021	<0.001	<0.001
C1s	48.7 ± 16 (n: 16)	61.7 ± 13.3 (n: 16)	78.5 ± 13.6 (n: 35)	95.6 ± 7.4 (n: 59)	0.007	<0.001	<0.001	<0.001
C2	62.5 ± 19.1 (n: 19)	73.2 ± 22.8 (n: 30)	79.4 ± 19.1 (n: 45)	101.9 ± 11.3 (n: 59)	NS	0.006	<0.001	<0.001
C3	48.5 ± 19.8 (n: 19)	63.1 ± 27 (n: 32)	71.5 ± 25.3 (n: 48)	96.4 ± 10.7 (n: 59)	NS	0.015	<0.001	<0.001
C4	56.3 ± 16.1 (n: 19)	56.6 ± 23.8 (n: 31)	72.7 ± 22 (n: 48)	99.4 ± 13.8 (n: 59)	NS	0.002	<0.001	<0.001
C5	59.6 ± 16.5 (n: 19)	70.4 ± 23 (n: 32)	70.1 ± 36.7 (n: 48)	96.6 ± 10.9 (n: 59)	NS	NS	<0.001	<0.001
C6	38.7 ± 19.3 (n: 16)	36.3 ± 12.9 (n: 16)	57.6 ± 14.3 (n: 35)	103.2 ± 11 (n: 59)	NS	<0.001	<0.001	<0.001
C7	72.7 ± 15.5 (n: 24)	75.2 ± 18.5 (n: 19)	94.8 ± 13.2 (n: 23)	102.5 ± 16.6 (n: 59)	NS	<0.001	<0.001	NS
C8	28.7 ± 8 (n: 24)	29.1 ± 10.7 (n: 18)	36.2 ± 8.1 (n: 28)	99.8 ± 11.3 (n: 59)	NS	0.003	<0.001	<0.001
C9	32.6 ± 28 (n: 13)	52.8 ± 35 (n: 10)	54.5 ± 6.7 (n: 15)	104.4 ± 18.3 (n: 59)	NS	NS	<0.001	<0.001

GA, gestational age (weeks); NS, not significant.

**P* value 1, preterm newborn (GA 28–33 weeks) vs preterm newborn (GA 34–36 weeks); *P* value 2, preterm newborn (GA 28–36 weeks) vs term newborn (GA 37–42 weeks); *P* value 3, preterm newborn (GA 28–36 weeks) vs adult; *P* value 4, term newborn (GA 37–42 weeks) vs adult.

Data expressed as a percentage of adult control (serum pooled from 15 adults).

From Wolach B, Dolfin T, Regev R, et al: The development of the complement system after 28 weeks' gestation. Acta Paediatr 1997;86:523.

adhesion molecule expression.[82] In addition to complement activation, proposed mechanisms that up-regulate endothelial adhesion molecules include the effects of cytokines, hypoxia, exogenous toxins such as endotoxin, and cell-mediated toxicity.[82, 83]

Adherence of neutrophils to endothelium is a physiologic prerequisite to migration across the endothelial barrier (i.e., transmigration) and movement directed toward a focus of infection (i.e., chemotaxis). Similarly, endothelial adherence of platelets must precede the formation of a hemostatic platelet plug. However, unrestricted adherence may result in pathologic endothelial injury because of release of proteolytic enzymes and reactive oxygen products from aggregated neutrophils.[84–87] Platelet aggregation and unrestricted induction of the coagulation cascade may then occur, causing an entrapment of erythrocytes in the microvascular lumen, local ischemia, amplification of the endothelial injury, interstitial capillary leakage of proteins, extension of injury into the surrounding tissues, and organ dysfunction. In the lung, sublethal complement-mediated endothelial injury is characterized by endothelial swelling, and lethality is associated with disruption of the cell membrane, lifting, necrosis, and then exposure of the basement membrane.[88]

Complement activation may enhance the adherence of neutrophils to endothelial cells by several different mechanisms. For example, C5a is released into the circulation of newborn infants after an event that initiates systemic complement activation such as bacterial sepsis, extracorporeal life support, or cardiopulmonary bypass during cardiac surgery.[26, 27] In vitro binding of C5a to C5a receptors on cultured endothelial cells or neutrophils results in the rapid up-regulation of adhesion molecules such as endothelial P-selectin and neutrophil CD11b/CD18 (i.e., CR3, Mo1, macrophage adhesion protein-1 [MAC-1], $\alpha_M\beta_2$-integrin). Consequently, the activated neutrophils adhere rapidly to endothelial cells.[89, 90] In neonates undergoing extracorporeal membrane oxygenation, complement activation occurs routinely and is associated with the rapid development of neutropenia, probably because of aggregation in the microvasculature.[26, 27]

In addition to observations made in vitro using cultured umbilical vein endothelial cells from human neonates, C5a-mediated neutrophil aggregation in the microvasculature with subsequent endothelial dysfunction has been demonstrated in vivo.[91] In animals infused with autologous plasma activated by incubation with zymosan or with renal dialyzer cellophane (both of which liberate C5a by activating the alternative complement pathway), histologically confirmed pulmonary vessel leukostasis developed and was associated with pulmonary artery hypertension and interstitial edema.[92] Moreover, in an in vivo animal model of postischemic reperfusion injury to skeletal muscle, the administration of the complement inhibitor sCR1 reduced leukocyte venular adherence, increased the number of reperfusing capillaries, and increased tissue viability of the postischemic muscle.[93] In humans, the intradermal injection of activated serum, but not activated C5-deficient serum, results in edema and adherence of neutrophils to the cutaneous vascular endothelium.[94]

C1q, the initial recognition and signaling component of the classic complement pathway, may also induce neutrophil adhesion to microvascular endothelial cells. After binding to circulating antigen-antibody complexes, C1q may then interact with a C1q-binding protein and the C1q receptor expressed by endothelial cells to induce up-regulation of adhesion molecules E-selectin, intercellular adhesion molecule-1 (ICAM-1), and vascular cell adhesion molecule-1. Neutrophils then adhere to the endothelial cells.[95]

Indirectly, the membrane attack complex of complement may augment adhesion of neutrophils to endothelial cells. Assembly of sublytic quantities of attack complexes on the surface of endothelial cells does not directly affect the adhesive properties of the cells. However, assembly of these complexes enhances the endothelial response to tumor necrosis factor-α, which induces expression of the adhesion molecules E-selectin and ICAM-1 on the cell surface.[96]

In addition to serving a signaling function for the up-regulation of adhesion molecules, complement proteins may serve as primary binding sites for neutrophils on endothelial cells. After activation of complement, complement cleavage products such as iC3b may be deposited on endothelial cells.[97] For example, iC3b is deposited on apoptotic human umbilical cord endothelial cells that activate the alternative pathway[98] and on xenogeneic endothelium after antibody-mediated activation of the classic pathway.[99] iC3b serves as a ligand for phagocytes that express CR3, such as neutrophils. Membrane attack complexes (C5b-9) have been identified on the surface of postischemic cardiac endothelial cells in experimental animals.[35] Adherent neutrophils and the assembled membrane attack complexes may then mediate injury to the endothelium.

Complement activation may also promote microvascular sequestration of neutrophils by mechanisms distinct from augmentation of adherence. Zymosan-activated serum, which contains complement activation products such as C5a, rapidly decreases the deformability of rabbit polymorphonuclear neutrophils, probably by inducing polymerization of F-actin. Stiffening reduces the capacity of neutrophils to pass through narrow blood vessels, thereby facilitating rapid in vivo margination of the cells in the capillary bed.[100]

Complement-mediated microvascular aggregation of neutrophils has been demonstrated or implicated in the pathogenesis of several different and apparently unrelated conditions. Examples include postischemic reperfusion injury to the myocardium,[101] skeletal muscle,[93, 102] and intestines[103]; acute respiratory decompensation after the institution of extracorporeal life support in human neonates[27]; and remote lung injury after a variety of insults, including experimental limb ischemia,[102] ischemia of the intestines,[103] thermal cutaneous injury,[104] peritonitis,[104] pancreatitis,[84] endotoxemia,[105] septic shock,[106] and hypovolemic shock.[107]

Complement activation is only one of several possible mechanisms that may augment the adherence of neutrophils to microvascular endothelial cells.[82] The relative importance of complement activation in the genesis of pathologic neutrophil aggregation is unknown, but development of the various conditions described depends on an intact complement system, has been associated with activation of complement, and can be ameliorated with the administration of agents that inhibit the activity of complement. It is tempting to speculate that in selected disease states, complement inhibition with new agents such as sCR1 might reduce microvascular neutrophil aggregation, thereby providing protection to the affected organs in human neonates. Basic and clinical investigations are under way to test this theory.

Chemotaxis

Activation of the complement system results in the liberation of chemoattractants, particularly C5a, that influence the directed migration of leukocytes toward sites of infection, inflammation, or tissue injury. Several different chemotaxins other than complement proteins have been identified.[82] However, the chemoattractant activity of serum is primarily attributable to the capacity of serum to generate C5a.[108] Compared with adult serum, the capacity of neonatal serum to generate chemotactic activity is impaired. Moreover, the capacity of neutrophils from neonates to respond to chemoattractants is restricted, especially if the cells are isolated from septic premature neonates.[109–114] The chemotactic deficiency of neonatal serum in part results from a limited capacity to generate chemoattractant complement activation products and cannot be attributed solely to a deficiency of specific antibody or to the presence of chemotactic inhibitors.[108, 112]

C5a may mediate chemotaxis directly by binding to C5a receptors on the surface of leukocytes[115, 116] or indirectly by mediating the release of IL-8,[117] a chemotactically active chemokine.[118] Studies using animals indicate that complement activation, C5a generation, and C5a-mediated neutrophil recruitment occur at the onset of experimental infection, sterile inflammation, or postischemic reperfusion. The subsequent appearance of chemotactically active IL-8 occurs after a delay of several hours.[119–121] The IL-8 is synthesized and secreted in part by C5a-activated neutrophils that had been initially recruited to the site.[117, 120, 122] C5a also attracts monocytes and stimulates monocytes to produce IL-8.[116, 117]

The importance of C5a in host defense is underscored by the observations that some organisms, such as group B streptococci, *Serratia marcescens*, and *Entamoeba histolytica*, have developed the virulence-enhancing capability to express a protease that cleaves C5a.[123–126] Moreover, animals that lack the C5a receptor are unable to clear intrapulmonary *Pseudomonas aeruginosa*.[127]

The importance of C5a in the pathogenesis

of complement-mediated tissue injury has also been demonstrated. In animal models, the administration of anti-C5a antibodies attenuates postischemic myocardial reperfusion injury and reduces pulmonary injury resulting from *E. coli* sepsis or the rapid intravenous administration of cobra venom factor, conditions known to cause systemic complement activation.[128–137]

The injection of C5a into animals reproduces many of changes in neutrophil kinetics observed when systemic complement activation is induced by an event such as the initiation of extracorporeal membrane oxygenation or the development of bacterial sepsis. Within 5 minutes of receiving intravenous C5a, the blood is essentially devoid of neutrophils. The initial period of neutropenia is followed within 1 to 1.5 hours by neutrophilia (250% to 400% of baseline) accompanied by a relative increase in the number of nonsegmented neutrophils (i.e., bands). These observations are consistent with a rapid C5a-mediated up-regulation of adhesion molecules on neutrophils and endothelial cells resulting in microvascular margination of the neutrophils, followed by C5a-mediated release of bone marrow reserves.[138] C5a promotes several actions that result in the migration of neutrophils from the bone marrow to sites of infection or tissue injury—bone marrow release, adherence, and chemotaxis.

Various therapies employed in newborn infants may affect neutrophil chemotaxis by modulating the generation of C5a in serum or affecting the host response to C5a. The initiation of extracorporeal membrane oxygenation is associated with an abrupt increase in the C5a plasma concentration. This phenomenon may account in part for the neutropenia and acute cardiopulmonary decompensation sometimes observed at the initiation of therapy.[139–142] In vitro, glucose-based dialysis solutions inhibit chemotaxis of human neutrophils toward C5a.[143] Animal studies in vivo reveal that the administration of dexamethasone inhibits neutrophil migration toward intraperitoneally injected zymosan-activated plasma, a source of C5a and the chemotactically active degradation product C5a desArg.[144] Possibly, in newborn infants undergoing peritoneal dialysis or receiving glucocorticoids, impairment of C5a-mediated chemotaxis of their neutrophils may be one of the conditions that predisposes them to the development of infectious complications such as peritonitis and bacterial sepsis.

C3a, like C5a, is a chemotactic complement cleavage product that is generated during activation of the classic or alternative pathway of complement. Human neutrophils express receptors for C5a but not C3a. In contrast, eosinophils express distinct receptors for C3a and C5a.[145] C3a is directly chemotactic for eosinophils but not neutrophils. However, C3a induces eosinophils to secrete an unidentified substance that is chemotactic for neutrophils. The chemotactic activity of C3a on neutrophils is indirect and requires the presence of intermediary cells such as eosinophils. Earlier reports that C3a activates human neutrophils may have resulted from contamination of the experimental neutrophil preparations with eosinophils.[145]

The assembly of sublytic concentrations of membrane attack complexes on endothelial cells may also indirectly modulate chemotaxis by inducing the synthesis and secretion of chemokines. In vitro, neutrophil and monocyte chemotaxis is enhanced by membrane attack complex–induced endothelial secretion of IL-8 and monocyte chemoattractant protein-1.[146]

By the various direct and indirect mechanisms described, C5a, C3a, and the membrane attack complex of complement may participate in the generation of chemotactic activity that accompanies complement activation. In the early phase of an invasive infection, complement-mediated chemotaxis represents an important facet of host resistance. However, in advanced conditions such as septic shock, severe ischemia-reperfusion (e.g., after asphyxia), and the initiation of extracorporeal membrane oxygenation, systemic complement activation may generate excessive cellular adherence and chemotactic activity. Subsequent microvascular leukoagglutination, especially in the lung, may further compromise tissue perfusion and thereby perpetuate the underlying pathologic process.

Cytolysis

The complement system may participate in the lytic destruction of foreign or host cells in two predominant ways. Assembly of a sufficient number of pore-forming membrane attack complexes on the surface of a cell may result in death of the cell in part by means of osmotic lysis.[51, 52] The surface deposition of opsonically active C3 cleavage products on target cells may serve as ligands for phagocytes that ingest and destroy cells (i.e., intracellular lysis).

Compared with adult serum, neonatal serum demonstrates impaired cytolytic activity mediated by the membrane attack complex of complement.[61, 147, 148] This deficiency appears to be one of several immunologic defects that predispose neonates to invasion by bacteria such as *E. coli*.[58] However, the cytolytic activity of complement is a double-edged sword that, if directed toward host cells, can induce tissue injury. It is theoretically possible that inefficient cytolytic activity is a protective mechanism limiting complement-mediated tissue injury in neonates during perinatal insults such as postasphyxial ischemia-reperfusion. Nevertheless, neonatal serum does contain sufficient complement-mediated cytolytic activity to lyse sensitized erythrocytes and kill susceptible strains of bacteria, albeit less efficiently and less rapidly compared with serum from adults.[61, 147, 148]

Cells vary tremendously with respect to their capacity to resist complement cytolytic attack. For instance, only one membrane attack complex is sufficient to lyse an erythrocyte,[149] but multiple complexes are required to kill bacteria or nucleated cells.[150, 151] The assembly of sublytic quantities of membrane attack complexes on the surfaces of leukocytes or endothelial cells results in cell activation rather than cell lysis.[152] Several mechanisms account for the variable sensitivity of cells to complement-mediated lysis. For example, the content of sialic acid in the cell wall or capsule of erythrocytes and bacteria inhibits direct activation of complement through the alternative pathway.[46, 153]

Mammalian cell membranes contain complement regulatory proteins that inhibit C3 deposition and promote degradation of C3 cleavage products on the cell surface. These regulators include CR1, decay accelerating factor, and membrane cofactor protein.[3] Homologous restriction factor and CD59 (i.e., protectin) are membrane-bound proteins that inhibit the assembly of the membrane attack complex.[154, 155] Nucleated mammalian cells such as neutrophils also possess the capacity to extrude membrane attack complexes into the surrounding environment by shedding plasma-membrane vesicles from the cell surface.[152, 156]

Circulating proteins such as vitronectin (complement S-protein) and clusterin (SP-40,40) also regulate complement-mediated cytolysis. Both molecules inhibit the assembly of membrane attack complexes by binding to and solubilizing precursors such as C5b67 that have not yet become attached to the cell membrane and also by inhibiting the incorporation of C9 into the complexes.[63, 157–159] C5b67, like C3b, may bind to any nearby cell. Subsequent lysis may occur when C8 and C9 bind to the C5b67 to form complete membrane attack complexes.[160] If the cell is a circulating erythrocyte, intravascular hemolysis could occur. Vitronectin and clusterin are probably important in the prevention of injury to "innocent bystander" host cells at localized sites of complement activation and also in the setting of systemic complement activation. The roles of vitronectin and clusterin have not been investigated in neonates.

In some circumstances, complement-mediated cytolysis may participate in the development of hemolytic anemia, neutropenia, and thrombocytopenia. Focal or systemic activation of complement from any cause may result in the generation of C3b and C5b67. Antibody-independent deposition of these molecules onto the surface of nearby erythrocytes may facilitate the ingestion and intracellular lysis of the cells by phagocytic leukocytes[161] and may induce cytolysis mediated by the subsequent assembly of membrane attack complexes. However, the most common examples of hemolysis encountered in the neonatal period are antibody mediated.

Although antibodies may mediate hemolysis by phagocytic leukocytes in the absence of complement activation,[162] the hemolytic activity of antierythrocyte antibodies is augmented by the deposition of complement cleavage products on the target cell.[13, 16, 17] For example, anti-A, anti-B, and anti-D antibodies of the IgG class mediate complement activation, resulting in the deposition of complement cleavage products on the surface of erythrocytes. The deposited complement proteins augment the hemolytic activity of these antibodies and reduce the number of antibodies required per erythrocyte to effect lysis.[16] When the concentration of complement components is limiting (possibly in the newborn infant), the susceptibility of erythrocytes to complement-mediated lysis depends on the concentration of sensitizing antibody.[163]

Complement activation may also participate in the pathophysiology of antibody-mediated neutropenia, which may be encountered in systemic lupus erythematosus, after the administration of some medications, and in otherwise healthy newborn infants. In patients with systemic lupus erythematosus, the degree of autoimmune neutropenia correlates with the capacity of their serum to fix C3 onto neutrophils.[18] Complement-dependent antibody-mediated neutropenia may also complicate the administration of medications in some patients.[164] In newborn infants, transplacental transfer of maternal autoimmune or alloimmune antineutrophil IgG antibodies may result in neutropenia if the antibodies possess specificity for one or more surface antigens on the infant's neutrophils.[165] However, the relative role of complement activation in the pathophysiology of neonatal immune neutropenias has not been studied.

Similarly, the role of complement activation in the pathogenesis of thrombocytopenia has not been specifically addressed in the newborn infant. However, studies in adult humans and animals have been informative. In some patients, complement activation undoubtedly participates in the development of thrombocytopenia. Complement proteins have been detected consistently on the surface of platelets obtained from patients who have immune thrombocytopenia.[166–174] Complement-dependent antibody-mediated agglutination, fragmentation, and lysis of platelets have been demonstrated.[14, 15] Platelet agglutination induced by human leukocyte antigen (HLA)–related antibodies depends on the activity of C8 and C9, suggesting a role for the membrane attack complex of complement.[14]

In addition to diminished platelet numbers, complement-dependent antibody-mediated platelet lysis may result in the liberation of thrombogenic platelet microparticles, perhaps explaining in part the paradoxical thrombosis sometimes observed in patients with immune thrombocytopenia.[15] Although antibodies in IgG and IgM classes mediate complement-dependent lysis, IgM antibodies are more potent in the promotion of platelet lysis.[15] In patients with idiopathic thrombocytopenic purpura (ITP), the presence of IgM and C3 on their platelets is associated with the development of severe thrombocytopenia.[175] Because neither IgM nor C3 have been shown to cross the placenta,[53, 54, 66, 176] these observations may explain why some infants have normal platelet counts despite being born to mothers with severe autoimmune thrombocytopenia.

Thrombocytopenia occurs commonly during pregnancy. Approximately 3.6% of pregnant women become newly thrombocytopenic during the pregnancy, and platelet-associated IgG, IgM, and C3 are found on maternal platelets in gestational thrombocytopenia (transient) and ITP (persistent).[177, 178] Transplacental passage of maternal autoimmune or alloimmune IgG antiplatelet antibodies may result in fetal and neonatal immune thrombocytopenia.[179] Antiplatelet antibodies (i.e., anti-P1^{A1}, anti-HLA, ITP autoantibodies, antiphospholipid antibodies, and drug-dependent platelet antibodies) may activate complement, resulting in the deposition of C4, C3, and the C5b-9 complex, thereby mediating platelet lysis.[171, 180–182] C3 is frequently present on the surface of platelets from patients with immune thrombocytopenia and may serve as an opsonic ligand that promotes ingestion of the sensitized platelets by phagocytes, particularly in the spleen and liver.[166–174] High concentrations of nonspecific IgG restrict plasma complement component deposition by serving as a preferred acceptor for the activation fragments C3b and C4b.[183–185] In one study, the administration of IVIG to patients with ITP resulted in a significant decrease in platelet-associated C3 levels. The quantity of C3 deposited on the platelets was inversely correlated with the platelet counts.[186]

The sera of subjects with ITP also contains antibodies that bind to megakaryocyte progenitors and may thereby participate in the development of thrombocytopenia. The megakaryocyte toxicity of these antibodies and the capacity of these antibodies to suppress megakaryocyte formation is complement dependent.[187]

Hemostasis

Interactions between the coagulation and complement systems are complex and only partially understood.[188–192] C1 inhibitor (C1-INH) represents a point of convergence of the contact system of coagulation and the classic pathway of complement activation. C1-INH is the major inhibitor of coagulation factor XIIa and is the only plasma protease inhibitor of activated C1r and C1s, which are subcomponents of the first component of complement.[189] Consequently, attacks of angioedema in patients with hereditary deficiency of C1-INH are characterized by activation of the contact and complement systems.[193] In experimental endotoxemia, the administration of C1-INH attenuates the consumption of antithrombin III, reduces microvascular deposition of fibrin, improves blood pressure and oxygenation, and in C3- or C4-deficient mice improves survival.[20, 194] In septic humans, the likelihood of death is positively correlated with the development of disseminated intravascular coagulation and with the intensity of complement activation and consumption.[195, 196] Because the functional activity of C1-INH is diminished during bacterial sepsis, C1-INH substitution therapy has been proposed as a novel strategy to attenuate activation of the contact and complement systems and to improve clinical outcome.[197]

The complement and blood coagulation systems are also linked by the interaction between C4b-binding protein (C4BP) and protein S.[190] C4BP is a circulating plasma protein that possesses seven α-chain subunits, each of which expresses a binding site for C4b.[188, 198] C4BP inhibits activity of the classic pathway by binding to fluid-phase C4b and serving as a cofactor in the factor I–mediated degradation of membrane-bound C4b.[3, 199] Each C4BP molecule also contains a β chain that possesses an independent single binding site for protein S, which participates in the regulation of the protein C and protein S system of endogenous anticoagulation.[200–202]

Protein S (not to be confused with the unrelated complement S-protein, also known as vitronectin) is a vitamin K–dependent plasma protein that serves as a cofactor for protein C in the inactivation of coagulation factors Va and VIIIa and the consequent inhibition of thrombin generation. In plasma, protein S exists as functionally active free protein (30% to 40%) or as functionally inactive protein reversibly bound to C4BP in an equimolar relationship.[188, 203, 204] The concentration of protein S depends on the concentration of C4BP, an acute-phase protein synthesized in the liver. During bacterial sepsis, protein C activity is significantly reduced and protein S is inhibited by an increased plasma concentration of C4BP. These conditions may possibly exacerbate endothelial procoagulant activity and consumptive coagulopathy and provide a rationale for the proposed use of coagulation inhibitor substitution in the treatment of sepsis.[205]

The significance of C4BP and protein S interactions is underscored by the existence of hereditary protein S deficiency type III. Protein S deficiency results in a predisposition to thrombosis. In the type III variant, the plasma concentration of protein S is normal, but the binding of circulating C4BP to protein S is of such high affinity that the concentration of free protein S is significantly reduced.[204]

In addition to its role as a natural anticoagulant, protein S may influence the complement regulatory activity of C4BP. In the presence of protein S, the number of C4BP molecules that spontaneously bind to the surface of neutrophils is approximately doubled. In areas of inflammation, an increased quantity of C4BP on neutrophils could possibly facilitate the degradation and inactivation of C4b randomly deposited on the cell surface, thereby protecting the neutrophils from "bystander" injury.[206]

The C4BP and protein S interactions are probably important in the regulation of the complement and coagulation systems in newborn infants. However, these interactions have not been studied specifically in human or animal neonates.

Hemostasis is also affected by the procoagulant activity of C3a and C5a generated during complement activation. C5a induces human umbilical vein endothelial cells to synthesize and express tissue factor, an integral membrane glycoprotein that serves as a cofactor for the blood coagulation factor VIIa.[207] Binding of C3a or C5a to their respective receptors on platelets results in platelet activation and aggregation.[208–210] The effect of C5a and C5a-desArg on platelets may also be indirect, requiring the presence of neutrophils. Binding of C5a and C5a-desArg stimulates polymorphonuclear neutrophils to release cathepsin G and platelet-activating factor, which promote activation and aggregation of nearby platelets.[211, 212] At the initiation of extracorporeal membrane oxygenation in the neonate, C3a and C5a generation coincide with activation of the contact system of coagulation and the consumption of platelets.[27] During intraoperative cardiopulmonary bypass or experimental extracorporeal circulation, C3a and C5a plasma concentrations and the consumption of platelets are reduced by bonding heparin to the circuit, administering anti-C5 antibodies, and applying blood ultrafiltration, which enhances clearance of C5a and C3a.[141, 213, 214]

The C5b-9 membrane attack complex of complement also participates in the modulation of hemostatic mechanisms. Complement activation with the subsequent assembly of membrane attack complexes on platelets or endothelial cells induces cellular procoagulant activity by stimulating the endothelial secretion of von Willebrand factor and by up-regulating surface expression of prothrombinase.[191, 215, 216] Moreover, the subsequent generation of thrombin on the platelet surface provides positive feedback of complement-mediated platelet activation. Thrombin interaction with its receptor on the platelet surface induces platelet secretion of the terminal complement components C5, C6, C7, C8, and C9.[217, 218] The membrane attack complex may participate indirectly in thrombogenesis. For instance, platelet aggregation induced by *Streptococcus sanguis*, a major etiologic agent of infective endocarditis, depends on the assembly of membrane attack complexes on the bacterial surface.[219]

Although the products of complement activation have been clearly shown to affect hemostatic mechanisms and could in theory participate in the pathogenesis of a variety of disorders observed in newborn infants, the procoagulant activity of complement has not been investigated in neonates.

NEONATAL MANIFESTATIONS OF COMPLEMENT DISORDERS

Unregulated complement activation and deficiencies of complement proteins participate in a variety of acute neonatal diseases of interest to the hematologist. However, hematologic manifestations of primary disorders of the complement system have rarely been reported in neonates. The list of primary diseases of the complement system with manifestations reported in newborn infants (Table 15–4) is distinguished by its brevity. As the role of complement in the pathogenesis of neonatal disease becomes better defined, the recognition and reporting of complement system disorders in neonates probably will increase. The diagnosis of each tabulated disorder depends on recognition of clinical signs consistent with the disorder and measurement of the deficient complement protein in the mother or newborn infant. Treatment is symptomatic.

Table 15–4. **Neonatal Clinical Manifestations of Complement Protein Deficiencies**

Clinical Manifestations	Deficiency
Complete heart block[220, 221] or photosensitive dermatitis[222] (neonatal lupus syndrome)	Maternal C1q, C2, or C4 deficiency with systemic lupus erythematosus[223–227]
Hematuria, hypocomplemententemic glomerulonephritis	Inherited abnormal form of C3[228]
Extensive dermatitis, diarrhea, failure to thrive	C5 deficiency (Leiner's disease)[229–231]
Recurrent pyogenic infections, maculopapular rash, progressive respiratory symptoms, malnutrition, leukocytosis, eosinophilia	Leukocyte CR1 deficiency (hyperimmunoglobulin E [Job's] syndrome)[232]
Omphalitis, delayed umbilical cord separation, recurrent pyogenic infections, lymphopenia, lymphoid tissue hypoplasia	Leukocyte CR3 deficiency (leukocyte adhesion deficiency)[82, 233–235]

Reported primary complement disorders in neonates are rare in part because of an estimated prevalence of inherited diseases of complement of only 0.03%.[236] Although acquired chronic diseases of the complement system are relatively common, these conditions almost invariably become symptomatic after the neonatal period. The assays of complement activity in specimens obtained from newborn infants are difficult to interpret. The concentration or function of most complement proteins is diminished in neonates compared with other age groups (see Table 15–3), and normal reference values are frequently unavailable or relatively inaccessible. Primary disorders of the complement system probably are under-recognized in the neonate.

FUNCTIONAL AND QUANTITATIVE ASSAYS OF COMPLEMENT

Larger reference laboratories in the United States offer more than 40 different complement tests for evaluation of the complement system. Many of these procedures are for investigational use and not recommended for diagnostic purposes. Of the procedures licensed for in vitro diagnostic use, most are available in clinical immunology or serology laboratories. There are two general categories of complement assays: tests that detect a biologic effect to measure functional activity or complement system activation and quantitative measurements of individual protein components, their fragments, or complexes.

Functional studies exploit the capacity of activated complement components to lyse erythrocytes. The functional tests most widely used in the clinical immunology laboratory are the 50% hemolytic assay (CH50) for evaluation of classic pathway function and the corresponding AH50 for evaluation of the alternative pathway.[237] Newer enzyme-linked immunosorbent assay (ELISA) procedures for initial screening evaluations are in various stages of release for commercial and diagnostic use and may ultimately replace the AH50 and CH50 techniques.

The CH50 test measures total hemolytic complement activity in serum or other fluids that is mediated by activation of the classic pathway. Sheep erythrocytes (E) coated with anti-sheep E antibodies are lysed by sequential activation of the components of the classic complement pathway[238] (C1-C4), followed by deposition of the terminal components (C5-C9), to form membrane attack complexes (see Fig. 15–1).[52] These pore-forming complexes penetrate the cell wall, permitting quantifiable leakage of hemoglobin molecules into the surrounding medium. There is a positive linear correlation of the quantity of released hemoglobin with the number of lysed erythrocytes. The number of CH50 units per 1 mL is calculated by determining the dilution of serum that can lyse 50% of the sensitized erythrocytes. If one of the classic pathway or terminal components is absent, CH50 activity should be zero.

The AH50 test measures the functional activity of C3 that is shared with the classic pathway and factors D, B and P, which are unique to the alternative pathway (see Fig. 15–1). In the AH50 assay, native (unsensitized) rabbit erythrocytes are lysed if the factors of the alternative pathway[239] and the terminal components are present in adequate concentrations.

Proper sample collection and storage before testing are critical to achieve accuracy in any functional assay of complement activity. C2 and factor B are heat labile, and repeated freeze-thaw cycles cause degradation of critical functional sites, especially the internal thiolester bond of C3.[240] An amount of blood sufficient to yield 0.5 mL of serum should be collected and allowed to clot for 30 to 60 minutes at room temperature or 37°C. It should be centrifuged under temperature-controlled conditions to separate the clot and the serum transferred to a clean plastic tube and frozen at −70°C until assayed. If the sample will be used in multiple assays at different times, it should be divided into single-use aliquots and stored in separate tubes at −70°C to avoid thawing and refreezing. Many laboratories recommend confirmation of any abnormally low CH50 or AH50 result on a freshly collected sample because of the clinical implications and the additional testing indicated by these results.

The CH50 and AH50 tests screen the classic and alternative complement pathways and the terminal components. They cannot detect deficiencies of the circulating regulatory proteins (i.e., factors H and I, C1 inhibitor, C4b binding protein, vitronectin, and clusterin), which must be investigated by other methods.[241] For example, quantitative and functional assays are available to detect genetic and acquired deficiencies of C1 inhibitor, which produce the syndrome of hereditary angioneurotic edema.

CH50 and AH50 tests are limited in detecting clinically significant complement activation that may accompany inflammation or tissue injury. Considerable complement consumption must occur before the CH50 or AH50 are altered.[242] However, even in the absence of significant consumption of components, complement activation can be detected by quantitative measurement of the complement cleavage products, such as C5a, whose concentration may reflect the intensity of the inflammatory process.[243] Reagents in kit form to measure the complement split products C3a desArg, C4a desArg, C5a desArg, iC3b, C4d, Bb and SC5b-9 are commercially available but are restricted to investigational use. Sample quality is critical, because complement activation in vitro during the collection or storage process may generate these cleavage products.

The second category of complement tests, quantitative assays, use specific polyclonal or monoclonal antibodies. C3, C4, C1-INH, and factor B are usually analyzed by radial immunodiffusion or automated nephelometry. More sensitive ELISAs or radioimmunoassays are used for proteins whose plasma concentration is normally low.[237]

Many cell types, including platelets, leukocytes, vascular endothelial cells, erythrocytes, and fibroblasts, have receptors for complement components. Methods using monoclonal antibodies and flow cytometry to quantify membrane-bound complement receptors are available, primarily for investigational purposes.[244]

Studies of complement genes have application in the study of autoimmune diseases, as an adjunct to HLA typing in transplantation and paternity testing, and to confirm inherited deficiencies of the complement system. The genetic polymorphism exhibited by some complement proteins can be detected by a variety of electrophoretic methods or molecular procedures using Southern blot or polymerase chain reaction–based analyses.[245]

Interpretation of data obtained with complement assays can be problematic. Multiple host-related and methodologic factors affect the conclusions drawn from test results. Paramount to the difficulty in interpretation has been the lack of established age-related ranges for preterm and newborn infants. This problem was alleviated with the publication of reference ranges for preterm and term infants for CH50, AH50, factors P and B, and C1-C9 (see Table 15–3).[246]

The reported results of complement assays can additionally be influenced by the specificity of antisera for the native form or split products, the presence of autoantibodies in patient serum, and polymorphism in the genes coding for some of the complement components.[237] Test results are also affected by host factors, such as decreased synthesis of complement components related to nutritional status, and the increases in some complement proteins during the acute-phase response.

Evaluations of the complement system usually begin with CH50 and AH50 tests. As indicated by the results of these screening tests, the investigation proceeds systematically to assays of individual proteins. Algorithms to identify specific complement deficiencies can be found in standard immunology manuals.[237, 241] Because both pathways activate C3 and the terminal components (C5-C9), low values in CH50 and AH50 suggest an abnormality in one of these components. An abnormal CH50 with a normal AH50 implies a defect in the early components of the classic pathway. A defect in the alternative pathway is indicated by a normal CH50 or an abnormal AH50. A CH50 or AH50 value of zero usually indicates a complete absence of a complement component. A value between zero and the lower range of normal is most likely associated with in vivo activation. Quantitative levels or functional assays of specific complement components can then be performed sequentially as indicated.

FUTURE RESEARCH

It may be possible to benefit newborn infants by controlling the complement system. For diseases caused or exacerbated by complement activation, complement inhibition may possibly represent a useful addition to currently available therapies. For diseases caused by or exacerbated by complement deficiency, up-regulation of complement synthesis or the administration of complement proteins may represent useful therapeutic adjuncts. To develop these new approaches, research must be conducted to determine the molecular mechanisms that regulate the neonatal complement system.

Investigations to define the pathogenic role of complement probably will result in novel therapeutic strategies to improve the clinical outcome of newborn infants with a variety of lethal and debilitating conditions. For instance, specific complement inhibitors are being used experimentally to study the pathologic effects of complement activation. These investigations may reveal a role for complement inhibitors in the prevention and treatment of neonatal diseases in which the pathogenesis includes complement activation. In our laboratory, studies have been initiated to determine whether the administration of sCR1 enhances the survival of neurons and oligodendrocytes in a neonatal model of hypoxic-ischemic cerebral injury. A list of candidate hematologic disorders is provided in Table 15–2.

In theory, antibacterial defense could be enhanced in the neonatal host by up-regulating complement synthesis. It is known that various cytokines participate in the regulation of complement protein synthesis,[63, 64, 247–251] but the complement regulatory role of cytokines in the newborn infant has not been studied. In our laboratory, studies have been initiated to identify one or more cytokines that stimulate the hepatic synthesis of plasma complement components in the neonate to enhance bacterial opsonization, bacteriolysis, and neutrophil activation, adherence, and chemotaxis. It is conceivable that the administration of cytokines with these characteristics may be useful in the prevention of nosocomial sepsis in the newborn intensive care unit, perhaps in conjunction with other measures such as the prophylactic administration of IVIG.

Research is needed to better define the role of complement in coagulopathic states such as disseminated intravascular coagulation associated with bacterial sepsis, particularly in the newborn infant. Substitution therapy with the classic pathway inhibitor and natural anticoagulant C1-INH has shown promise.[20, 194] However, this strategy is of unproved clinical efficacy and has not been studied in animal or human neonates. Similarly, studies designed to assess C4BP interactions with S-protein in neonates may yield useful information that could be therapeutically exploited.

Since the first descriptions of the complement system more than 100 years ago, an immense body of information has been compiled. This information probably will take form in new therapeutic interventions to combat the deleterious consequences of unregulated complement activation or to enhance host immunity. The newborn infant should prove to be a major beneficiary.

References

1. Berger M, Frank MM: The serum complement system. In Stiehm ER (ed): Immunologic Disorders in Infants and Children, 4th ed. Philadelphia: WB Saunders, 1996, pp 133–158.
2. Frank MM: The complement system. In Frank MM, Austen KF, Claman HN, Unanue ER (eds): Sampter's Immunologic Diseases, 5th ed. Boston: Little, Brown, 1995, pp 331–352.
3. Morgan BP: The complement system. In Morgan BP (ed): Complement: Clinical Aspects and Relevance to Disease. London: Academic Press, 1990, pp 1–35.
4. Ross GD (ed). Immunobiology of the Complement System: An Introduction for Research and Clinical Medicine. London: Academic Press Limited, 1986.
5. Rother K, Till GO (eds): The complement system. Berlin: Springer-Verlag, 1988.
6. Winkelstein JA: The complement system of the fetus and newborn. In Polin RA, Fox WW (eds): Fetal and Neonatal Physiology, 2nd ed. Vol. 2. Philadelphia: WB Saunders, 1998, pp 1961–67.
7. Adamkin D, Stitzel A, Urmson J, et al: Activity of the alternative pathway of complement in the newborn infant. J Pediatr 1978;93:604.
8. Ballow M, Fang F, Good RA, et al: Developmental aspects of complement components in the newborn: the presence of complement components and C3 proactivator (properdin factor B) in human colostrum. Clin Exp Immunol 1974;18:257.
9. Feinstein PA, Kaplan SR: The alternative pathway of complement activation in the neonate. Pediatr Res 1975;9:803.
10. Miller ME: Phagocytosis in the newborn infant: humoral and cellular factors. J Pediatr 1969;74:255.
11. Stossel TP, Alper CA, Rosen FS: Opsonic activity in the newborn: role of properdin. Pediatrics 1973;52:134.
12. Ross GD: Introduction and history of complement research. In Ross GD (ed): Immunobiology of the Complement System: An Introduction for Research and Clinical Medicine. London: Academic Press, 1986, pp 1–19.
13. Bakacs T, Totpal K, Ringwald G, et al: Comparison of monocyte and complement mediated haemolysis of human A1 erythrocytes: the relationship between antibody, target and effector concentrations in the induction of lysis. J Clin Lab Immunol 1988;25:53.
14. Brant JT, Julius CJ, Osborne JM, et al: The mechanism of platelet aggregation induced by HLA-related antibodies. Thromb Haemost 1996;76:774.
15. Horstman LL, Jy W, Schultz DR, et al: Complement-mediated fragmentation and lysis of opsonized platelets: gender differences in sensitivity. J Lab Clin Med 1994;123:464.
16. Kurlander RJ, Rosse WF, Logue GL: Quantitative influence of antibody and complement coating of red cells on monocyte-mediated cell lysis. J Clin Invest 1978;61:1309.
17. Rothlein R, Springer TA: Complement receptor type three-dependent degradation of opsonized-erythrocytes by mouse macrophages. J Immunol 1985;135:2668.
18. Rustagi PK, Currie MS, Logue GL: Complement-activating antineutrophil antibody in systemic lupus erythematosus. Am J Med 1985;78:971.
19. Kawamata M, Miyabe M, Omote K, et al: Acute pulmonary edema associated with transfusion of packed red blood cells. Intensive Care Med 1995;21:443.
20. Scherer RU, Giebler RM, Schmidt U, et al: The influence of C1-esterase inhibitor substitution on coagulation and cardiorespiratory parameters in an endotoxin-induced rabbit model of hypercoagulability. Semin Thromb Hemost 1996;22:357.
21. Bengtsson A, Redl H, Paul E, et al: Complement and leukocyte activation in septic baboons. Circulatory Shock 1993;39:83.
22. Rother U: Shock and shock fragments. In Rother K, Till GO (eds): The Complement System. Berlin: Springer-Verlag, 1988, pp 504–510.
23. Kilgore KS, Friedrichs GS, Homeister JW, et al: The complement system in myocardial ischaemia/reperfusion injury. Cardiovasc Res 1994;28:437.
24. Vakeva A, Laurila P, Meri S: Loss of expression of protectin (CD59) is associated with complement membrane attack complex deposition in myocardial infarction. Lab Invest 1992;67:608.
25. Miller CG, Cook DN, Kotwal GJ: Two chemotactic factors, C5a and MIP-1 alpha, dramatically alter the mortality from zymosan-induced multiple organ dysfunction syndrome (MODS): C5a contributes to MODS while MIP-1 alpha has a protective role. Mol Immunol 1996;33:1135.

26. Seghaye MC, Grabitz RG, Duchateau J, et al: Inflammatory reaction and capillary leak syndrome related to cardiopulmonary bypass in neonates undergoing cardiac operations. J Thoracic Cardiovasc Surg 1996;112:687.
27. Plotz FB, van Oeveren W, Bartlett RH, et al: Blood activation during neonatal extracorporeal life support. J Thoracic Cardiovasc Surg 1993;105:823.
28. Pratt JR, Hibbs MJ, Laver AJ, et al: Effects of complement inhibition with soluble complement receptor-1 on vascular injury and inflammation during renal allograft rejection in the rat. Am J Pathol 1996;149:2055.
29. Pruitt SK, Bollinger RR: The effect of soluble complement receptor type 1 on hyperacute allograft rejection. J Surg Res 1991;50:350.
30. Ryan US: Complement inhibitory therapeutics and xenotransplantation. Nat Med 1995;1:967.
31. Scoazec JY, Borghi-Scoazec G, Durand F, et al: Complement activation after ischemia-reperfusion in liver allografts: incidence and pathophysiological relevance. Gastroenterology 1997;112:908.
32. Xia W, Fearon DT, Moore FD Jr, et al: Prolongation of guinea pig cardiac xenograft survival in rats by soluble human complement receptor type 1. Transplant Proc 1992;24:479.
33. Buerke M, Murohara T, Lefer AM: Cardioprotective effects of a C1 esterase inhibitor in myocardial ischemia and reperfusion. Circulation 1995;91:393.
34. Thomas TC, Rollins SA, Rother RP, et al: Inhibition of complement activity by humanized anti-C5 antibody and single-chain Fv. Mol Immunol 1996; 33:1389.
35. Weisman HF, Bartow T, Leppo MK, et al: Soluble human receptor type 1: in vivo inhibitor of complement suppressing postischemic myocardial inflammation and necrosis. Science 1990;249:146.
36. Ryan US: Complement inhibition by sCR1 in clinical trials (abstract). Program of the International Business Communications Annual Conference on Controlling the Complement System for Novel Drug Development; San Diego, CA: International Business Communications, 1996, p 3.
37. Hughes-Jones NC: The classical pathway. In Ross GD (ed): Immunobiology of the Complement System: an Introduction for Research and Clinical Medicine. London: Academic Press, 1986, pp 21–44.
38. Lachmann PJ, Hughes-Jones NC: Initiation of complement activation. Semin Immunopathol 1984;7:143.
39. Pangburn MK, Schreiber RD, Mhller-Eberhard HJ: Formation of the initial C3 convertase of the alternative complement pathway. J Exp Med 1981;154:856.
40. Cheung AK, Parker CJ, Wilcox L, et al: Activation of the alternative pathway of complement by cellulosic hemodialysis membranes. Kidney Int 1989;36:257.
41. Pertosa G, Tarantino EA, Gesualdo L, et al: C5b-9 generation and cytokine production in hemodialyzed patients. Kidney Int 1993;41:S221.
42. Tamiya T, Yamasaki M, Maeo Y, et al: Complement activation in cardiopulmonary bypass, with special reference to anaphylatoxin production in membrane and bubble oxygenators. Ann Thorac Surg 1988;46:47.
43. Pangburn MK: The alternative pathway. In Ross GD (ed): Immunobiology of the Complement System: An Introduction for Research and Clinical Medicine. London: Academic Press, 1986, pp 45–86.
44. Göetz O: The alternative pathway of activation. In Rother K, Till GO (eds): The Complement System. Berlin: Springer-Verlag, 1988, pp 154–168.
45. Edward MS, Nicholson-Weller A, Baker CJ, et al: The role of specific antibody in alternative complement pathway-mediated opsonophagocytosis of type III, group B streptococcus. J Exp Med 1980;151:1275.
46. Edward MS, Kasper DL, Jennings HJ, et al: Capsular sialic acid prevents activation of the alternative complement pathway by type III, group B streptococci. J Immunol 1982;128:1278.
47. Fleer A, Gerards LJ, Aerts P, et al: Opsonic defense to *Staphylococcus epidermidis* in the premature neonate. J Infect Dis 1985;5:930.
48. Givner LB, Edward MS, Anderson DC, et al: Immune globulin for intravenous use: enhancement of in vitro opsonophagocytic activity of neonatal serum. J Infect Dis 1985;151:217.
49. Lassiter H, Christensen RD, Parker CJ: Immunological regulation of *E. coli* K1 by serum from neonatal rats is enhanced following intraperitoneal administration of human IgG. J Infect Dis 1989;159:518.
50. Stevens P, Huang SN-Y, Welch WK, et al: Restricted complement activation by *Escherichia coli* with the K-1 capsular serotype: a possible role in pathogenicity. J Immunol 1978;121:2174.
51. Esser AF: The membrane attack complex of complement. Yearbook Immunol 1990;6:229.
52. Esser AF: The membrane attack complex of complement. Assembly, structure and cytolytic activity. Toxicology 1994;87:229.
53. Gitlin D, Biasucci A: Development of gamma-G, gamma-A, gamma-M, beta 1C/beta 1A, C1esterase inhibitor, ceruloplasmin, transferrin, hemopexin, haptoglobin, fibrinogen, plasminogen, alpha 1-antitrypsin, orosomucoid, beta-lipoprotein, alpha 2-macroglobulin, and prealbumin in the human conceptus. J Clin Invest 1969;48:1422.
54. Kohler PF: Maturation of the human complement system. I. Onset time and sites of fetal C1q, C4, C3, and C5 synthesis. J Clin Invest 1973;52:671.
55. Wurzner R, Joysey, Lachmann PJ: Complement component C7: Assessment of in vivo synthesis after liver transplantation reveals that hepatocytes do not synthesize the majority of C7. J Immunol 1994;152:4624.
56. Kai C, Yoshikawa Y, Yamanouchi K, et al: Ontogeny of the third component of complement of Japanese quails. Immunology 1985;54:463.
57. Abe T, Komatsu M, Oishi T, et al: Development and genetic differences of complement activity in rabbits. Anim Blood Groups Biochem Genet 1979;10:19.
58. Lassiter HA, Walz BM, Wilson JL, et al: The administration of complement component C9 enhances the survival of neonatal rats with *Escherichia coli* sepsis. Pediatr Res 1997;42:128.
59. Tyler JW, Cullor JS, Douglas VL, et al: Ontogeny of the third component of complement in swine. Am J Vet Res 1989;50:1141.
60. Davis CA, Vallota EH, Forristal J: Serum complement levels in infancy: age related changes. Pediatr Res 1979;13:1043.
61. Notarangelo LD, Chirico G, Chiara A, et al: Activity of the classical and alternative pathways of complement in preterm and small for gestational age infants. Pediatr Res 1984;18:281.
62. Colten HR: Genetics and synthesis of components of the complement system. In Ross GD (ed): Immunobiology of the Complement System. London: Academic Press, 1986, pp 163–181.
63. Berge V, Johnson E, Berge KE: Interleukin-1 alpha, interleukin 6, and tumor necrosis factor alpha increase the synthesis and expression of the functional alternative and terminal complement pathways by human umbilical vein endothelial cells in vitro. APMIS 1996;104:213.

64. Kawakami Y, Watanabe Y, Yamaguchi M, et al: TNF-alpha stimulates the biosynthesis of complement C3 and factor B by human umbilical cord vein endothelial cells. Cancer Lett 1997;116:21.
65. Baker CJ, Kasper DL: Correlation of maternal antibody deficiency with susceptibility to neonatal group B streptococcal infection. N Engl J Med 1976;294:753.
66. Ballow M, Cates LK, Rowe JC, et al: Development of the immune system in very low birth weight (less than 1500 g) premature infants: concentrations of plasma immunoglobulins and patterns of infections. Pediatr Res 1986;20:899.
67. Dossett JH, Williams RD, Quie PG: Studies on the interaction of bacteria, serum factors and polymorphonuclear leukocytes in mothers and newborns. Pediatrics 1969;44:49.
68. Hyvarinen M, Zeltzer P, Oh W, et al: Influence of gestational age on serum levels of alpha-1-fetoprotein, IgG globulin, and albumin in newborn infants. J Pediatr 1973;82:430.
69. Lassiter HA, Speranza MJ, Hall RT, et al: Complement C3 deposition onto bacteria by neonatal serum is not enhanced after the infusion of intravenous immunoglobulin. J Perinatol 1990;10:27.
70. Lassiter HA, Robinson TW, Brown MS, et al: Effect of intravenous immunoglobulin G on the deposition of immunoglobulin G and C3 onto type III group B streptococcus and *Escherichia coli* K1. J Perinatol 1996;16:346.
71. Zach TL, Hostetter MK: Biochemical abnormalities of the third component of complement in neonates. Pediatr Res 1989;26:116.
72. Bruce MC, Baley JE, Medvik KA, et al: Impaired surface membrane expression of C3bi but not C3b receptors on neonatal neutrophils. Pediatr Res 1987;21:306.
73. Smith JB, Campbell DE, Ludormirsky A, et al: Expression of the complement receptors CR1 and CR3 and the type III Fc receptor on neutrophils from newborn infants and from fetuses with Rh disease. Pediatr Res 1990;28:120.
74. Torok C, Lundahl J, Hed J, et al: Diversity of adhesion molecules (Mac-1 and L-selectin) in monocytes and neutrophils from neonates and adults. Arch Dis Child 1993; 68:561.
75. Al-Hadithy H, Addison IE, Goldstone AH, et al: Defective neutrophil function in low-birth-weight premature infants. J Clin Pathol 1981;34:366.
76. Anderson DC, Pickering LK, Feigin RD: Leukocyte function in normal and infected neonates. J Pediatr 1974;85:420.
77. Chirico G, Marconi M, De Amici M, et al: Deficiency of neutrophil bactericidal activity in term and preterm infants: a longitudinal study. Biol Neonate 1985;47:125.
78. Forman ML, Stiehm ER: Impaired opsonic activity but normal phagocytosis in low-birth-weight infants. N Engl J Med 1969;281:926.
79. Shigeoka AO, Santos JI, Hill HR: Functional analysis of neutrophil granulocytes from healthy, infected, and stressed neonates. J Pediatr 1979;95:454.
80. Wright WC, Ank BJ, Herbert J, et al: Decreased bactericidal activity of leukocytes of stressed newborn infants. Pediatrics 1975;56:579.
81. Kocherlakota P, La Gamma EF, Fleit H, et al: Recombinant human granulocyte colony stimulating factor (rhGCSF) alters surface expression of Fcγ & complement receptors in neutropenic neonates (Abstract 1318). Pediatr Res 1996;39:222A.
82. Mariscalco MM, Smith CW: Integrins and cell adhesion molecules. In Polin RA, Fox WW (eds): Fetal and Neonatal Physiology, 2nd ed. Vol 2. Philadelphia: WB Saunders, 1998, p 1980–2001.
83. Palmer C: Ischemia-reperfusion injury. In Stevensen DK, Sunshine P (eds): Fetal and Neonatal Brain Injury. Oxford, Oxford University Press, 1997, pp 38–58.
84. Guice KS, Oldham KT, Caty MG, et al: Neutrophil-dependent, oxygen radical mediated lung injury associated with pancreatitis. Ann Surg 1989;210:740.
85. Hardy MM, Flickinger AG, Riley DP, et al: Superoxide dismutase mimetics inhibit neutrophil-mediated human aortic endothelial cell injury in vitro. J Biol Chem 1994;269:18535.
86. Sacks T, Moldow CF, Craddock PR, et al: Oxygen radicals mediate endothelial damage by complement-stimulated granulocytes: an in vitro model of immune vascular damage. J Clin Invest 1978;61:1161.
87. Smedly LA, Tonnesen MG, Sandhaus RA, et al: Neutrophil-mediated injury to endothelial cells: enhancement by endotoxin and essential role of neutrophil elastase. J Clin Invest 1986;77:1233.
88. Baker JR, Bullock GR, Butler KD, et al: An ultrastructural analysis of the vascular damage in the lethal and sublethal Forssman reaction in the guinea-pig. Br J Exp Pathol 1985;66:709.
89. Foreman KE, Vaporciyan AA, Bonish BK, et al: C5a-induced expression of P-selectin in endothelial cells. J Clin Invest 1994;94:1147.
90. Foreman KE, Glovsky MM, Warner RL, et al: Comparative effect of C3a and C5a on adhesion molecule expression on neutrophils and endothelial cells. Inflammation 1996;20:1.
91. Hammerschmidt DE, Harris PD, Wayland JH, et al: Complement-induced granulocyte aggregation in vivo. Am J Pathol 1981;102:146.
92. Craddock PR, Fehr J, Brigham KL, et al: Complement and leukocyte-mediated pulmonary dysfunction in hemodialysis. N Engl J Med 1977;296:769.
93. Pemberton M, Anderson G, Vetvicka V, et al: Microvascular effects of complement blockade with soluble recombinant CR1 on ischemia/reperfusion injury of skeletal muscle. J Immunol 1993;150:5104.
94. Williamson LM, Sheppard K, Davies JM, et al: Neutrophils are involved in the increased vascular permeability produced by activated complement in man. Br J Haematol 1986;64:357.
95. Lozada C, Levin RI, Hie M, et al: Identification of C1q as the heat-labile serum cofactor required for immune complexes to stimulate endothelial expression of the adhesion molecules E-selectin and intercellular and vascular cell adhesion molecules 1. Proc Nat Acad Sci U S A 1995;92:8378.
96. Kilgore KS, Shen JP, Miller BF, et al: Enhancement by the complement membrane attack complex of tumor necrosis factor-alpha–induced endothelial cell expression of E-selectin and ICAM-1. J Immunol 1995;1434.
97. Marks RM, Todd RF, Ward PA: Rapid induction of neutrophil-endothelial adhesion by endothelial complement fixation. Nature 1989;339:314.
98. Tsuji S, Kaji K, Nagasawa S: Activation of the alternative pathway of human complement by apoptotic human umbilical vein endothelial cells. J Biochem 1994;116:794.
99. Vercellotti GM, Platt JL, Bach FH, et al: Neutrophil adhesion to xenogeneic endothelium via iC3b. J Immunol 1991;146:730.
100. Inano H, English D, Doerschuk CM: Effect of zymosan-activated plasma on the deformability of rabbit polymorphonuclear leukocytes. J Appl Physiol 1992;73:1370.

101. Lucchesi BR: Complement activation, neutrophils, and oxygen radicals in reperfusion injury. Stroke 1993;24(Suppl 12):I41.
102. Lindsay TF, Hill J, Ortiz F, et al: Blockade of complement activation prevents local and pulmonary albumin leak after torso ischemia-reperfusion. Ann Surg 1992;216:677.
103. Hill J, Lindsay TF, Ortiz F, et al: Soluble complement receptor type 1 ameliorates local and remote organ injury after intestinal ischemia-reperfusion in the rat. J Immunol 1992;149:1723.
104. Mulligan MS, Yeh CG, Rudolph AR, et al: Protective effects of soluble CR1 in complement- and neutrophil-mediated tissue injury. J Immunol 1992;148:1479.
105. Uchiba M, Okajima K, Murakami K, et al: Endotoxin-induced pulmonary vascular injury is mainly mediated by activated neutrophils in rats. Thromb Res 1995;78:117.
106. Sakai A: Protection against septic shock in mice with SJC13, an azaindolidine derivative that is a cell adhesion inhibitor. Inflamm Res 1996;45:448.
107. Lindsay TF, Walker PM, Romaschin A: Acute pulmonary injury in a model of ruptured abdominal aortic aneurysm. J Vasc Surg 1995;22:1.
108. Anderson DC, Hughes BJ, Edward MS, et al: Impaired chemotaxigenesis by type III group B streptococci in neonatal sera: relationship to diminished concentration of specific anticapsular antibody and abnormalities of serum complement. Pediatr Res 1983;17:496.
109. Boner A, Zeligs BJ, Bellanti JA: Chemotactic responses of various differentiational stages of neutrophils from human cord and adult blood. Infect Immun 1982;35:922.
110. Klein RB, Fischer TJ, Gard SE, et al: Decreased mononuclear and polymorphonuclear chemotaxis in human newborns, infants and young children. Pediatrics 1977;60:467.
111. Laurenti F, Ferro R, Marzetti G, et al: Neutrophil chemotaxis in preterm infants with infections. J Pediatr 1980;96:468.
112. Maródi L, Jezérniczky J, Csorba S, et al: Chemotactic and random movement of cord-blood granulocytes. Experientia 1984;40:1407.
113. Miller ME: Chemotactic function in the human neonate: humoral and cellular aspects. Pediatr Res 1971;5:487.
114. Pahwa SG, Pahwa R, Grimes E, et al: Cellular and humoral components of monocyte and neutrophil chemotaxis in cord blood. Pediatr Res 1977;11:677.
115. Gerard NP, Gerard C: The chemotactic receptor for human C5a anaphylatoxin. Nature 1991;349:614.
116. Katona IM, Ohura K, Allen JB, et al: Modulation of monocyte chemotactic function in inflammatory lesions: role of inflammatory mediators. J Immunol 1991;146:708.
117. Ember JA, Sanderson SD, Hugli TE, et al: Induction of interleukin-8 synthesis from monocytes by human C5a anaphylatoxin. Am J Pathol 1994;144:393.
118. Quan JM, Martin TR, Rosenberg GB, et al: Antibodies against the N-terminus of IL-8 receptor A inhibit neutrophil chemotaxis. Biochem Biophys Res Commun 1996;219:405.
119. Collins PD, Jose PJ, Williams TJ: The sequential generation of neutrophil chemoattractant proteins in acute inflammation in the rabbit in vivo: relationship between C5a and proteins with the characteristics of IL-8/neutrophil-activating protein 1. J Immunol 1991;146:677.
120. Ivey CL, Williams FM, Collins PD, et al: Neutrophil chemoattractants generated in two phases during reperfusion of ischemic myocardium in the rabbit. Evidence for a role for C5a and interleukin-8. J Clin Invest 1995;95:2720.
121. Shuster DE, Kehrli ME Jr, Rainard P, et al: Complement fragment C5a and inflammatory cytokines in neutrophil recruitment during intramammary infection with *Escherichia coli*. Infect Immun 1997;65:3286.
122. Kuhns DB, Gallin JI: Increased cell-associated IL-8 in human exudative and A23187-treated peripheral blood neutrophils. J Immunol 1995;154:6556.
123. Bohnsack JF, Mollison KW, Buko AM, et al: Group B streptococci inactivate complement component C5a by enzymatic cleavage at the C-terminus. Biochem J 1991;273:635.
124. Bohnsack JF, Widjaja K, Ghazizadeh S, et al: A role for C5 and C5a-ase in the acute neutrophil response to group B streptococcal infections. J Infect Dis 1997;175:847.
125. Oda T, Kojima Y, Akaike T, et al: Inactivation of chemotactic activity of C5a by the serratial 56-kilodalton protease. Infect Immun 1990;58:1269.
126. Reed SL, Ember JA, Herdman DS, et al: The extracellular proteinase of *Entamoeba histolytica* degrades anaphylatoxins C3a and C5a. J Immunol 1995;155:266.
127. Hopken UE, Lu B, Gerard NP, et al: The C5a chemoattractant receptor mediates mucosal defense to infection. Nature 1996;383:86.
128. Amsterdam EA, Stahl GL, Pan HL, et al: Limitation of reperfusion injury by a monoclonal antibody to C5a during myocardial infarction in pigs. Am J Physiol 1995;268:H448.
129. de Boer JP, Wolbink GJ, Thijs LG, et al: Interplay of complement and cytokines in the pathogenesis of septic shock. Immunopharmacol 1992;24:135.
130. Gewurz H, Shin HS, Mergenhagen SE: Interactions of the complement system with endotoxic lipopolysaccharide: consumption of each of the six terminal complement components. J Exp Med 1968;128:1049.
131. Göetz O, Müller-Eberhard HJ: The C3-activator system: an alternative pathway of complement activation. J Exp Med 1971;134:90s.
132. McCabe W: Serum complement levels in bacteremia due to gram-negative sepsis. N Engl J Med 1973;288:21.
133. Mulligan MS, Schmid E, Beck-Schimmer B, et al: Requirement and role of C5a in acute lung inflammatory injury in rats. J Clin Invest 1996;98:503.
134. Padalino P, Gardinali M, Pallavicini J, et al: Complement activation and endotoxin in sepsis. Prog Clin Biol Res 1989;308:277.
135. Shin HS, Gewurz H, Snyderman R: Reaction of cobra venom factor with guinea pig complement and generation of an activity chemotactic for polymorphonuclear leukocytes. Proc Soc Exp Biol Med 1969;131:203.
136. Stevens JH, O'Hanley P, Shapiro JM, et al: Effects of anti-C5a antibodies on the adult respiratory distress syndrome. J Clin Invest 1986;77:1812.
137. Till GO, Ward PA: Systemic complement activation and acute lung injury. Fed Proc 1986;45:13.
138. Jagels MA, Hugli TE: Neutrophil chemotactic factors promote leukocytosis: a common mechanism for cellular recruitment from bone marrow. J Immunol 1992;148:1119.
139. Hocker JR, Wellhausen SR, Ward RA, et al: Effect of extracorporeal membrane oxygenation on leukocyte function in neonates. Artif Organs 1991;15:23.
140. Martin GR, Short BL, Abbot C, et al: Cardiac stun in infants undergoing extracorporeal membrane oxygenation. J Cardiovasc Surg 1991;101:607.

141. Rinder CS, Rinder HM, Smith BR, et al: Blockade of C5a and C5b-9 generation inhibits leukocyte and platelet activation during extracorporeal circulation. J Clin Invest 1995;96:1564.
142. Taylor GA, Lotze A, Kapur S, et al: Diffuse pulmonary opacification in infants undergoing extracorporeal membrane oxygenation: clinical and pathologic correlation. Radiology 1986;161:347.
143. Dobos GJ, Andre M, Bohler J, et al: Inhibition of C5a-induced actin polymerization, chemotaxis, and phagocytosis of human polymorphonuclear neutrophils incubated in a glucose-based dialysis solution. Adv Perit Dial 1993;9:307.
144. Ribeiro RA, Souza-Filho MV, Souza MH, et al: Role of resident mast cells and macrophages in the neutrophil migration induced by LTB_4, fMLP, and C5a desArg. International Arch Allergy Immunol 1997;112:27.
145. Daffern PJ, Pfeifer PH, Ember JA, et al: C3a is a chemotaxin for human eosinophils but not for neutrophils. I. C3a stimulation of neutrophils is secondary to eosinophil activation. J Exp Med 1995;181:2119.
146. Kilgore KS, Flory CM, Miller BF, et al: The membrane attack complex of complement induces interleukin-8 and monocyte chemoattractant protein-1 secretion from human umbilical vein endothelial cells. Am J Pathol 1996;149:953.
147. Lassiter HA, Watson SW, Seifring ML, et al: Complement factor 9 deficiency in the serum of human neonates. J Infect Dis 1992;166:53.
148. Lassiter HA, Wilson JL, Feldhoff RC, et al: Supplemental complement component C9 enhances the capacity of neonatal serum to kill multiple isolates of pathogenic *Escherichia coli*. Pediatr Res 1994;35:389.
149. Rommel FA, Mayer MM: Studies of guinea pig complement component C9: reaction kinetics and evidence that lysis of EAC1-8 results from a single membrane lesion caused by one molecule of C9 J Immunol 1973;110:637.
150. Born J, Bhakdi S: Does complement kill *E. coli* by producing transmural pores? Immunology 1986; 59:139.
151. Koski CL, Ramm LE, Hammer CH, et al: Cytolysis of nucleated cells by complement: cell death displays multi hit characteristics. Proc Natl Acad Sci U S A 1983;80:3816.
152. Morgan BP: Complement membrane attack on nucleated cells: resistance, recovery and non-lethal effect. Biochem J 1989;264:1.
153. Fearon DT: Regulation by membrane sialic acid of β1H-dependent decay-dissociation of amplification C3 convertase of the alternative complement pathway. Proc Natl Acad Sci U S A 1978;75:1971.
154. Davies A, Lachmann PJ: Membrane defense against complement lysis: the structure and biological properties of CD59. Immunol Res 1993;12:258.
155. Whitlow MB, Iida K, Stefanova I, et al: H19, a surface membrane molecule involved in T-cell activation, inhibits channel formation by human complement. Cell Immunol 1990;126:176.
156. Stein JM, Luzio JP: Ectocytosis caused by sublytic autologous complement attack on human neutrophils: the sorting of endogenous plasma-membrane proteins and lipids into shed vesicles. Biochem J 1991;274:381.
157. Johnson E, Berge V, Hogasen K: Formation of the terminal complement complex on agarose beds: further evidence that vitronectin (complement S-protein) inhibits C9. Scand J Immunol 1994;39:281.
158. McDonald JF, Nelsestuen GL: Potent inhibition of terminal complement assembly by clusterin: characterization of its impact on C9 polymerization. Biochem 1997;36:7464.
159. Sheehan M, Morris CA, Pussell BA, et al: Complement inhibition by human vitronectin involves non-heparin binding domains. Clin Exp Immunol 1995;101:136.
160. Milis L, Morris CA, Sheehan MC, et al: Vitronectin-mediated inhibition of complement: evidence for different binding sites for C5b-7 and C9. Clin Exp Immunol 1993;92:114.
161. Sererling M, Hahn H, Opferkuch W: Phagocytosis of C3b-coated sheep red blood cells by guinea-pig macrophages in the absence of antibody. Immunobiology 1982;162:39.
162. Woolley PV 3rd, Sacher RA, Priego VM, et al: Methotrexate-induced immune haemolytic anaemia. Br J Haematol 1983;54:543.
163. Bakacs T, Ringwald G, Kimber I: Differential susceptibility of haemolysin-sensitized erythrocytes to complement-mediated cytotoxicity: a biological manifestation of the relationship between antibody availability and complement fixation. J Clin Lab Immunol 1989;30:61.
164. Weitzman SA, Stossel TP: Drug-induced immunological neutropenia. Lancet 1978;1:1068.
165. Al-Mulla ZS, Christensen RD: Neutropenia in the neonate. Clin Perinatol 1995;22:711.
166. Cines DB, Schreiber AD: Immune thrombocytopenia. Use of a Coombs antiglobulin test to detect IgG and C3 on platelets. N Engl J Med 1979;300:106.
167. Freedman J, Cheong T, Garvey MB: Use of the indirect platelet antiglobulin test with anti-IgG and anti-C3 in immune and nonimmune thrombocytopenias. Am J Hematol 1985;18:297.
168. Handin RI, Stossel TP: Effect of corticosteroid therapy on the phagocytosis of antibody-coated platelets by human leukocytes. Blood 1978;51:771.
169. Hauch TW, Rosse WF: Platelet-bound complement (C3) in immune thrombocytopenia. Blood 1997; 50:1129.
170. Hedge UM, Bowes A, Roter BL: Platelet associated complement components (PAC3c and PAC3d) in patients with autoimmune thrombocytopenia. Br J Haematol 1985;60:49.
171. Kernoff LM, Malan E: Complement (C3) binding to platelets in autoimmune thrombocytopenia. Clin Lab Haematol 1983;5:1.
172. Panzer S, Niessner H, Lechner K, et al: Platelet-associated immunoglobulins IgG, IgM, IgA, and complement C3c in sequestration pattern of ^{111}indium labeled platelets. Scand J Haematol 1986;37:97.
173. Panzer S, Szamait S, Bodeker RH, et al: Platelet-associated immunoglobulins IgG, IgM, IgA and complement C3 in immune and nonimmune thrombocytopenic disorders. Am J Hematol 1986;23:89.
174. Zucker-Franklin D, Karpatkin S: Red-cell and platelet fragmentation in idiopathic autoimmune thrombocytopenic purpura. N Engl J Med 1977;297:517.
175. Nomura S, Yanabu M, Soga T, et al: Analysis of idiopathic thrombocytopenia purpura patients with antiglycoprotein IIb/IIIa or Ib autoantibodies. Acta Haematol 1991;86:25.
176. Fink CW, Miller WE Jr, Dorward B, et al: The formation of macroglobulin antibodies. II. Studies on neonatal infants and older children. J Clin Invest 1962;41:1422.
177. Lescale KB, Eddleman KA, Cines DB, et al: Antiplatelet antibody testing in thrombocytopenic pregnant women. Am J Obstet Gynecol 1996;174:1014.
178. Matthews JH, Benjamin S, Gill DS, et al: Pregnancy-

associated thrombocytopenia: definition, incidence and natural history. Acta Haematol 1990;84:24.
179. Burrows RF, Kelton JG: Perinatal thrombocytopenia. Clin Perinatol 1995;22:779.
180. Christie DJ, Diaz-Arauzo H, Cook JM: Antibody-mediated platelet destruction by quinine, quinidine, and their metabolites. J Lab Clin Med 1988;112:92.
181. Stewart MW, Etches WS, Gordon PA: Antiphospholipid antibody-dependent C5b-9 formation. Br J Haematol 1997;96:451.
182. Tsubakio T, Tani P, Curd JG, et al: Complement activation in vitro by antiplatelet antibodies in chronic immune thrombocytopenic purpura. Br J Haematol 1986;63:293.
183. Basta M, Langlois PF, Marques M, et al: High-dose intravenous immunoglobulin modifies complement-mediated in vivo clearance. Blood 1989;74:326.
184. Basta M, Kirshbom P, Frank MM, et al: Mechanism of therapeutic effect of high-dose intravenous immunoglobulin: attenuation of acute, complement-dependent immune damage in a guinea pig model. J Clin Invest 1989;84:1974.
185. Basta M, Fries LF, Frank MM: High doses of intravenous Ig inhibit in vitro uptake of C4 fragments onto sensitized erythrocytes. Blood 1991;77:376.
186. Follea G, Souillet G, Clerc M, et al: Intravenous plasmin-treated gamma-globulin therapy in idiopathic thrombocytopenia purpura: results in 40 patients. Nouv Rev Fr Hematol 1985;27:5.
187. Usuki Y, Kohsaki M, Nagai K, et al: Complement-dependent cytotoxic factor to megakaryocyte progenitors in sera from patients with idiopathic thrombocytopenic purpura. Int J Cell Cloning 1986;46:447.
188. Dahlback B: Protein S and C4b-binding protein: components involved in the regulation of the protein C anticoagulant system. Thromb Haemost 1991;66:49.
189. Davis AE 3d: Hereditary and acquired deficiencies of C1 inhibitor. Immunodefic Rev 1989;1:207.
190. Hessing M: The interaction between complement component C4b-binding protein and the vitamin K-dependent protein S forms a link between blood coagulation and the complement system. Biochem J 1991;277:581.
191. Sims PJ, Wiedmer T: Induction of cellular procoagulant activity by the membrane attack complex of complement. Semin Cell Biol 1995;6:275.
192. Sundsmo JS, Fair DS: Relationships among the complement, kinin, coagulation, and fibrinolytic systems. Springer Semin Immunopathol 1983;6:231.
193. Cugno M, Cicardi M, Bottasso B, et al: Activation of the coagulation cascade in C1-inhibitor deficiencies. Blood 1997;89:3213.
194. Fischer MB, Prodeus AP, Nicholson-Weller A, et al: Increased susceptibility to endotoxin shock in complement C3- and C4-deficient mice is corrected by C1 inhibitor replacement. J Immunol 1997;159:976.
195. Cairo MS, Worcester C, Rucker R, et al: Role of circulating complement and polymorphonuclear leukocyte transfusion in treatment and outcome in critically ill neonates with sepsis. J Pediatr 1987;110:935.
196. Nakae H, Endo S, Inada K, et al: Chronological changes in the complement system in sepsis. Surg Today 1996;26:225.
197. Hack CE, Ogilvie AC, Eisele B, et al: C1-inhibitor substitution therapy in septic shock and in the vascular leak syndrome induced by high doses of interleukin-2. Intensive Care Med 1993;19(Suppl 1):S19.
198. Hardig Y, Hillarp A, Dahlbach B: The amino-terminal module of the C4b-binding protein alpha-chain is crucial for C4b binding and factor I-cofactor function. Biochem J 1997;323:469.
199. Scharfstein J, Ferreira A, Nussenzweig V: Human C4 binding protein. I. Isolation and characterization. J Exp Med 1978;148:207.
200. Fernandez JA, Griffin JH: A protein S binding site on C4b-binding protein involves beta chain residues 31–45. J Biol Chem 1994;269:2535.
201. Hardig Y, Rezaie A, Dahlback B: High affinity binding of human vitamin K–dependent protein S to a truncated recombinant beta-chain of C4b-binding protein expressed in *Escherichia coli*. J Biol Chem 1993; 268:3033.
202. Hardig Y, Dahlback B: The amino-terminal module of the C4b-binding protein beta-chain contains the protein S-binding site. J Biol Chem 1996;271:20861.
203. Dahlback B, Frohm B, Nelsestuen G: High affinity interaction between C4b-binding protein and vitamin K–dependent protein S in the presence of calcium. Suggestion of a third component in blood regulating the interaction. J Biol Chem 1990;265:16082.
204. Zoller B, Garcia de Frutos P, Dahlback B: Evaluation of the relationship between protein S and C4b-binding protein isoforms in hereditary protein S deficiency demonstrating type I and type III deficiencies to be phenotypic variants of the same genetic disease. Blood 1995;85:3524.
205. Fourrier F, Jourdain M, Tournois A, et al: Coagulation inhibitor substitution during sepsis. Intensive Care Med 1995;21:S264.
206. Furmaniak-Kazmierczak E, Hu CY, Esmon CT: Protein S enhances C4b binding protein interaction with neutrophils. Blood 1993;81:405.
207. Ikeda K, Nagasawa K, Horiuchi T, et al: C5a induces tissue factor activity on endothelial cells. Thromb Haemost 1997;77:394.
208. Fukuoka Y, Tachibana T, Yasui A: Anaphylatoxin C3a induces rapid protein phosphorylation in guinea pig platelets. Immunopharmacology 1994;28:95.
209. Kretzschmar T, Kahl K, Rech K, et al: Characterization of the C5a receptor on guinea pig platelets. Immunobiology 1991;183:418.
210. Watanabe H, Kuraya M, Kasukawa R, et al: Analysis of C5a receptor by monoclonal antibody. J Immunol Methods 1995;185:19.
211. Damerau B, Meyer B, Vogt W: Formation of mixed aggregates of human polymorphonuclear leukocytes and platelets by C5a-desArg. Complement Inflamm 1991;8:25.
212. Stahl GL, Morse DS, Martin SL: Eicosanoid production from porcine neutrophils and platelets: differential production with various agonists. Am J Physiol 1997;272:C1821.
213. Andreasson S, Gothberg S, Berggen H, et al: Hemofiltration modifies complement activation after extracorporeal circulation in infants. Ann Thorac Surg 1993;56:1515.
214. Horimoto H, Kondo K, Asada K, et al: Heparin-coated cardiopulmonary bypass circuits in coronary bypass surgery. Artif Organs 1996;20:936.
215. Hamilton KK, Ji Z, Rollins S, et al: Regulatory control of the terminal complement proteins at the surface of human endothelial cells: neutralization of a C5b-9 inhibitor by antibody to CD59. Blood 1990;76:2572.
216. Sims PJ, Rollins SA, Wiedmer T: Regulatory control of complement on blood platelets: modulation of platelet procoagulant responses by a membrane inhibitor of the C5b-9 complex. J Biol Chem 1989; 264:19228.
217. Houle JJ, Leddy JP, Rosenfeld SI: Secretion of the terminal complement proteins, C5–C9, by human platelets. Clin Immunol Immunopathol 1989;50:385.

218. Polley MJ, Nachman RL: Human complement in thrombin-mediated platelet function: uptake of the C5b-C9 complex. J Exp Med 1979;150:633.
219. Ford I, Douglas CW, Heath J, et al: Evidence for the involvement of complement proteins in platelet aggregation by *Streptococcus sanguinis*. Br J Haematol 1996;94:729.
220. Agarwala B, Sheikh Z, Cibils LA: Congenital heart block. J Natl Med Assoc 1996;88:725.
221. Buyon JP: Congenital complete heart block. Lupus 1993;2:291.
222. Watson RM, Lane AT, Barnett NK, et al: Neonatal lupus erythematosus: a clinical, serological and immunogenic study with review of the literature. Medicine (Baltimore) 1984;63:362.
223. Bowness P, Davies KA, Norsworthy PJ, et al: Hereditary C1q deficiency and systemic lupus erythematosus. Q J Med 1994;87:455.
224. Meyer O, Hauptmann G, Tappeiner G, et al: Genetic deficiency of C4, C2, or C1q and lupus syndromes. Association with anti-Ro (SS-A) antibodies. Clin Exp Immunol 1985;62:678.
225. Provost TT, Arnett FC, Reichlin M: Homozygous C2 deficiency, lupus erythematosus and anti Ro (SS-A) antibodies. Arthritis Rheum 1983;26:1279.
226. Reichlin M, Harley JB: Antibodies to Ro (SSA) and the heterogeneity of systemic lupus erythematosus. J Rheumatol 1987;14 (Suppl 13):112.
227. Sullivan KE, Petri MA, Schmeckpeper BJ, et al: Prevalence of a mutation causing C2 deficiency in systemic lupus erythematosus. J Rheumatol 1994;21:1128.
228. Linsaw MA, Stapleton FB, Cuppage FE, et al: Hypocomplementemic glomerulonephritis in an infant and mother: evidence for an abnormal form of C3. Am J Nephrol 1987;7:470.
229. Miller ME, Koblenzer PJ: Leiner's disease and deficiency of C5. J Pediatr 1972;80:879.
230. Ammann AJ: Leiner's disease and C5 deficiency. J Pediatr 1972;81:1221.
231. Jacobs JC, Miller ME: Fatal familial Leiner's disease: a deficiency of opsonic activity of serum complement. Pediatrics 1972;49:225.
232. Gaither TA, Gallin JL, Lida K, et al: Deficiency in C3b receptors on neutrophils of patients with chronic granulomatous disease and hyperimmunoglobulin-E recurrent infection (Job's) syndrome. Inflammation 1984;8:429.
233. Nunoi H, Yanabe Y, Higuchi S, et al: Severe hypoplasia of lymphoid tissues in Mo1 deficiency. Hum Pathol 1988;19:753.
234. Ross GD: Clinical and laboratory features of patients with an inherited deficiency of neutrophil membrane complement receptor type 3 (CR3) and the related membrane antigens LFA-1 and p150,95. J Clin Immunol 1986;6:107.
235. Mazzone A, Ricevuti G: Leucocyte CD11/CD18 integrins: biological and clinical relevance. Haematologica 1995;80:161.
236. Ross SC, Densen P: Complement deficiency states and infection: epidemiology, pathogenesis and consequences of neisserial and other infections in an immune deficiency. Medicine (Baltimore) 1984;63:243.
237. Giclas P: Complement tests. In Rose N, de Macario E, Folds J, et al (eds): Manual of Clinical Laboratory Immunology, 5th ed. Washington, DC: ASM Press, 1997, pp 181–186.
238. Fine DP, Marney SR Jr, Colley DG, et al: C3 shunt activation in human serum chelated with EGTA. J Immunol 1972;109:807.
239. Platts-Mills TAE, Ishizaka K: Activation of the alternative pathway of human complement by rabbit cells. J Immunol 1974;113:348.
240. Isenman DE, Kells DI, Cooper NR, et al: Nucleophilic modification of human complement protein C3: correlation of conformational changes with acquisition of C3b-like functional properties. Biochemistry 1981;20:4458.
241. McLean R, Welch T: Complement. In Leffel M, Donnenberg A, Rose N (eds): Handbook of Human Immunology. Boca Raton: CRC Press, 1997, pp 267–318.
242. Rabson A: Complement activation. In Rose N, de Macario E, Folds J, et al (eds): Manual of Clinical Laboratory Immunology, 5th ed. Washington, DC: ASM Press, 1997, p 187–191.
243. Peakman M, Senaldi G, Vergani D: Review: assessment of complement activation in clinical immunology laboratories: time for reappraisal? J Clin Pathol 1989;42:1081.
244. Holers VM: Complement receptors. In Rose N, de Macario E, Folds J, et al (eds): Manual of Clinical Laboratory Immunology, 5th ed. Washington, DC: ASM Press, 1997, pp 192–202.
245. Moulds J: Genetic typing of the complement system. In Rose N, de Macario E, Folds J, et al (eds): Manual of Clinical Laboratory Immunology, 5th ed. Washington, DC: ASM Press, 1997, p 203–207.
246. Wolach B, Dolfin T, Regev R, et al: The development of the complement system after 28 weeks' gestation. Acta Paediatr 1997;86:523.
247. Mitchell TJ, Naughton M, Norsworthy P, et al: γ-interferon upregulates expression of C3 and C4 by stabilization of mRNA. J Immunol 1996;156:4429.
248. Perissutti S, Tedesco F: Effect of cytokines on the secretion of the fifth and eighth complement components by HepG2 cells. Int J Clin Lab Res 1994:24:45.
249. Phillips DJ, Novinger MS, Evatt BL, et al: TNF-α suppresses IL-β and IL-6 up-regulation of C4b-binding protein in HepG2 hepatoma cells. Thromb Res 1996:81:307.
250. Spath GM, Ramadori G, Rittner C, et al: Expression of the complement C8 genes during IL-6-mediated in vitro induction of the acute-phase response. Exp Clin Immunogenet 1995;12:53.
251. Vincent F, de la Salle H, Bohbot A, et al: Synthesis and regulation of complement components by human monocytes/macrophages and by acute monocytic leukemia. DNA Cell Biol 1993;12:415.

CHAPTER 16

Hemoglobin Synthesis and Metabolism During the Neonatal Period

Harry Bard, M.D.

HEMOGLOBIN STRUCTURE AND FUNCTION

Structure

Hemoglobin is a tetrameric molecule comprising two pairs of polypeptide subunits, each encoded by a different family of genes, the α-like globin genes found on chromosome 16 and the β-like globin genes on chromosome 11. The α-globin chains are made up of 141 amino acids, and the β-globin chains are made up of 146. Each subunit consists of a protoheme to which oxygen binds and a globin chain made up of amino acids arranged in a definite sequential and spatial pattern. The two α-globin chains and the two non-α-globin chains fit together specifically to form a hemoglobin tetramer with a molecular mass of about 65 kd.

Each heme group contains a porphyrin ring and a ferrous atom capable of reversibly binding one oxygen molecule. The globin units of deoxyhemoglobin are tightly held by electrostatic bonds in a tense (T) conformation with a relatively low affinity for oxygen. Binding of oxygen imposes chemical and mechanical stresses that break these electrostatic bonds, leading to a relaxed (R) conformation in which the remaining binding sites become more available. Because conformational changes lead to cooperativity among binding sites, binding of one oxygen molecule to deoxyhemoglobin increases the oxygen affinity of the remaining binding sites on the same hemoglobin molecule. The binding curve assumes a sigmoid shape, reflecting the transition from low to high affinity as more binding sites become occupied.[1] The properties of an allosteric protein such as hemoglobin include multiple interacting binding sites, reversible noncovalent binding to a primary ligand, quaternary conformational changes induced by ligand binding (i.e., homotropic effects), and modulation of ligand binding by secondary effectors (i.e., heterotropic effects).[2]

The major heterotropic effectors of hemoglobin are hydrogen ion, carbon dioxide, and red blood cell 2,3-diphosphoglycerate (2,3-DPG). These effectors decrease the affinity of hemoglobin for oxygen by strengthening the salt bridges that maintain the molecule in the T conformation. Some abnormal hemoglobins with intrinsically high oxygen affinity occur as a result of an amino acid substitution that causes the loss of bonds that stabilize the tetramer in the T configuration.

Functional Properties

Solubility

A physiologically important property of hemoglobin is its high degree of solubility. The solubility of hemoglobin is critical because precipitated hemoglobin, globin, and their catabolic byproducts are deleterious to erythrocytes. These materials oxidize delicate cellular components, adhere to membrane cytoskeletal proteins, or both, leading ultimately to altered membrane surfaces, increased viscosity, and deranged shapes that result in recognition and premature destruction (i.e., hemolysis) of the affected red blood cells by macrophages of the reticuloendothelial system. Mutations that alter hemoglobin stability (i.e., unstable hemoglobins) are often characterized by various degrees of hemolytic anemia, which can be exacerbated by exposure to oxidative agents.

Hemoglobin Binding of Nitric Oxide

In addition to carrying oxygen, hemoglobin acts as a carrier of nitric oxide. Hemoglobin scavenges nitric oxide through the high-affinity ferrous binding sites on heme, which have an affinity for nitric oxide 8000 times their affinity for oxygen. A second binding site was reported at the β93 cysteine residue on the globin chain, where nitric oxide binds in the form of *S*-nitrosothiol.[3] The transfer of nitric oxide from *S*-nitrosothiol to hemoglobin is allosterically regulated and functionally linked to the binding of oxygen to hemoglobin. As hemoglobin binds oxygen in the lungs, its binding affinity for *S*-nitrosothiol is increased. As hemoglobin releases oxygen in the periphery, its affinity for *S*-nitrosothiol is reduced, and nitric oxide is released into the tissues. The thiol group of *S*-nitrosothiol protects nitric oxide from being scavenged by the binding site on heme. The enhanced release of nitric oxide from nitrosohemoglobin in hypoxic tissue reduces the regional vascular resistance.[4] These findings are an example of the allosteric properties of hemoglobin that enhances oxygen transport by improving the matching of regional oxygen requirements to blood flow.

ORGANIZATION AND STRUCTURE OF THE GLOBIN GENES

Normal red blood cells in adults contain at least three different types of hemoglobin, including Hb A ($\alpha_2\beta_2$), Hb A_2 ($\alpha_2\delta_2$), and Hb F ($\alpha_2\gamma_2$). Hb A refers to the predominant hemoglobin in adult blood and Hb A_2 to the minor component that constitutes about 2.5% of the total hemoglobin. Hb F is the major hemoglobin in red blood cells of the fetus and newborn infant and is present in trace amounts (usually $<2\%$) in the adult.

The type of hemoglobin produced at any given gestational age during human fetal development is determined by the selective expression of globin genes. These genes are organized into two tightly linked clusters. The α-gene cluster, which contains two coexpressed adult α-globin genes, two embryonic α-globin-like genes (ζ-globin), and one or more nonfunctional α-globin-like gene remnants (i.e., products of pseudogenes), is located on chromosome 16.[5,6] The β-globin gene cluster, which contains the adult β-globin gene, the minimally expressed δ-globin gene, two coexpressed fetal γ-globin genes, the embryonic ϵ-globin genes, and β-globin–related pseudogenes, is found on chromosome 11.[5,6]

The genes within each family are expressed according to a strict ontogenic schedule, and the quantitative expression of genes from each of these two families is strictly balanced and coordinated.[7] Such intrachromosomal and interchromosomal control of gene expression implies complex regulatory mechanisms. Fetal Hb F ($\alpha_2\gamma_2$), the major hemoglobin of intrauterine life, and adult Hb A ($\alpha_2\beta_2$) are assembled by the combination of two α-globin chains with two γ-chains and two β-chains, respectively.[7]

The perinatal period in humans is characterized by a major switch in hemoglobin composition. Expression of the γ-globin gene begins in early embryogenesis, peaks during mid-gestation, and declines rapidly during the last month of fetal development. As the γ-globin gene expression declines, the proportion of β-globin gene expression increases.[8]

Concomitant with the changes in γ- and β-globin gene expression, changes in α-globin gene expression occur. In the human two adjacent globin genes, α_1 and α_2, encode identical α-globin products. Despite their remarkable level of structural similarity, the α_2-globin locus is dominant in the human adult, and α_2-globin mRNA is twofold to threefold more abundant than α_1-globin mRNA.[9–11] The dominance of the 5′ or α_2-globin gene over the 3′ or α_1-globin gene has also been demonstrated in other species.[12] The levels of mRNA encoded by the two α-globin loci are equal in the human embryo and subsequently shift toward the dominant expression of the α_2-globin form at 8 weeks' gestation.[13]

The general organization of the human globin gene clusters; the genes expressed; the hemoglobins produced during the embryonic, fetal, and adult developmental periods; and the site of erythropoiesis are shown in Figure 16–1. The globin genes are arranged from 5′ to 3′ according to the order of their expression during ontogeny. Two genes of the β-globin locus, $^G\gamma$ and $^A\gamma$, are structurally identical products of gene duplication and gene conversion. The two types of γ-chains can be distinguished only at amino acid position 136, where the $^G\gamma$ gene encodes for glycine and the $^A\gamma$ gene encodes for alanine.[8] The relative amounts of $^G\gamma$ and $^A\gamma$ differ in the fetus compared with the adult. The $^G\gamma$ to $^A\gamma$ ratio of 3:1 found in fetal red blood cells becomes 2:3 in adult red blood cells.[14–16]

The nucleotide sequences of each of these genes and the intragenic DNA have been determined. All globin genes (across most species) are in the same 5′ to 3′ orientation, and the genes are arranged in order of appearance during developmental expression. All globins characterized have 3 exons (coding regions) and two introns (noncoding regions). The α-like cluster extends over a 40-kb range and the β-like segment over a 60-kb range. In the α-globin gene cluster, two α-globin structured genes[11] are located at the 3′ end. The nucleotide sequences of the coding portions of the two genes are identical. Minor differences in the sequence of the second intron have been detected. The genes within each cluster are expressed according to a strict ontogenic schedule, and the quantitative expression of genes from each of these two families is strictly balanced and coordinated. Such intrachromosomal and interchromosomal control of gene expression implies complex regulatory mechanisms.

HEMOGLOBIN DURING FETAL DEVELOPMENT

Hemoglobin synthesis undergoes several developmental changes during the perinatal pe-

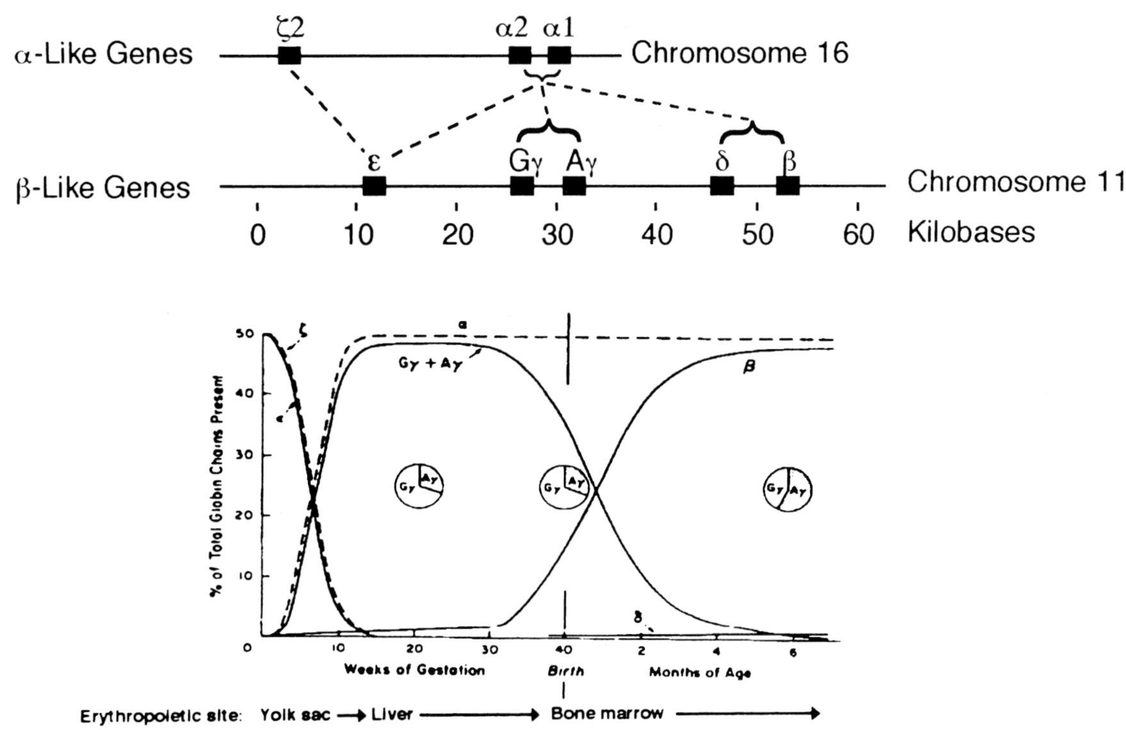

Figure 16–1. Location of the hemoglobin genes and the hemoglobin produced, changes in the expression of globin genes, relative portion of $^G\gamma$- and $^A\gamma$-chains in fetal hemoglobin, and sites of hematopoiesis during different stages of human development. (Adapted from Stamatoyannopoulos G, Nienhuis AW: Hemoglobin switching. In Collins FS, Weissman SM [eds]: The Molecular Basis of Blood Diseases, 2nd ed. Philadelphia: WB Saunders, 1994, p 108, and Collins FS, Weissman SM: The molecular genetics of human hemoglobin. Prog Nucleic Acid Res Mol Biol 1993;31:315.)

riod. The production of α-like and β-like chains is balanced throughout human development. In the early embryo, hemoglobin is composed of two ζ-chains and two ε-chains and is designated Hb Gower I. As the synthesis of the embryonic chain is phased out, synthesis of the α-chains and γ-chains begin. During a transition period, two other embryonic hemoglobins, Hb Gower II ($\alpha_2\epsilon_2$) and Hb Portland ($\zeta_2\gamma_2$), can be detected.

By 12 weeks' gestation, Hb F ($\alpha_2\gamma_2$) accounts for almost the entire amount of hemoglobin. Between 12 and 34 weeks' gestation, the relative proportion of Hb F synthesis decreases gradually from about 100% to 85%, and from then on, the decrease is more rapid until the postconceptional age of 56 weeks, when the remaining amount of Hb F again decreases gradually, reaching 1% to 2% at 1 year of age. A corresponding increase in Hb A occurs throughout the decrease in Hb F. The level of Hb F is primarily determined by postconceptional age. The δ-globin gene is only activated toward the end of gestation. Hb A_2 ($\alpha_2\delta_2$) is detected in trace amounts at term and then increases gradually to a maximum of about 2.5%.

Regulation of Hemoglobin Switching

Hemoglobin production in humans is characterized by several "switches" in the hemoglobin composition of red blood cells.[17] During the first 3 months of gestation, human red blood cells contain embryonic hemoglobins, whereas during the last 6 months of gestation, red blood cells contain predominantly fetal hemoglobin. The major transition from fetal to adult hemoglobin occurs in the perinatal period, and by the end of the first year, red blood cells have a hemoglobin composition that subsequently remains stable.

In the human fetus, the switch from ε-globin to γ-globin production begins very early in gestation; Hb F is readily detected in 5-week human embryos, and the switch is completed well before 10 weeks of gestation.[18–20] Globin expression starts early in human development, and small amounts of Hb A can be detected by biosynthetic or immunochemical methods even in the smallest human fetus studies.[21–23] During intrauterine development, β-chain synthesis in-

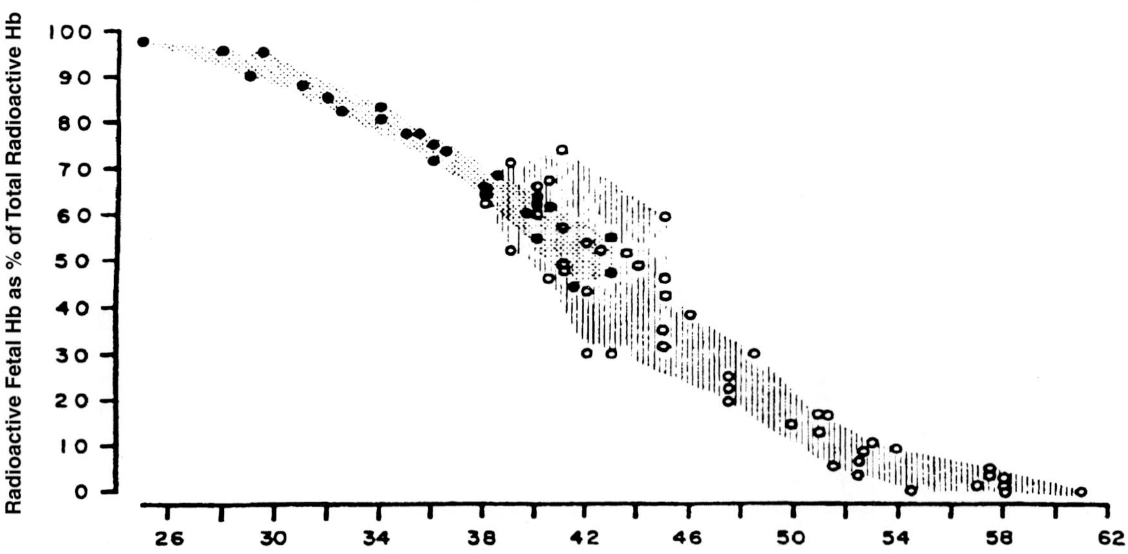

Figure 16–2. Decline in fetal hemoglobin synthesis as a function of gestational age. Solid dots indicate cord blood samples from preterm infants, and open circles indicate samples from infants considered to have been delivered at term. (From Bard H: The postnatal decline of hemoglobin F synthesis in normal full-term infants. J Clin Invest 1975;55:395. Reproduced from The Journal of Clinical Investigation by copyright permission of the American Society for Clinical Investigation.)

creases progressively to approximately 10% of total globin chain synthesis by 32 weeks. Afterward, the β-chain synthesis increases sharply, but γ-chain production falls. At birth, Hb F composes 60% to 80% of the total hemoglobin. At 16 to 20 weeks after term birth, Hb F constitutes about 3% of all hemoglobin synthesized (Fig. 16–2).[8]

Three types of γ-chain normally compose fetal hemoglobin. They are coded by two closely linked γ-genes, $^{G}\gamma$ and $^{A}\gamma$, present in the β-gene cluster on chromosome 11. At position 136, the $^{G}\gamma$ chain has glycine, whereas the $^{A}\gamma$ has alanine. The $^{A}\gamma$ chain is polymorphic, with residue 75 occupied by isoleucine ($^{A}\gamma^{I}$-chain) or threonine ($^{A}\gamma^{T}$-chain).[24, 25] The relative amount of the $^{G}\gamma$-chain to total γ-chains ($^{G}\gamma/^{A}\gamma + {}^{G}\gamma$) produced during the second and third trimester of fetal life is 70%, whereas the small amount of Hb F synthesized during adult life is made up of 40% $^{G}\gamma$-chains.[20, 26, 27] However, the timing of the $^{G}\gamma$ to $^{A}\gamma$ switch is not the same as the γ to β switch. During fetal life, the ratio is approximately 3:1, but after 44 weeks' postconceptional age, the values begin to change toward the normal adult ratio of 2:3.[16]

The proportion of Hb F in newborns is related to their age from conception rather than to birth itself. Premature newborns have very high levels of Hb F; such newborns switch to Hb A at a time corresponding to the end of their normal gestational period.[28] This observation favors the concept that the switch is developmentally determined independent of the intrauterine or extrauterine status of the individual; rather, the degree of developmental maturity of the fetus determines the rate and timing of the γ to β switch.

The γ-globin to β-globin switch has been documented at the mRNA level.[29] This was possible because of the extraordinary stability of the α-, β-, and γ-globin mRNA chains, which have a stable half-life of 30 to 50 hours.[30, 31] When the globin gene activity was assessed by determining mRNA levels throughout the last trimester of human development, the relative amounts of γ-globin to non-α-globin synthesis was directly related to the amount of γ to non-α-globin mRNAs in the erythroid cells. The proportion of $^{G}\gamma$- and $^{A}\gamma$-globin mRNAs was similar to the proportion of $^{G}\gamma$- and $^{A}\gamma$-globin chain synthesis. The determination of γ-globin mRNA as a percentage of non-α-globin mRNAs can be considered an accurate measure of Hb F synthesis (Fig. 16–3).

Transcriptional Regulation of Globin Gene Expression

The most widely studied changes during red blood cell ontogeny are the switches in globin types. Beyond its biologic interest, research in this area has been stimulated by the possibility of manipulating globin switching to ameliorate the clinical symptoms and disorders of hemoglobinopathies related to the β-globin locus (e.g., sickle cell anemia, thalassemia).

The erythroid populations that follow each other developmentally have distinct phenotypes and intrinsic programs that depend on gestational time and not on the sites at which they mature. The sequential activation of globin genes occurs in the order of their location on chromosome 11 or 16 and is thought to be mediated through interaction between stage-specific transcriptional factors and *cis*-regulatory sequences within the globin loci. The major

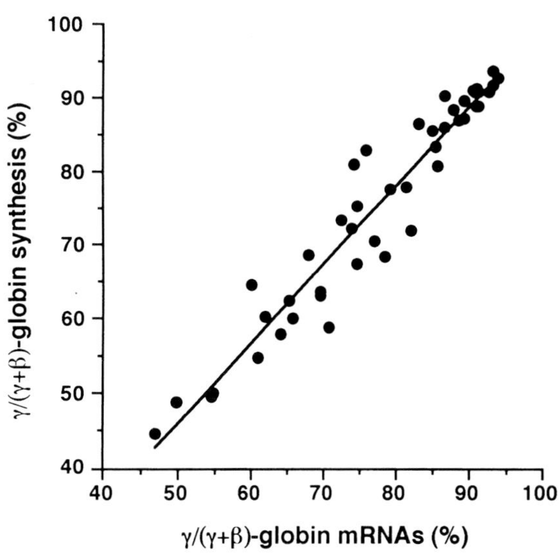

Figure 16–3. Correlation between proportion of hemoglobin (Hb F) measured as de novo synthesized globin by radiolabeling, high-performance liquid chromatography separation and quantitation, and mRNA encoding Hb F by an RNase protection assay. $R^2 = 0.924$ ($n = 45$; $P < .001$). (From Peri K, Gagnon C, Bard H: Quantitative correlation between globin mRNAs and synthesis of fetal and adult hemoglobins during hemoglobin switchover in the perinatal period. Pediatr Res 1998;43:506.)

molecular elements mediating regulation are protein transcription factors and short specialized regions of DNA sequences that are recognized by some of these transcription factors. The interaction causes these DNA elements to act as promoters, enhancers, or silences of gene activity.

Much is known about the structure and molecular pathology of human hemoglobin genes, but it is still not clear how their differential expression during normal development is regulated. The process of globin gene switching involves complex interactions of stage-specific transcription factors, chromosomal gene order, gene proximity to the globin locus control region, *cis*-acting sequences, and *trans*-acting factors.[32] The interaction causes these DNA elements to act as promoters, enhancers, or silencers of gene activity.

Nuclear proteins that interact with the globin gene clusters include DNA-binding proteins and proteins that interact with the DNA-binding proteins by means of specific protein-protein interactions. These domains, with respect to access to transcriptional activating elements, appear to be under the influence of an enhancer sequence, the locus control region (LCR). Each is located several tens of kilobases upstream of the ϵ-gene on chromosome 11 and the ζ-gene on chromosome 16. LCRs are modular DNA sequence elements. The LCR is required for the quantitatively high rates of globin gene expression during erythroid differentiation. The mechanism of how LCR determines the tissue specificity of globin gene expression in other tissues or the sequential activation and silencing of genes during hemoglobin switching remains unclear.

Associations of the LCR and the individual promoters, enhancers, and silencers during erythroid differentiation and hemoglobin switching require clarification. It appears that tissue and developmental specificity and highly active and efficient expression of individual globin genes require interaction between the LCR and the individual promoter or enhancer elements flanking the globin gene selected for expression. The essential role of promoters and enhancers located near the globin genes is suggested by the discovery of mutations in these regions that affect hemoglobin switching or that cause thalassemia-like syndromes; physical interactions between multiple protein-DNA complexes bound to individual gene promoters and the LCR are postulated to be involved.[33, 34]

The nuclei of erythroid cells contain numerous proteins that have been identified as transcription factors. Many of these are found in a wide variety of tissues. At least two factors, GATA-binding protein-1 (GATA-1) and erythroid-derived nuclear factor–2 (NF-E2), are much more restricted in their range of expression and have been implicated as particularly important for globin gene expression. Neither GATA-1 nor NF-E2 alone can be the sole determinants of tissue specificity of the globin genes. However, each of these proteins is indispensable for globin gene expression and erythropoiesis.[35, 36]

GATA-1 and NF-E2 are thought to interact with each other directly or by means of binding to intermediary proteins, activating the expression of globin genes and other genes necessary for erythroid maturation. Several other proteins have been identified as binding to various control elements in the globin gene cluster. Some of these appear to be stage-specific selector elements that bind predominantly to the γ- or β-globin gene enhancers and promoters. Others are generic transcription factors. The potential for expression of γ- and β-genes is determined in primitive erythroid stem cells (i.e., burst-forming unit–erythroid), long before actual expression of the globin genes is initiated at a later stage of differentiation.

Among the genetic factors known to affect Hb F production in adults are DNA sequence variations within the β-globin gene cluster, particularly the C→T variation at position −158 upstream of the $^{G}\gamma$-globin gene, which is detectable by the restriction enzyme *Xmn*I. This sequence variation has been shown to increase Hb F levels in β-thalassemia and sickle cell anemia.[37] Normal adults heterozygous or homozygous for this polymorphism have higher Hb F levels than controls without this variation.[38] An increase in Hb F has also been documented in the presence of this polymorphism during pregnancy[39] and in persons with Fanconi's anemia[40] or leukemia.[41]

The relationship of *Xmn*I polymorphism and Hb F has been studied in adult populations; however, it is not clear whether the presence (+) or absence (−) of an *Xmn*I restriction site can modulate the level of Hb F production during the switch from Hb F to Hb A. When human fetal development reaches the maturation that corresponds to term gestation, the switch from fetal to adult hemoglobin synthesis is near the midpoint of completion. Despite the same postconceptional age, the relative amounts of Hb F synthesized during this period of gestation can vary over a wide range (30% to 60%).[8] This dispersion of Hb F production exists in these newborn infants despite the fact that they are at the same stage of their maturational development.

The level of Hb F synthesis and $^{G}\gamma$-globin chain production is greater in term newborns with the *Xmn*I genotype. The ratio of $^{G}\gamma$-globin is increased in the presence of the (C→T) variation.[42] A DNA polymorphism of the *Xmn*I restriction site at −158 bp from the cap site of the $^{G}\gamma$-gene is associated with a delayed switch from Hb F to Hb A during the perinatal period.

Erythroid Precursor Cells

The burst-forming and colony-forming erythroid progenitor cells (BFU-E and CFU-E) are defined by morphologic criteria. The earliest recognizable erythroid cell is the proerythroblast that, after four to five mitotic divisions and serial morphologic changes, gives rise to mature erythroid cells. Their morphologic characteristics reflect the accumulation of erythroid specific proteins (e.g., hemoglobin) and the decline in nuclear activity. The deviation from the normal orderly maturation sequence is thought to be dictated by the level of erythropoietin. In response to an acute demand for red blood cell production (e.g., hypoxemia, blood lost, hemolysis), the kinetics of the formation of new reticulocytes are more rapid, resulting in skipped divisions and in larger cells containing increased amounts of Hb F.

The quantity of Hb F in the red blood cell is determined in the BFU-E and throughout the CFU-E period. In vitro, most BFU-Es have the potential to express high levels of Hb F, whereas in vivo, the proportion of Hb F that is expressed depends on the developmental age of the individual source from which the cell is derived. This potential appears to be lost during normal cell differentiation and maturation in vivo. This concept links the potential for increased Hb F expression to the pathway of erythroid differentiation and may have implications for interpreting the reactivation of Hb F synthesis that occurs in the perinatal period under diverse pathologic conditions (e.g., intrauterine growth retardation, infant of diabetic mother, anemia, congenital cyanotic heart disease). These circumstances influence Hb F levels by modifying the kinetics of the normal differentiation and maturation.

Stress Erythropoiesis

Studies have shown that hypoxia can increase Hb F synthesis in juvenile baboons[43] and in hyperglycemic fetal lambs.[44] Increased levels of Hb F synthesis have been documented in human newborns with prenatal complications associated with maternal hypoxemia,[45] placental insufficiency,[46] and diabetes.[47] In human studies, infants with oxygen-dependent bronchopulmonary dysplasia,[48] infants with severe anemia of prematurity,[49] and children with congenital cyanotic heart disease synthesized greater amounts of Hb F compared with controls.[50] In a study using fetal lambs late in gestation, hypoxemia, without any additional complicating factors, resulted in higher amounts of fetal hemoglobin being synthesized than could be expected for the time in gestation.[51] These important observations led to the hypotheses that hypoxemia increases the synthesis of Hb F and that reactivation of Hb F synthesis could be used as a marker for the detection of fetuses or infants at risk for hypoxic sequelae.

A group of conditions in which an altered hemoglobin pattern could possibly be of significance involves pregnancies in which the levels of Hb F in the cord blood are unusually high for the gestational age of the fetus. Infants who are small for gestational age as a result of placental insufficiency and have higher than normal levels of Hb F synthesis at birth rapidly adjust after birth, and by the age of 2 months, they are indistinguishable from normal-weight neonates in terms of the proportions of Hb F and Hb A synthesized.[46] This suggests that the higher Hb F levels at birth are a secondary effect and not the result of a change in the primary process of the switch. Fetal erythropoiesis is responsive to the hormone erythropoietin, the levels of which are regulated independently of the maternal circulation.[52]

The induction of increased Hb F has been

attributed to changes in the erythroid stem cell compartment induced by erythropoietic stimuli. The shift in source of reticulocytes to immature progenitors is thought to underline increased synthesis of Hb F. The programming of γ-gene expression is thought to be made at the level of the early erythroid progenitors, and the intrinsic potential of the early progenitors for Hb F synthesis is influenced by the stage of developmental maturation.

To explain the mechanisms involved, hematopoiesis at the cellular level must be described. Development of the pluripotent stem cell (CFU-S) leads to the production of erythrocytes, leukocytes, and platelets. The first cell committed to erythroid differentiation is a primitive progenitor, the BFU-E. A more mature erythroid progenitor is the CFU-E. These progenitors are mononuclear cells, which are not morphologically identifiable as erythroid. They are determined indirectly, based on their configuration and rate of colonies to which they give rise in vitro. Within these in vitro colonies or in the bone marrow in vivo are erythroid precursors that are in the various stages of morphologically recognizable nucleated erythroid cells, ranging from proerythroblasts to orthochromatophilic erythroblasts. These then mature into the definitive anucleate erythroid cells, reticulocytes, and erythrocytes. The hemoglobin synthesis programmed in the progenitors is determined by examination of hemoglobin synthesis in colonies derived from CFU-Es or BFU-Es. The relative proportions of Hb F and Hb A synthesis of the precursors are determined by the direct examination of peripheral blood, bone marrow, or liver obtained in vivo.

Many studies have determined hemoglobin synthesis in erythroid colonies grown from human cells obtained at various stages of development. In general, the results suggest that the pattern of hemoglobin synthesized in colonies produced by midgestation fetal cells closely resembles that produced by erythroid cells of intact animals of the same gestational development.[53] In colonies derived from cord blood cells that are in the process of switching, the pattern of synthesis in vitro is similar to that produced in vivo or shows slightly higher levels of γ-chain than β-chain synthesis, consistent with the fact that these cells are derived from precursors that in vivo would not differentiate into hemoglobin-synthesizing cells for another 1 to 2 weeks. Erythroid colonies derived from adult blood, however, consistently show increased proportions of Hb F synthesis, up to 30% of the total compared with a level of less than 2% in vivo. Analysis of colonies derived from precursor cells of increasing degrees of immaturity has shown a positive correlation between the proportion of Hb F synthesized (or proportion of Hb F-producing colonies) and the immaturity of the precursor.

These observations suggest a pattern of hemoglobin synthesis describing the maturation of the erythroid precursors; during erythroid differentiation, the maturation of the precursor cells obtained from adult sources have a decreasing capacity to produce Hb F.[54] The most primitive BFU-Es are programmed largely for Hb F production, whereas the more mature precursors are restricted to Hb A (or Hb F and Hb A) production, depending on the developmental age of the animal or human source of the cells.

The point in the maturation pathway at which the precursor cell becomes terminally committed to hemoglobin synthesis determines the type of hemoglobin in its progeny erythrocytes. In erythropoiesis of the normal, term newborn infant, most precursor cells complete the full program of maturation and produce approximately 50% Hb A and 50% Hb F. Conditions that promote the early commitment to hemoglobin synthesis of less mature BFU-E result in increased Hb F synthesis, and in vitro conditions using very high levels of erythropoietin may produce such an effect. If this concept is adapted to the perinatal period, in vivo situations in which there is likely to be increased recruitment of immature erythroid precursor cells should also be associated with increased Hb F production. This phenomenon is demonstrated in Figure 16–4. Such conditions are obtained in situations that stimulate acute erythroid expansion.

The possibility that erythropoiesis in the fetus has a different level of sensitivity to control factors needs further study, because differences in the behavior of fetal erythroid precursor cells (BFU-E and CFU-E) in vitro have been reported. These cells produce larger hemoglobinized colonies earlier in culture than their adult counterparts in mice,[55] sheep,[56] and humans,[57, 58] suggesting a shorter cell cycle time for the fetal cells. Moreover, the colonies appear

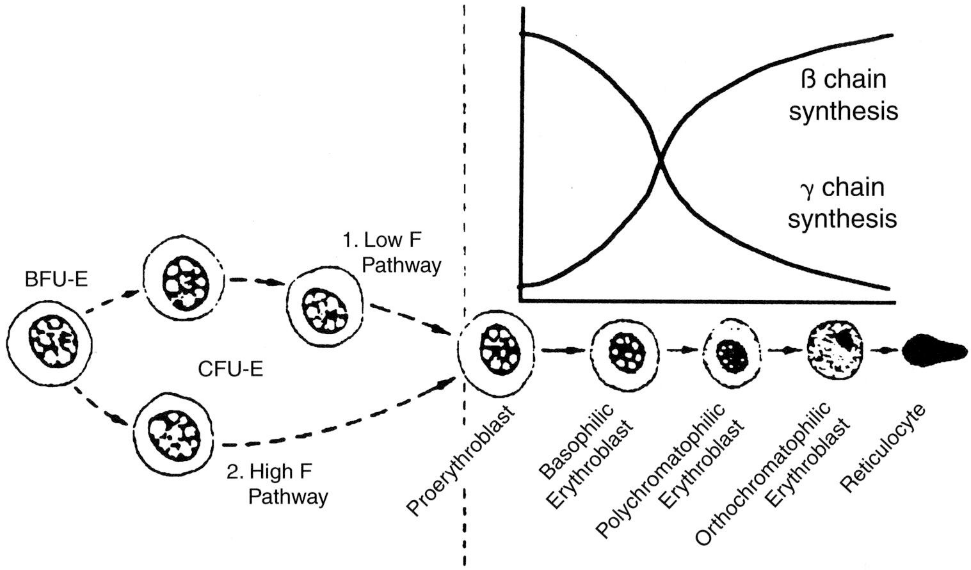

Figure 16–4. A model of the possible changes of hemoglobin (Hb F) synthesis during erythroid maturation and progenitor cell differentiation. Pathway 1 is that of normal progenitor differentiation and has a low chance for the production of increased Hb F. In pathway 2, premature commitment or skipping of divisions increases the likelihood of cells with increased Hb F synthesis. The diagram on the right illustrates the asynchronous synthesis of γ and β globin during the maturation of erythroblasts. (From Stamatoyannopoulos G, Nienhuis AW: Hemoglobin switching. In Collins FS, Weissman SM [eds]: The Molecular Basis of Blood Diseases, 2nd ed. Philadelphia: WB Saunders, 1994, p 135.)

at lower concentrations of exogenous erythropoietin. This may result from greater stimulation of the precursor cells in vivo, but it could imply that fetal cells are more sensitive to erythropoietin. The latter hypothesis may explain how the fetus is able to maintain its greater rate of red blood cell production when levels of circulating erythropoietin are low. These differences in the patterns of erythropoiesis could play a role in determining the type of hemoglobin produced.

Evidence suggesting that such a relationship may occur comes from the studies of hemoglobin synthesis in erythroid colonies in vitro and from the association of increased Hb F production with acute marrow expansion observed in vivo.[59–61] Experimental support for this concept has been provided by DeSimone and colleagues,[62] using the baboon as an animal model. Baboons subjected to acute anemia by injections of phenylhydrazine or placed in hypobaric chambers to stimulate an altitude of 23,000 feet respond to this acute erythroid demand by producing Hb F.[63] In adults, Hb F production appears to be restricted to a subpopulation of red blood cells, the F cells. These cells originate from the same progenitors as erythrocytes, which do not contain fetal hemoglobin. An impressive stimulation of F cell production in baboons treated with recombinant human erythropoietin was shown by pulsed administration of high levels of recombinant erythropoietin, which induced rapid erythroid regeneration and stimulated the formation of Hb F.[64]

Reactivation of Hemoglobin F

During stress erythropoiesis, when immature progenitors are forced to enter terminal differentiation rather than maturation pathways, a greater number of red blood cells that contain Hb F than is normally expected for the stage of development appear in the circulation. These cells are the product of premature differentiation of erythroid progenitors rather than the orderly production of reticulocytes from dividing and maturing proerythroblasts. The response of γ-gene expression to erythropoietin is thought to represent the effect of the hormone on recruitment of more immature progenitors into erythroblast colony formation.

When sudden accelerated demands for erythropoiesis occur, such as the demands of hypoxia or anemia, a massive influx of proerythroblasts derived from the progenitor pool can be demonstrated. It has been shown[65] that a need for reticulocytes during stress erythropoiesis is not met by a change in the division rate of erythroblasts but rather by an influx of new proerythroblasts from progenitors. Based on the results obtained from experiments using primates, cell cycle–specific drugs, acute bleeding, or recombinant erythropoietin, increase in Hb F production appears 3 to 4 days after treatment and peaks between 5 and 6 days after treatment.[66]

The phenomenon of stress erythropoiesis may explain the numerous reports proposing that elevated neonatal nucleated erythrocyte counts could be a marker of fetal hypoxia,[67] which in some cases is sufficient to cause central nervous system injury.[68] The influx of erythroblasts resulting from stress erythropoiesis triggered by fetal hypoxemia correlates with neurologically impaired infants. These studies have also correlated the elevation of the number of immature red blood cells with the presence of fetal asphyxia documented by abnormal umbilical artery Doppler measurements.[69]

Neonatal Red Blood Cell Survival

Because of frequent blood sampling, hemorrhagic complications, and anemia of prematurity, early preterm newborn infants represent a group of patients considered to be the most frequent recipients of blood transfusions. It is important for the clinical care of these infants to have a good estimate of the life span of the transfused red blood cells that they receive.

Earlier studies attempted to determine autologous newborn red blood cell survival. It is almost 3 decades since Pearson[70] provided some general conclusions about the red blood cell life span in the newborn infant. It is shorter in the term infant than in adults, and the shortness is more pronounced in preterm infants. The estimates of survival of transfused erythrocytes carried out in the 1940s,[71, 72] based on the Ashby differential agglutination technique,[73] were believed to carry a considerable error.

After the advent of radioisotopes, the Ashby method was quickly replaced by isotopic methods. The ^{51}Cr technique was the method of choice, and these studies[70] reported a mean ^{51}Cr half-life of erythrocytes from term infants of 23.3 days (range, 13 to 35 days) and a mean value for red blood cells from preterm infants of 16.6 days (range, 9 to 26 days). Conversion of these fetal red blood cell life spans for term infants from ^{51}Cr half-life to true red blood cell survival times indicated an actual life span of approximately 60 to 70 days. Similar calculations for the red blood cells of preterm infants provided values of 35 to 50 days.

Based on the studies that followed the changes in the levels of Hb A and Hb F in the peripheral circulation after a blood transfusion, the mean life span of adult red blood cells transfused to preterm infants was determined to be 56.4 $\pm$ 7 days (range, 46 to 68 days).[74] This length of survival is within the range of what has been generally accepted for labeled cord blood cells when transfused to newborns or adults, but it is much shorter than the 110 to 120 days expected for adult red blood cells transfused to adults. Fetal red blood cells have a shorter life span than adult red blood cells, possibly because of differences in physical properties related to surface charge, aggregation, deformability, filterability, and fragility.[75] However, the findings in this study may suggest the existence of unknown endogenous environmental factors specific to immature infants that affect the life span of autologous and allogenic erythrocytes. The red blood cell life span may be related to body weight; the red blood cells of large mammals live longer than those of small ones.[76]

The results obtained on the changes in the proportion of Hb F and Hb A after a transfusion[74] imply that the half-life (i.e., the number of days after of transfusion at which one half of the cells infused remain in the circulation) is about 30 days (i.e., a 1.7% elimination rate). This information could be a useful reference for guiding clinicians caring for preterm infants after a transfusion or an exchange transfusion and for those who are responsible for in utero fetal transfusions.

HEMOGLOBIN OXYGEN AFFINITY

In most mammals investigated, the oxygen affinity of fetal blood is higher than that of adult blood. After birth, the oxygen affinity gradually decreases to the adult levels. The time course of this decrease in oxygen affinity varies by species. Although the difference in oxygen affinity between human fetal and adult blood has been known since 1931,[77] the mechanism responsible has been clarified only during the past decade. The difference mainly reflects the intrinsic structure of the hemoglobin molecule, the specific action of 2,3-DPG on the hemoglobin molecule,[78, 79] and the unspecific effects of changes of the red blood cell pH.[80, 81]

The multiple molecular forms of hemoglobin in normal humans and other animals that have developed in the course of evolution appear to confer a physiologic advantage within the period of ontogeny during which that particular hemoglobin is present in high concentration. In humans, it is the switch from fetal to adult hemoglobin synthesis that has evolved as the main method for the change in red blood cell oxygen affinity from the fetal to the air environment.

The oxygen dissociation curve of normal fetal blood represents the reaction of the intracellular hemoglobin type (Hb A and Hb F) with oxygen as modified by the ligands present in the intracellular environment. The ligands of physiologic importance are hydrogen ions, 2,3-DPG, and carbon dioxide. The oxygen affinity of hemoglobin within the red blood cell strongly depends on the intrinsic properties of the type of hemoglobin. However, the position of the oxygen dissociation curve can be modified by a number of heterotopic modifiers such as temperature, pH, organic phosphates, and carbon dioxide concentration. The effect of these modifiers on the oxygen tension at which the hemoglobin molecule is half saturated (P_{50}) are shown in Figure 16–5.

The major intracellular modulator of hemoglobin's oxygen affinity in human erythrocytes is the organic phosphate, 2,3-DPG, an intermediate product of glycolysis present within the erythrocyte at concentrations equimolar to hemoglobin. The synthesis of 2,3-DPG is enzymatically regulated, and it is able to bind stereospecifically within the central cavity of the hemoglobin tetramer. In the absence of 2,3-DPG, hemoglobin has a very high oxygen af-

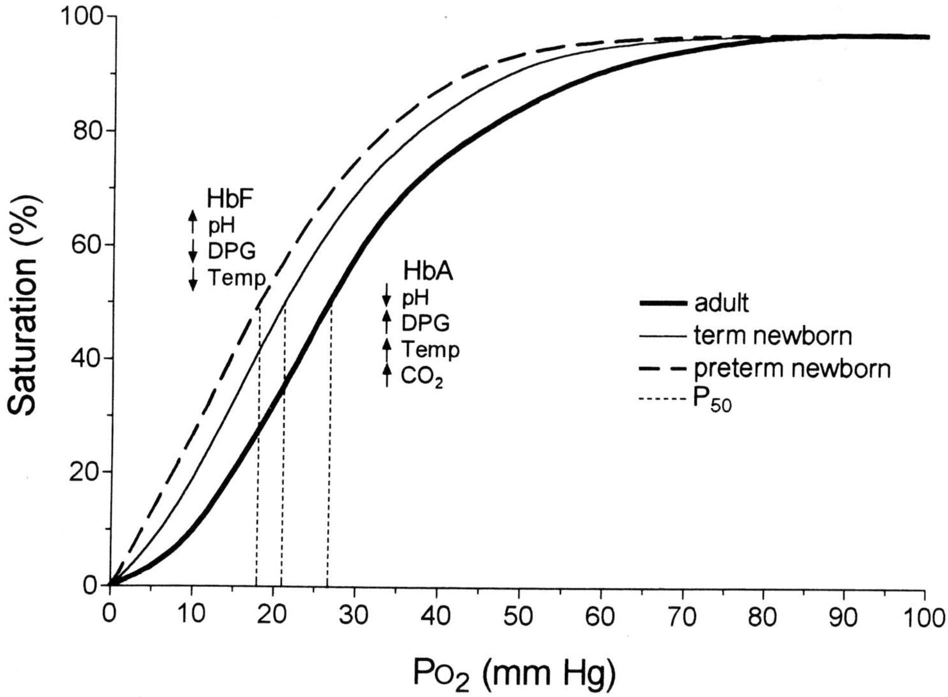

Figure 16–5. The oxygen dissociation curve of hemoglobin during different periods of development. The approximate P_{50} (i.e., oxygen tension at which the hemoglobin is 50% saturated) of adult blood is 27 mm Hg, that of a term newborn infant is 22 mm Hg, and that of a preterm newborn is 18 mm Hg. The heterotropic modifiers of hemoglobin function shown can increase (leftward shift) or decrease (rightward shift) hemoglobin oxygen affinity.

finity but, as 2,3-DPG is added to a hemoglobin solution, the oxygen affinity progressively decreases. DPG is a polyanion that binds strongly to the deoxygenated form of hemoglobin but poorly to its oxygenated or other ligand-bound forms. Specific amino acids (β-chain residues) are involved in the binding of 2,3-DPG.

Red blood cells containing high levels of fetal hemoglobin exhibit high oxygen affinity because Hb F binds 2,3-DPG poorly. Physiologically, this ensures that the hemoglobin of the fetus is oxygenated at the expense of the maternal Hb A. The high oxygen affinity of Hb F caused by its low affinity for 2,3-DPG is accounted for by a single change in its primary structure: the presence of a serine residue at helical position H21 in place of the histidine found in the β-globin chain. Mutations of the α- or β-globin chains that affect 2,3-DPG binding have been identified; these mutant hemoglobins have altered oxygen affinity.

In the human fetus, the decrease in oxygen affinity of fetal red blood cells during last trimester of gestation is mainly caused by the increase in the amount of adult-type hemoglobin. The changes in P_{50} as gestational age advances are shown in Figure 16–6. The P_{50} value correlates significantly with gestational age. The regression line increases from 17.8 mm Hg at 24 weeks to 22.5 mm Hg at 42 weeks of gestation.[82] The oxygen tension at which cord blood is 50% saturated (P_{50}) at term gestation is 19 to 22 mm Hg; this level is 6 to 8 mm Hg lower than that of normal adult blood. This shift is explained by the poor binding of 2,3-DPG to Hb F. The position of the oxygen dissociation curve is determined by the percentage of Hb A and the red blood cell content of 2,3-DPG.

The increased oxygen affinity of Hb F may confer a physiologic advantage to the fetus in facilitating the transfer of oxygen from the mother to the fetus. However, normal fetal development has been recorded when, because of maternal hemoglobinopathies, the maternal oxygen affinity may be decreased in relation to the fetus. As the relative proportion of Hb A increases, the oxygen dissociation curve of the newborn shifts toward that of the adult.[83]

The association between PaO_2 and 90% oxygen saturation of hemoglobin in the early preterm newborn has been described (Fig. 16–7).[84] The data obtained demonstrate the fetal nature

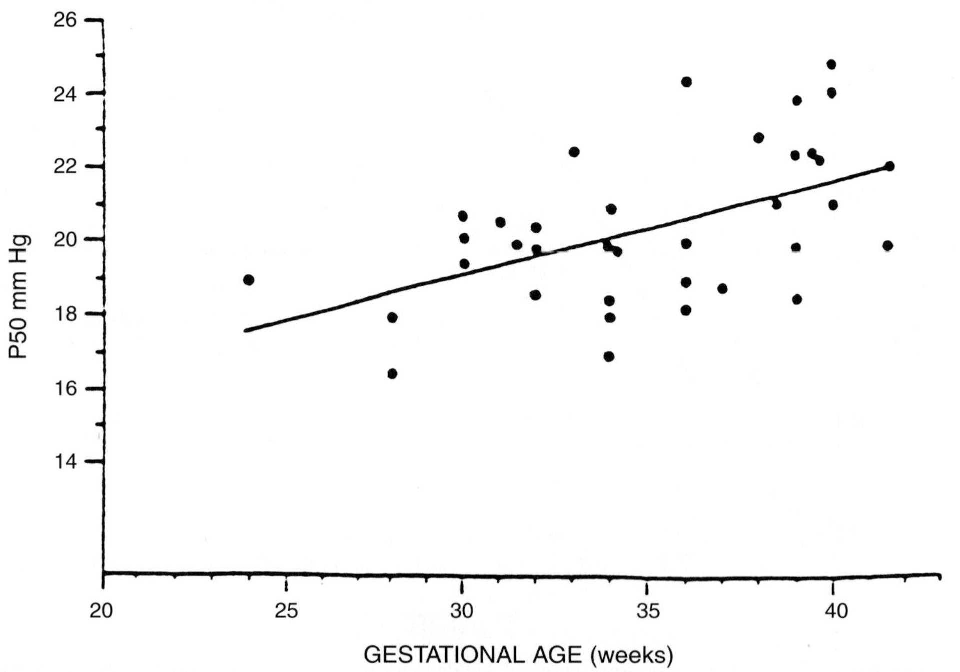

Figure 16–6. Blood P_{50} in relation to gestational age. The solid line is the calculated linear regression line ($r = 0.62$; $P < .001$). (From Bard H, Teasdale F: Red cell oxygen affinity, hemoglobin type, 2,3-diphosphoglycerate, and pH as a function of fetal development. Pediatrics 1979;64:483. Reproduced by permission of Pediatrics.)

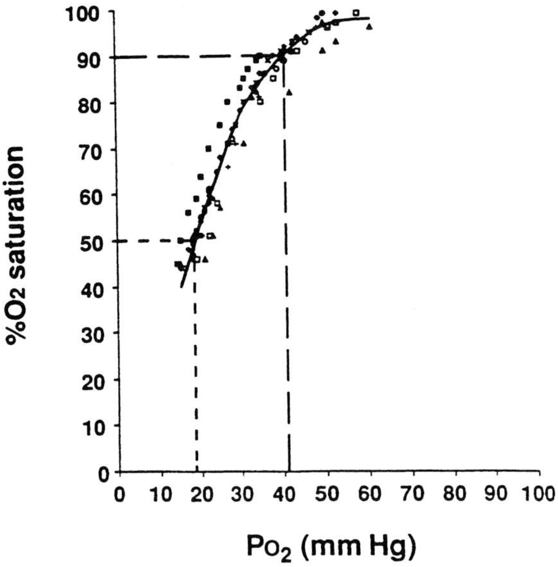

Figure 16–7. Mean hemoglobin-oxygen dissociation curve at a pH of 7.4 for newborns weighing less than 1000 g at birth after less than 30 weeks of gestation. Each type of symbol represents a different infant. The P_{50} was 18.3 mm Hg, and P_{90} was 40.8 mm Hg. (From Emond D, Lachance C, Gagnon C, et al: Arterial pressure of oxygen required to achieve 90% saturation of hemoglobin in very low birth weight newborns. Pediatrics 1993;91:602. Reproduced by permission of Pediatrics.)

of the oxygen dissociation curve of the very-low-birth-weight newborn, which reflects the virtual absence of adult-type hemoglobin early in gestation.[85] On the basis of this report, an increase in PaO_2 above 50 mm Hg can achieve very little in terms of oxygen content, because the hemoglobin is virtually completely saturated. The findings of this report show that a minimal PaO_2 of 41 mm Hg (5.5 kPa) could be adequate to saturate 90% of the hemoglobin at a physiologic pH.

During adult life in a variety of clinical states in which tissue oxygenation is impaired, the DPG levels rise, producing a decrease in red blood cell oxygen affinity.[86] However, a similar role for 2,3-DPG in utero may be detrimental to the fetus if the higher oxygen affinity of fetal blood favors the placental transfer of oxygen to the fetus. The observation by Novy and coworkers[87] that fetal anemia does not cause a rise in 2,3-DPG levels suggests that the ability for fetal red blood cells to increase 2,3-DPG in utero may be limited. The human fetus appears to respond to the stress of hypoxia by an increase in the synthesis of fetal hemoglobin and an increase of its red blood cell mass.[46]

HEMOGLOBINOPATHIES

Thalassemia Syndromes

The main characteristic of thalassemia syndromes is a decreased or absent synthesis of one or more globin chains. The α- and β-thalassemias refer to deficits in α- and β-globin production, respectively. Because the structural gene for α-globin is duplicated on chromosome 16, each diploid human cell contains four copies of the α-globin gene. The four α-thalassemia syndromes, which are silent carrier, α-thalassemia trait, Hb H disease, and hydrops fetalis, reflect the inheritance of molecular defects affecting the output of one, two, three, or four of the α-globin genes, respectively. More than 30 different mutations affecting one or both α-globin genes on a chromosome have been described.[88] Some mutations abolish expression of an α-globin gene (α°), whereas others reduce expression of the gene to a variable degree (α^+). Each of the four general categories of α-thalassemia has marked genetic and clinical heterogeneity. Heterogeneity arises because the syndrome in any given individual may represent the combination of 2 or more of the 30 mutations that have been described.

The β-thalassemias also include four clinical syndromes of increasing severity: silent carrier, thalassemia trait, thalassemia intermedia, and thalassemia major.[89–91] In contrast to the α-thalassemias, the four classes of β-thalassemia are not correlated with the number of functioning genes. Because a single functional β-globin gene resides on each chromosome 11, a diploid cell normally has two β-globin genes. The clinical heterogeneity of the β-thalassemias represents the diversity of specific mutations that variably affect β-globin gene expression. Many mutations eliminate β-globin gene expression (β°), whereas others variably decrease the level of β-globin gene expression (β^+).[90, 91] The capacity of individual patients to synthesize γ-globin affects the clinical severity because the severity of thalassemias is determined by the degree of globin chain imbalance rather than the absolute level of α- or β-globin synthesis.[92–95] An adequate amount of γ-globin synthesis in the immature red blood cells of β-thalassemic individuals lessens the extent of chain imbalance and improves red blood cell production.[96–98] Clinical severity in any individual patient represents the outcome of complex genetic interactions.

The clinical syndrome can be considered to be based on the consequences of inadequate hemoglobin accumulation and the unbalanced accumulation of globin subunits. The former causes hypochromia and microcytosis, and the latter produces ineffective erythropoiesis and hemolytic anemia. The clinical symptoms can range from asymptomatic hypochromia or microcytosis to severe anemia. Thalassemia represents the most common gene disorder known and, in many parts of the world, constitutes a major public health problem.

The most common form of thalassemia arises from the total absence or the partial reduction in the synthesis of structurally normal globin chains. It contrasts with the structural hemoglobinopathies (e.g., sickle cell anemia), which are characterized by the production of normal amounts of mutant globin chains having abnormal physical or chemical properties. The thalassemias are considered to be quantitative disorders. The primary lesion lies in the amount, but some rare forms of thalassemias are characterized by the production of structurally abnormal globin chains in reduced amounts.[99]

The pathophysiology and molecular biology of individual forms of thalassemia are interrelated. The primary lesion in all forms of thalassemia is reduced or absent production of one or more globin chains. The major impact on clinical well-being occurs only when these lesions affect the α- or β-globin chains necessary for the synthesis of Hb A ($\alpha_2\beta_2$). Severe impairment of γ-, ε-, or ζ-globin production is considered lethal in utero. One consequence of reduced globin chain production that is immediately apparent is the reduced production of functioning hemoglobin tetramers. As a result, hypochromia and microcytosis are characteristic of virtually all patients with thalassemia. In the milder forms of the disease, this phenomenon may be barely detectable.

The second consequence of impaired globin biosynthesis is unbalanced synthesis of the individual α- and β-subunits. Hemoglobin tetramers are highly soluble and have reversible oxygen-carrying properties exquisitely adapted for oxygen transport and delivery under physiologic conditions. Free α-, β-, and γ-globin chains are highly insoluble, are incapable of releasing oxygen normally, or both. The abnormal solubility or oxygen-carrying properties of these chains lead to a variety of physiologic abnormalities. In the severe forms of thalassemia, it is the unpaired globin chains accumulating in relative excess that dominates the pathophysiology of the severe forms of the thalassemia syndrome, rather than the mere underproduction of functioning hemoglobin tetramers. The precise complications of this pathophysiologic phenomenon are rather diverse, depending on the amount and the identity of the globin chain accumulating in excess. The thalassemias cause symptoms by underproduction of hemoglobin and by accumulation of unpaired globin subunits. The unpaired subunits are usually the major source of morbidity and mortality.

The predominant circulating hemoglobin at the moment of birth is Hb F ($\alpha_2\gamma_2$).[85] Although the switch from α- to β-globin biosynthesis begins before birth, the composition of hemoglobin in the peripheral blood changes much later because of the life span of normal circulating red blood cells. Because Hb F is slowly replaced by Hb A, the infants do not depend heavily on normal amounts and function of Hb A until they are 4 to 6 months of age. The pathophysiologic consequences of these considerations are that α-chain hemoglobinopathies tend to be symptomatic in utero and at birth, whereas individuals with β-chain abnormalities are asymptomatic until 4 to 6 months of age. These differences in the onset of phenotypic expression arise because α-chains are needed to form Hb F and Hb A, whereas β-chains are required only for Hb A.

Hereditary Persistence of Fetal Hemoglobin

Some mutations alter the patterns of fetal to adult hemoglobin switching. This condition is called hereditary persistence of fetal hemoglobin and usually is not associated with clinical symptoms. The mutations' importance lies in their roles as interesting models for investigating the molecular basis for gene regulation during human development.

Thalassemia Intermedia

Approximately 10% of patients with homozygous β-thalassemia exhibit a phenotype characterized by intermediate hematologic severity. This condition is called thalassemia intermedia.

β-*Thalassemia Minor*

β-Thalassemia minor, also called thalassemia trait, is caused by an inherited single β-thalassemia allele that results in a hypochromic microcytic anemia. Elevation in Hb A_2 and Hb F occurs during the early years of life.[100]

Hemoglobin Barts

Hydrops fetalis results from the homozygous state for the α-thalassemia 1-*cis* deletion. The α-globins are totally absent. There is no physiologically useful hemoglobin beyond the embryonic stage of development. Free γ-globulin accumulates, forming γ_4-tetramers called Hb Barts. Hb Barts has a very high hemoglobin oxygen affinity, and no oxygen is released at the tissue level, resulting in severe asphyxia, edema, congestive heart failure, and usually death in utero.

Thalassemic Structure of Variants

Specific structural hemoglobin variants are characterized by biosynthetic defects and abnormal structures, such as Hb Lepore ($\alpha_2[\gamma\delta\gamma\beta_2]$) or Hb E ($\alpha_2\beta_2^{26glu \rightarrow lys}$).

The successful prenatal diagnosis of α-thalassemia of the hydrops fetalis variety using solution hybridization methods to detect deficiency of α-globin genes in amniotic fluid cell DNA was first reported by Kan and associates in 1975.[101] Southern blot analysis rapidly supplanted this approach for the detection of gene deletion in α- or β-thalassemias.[102, 103]

Detection of mutations in DNA rapidly became the preferred strategy for prenatal diagnosis as mutations became defined in β-thalassemias.[104] The introduction of polymerase chain reaction methods further facilitated mutation detection and permitted the use of nonradioactive tests.[105] Coupled with chorionic villus biopsy, accurate and safe diagnoses can be accomplished within the first trimester of pregnancy.

Sickle Cell Disease

Characterization

An inherited multisystem disorder, the main features of sickle cell disease are chronic hemolytic anemia and recurrent painful episodes related to the presence of a mutant sickle cell anemia (Hb S) within the red blood cells. The A→T nucleotide substitution in the sixth codon of the β-globin gene and substitution of valine for glutamic acid on the outer surface of the Hb S molecule cause reduced solubility and polymerization of Hb S when deoxygenated, sickling and poor deformability of polymer-containing erythrocytes, and occlusion by sickle cells of the microvasculature. The syndromes and genotypes that compose sickle cell disease are mainly sickle cell anemia (Hb SS), sickle cell β°-thalassemia (Hb S-β° thal), Hb SC disease (Hb SC), sickle cell B + thal (Hb S-B + thal), and sickle trait (Hb AS), which causes no anemia or pain.

The pathologic basis of the disorder and its relation to the hemoglobin molecule were defined in 1927 by Hahn and Gillespie.[106] Pauling and coworkers,[107] Beet,[108] and Neel[109] defined the genetics of the disorder and clearly distinguished sickle trait, the heterozygous condition (AS), from sickle cell anemia, the homozygous state (SS). Ingram applied tryptic digestion, high-voltage electrophoresis, and paper chromatography to the isolated sickle hemoglobin and found that the amino acid substitution in sickle hemoglobin was a valine instead of a glutamic acid in the number 6 position of the β-chain. The α-chain is normal.[110] The chemical nomenclature for sickle hemoglobin is therefore $\alpha_2\beta_2^{6Glu \rightarrow Val}$. The milestones of sickle cell anemia have been reviewed elsewhere.[111]

The sickle gene is a common mutant that provides some protection to infants who may otherwise succumb to cerebral falciparum malaria, and its incidence in certain countries parallels the incidence of malaria. Whereas the average incidence of the sickle gene among American blacks is approximately 8%,[112] the frequency is much higher in inhabitants of certain areas of Africa.

In 1927, Hahn and Gillespie[106] showed that sickling, which is the change from a biconcave disk to the sickle form, depended on deoxygenation. Electron micrographs of sickled red blood cells reveal long, thin bundles of Hb S fibers that run parallel to the long axis of the cell or the abnormal protuberances. The ultrastructure of these Hb S fibers has been detailed by electron microscopy and image reconstruction.[113–115]

The polymerization of deoxy-Hb S is a highly complex process that results in the formation of gelled, aggregated Hb S tetramers in equilibrium with hemoglobin tetramers in solution. Perturbations in oxygen levels,[116, 117] temperature,[118–120] pH,[121, 122] ionic strength,[123] 2,3-DPG,[122, 124, 125] and carbon monoxide[126, 127] affect the formation of Hb S gels. This sol-gel transition of Hb S is the basic feature that leads to the viscosity changes, distortion of cell morphology, sludging, and organ infarction that are identified as the clinical manifestations of sickle cell disease.

The interaction with other hemoglobins supports a rational basis for the understanding of the clinical manifestations of the various sickle syndromes. Numerous investigators have carefully studied mixtures of Hb S with Hb F or Hb A to determine the effects on gelation and solubility.[121, 128–131] The kinetic data show that Hb A and Hb F have a profound, dose-related effect, increasing the delay time and decreasing Hb S polymer content in cells. The effect of Hb F is considerably larger than the effect of Hb A.

Fetal hemoglobin can be increased in patients with sickle cell anemia and presumably increase delay times and decrease polymer content within cells. In the interactions of Hb S with Hb F, increasing the amount of Hb F increases the delay time and solubility of Hb S. In sickle cell disease, 4-azacytidine[132–134] and hydroxyurea[135–137] have been used successfully to increase Hb F in SS individuals. Recombinant human erythropoietin in supraphysiologic doses has also transiently increased Hb F in adult sickle cell patients.[138] Administration of recombinant erythropoietin with hydroxyurea has inconsistently increased Hb F above levels obtained with hydroxyurea alone.[139, 140] Butyric acid analogues also increase fetal hemoglobin production in sickle cell patients, some thalassemia patients, and normal individuals.[141, 142] In addition to increasing Hb F, hydroxyurea has reduced the proportion of dense cells and increased the mean corpuscular volume and mean corpuscular hemoglobin concentration of sickle cells.[134–136] Epidemiologic data show that increases in Hb F from 4% to 16% can decrease vaso-occlusive crises by 50%.[143]

Methods of prenatal diagnosis for sickle cell anemia have improved rapidly in the past 2 decades. In 1978, Kan and Dozy[144] described DNA polymorphisms around the β-globin gene, leading to the first DNA-based method for prenatal diagnosis. Later, direct detection of the mutation became possible, because the A→T substitution in codon 6 responsible for the glutamic acid to valine change in β-globin altered the recognition site of restriction enzyme.[145–147] Wallace and coworkers[148] showed that specific synthetic oligonucleotides could be used to recognize homologous sequences; this finding led to the development of radioactive and nonradioactive probes that specifically bind to the normal β-globin gene or the mutant sickle gene.[149–152] Polymerase chain reaction amplification of specific DNA sequences produces a sufficient amount of DNA to be obtained from a few fetal cells. Chorionic villous biopsy offers an alternative to amniocentesis for obtaining fetal cells as early as 8 to 10 weeks' gestation.[153, 154]

The newborn with sickle cell anemia usually is not anemic and is asymptomatic because of the protective effect of fetal hemoglobin. The "sickle prep" and solubility tests are unreliable during the first few months of life. Death from bacterial sepsis or sequestration crisis is more likely for infants with sickle cell anemia after 2 to 3 months of age.

Because recognition of the disease in the newborn can lead to prevention of mortality and morbidity, all newborns at risk should be screened for sickle cell anemia.[155] Screening using starch gel electrophoresis and acid or alkaline electrophoresis was first done on a large scale by Schneider and Gilman and their associates.[156, 157] Screening combined with comprehensive follow-up care was first begun by Pearson in New Haven and Serjeant in Jamaica in the 1970s.[158, 159]

Current screening methodologies include acid and alkaline electrophoresis, high-performance liquid chromatography, and isoelectric focusing. These tests can be performed on cord blood or on a dried blood specimen blotted on filter paper. Diagnosis can also be performed using polymerase chain reaction amplification of DNA extracted from filter paper.[160] Several studies have confirmed that neonatal diagnosis and follow-up can reduce mortality of infants with sickle cell anemia and can be cost effective.[161–164]

Hb F has an inhibitory effect on Hb S polymerization and cellular sickling. The high fraction of Hb F at birth masks the expression of sickle cell disease until Hb S levels increase to more than 75% at about 6 months.

Pharmacologic Manipulation of Hemoglobin F Synthesis

Because of the compelling biochemical and clinical evidence that Hb F inhibits sickling, drugs that increase the production of Hb F can be expected to benefit patients with sickle cell disease. The first drug to be tested, 5-azacytidine, an antineoplastic drug that inhibits maintenance methylation of DNA, caused a marked increase in Hb F in baboons.[165] These results prompted limited clinical trials that demonstrated significant, but not dramatic, induction of Hb F production in patients with sickle cell disease.[134, 166] Subsequently, other antitumor drugs, particularly hydroxyurea, were shown to increase the production of Hb F in nonhuman primates and in patients with SS disease.[135, 136] The molecular mechanism through which these agents stimulate Hb F production is unknown.

There is considerable interest in the physiologic and pharmacologic roles of butyric acid and its analogues in the regulation of Hb F production. In infants of diabetic mothers, the switch from Hb F to Hb A is delayed.[47, 167] This delay is associated with increased serum concentrations of amino-*n*-butyric acid.[168] This metabolite and sodium butyrate enhance the expression of the γ-globin gene in erythroid progenitors from patients with sickle cell disease or β-thalassemia.[169] Infusions of butyrate in sheep fetuses[170] and normal baboons[171] resulted in increased Hb F production. However, the data disagree about the efficacy of butyrate therapy in patients with β-thalassemia or sickle cell disease.[141]

Unstable Hemoglobins

Other than sickle cell anemia and thalassemias, the major hemoglobinopathies producing clinical symptoms are caused by hemoglobins exhibiting altered solubility (i.e., unstable hemoglobins), hemoglobins with increased oxygen affinity, hemoglobins with decreased oxygen affinity, and methemoglobins. The abnormal functional properties of most mutant hemoglobins do not produce laboratory or clinical abnormalities relevant to clinical practice.

The term *unstable hemoglobins* has been applied to hemoglobins exhibiting reduced solubility or higher susceptibility to oxidation of amino acid residues within the individual globin chains. More than 100 structurally different unstable hemoglobin mutants have been documented.[172] Most exhibit only mild instability by means of in vitro laboratory tests and do not generate significant clinical manifestations. Both α- and β-globin variants can cause this condition, but about 75% of the mutations described are β-globin variants.

The clinical symptoms of unstable hemoglobins depend in part on the quantitative proportion of the abnormal hemoglobin. Because the α-globin genes are duplicated, mutation in a single locus usually produces only 25% to 35% abnormal globin. In contrast, a simple heterozygote at the single β-globin locus produces 50% of the abnormal variant.

The mechanisms by which unstable hemoglobin mutations produce hemoglobin precipitation remain incompletely understood. The fundamental step in the pathogenesis appears to be derangement of the normal linkages between heme and globins. Loss of appropriate globin chain folding and interaction may ultimately destabilize the heme-globin linkage or lead to partial proteolysis of the chain, thereby releasing heme from that linkage. The freed heme probably binds nonspecifically to other regions of the globin molecule, forming precipitated hemichromes, which lead to further denaturation and aggregation of the globin subunits to form a precipitate containing α- and β-globin chains, globin fragments, and heme, called the Heinz body.[173, 174]

Heinz bodies interact with red blood cell membrane components, thereby reducing red blood cell deformability. These cells tend to be trapped in the splenic microcirculation and "pitted," reflecting attempts by the splenic macrophages to remove the Heinz bodies. Several biochemical perturbations correlate with the presence of free heme, including generation of reactive oxidants such as hydrogen peroxide, superoxide, and hydroxyl radicals. The end result of this process is premature destruction of the red blood cell, producing hemolytic anemia. Individual unstable hemoglobins vary considerably in their propensity to generate Heinz bodies and hemolysis. An example of this variability is the Hb Zurich variant, which exhibits relatively mild insolubility and virtually absent hemolysis. Hemolysis may become clinically apparent only with additional oxidant stresses, such as infection and fever, or after ingestion of oxidant drugs.[175]

Unstable hemoglobins are usually inherited as autosomal dominant disorders. However, the rate of spontaneous mutation appears to be high, so that the absence of affected parents or siblings does not exclude the presence of an unstable hemoglobin in a family. A positive family history can be a useful adjunct to diagnosis and should prompt consideration of an unstable hemoglobin as the cause of the familial hemolytic diathesis.

The clinical syndrome associated with unstable hemoglobin disorders is often called *congenital Heinz body hemolytic anemia*. This term is derived from the fact that only the most severe cases were detected before the widespread availability of advanced methods for detecting and characterizing abnormal hemoglobins. Clinical manifestations range from a virtually asymptomatic state in the absence of environmental stressors to severe hemolytic anemia manifesting at birth. Unstable hemoglobin should be suspected in infants with one or more stigmata of accelerated red blood cell destruction: chronic or intermittent hemolytic anemia or jaundice, unexplained reticulocytosis, or bouts of intermittent symptoms that can be related to exposure to oxidant drugs or infections. Other symptoms include dark urine and transient jaundice.

Laboratory diagnosis depends on identification of a mutant hemoglobin that precipitates more easily than normal hemoglobin. The peripheral blood smear may or may not show evidence of hemolysis (i.e., poikilocytosis, polychromasia, or shift cells). The morphologic evidence for precipitated hemoglobin is the Heinz body, the intraerythrocytic inclusion body detected by staining the peripheral blood smear with a supravital dye, such as brilliant cresyl blue or new methylene blue. The spleen removes Heinz bodies efficiently, especially if hemolysis is not particularly acute or brisk. Heinz bodies may not be demonstrable at all times.

Hemoglobin electrophoresis should be performed but should not be relied on as the major diagnostic criterion for confirming or excluding a hemoglobinopathy. Many amino acid substitutions that have important effects on solubility do not change the overall charge on the hemoglobin molecule. If the clinical picture or family history supports the diagnosis, a normal electrophoresis result should not be regarded as evidence against the possibility of a mutant hemoglobin.

The severity of the clinical complications of unstable hemoglobins varies enormously. Many infants can be managed adequately by observation and parental education to avoid oxidant drugs that provoke hemolysis. Some patients may require transfusions during bouts of severe acute hemolytic anemia. Children with severe hemolysis may require transfusion support until they are old enough (3 or 4 years of age) to undergo splenectomy without unacceptable immunologic compromise. Splenectomy is usually effective for abolition or reduction of symptoms. Infection often exacerbates hemolysis. Fever should therefore prompt close monitoring of patients for evidence of hemolysis or anemia.

HEMOGLOBIN VARIANTS WITH ABNORMAL OXYGEN BINDING

Oxygen transport by hemoglobin depends on the sigmoidal shape of the hemoglobin–oxygen affinity curve. During the transition from the fully deoxygenated (T) to the fully oxygenated (R) state, the initial oxygenation steps occur with difficulty. The act of binding the first oxygen molecule increases the affinity of the molecule for subsequent oxygen binding events, creating the sigmoidal shape of the curve. The necessary intramolecular reorganization occurs only when the proper arrangement of hydrogen bonds, hydrophobic interactions, and salt bridges is broken and formed in the proper sequence during R-T transitions.

Mutant hemoglobins exhibiting altered oxygen affinity arise from amino acid substitutions at the interface between α- and β-chains or in regions affecting the hydrogen bonds, hydrophobic interactions, or salt bridges that influence the interaction of heme with oxygen. A second major class of mutations alters binding to 2,3-DPG, which alters oxygen affinity when bound to hemoglobin.

Hemoglobin with Increased Oxygen Affinity

High-affinity hemoglobins exhibit higher affinity for oxygen, causing the oxygen dissociation curve to shift to the left. These hemoglobins bind oxygen more readily than normal and retain the oxygen at lower PO_2 levels. At normal capillary PO_2, high-affinity hemoglobins may deliver less oxygen. At physiologic hematocrits, a mild tissue hypoxia can occur that stimulates an increase in erythropoietin production, causing elevated red blood cell production and polycythemia. Some affected mothers have had normal term pregnancies.[176, 177] The oxygen affinity of the maternal blood was greater than that of the fetus, but no fetal complications were reported for any of these cases.[176, 177]

High-affinity hemoglobins cause unexplained erythrocytosis, especially if there is a positive family history. Functional testing of the hemoglobin is the key to diagnosis. Oxygen affinity is usually measured as P_{50}, the partial pressure of oxygen at which hemoglobin is 50% saturated with oxygen. Infants with high-affinity hemoglobins have mild erythrocytosis; they do not require intervention. Rarely, the hematocrit can be very high. The blood viscosity is then sufficiently elevated to require therapeutic phlebotomy.

Hemoglobins with Decreased Oxygen Affinity

Low-affinity hemoglobin variants arise from mutations that impair hemoglobin-oxygen binding or reduce cooperation. Most low-affinity variants possess enough oxygen affinity to become fully saturated in the normal lung. At the low capillary PO_2 in other tissues, these hemoglobins deliver higher than normal mounts of oxygen. They become more desaturated than normal hemoglobins.

Two abnormalities result from this high level of oxygen delivery. First, because tissue oxygen delivery is so efficient, normal oxygen requirements can be met by lower than normal hematocrits. In this condition, infants are completely normal despite a low hematocrit. Second, cyanosis is usually associated with these variants. This finding is entirely misleading in these infants, because it reflects no morbidity.

Infants with cyanosis who appear to be entirely well in all other respects should be evaluated, especially if there is a positive family history. Infants with low-affinity hemoglobins are invariably asymptomatic. No treatment is required. It is important to document that a low-affinity hemoglobin is the cause of an apparent anemia or cyanosis to preempt inappropriate work-ups and provide reassurance to the parents.

METHEMOGLOBINEMIAS

Methemoglobin results from oxidation of the iron moieties in hemoglobin from the ferrous (Fe^{2+}) to the ferric (Fe^{3+}) state. Normal oxygenation of hemoglobin causes a partial transfer of an electron from the iron to the bound oxygen. Iron in this state resembles ferric iron, and the oxygen resembles superoxide (O_2^-). Deoxygenation returns the electron to the iron, with release of oxygen. Methemoglobin forms if the electron is not returned.

Methemoglobin constitutes 3% or less of the total hemoglobin in normal humans. Methemoglobin levels in humans are maintained at 1% or less by the methemoglobin reductase enzyme system (nicotinamide adenine dinucleotide [NADH] dehydratase, NADH diaphorase, erythrocyte cytochrome b_3). This enzyme reduces hemoglobin iron by transfer of an electron from NADH to oxidize cytochrome b_3; cytochrome b_3 then converts ferric to ferrous iron by direct interaction with hemoglobin. The generation of NADH depends on the glycolytic pathway.[178]

A second reducing enzyme, nicotinamide adenine dinucleotide phosphate (NADPH)–dependent methemoglobin reductase, does not normally function in erythrocytes because no electron carrier is available in erythrocytes to interact with NADPH. Exogenous electron carriers, such as methylene blue, can provide the missing activity. Agents such as methylene blue can therefore serve as pharmacologic agents for the treatment of methemoglobinemia.

Abnormal hemoglobins producing methemoglobinemia (M hemoglobins) can arise from mutations that stabilize the heme iron in the ferric state. Classically, a histidine in the vicinity of the heme pocket is replaced by a tyrosine; the hydroxyl group of the tyrosine forms a complex that stabilizes the iron in the ferric state. The oxidized heme iron is relatively resistant to reduction by the methemoglobin reductase system. This group of abnormalities also can contain a rare hereditary methemoglobinemia resulting from methemoglobin reductase deficiency.[179] A third toxic form of methemoglobinemia is caused by exposure to certain chemical agents and drugs that accelerate the oxidation of methemoglobin. Nitrates are a frequent environmental cause of toxic methemoglobinemia. In general, substantial intake of these agents is required before significant amounts of methemoglobin are generated.

Nitric oxide is being used as a novel selective pulmonary vasodilator in newborn infants with hypoxic respiratory failure and persistent pulmonary hypertension. Methemoglobinemia sufficient to cause significant impairment of oxygen-carrying capacity can result from an overdose of inhaled nitric oxide.[180] Very young infants are more susceptible to these agents than are adults, but all age groups are at risk given sufficient exposure. Acquired methemoglobinemia is virtually the only situation in which life-threatening amounts of methemoglobin accumulate. The symptoms reflect a true lack of oxygen availability at the tissue level. Methemoglobin is a markedly left-shifted hemoglobin that delivers little oxygen to the tissues. When methemoglobin is more than 50% of the total hemoglobin concentration, loss of consciousness, coma, and death can rapidly ensue. At this level, the blood is chocolate brown.

Methemoglobinemia should be suspected in infants with unexplained cyanosis. Infants with M hemoglobins are usually asymptomatic and require no management. Patients with deficiency of the reductase system generally do not require treatment. Emergency treatment of high levels of toxic methemoglobinemia begins with 1 to 2 mg/kg of intravenous methylene blue as a 1% solution in saline. It is usually infused rapidly (10 to 15 minutes). The dose may be repeated if necessary. This treatment is usually effective.

References

1. Lehninger AL, Nelson DL, Cox MM: Principles of biochemistry, 2nd ed. New York: Worth, 1993.
2. Imai K: Allosteric effects in haemoglobin. Cambridge: England: Cambridge University Press, 1982.
3. Jia L, Bonaventura C, Bonaventura J, et al: *S*-nitrosohaemoglobin: a dynamic activity of blood involved in vascular control. Nature 1996;380:221.
4. Stamler JS, Jia L, Eu JP, et al: Blood flow regulation by *S*-nitrosohemoglobin in the physiological oxygen gradient. Science 1997;276:2034.
5. Stamatoyannopoulos G, Nienhuis AW: Hemoglobin switching. In Stamatoyannopoulos G, Nienhuis AW, Majerus PW, Varmus HV (eds): The Molecular Basis of Blood Diseases. Philadelphia: WB Saunders, 1994.
6. Steinberg HM, Benz EJ Jr: Hemoglobin synthesis, structure, and function. In Hoffman R, Benz EJ Jr, Shattil SJ, et al (eds): Hematology: Basic Principles and Practice, 2nd ed. New York: Churchill Livingstone, 1995, p 458.
7. Bunn H, Forget BG, Ranney HM: Hemoglobin biosynthesis. In Bunn H, Forget BG, Ranney HM (eds): Human Hemoglobins. Philadelphia: WB Saunders, 1977, p 101.
8. Bard H: The postnatal decline of hemoglobin F synthesis in normal full-term infants. J Clin Invest 1975;55:395.
9. Orkin SH, Goff SC: The duplicated human alpha-globin genes: their relative expression as measured by RNA analysis. Cell 1981;24:345.
10. Liebhaber SA, Kan YW: Differentiation of the mRNA transcripts originating from the $alpha_1$- and $alpha_2$-globin loci in normals and alpha-thalassemics. J Clin Invest 1981;68:439.
11. Higgs DR, Vickers MA, Wilkie AO, et al: A review of the molecular genetics of the human alpha-globin gene cluster. Blood 1989;73:1081.
12. Snyder LGR: Closely linked alpha-chain hemoglobin loci in *Peromyscus* and other animals: speculation on the evolution of duplicate loci. Evolution 1980;34:1077.
13. Albitar M, Cash FE, Peschle C, et al: Developmental switch in the relative expression of the $alpha_1$- and $alpha_2$-globin genes in humans and in transgenic mice. Blood 1992;79:2471.
14. Huisman TH, Harris H, Gravely M: The chemical heterogeneity of the fetal hemoglobin in normal newborn infants and in adults. Mol Cell Biochem 1977;17:45.
15. Schroeder WA: The synthesis and chemical heterogeneity of human fetal hemoglobin: overview and present concepts. Hemoglobin 1980;4:431.
16. Bard H, Widness JA, Ziegler EE, et al: The proportions of $^{G}\gamma$ and $^{A}\gamma$ globins in the fetal hemoglobin synthesized in preterm and term infants. Pediatr Res 1995;37:361.
17. Collins FS, Weissman SM: The molecular genetics of human hemoglobin. Prog Nucleic Acid Res Mol Biol 1984;31:315.
18. Huehns ER, Dance N, Beaven GH, et al: Human embryonic haemoglobins. Nature 1964;201:1095.
19. Hecht F, Motulsky AG, Lemire RJ, et al: Predomi-

nance of hemoglobin Gower 1 in early human embryonic development. Science 1966;152:91.
20. Gale RE, Clegg JB, Huehns ER: Human embryonic haemoglobins Gower 1 and Gower 2. Nature 1979;280:162.
21. Papayannopoulou TH, Shepard TH, Stamatoyannopoulos G: Studies of hemoglobin expression in erythroid cells of early human fetuses using anti-γ and anti-β-globin chain fluorescent antibodies. In Stamatoyannopoulos G, Nienhuis A (eds): Globin Gene Expression and Hemopoietic Differentiation. New York: Alan R Liss, 1983, p 421.
22. Kazazian HH Jr, Woodhead AP: Hemoglobin A synthesis in the developing fetus. N Engl J Med 1973;289:58.
23. Cividalli G, Nathan DG, Kan YW, et al: Relation of beta to gamma synthesis during the first trimester: an approach to prenatal diagnosis of thalassemia. Pediatr Res 1974;8:553.
24. Schroeder WA, Huisman TH, Shelton JR, et al: Evidence for multiple structural genes for the gamma chain of human fetal hemoglobin. Proc Natl Acad Sci U S A 1968;60:537.
25. Nute PE, Pataryas HA, Stamatoyannopoulos G: The $^{G}\gamma$ and $^{A}\gamma$ hemoglobin chains during human fetal development. Am J Hum Genet 1973;25:271.
26. Schroeder WA, Shelton JR, Shelton JB, et al: Worldwide occurrence of nonallelic genes for the γ-chain of human foetal haemoglobin in newborns. Nat New Biol 1972;240:273.
27. Alter BP: The G gamma:A gamma composition of fetal hemoglobin in fetuses and newborns. Blood 1979;54:1158.
28. Bard H, Prosmanne J: The postnatal fetal and adult hemoglobin synthesis in preterm infants whose birth weight was less than 1000 g. J Clin Invest 1982;70:50.
29. Peri KG, Gagnon C, Bard H: Quantitative correlation between globin mRNAs and synthesis of fetal and adult hemoglobins during hemoglobin switchover in the perinatal period. Pediatr Res 1998;43:504.
30. Ross J, Sullivan D: Half-lives of beta and gamma globin messenger RNAs and of protein synthetic capacity in cultured human reticulocytes. Blood 1985;66:1149.
31. Weiss IM, Liebhaber SA: Erythroid cell-specific determinants of alpha-globin mRNA stability. Mol Cell Biol 1994;14:8123.
32. Cunningham JM, Jane SM: Hemoglobin switching and fetal hemoglobin reactivation. Semin Hematol 1996;33:9.
33. Orkin SH: Globin gene regulation and switching: circa 1990. Cell 1990;63:665.
34. Choi O-R, Engel JD: Developmental regulation of beta-globin gene switching. Cell 1988;55:17.
35. Orkin SH: GATA-binding transcription factors in hematopoietic cells. Blood 1992;80:575.
36. Andrews NC, Erdjument-Bromage H, Davidson MB, et al: Erythroid transcription factor NF-E2 is a hematopoietic-specific basic-leucine zipper protein. Nature 1993;362:722.
37. Gilman JG, Huisman TH: DNA sequence variation associated with elevated fetal G gamma globulin production. Blood 1985;66:783.
38. Sampietro M, Thein SL, Contreras M, et al: Variation of Hb F and F-cell number with the G-gamma Xmn I (C→T) polymorphism in normal individuals. Blood 1992;79:832.
39. Lolis D, Georgiou I, Loizou P, et al: High Hb F in pregnancy is associated with the Xmn I polymorphism at the −158bp of the G gamma-globin gene. Eur J Obstet Gynecol Reprod Biol 1995;60:153.
40. Rosatelli MC, Altay C, Oner R, et al: Beta-globin haplotype and Xmn I polymorphism at position G (gamma) −158 and Hb F production in Fanconi's anemia. Haematologica 1992;77:106.
41. Shimizu K, Keino H, Terasawa T, et al: Elevated haemoglobin F in juvenile and adult chronic myelogenous leukaemia. Acta Haematol 1988;80:28.
42. Peri KG, Gagnon J, Gagnon C, et al: Association of −158(C→T) (*XmnI*) DNA polymorphism in $^{G}\gamma$-globin promoter with delayed switchover from fetal to adult hemoglobin synthesis. Pediatr Res 1997;41:214.
43. DeSimone J, Biel SI, Heller P: Stimulation of fetal hemoglobin synthesis in baboons by hemolysis and hypoxia. Proc Natl Acad Sci U S A 1978;75:2937.
44. Bard H, Fouron JC, Prosmane J: The increase in fetal hemoglobin synthesis in fetal lamb during hyperglycemic hypoxemia. Am J Obstet Gynecol 1988;159:1269.
45. Bromberg YM, Abrahmov A, Salzverger M: The effect of maternal anoxaemia on the foetal haemoglobin of the newborn. J Obstet Br Emp 1956;63:875.
46. Bard H: The effect of placental insufficiency on fetal and adult hemoglobin synthesis. Am J Obstet Gynecol 1974;120:67.
47. Bard H, Prosmanne J: Relative rates of fetal and adult hemoglobin synthesis in cord blood of infants of insulin-dependent diabetic mothers. Pediatrics 1985; 75:1143.
48. Bard H, Prosmanne J: Elevated levels of fetal hemoglobin synthesis in infants with chronic bronchopulmonary dysplasia. Pediatrics 1990;86:193.
49. Bard H, Lachance C, Widness JA, et al: The reactivation of fetal hemoglobin synthesis during anemia of prematurity. Pediatr Res 1994;36:253.
50. Bard H, Fouron JC, Gagnon C, et al: Hypoxemia and increased fetal hemoglobin synthesis. J Pediatr 1994;124:941.
51. Bard H, Fouron JC, Prosmanne J, et al: Effect of hypoxemia on Hb F synthesis during late gestation. Pediatr Res 1992;31:483.
52. Zanjani ED, Peterson EN, Gordon AS, et al: Erythropoietin production in the fetus: role of the kidney and maternal anemia. J Lab Clin Med 1974;83:281.
53. Peschle C, Migliaccio AR, Migliaccio G, et al: Regulation of Hb synthesis in ontogenesis and erythropoietic differentiation: in vitro studies on fetal liver, cord blood, normal adult blood or marrow, and blood from HPFH patients. In Stamatoyannopoulos G, Nienhuis AW (eds): Hemoglobins in Development and Differentiation. New York: Alan R Liss, 1981, pp 359–371.
54. Stamatoyannopoulos G, Papayannopoulou T: Fetal hemoglobin and the erythroid stem cell differentiation process. In Stamatoyannopoulos G, Nienhuis AW (eds): Cellular and Molecular Regulation of Hemoglobin Switching. New York: Grune & Stratton, 1979, p 323.
55. Rich IN, Kubanek B: The ontogeny of erythropoiesis in the mouse detected by the erythroid colony-forming technique. I. Hepatic and maternal erythropoiesis. J Embryol Exp Morphol 1979;50:57.
56. Darbre PD, Adamson JW, Wood WG, et al: Patterns of globin chain synthesis in erythroid colonies grown from sheep marrow of different developmental stages. Br J Haematol 1979;41:459.
57. Hassan MW, Lutton JD, Levere RD, et al: In vitro culture of erythroid colonies from human fetal liver and umbilical cord blood. Br J Haematol 1979;41:477.
58. Stamatoyannopoulos G, Rosenblum BB, Papayannopoulou T, et al: Hb F and Hb A production in erythroid cultures from human fetuses and neonates. Blood 1979;54:440.

59. Alter BP, Rappeport JM, Huisman TH, et al: Fetal erythropoiesis following bone marrow transplantation. Blood 1976;48:843.
60. Papayannopoulou TH, Vichinsky E, Stamatoyannopoulos G: Fetal Hb production during acute erythroid expansion. I. Observations in patients with transient erythroblastopenia and post-phlebotomy. Br J Haematol 1980;44:535.
61. Dover GJ, Boyer SH, Zinkham WH: Production of erythrocytes that contain fetal hemoglobin in anemia: transient in vivo changes. J Clin Invest 1979;63:173.
62. DeSimone J, Heller P, Amsel J, et al: Magnitude of the fetal hemoglobin response to acute hemolytic anemia in baboons is controlled by genetic factors. J Clin Invest 1980;65:224.
63. DeSimone J, Biel M, Heller P: Maintenance of fetal hemoglobin (Hb F) elevations in the baboon by prolonged erythropoietic stress. Blood 1982;60:519.
64. Al-Khatti A, Veith RW, Papayannopoulou T, et al: Stimulation of fetal hemoglobin synthesis by erythropoietin in baboons. N Engl J Med 1987;317:415.
65. Alpen EL, Cranmore D: Observations on the regulation of erythropoiesis and on cellular dynamics by Fe^{59} autoradiography. In Stohlman F Jr (ed): The Kinetics of Cellular Proliferation. New York: Grune & Stratton, 1959, p 290.
66. Stamatoyannopoulos G, Veith R, Al-Khatti A, et al: On the induction of fetal hemoglobin in the adult: stress erythropoiesis, cell cycle-specific drugs, and recombinant erythropoietin. Prog Clin Biol Res 1987;251:443.
67. Green DW, Mimouni F: Nucleated erythrocytes in healthy infants and in infants of diabetic mothers. J Pediatr 1990;116:129.
68. Phelan JP, Ahn MO, Korst LM, et al: Nucleated red blood cells: a marker for fetal asphyxia? Am J Obstet Gynecol 1995;173:1380.
69. Bernstein PS, Minior VK, Divon MY: Neonatal nucleated red blood cell counts in small-for-gestational-age fetuses with abnormal umbilical artery Doppler studies. Am J Obstet Gynecol 1997;177:1079.
70. Pearson HA: Life-span of the fetal red blood cell. J Pediatr 1967;70:166.
71. Mollison PL: The survival of transfused erythrocytes in haemolytic disease of the newborn. Arch Dis Child 1943;18:161.
72. Mollison PL: Physiological jaundice of the newborn. Lancet 1948;1:513.
73. Ashby W: The determination of the length of life of transfused blood corpuscles in man. J Exp Med 1919;29:267.
74. Bard H, Widness JA: The life span of erythrocytes transfused to preterm infants. Pediatr Res 1997;42:9.
75. Stockman JA III: Physical properties of the neonatal red blood cell. In Stockmann III JA, Pochedly C (eds): Developmental and Neonatal Hematology. New York: Raven Press, 1988, p 297.
76. Vácha J, Znohl V: The allometric dependence of the life span of erythrocytes on body weight in mammals. Comp Biochem Physiol 1981;69A:357.
77. Haselhorst G, Stromberger K: Über den Gasgehalt des Nabelschnurblutes vor und nach der Geburt des Kindes und über den Gastausch in der Placenta. Z Geburtshilfe Gynaekol 1931;100:48.
78. Bauer CH, Ludwig I, Ludwig M: Different effects of 2,3-diphosphoglycerate and adenosine triphosphate on the oxygen affinity of adult and foetal human hemoglobin. Life Sci 1968;7:1339.
79. Tyuma I, Shimizu K: Different response to organic phosphates of human fetal and adult hemoglobins. Arch Biochem Biophys 1969;129:404.
80. Bellingham AJ, Detter JC, Lenfant C: Regulatory mechanisms of hemoglobin oxygen affinity in acidosis and alkalosis. J Clin Invest 1971;50:700.
81. Astrup P, Rorth M, Thorshauge C: Dependency on acid-base status of oxyhemoglobin dissociation and 2,3-diphosphoglycerate level in human erythrocytes. II. In vivo studies. Scand J Clin Lab Invest 1970;26:47.
82. Bard H, Teasdale F: Red cell oxygen affinity, hemoglobin type, 1,3-diphosphoglycerate, and pH as a function of fetal development. Pediatrics 1979;64:483.
83. Oski FA, Delivoria-Papadopoulos M: The red cell, 2-3-diphosphoglycerate, and tissue oxygen release. J Pediatr 1970;77:941.
84. Émond D, Lachance C, Gagnon J, et al: Arterial partial pressure of oxygen required to achieve 90% saturation of hemoglobin in very low birth weight newborns. Pediatrics 1993;91:602.
85. Bard H, Makowski EL, Meschia G, et al: The relative rates of synthesis of hemoglobins A and F in immature red cells of newborn infants. Pediatrics 1970;45:766.
86. Bunn HF, Forget GB, Ranney HM: Human Hemoglobins. Philadelphia: WB Saunders, 1977, p 79.
87. Novy MJ, Frigoletto FD, Easterdy CL, et al: Changes in umbilical-cord blood oxygen affinity after intrauterine transfusions for erythroblastosis. N Engl J Med 1971;285:589.
88. Rosatelli C, Falchi AM, Scalas MT, et al: Hematological phenotype of the double heterozygous state for alpha and beta thalassemia. Hemoglobin 1984;8:25.
89. Weatherall DJ, Clegg JB: The Thalassemia Syndromes, 3rd ed. Oxford: Blackwell Scientific, 1981.
90. Weatherall DJ: The thalassemias. In Stamatoyannopoulos G, Nienhuis AW, Majerus PW, Varmus HE (eds): Molecular Basis of Blood Diseases, 2nd ed. Philadelphia: WB Saunders, 1993, p 157.
91. Engle MA: Cardiac involvement in Cooley's anemia. Ann N Y Acad Sci 1964;119:694.
92. Borow KM, Propper R, Bierman FZ, et al: The left ventricular end-systolic pressure-dimension relation in patients with thalassemia major: a new noninvasive method for assessing contractile state. Circulation 1982;66:980.
93. Stanfield JB: Acute benign pericarditis in thalassemia major. Proc R Soc Med 1962;55:236.
94. Wasi P: Streptococcal infection leading to cardiac and renal involvement in thalassaemia. Lancet 1971;1:949.
95. Secchi GC, Scotti PG, Cambiaghi G, et al: Respiratory function tests in adolescents with beta-thalassemia major. Haematologica 1982;67:23.
96. Hoyt RW, Scarpa N, Wilmott RW, et al: Pulmonary function abnormalities in homozygous beta-thalassemia. J Pediatr 1986;109:452.
97. Keens TG, O'Neal MH, Ortega JA, et al: Pulmonary function abnormalities in thalassemia patients on a hypertransfusion program. Pediatrics 1980;65:1013.
98. Cooper DM, Hyman CB, Weiler-Ravell D, et al: Gas exchange during exercise in children with thalassemia major and Diamond-Blackfan anemia. Pediatr Res 1985;19:1215.
99. Adams JG, Coleman MB: Structural hemoglobin variants that produce the phenotype of thalassemia. Semin Hematol 1990;27:229.
100. Metaxotou-Mavromati AD, Antonopoulou HK, Laskari SS, et al: Developmental changes in hemoglobin F levels during the first two years of life in normal and heterozygous beta-thalassemia infants. Pediatrics 1982;69:734.
101. Kan YW, Golbus MS, Klein P, et al: Successful application of prenatal diagnosis in a pregnancy at risk for homozygous beta-thalassemia. N Engl J Med 1975;292:1096.

102. Orkin SH, Alter BP, Altay C, et al: Application of endonuclease mapping to the analysis and prenatal diagnosis of thalassemias caused by globin-gene deletion. N Engl J Med 1978;299:166.
103. Dozy AM, Forman EN, Abuelo DN, et al: Prenatal diagnosis of homozygous alpha thalassemia. JAMA 1979;241:1610.
104. Kazazian HH Jr: The thalassemia syndromes: Molecular basis and prenatal diagnosis in 1990. Semin Hematol 1990;27:209.
105. Saiki RK, Walsh PS, Levenson CH, et al: Genetics analysis of amplified DNA with immobilized sequence-specific oligonucleotide probes. Proc Natl Acad Sci U S A 1989;86:6230.
106. Hahn EV, Gillespie EB: Sickle-cell anemia: report of a case greatly improved by splenectomy. Arch Intern Med 1927;39:233.
107. Pauling L, Itano HA, Singers SJ, et al: Sickle cell anemia: a molecular disease. Science 1949;10:543.
108. Beet EA: Genetics of the sickle cell trait in a Bantu tribe. Ann Eugen 1949;14:279.
109. Neel JV: Inheritance of the sickling phenomenon with particular reference to sickle-cell disease. Blood 1951;6:389.
110. Ingram VM: Gene mutations in human haemoglobin: the chemical difference between normal and sickle cell haemoglobin. Nature 1957;180:326.
111. Ranney HM: Historical milestones. In Emburry SH, Hebbel RP, et al (eds): Sickle Cell Disease: Basic Principles and Clinical Practice. New York: Raven Press, 1994, pp 1–5.
112. Motulsky AG: Frequency of sickling disorders in U.S. blacks. N Engl J Med 1973;288:31.
113. Dykes GW, Crepeau RH, Edelstein SJ: Three-dimensional reconstruction of the fibers of sickle cell hemoglobin. Nature 1978;272:506.
114. Garrell RL, Crepeau RH, Edelstein SJ: Cross-sectional views of hemoglobin S fibers by electron microscopy and computer modeling. Proc Natl Acad Sci U S A 1979;76:1140.
115. Dykes G, Crepeau RH, Edelstein SJ: Three-dimensional reconstruction of the 14-filament fibers of hemoglobin S. J Mol Biol 1979;130:451.
116. Gill SJ, Spokane R, Benedict RC, et al: Ligand-linked phase equilibria of sickle cell hemoglobin. J Mol Biol 1980;140:299.
117. Sunshine HR, Hofrichter J, Ferrone FA, et al: Oxygen binding by sickle cell hemoglobin polymers. J Mol Biol 1982;158:251.
118. Ross PD, Hofrichter J, Eaton WA: Calorimetric and optical characterization of sickle cell hemoglobin gelation. J Mol Biol 1975;96:239.
119. Ross PD, Hofrichter J, Eaton WA: Thermodynamics of gelation of sickle cell deoxyhemoglobin. J Mol Biol 1977;115:111.
120. Magdoff-Fairchild B, Poillon WN, Li T, et al: Thermodynamic studies of polymerization of deoxygenated sickle cell hemoglobin. Proc Natl Acad Sci U S A 1976;73:990.
121. Goldberg MA, Husson MA, Bunn HF: The participation of hemoglobins A and F in polymerization of sickle hemoglobin. J Biol Chem 1977;252:3414.
122. Briehl RW: Gelation of sickle cell hemoglobin. IV. Phase transitions in hemoglobin S gels: separate measures of aggregation and solution-gel equilibrium. J Mol Biol 1978;123:521.
123. Poillon WN, Bertles JF: Deoxygenated sickle hemoglobin. Effects of lyotropic salts on its solubility. J Biol Chem 1979;254:3462.
124. Swerdlow PH, Bryan RA, Bertles JF, et al: Effect of 2,3-diphosphoglycerate on the solubility of deoxysickle hemoglobin. Hemoglobin 1977;1:527.
125. Poillon WN, Kim BC, Walder JA: Deoxygenated sickle hemoglobin: the effects of 2,3-diphosphoglycerate and inositol hexaphosphate on its solubility. In Beuzard Y, Charache S (eds): Approaches to Therapy of Sickle Cell Anemia. Paris: INSERM, 1986, p 89.
126. Hofrichter J, Ross PD, Eaton WA: Supersaturation in sickle cell hemoglobin solutions. Proc Natl Acad Sci U S A 1976;73:3035.
127. Hofrichter J: Ligand binding and the gelation of sickle cell hemoglobin. J Mol Biol 1979;128:335.
128. Sunshine HR, Hofrichter J, Eaton WA: Gelation of sickle cell hemoglobin in mixtures with normal adult and fetal hemoglobins. J Mol Biol 1979;133:435.
129. Behe MJ, Englander SW: Mixed gelation theory. Kinetics, equilibrium and gel incorporation in sickle hemoglobin mixtures. J Mol Biol 1979;133:137.
130. Adachi K, Ozguc M, Asakura T: Nucleation-controlled aggregation of deoxyhemoglobin S. Participation of hemoglobin A in the aggregation of deoxyhemoglobin S in concentrated phosphate buffer. J Biol Chem 1980;255:3092.
131. Benesch RE, Edalji R, Benesch R, et al: Solubilization of hemoglobin S by other hemoglobins. Proc Natl Acad Sci U S A 1980;77:5130.
132. Ley TJ, DeSimone J, Anagnou NP, et al: 5-Azacytidine selectively increases gamma-globin synthesis in a patient with beta-thalassemia. N Engl J Med 1982;307:1469.
133. Charache S, Dover G, Smith K, et al: Treatment of sickle cell anemia with 5-azacytidine results in increased fetal hemoglobin production and is associated with non-random hypomethylation of DNA around the gamma-delta-beta-globin gene complex. Proc Natl Acad Sci U S A 1983;80:4842.
134. Ley TJ, DeSimone J, Noguchi CT, et al: 5-Azacytidine increases gamma-globin synthesis and reduces the proportion of dense cells in patients with sickle cell anemia. Blood 1983;62:370.
135. Platt OS, Orkin SH, Dover G, et al: Hydroxyurea enhances fetal hemoglobin production in sickle cell anemia. J Clin Invest 1984;74:652.
136. Charache S, Dover GJ, Moyer MA, et al: Hydroxyurea-induced augmentation of fetal hemoglobin production in patients with sickle cell anemia. Blood 1987;69:109.
137. Rodgers GP, Dover GJ, Noguchi CT, et al: Hematological responses of patients with sickled cell disease treated with hydroxyurea. N Engl J Med 1990; 322:1037.
138. Stamatoyannopoulos G, Umemura T, Al-Khatti A, et al: Modulation of fetal hemoglobin production by erythropoietin. In Stamatoyannopoulos G, Nienhuis AW (eds): Hemoglobin Switching, Part B: Cellular and Molecular Mechanisms. New York: Alan R Liss, 1989, p 269.
139. Goldberg MA, Brugnara C, Dover GJ, et al: Treatment of sickle cell anemia with hydroxyurea and erythropoietin. N Engl J Med 1990;323:366.
140. Rodgers GP, Dover GJ, Uyesaka N, et al: Augmentation by erythropoietin of fetal hemoglobin response to hydroxyurea in sickle cell disease. N Engl J Med 1993;328:73.
141. Perrine SP, Ginder GD, Faler DV, et al: A short-term trial of butyrate to stimulate fetal-globin-gene expression in the beta-globin disorders. N Engl J Med 1993;328:81.
142. Dover GJ, Brusilow S, Charache S: Induction of fetal hemoglobin production in subjects with sickle cell

anemia by oral sodium phenylbutyrate. Blood 1994;84:339.
143. Platt OS, Thorington BD, Brambilla DJ, et al: Pain in sickle cell disease: rates and risk factors. N Engl J Med 1991;325:11.
144. Kan YW, Dozy AM: Polymorphism of DNA sequence adjacent to human beta-globin structural gene: relationship to sickle mutation. Proc Natl Acad Sci U S A 1978;75:5631.
145. Wilson JT, Milner PF, Summer ME, et al: Use of restriction endonucleases for mapping the allele for beta S-globin. Proc Natl Acad Sci U S A 1982;79:3628.
146. Chang JC, Kan YW: A sensitive new prenatal test for sickle cell anemia. N Engl J Med 1982;307:30.
147. Orkin SH, Little PF, Kazazian HH Jr, et al: Improved detection of the sickle mutation by DNA analysis: application to prenatal diagnosis. N Engl J Med 1982;307:32.
148. Wallace RB, Schold M, Johnson MJ, et al: Oligonucleotide directed mutagenesis of the human beta-globin gene: a general method for producing specific point mutations in cloned DNA. Nucleic Acids Res 1981;9:3647.
149. Conner BJ, Reyes AA, Morin C, et al: Detection of sickle cell beta S-globin allele by hybridization with synthetic oligonucleotides. Proc Natl Acad Sci U S A 1983;80:278.
150. Studencki AB, Conner BJ, et al: Prenatal diagnosis of beta-thalassemia: detection of a single mutation in DNA. N Engl J Med 1983;309:284.
151. Saiki RK, Chang CA, Levenson CH, et al: Diagnosis of sickle cell anemia and beta-thalassemia with enzymatically amplified DNA and non-radioactive allele specific oligonucleotide probes. N Engl J Med 1988;319:537.
152. Chehab FF, Kan YW: Detection of sickle cell anemia by colour DNA amplification. Lancet 1990;335:15.
153. Goossens M, Dumez Y, Kaplan L, et al: Prenatal diagnosis of sickle-cell anemia in the first trimester of pregnancy. N Engl J Med 1983;309:831.
154. Old JM, Fitches A, Heath C, et al: First-trimester fetal diagnosis for haemoglobinopathies: report on 200 cases. Lancet 1986;2:763.
155. Newborn Screening for Sickle Cell Disease and Other Hemoglobinopathies. Consensus Development Conference Statement. Bethesda: National Institutes of Health, 1987.
156. Schneider RG, Gustafson LP, Haggard ME: The incidence of genetically determined abnormalities in 11,427 cord blood samples. Presented at the 13th International Congress of Haematology; Munich, August 1970.
157. Gilman PA, McFarlane JM, Huisman TJ: Natural history of sickle cell anemia: re-evaluation of a 15 year cord blood testing program. Pediatr Res 1976;10:376.
158. Serjeant G, Grandison Y, Lowrie Y, et al: The development of hematological changes in homozygous sickle cell disease: a cohort study from birth to six years. Br J Haematol 1981;48:533.
159. Pearson HA: A neonatal program for sickle cell anemia. Adv Pediatr 1986;33:381.
160. Jinks DC, Minter M, Tarver DA, et al: Molecular genetic diagnosis of sickle cell disease using dried blood specimens on blotters used for newborn screening. Hum Genet 1989;81:363.
161. Powars D: Diagnosis at birth improves survival of children with sickle cell anemia. Pediatrics 1989;83(5 Pt 2):830.
162. Grover R: Newborn screening for sickle cell disease and other hemoglobinopathies: newborn screening in New York City. Pediatrics 1989;83(5 Pt 2):819.
163. Gill FM, Brown A, Gallagher D, et al: Newborn experience in the cooperative study of sickle cell disease. Pediatrics 1989;83(5 Pt 2):827.
164. Sprinkle RH, Hynes DM, Konrad TR: Is universal neonatal hemoglobinopathy screening cost-effective? Arch Pediatr Adolesc Med 1994;148:461.
165. DeSimone J, Heller P, Hall L, et al: 5-Azacytidine stimulates fetal hemoglobin synthesis in anemic baboons. Proc Natl Acad Sci U S A 1982;79:4428.
166. Dover GJ, Charache S, Boyer SH, et al: 5-Azacytidine increases fetal hemoglobin production in a patient with sickle cell disease. Prog Clin Biol Res 1983;134:475.
167. Perrine SP, Greene MF, Faller DV: Delay in the fetal globin switch in infants of diabetic mothers. N Engl J Med 1985;312:334.
168. Perrine SP, Miller BA, Faller DV, et al: Sodium butyrate enhances fetal globin gene expression in erythroid progenitors of patients with Hb SS and beta thalassemia. Blood 1989;74:454.
169. Perrine SP, Rudolph A, Faller DV, et al: Butyrate infusions in the ovine fetus delay the biologic clock for globin gene switching. Proc Natl Acad Sci U S A 1988;85:8540.
170. Constantoulakis P, Knitter G, Stamatoyannopoulos G: On the induction of fetal hemoglobin by butyrates: in vivo and in vitro studies with sodium butyrate and comparison of combination treatments with 5-azaC and araC. Blood 1989;74:1963.
171. Sher GD, Ginder GD, Little J, et al: Extended therapy with intravenous arginine butyrate in patients with beta-hemoglobinopathies. N Engl J Med 1995; 332:1606.
172. Carver MF, Huisman TH: International Hemoglobin Information Center variant list. Hemoglobin 1996;20:213.
173. Rachmilewitz EA: Denaturation of the normal and abnormal hemoglobin molecule. Semin Hematol 1974;11:441.
174. Winterbourn CC, Carrell RW: Characterization of Heinz bodies in unstable hemoglobin haemolytic anemia. Nature 1972;240:150.
175. Flynn TP, Allen DW, Johnson GJ, et al: Oxidant damage of the lipids and proteins of the erythrocyte membranes in unstable hemoglobin disease: evidence for the role of lipid peroxidation. J Clin Invest 1983;71:1215.
176. Bard H, Rosenberg A, Huisman T: Hemoglobinopathies affecting maternal-fetal oxygen gradient during pregnancy: molecular, biochemical and clinical studies. Am J Perinatol 1998;15:389.
177. Charache S, Catalano P, Burns S, et al: Pregnancy in carriers of high-affinity hemoglobins. Blood 1985;65:713.
178. Kiese M: Die Reduktion des Hämoglobins. Biochem Zeitschr 1943;316:264.
179. Scott EM, Hoskins DD: Hereditary methemoglobinemia in Alaskan Eskimos and Indians. Blood 1958;13:795.
180. Heal CA, Spencer SA: Methaemoglobinaemia with high-dose nitric oxide administration. Acta Paediatr 1995;84:1318.

CHAPTER 17

Use of Hematologic Data to Evaluate Infections in Neonates

Paola Papoff, M.D.

The early diagnosis of neonatal sepsis is difficult to establish because of the subtle nature of the signs and symptoms. Given the high mortality, however, treatment cannot be delayed. Treatment based on risk factors results in many neonates receiving unneeded antibiotic therapy. Hammerschlag found in a prospective study that, for each infant with positive blood cultures, approximately 30 infants were treated with antibiotics.[1] Although this approach seems reasonable given the dire outcome of a missed diagnosis, improvement in diagnostic accuracy should diminish the exposure of healthy neonates to the risks of unwarranted antibiotic treatment, decrease antibiotic resistances, and reduce the length and cost of hospital stays.

The isolation of bacteria from a central body fluid is considered the standard and most specific tool to diagnose neonatal sepsis,[2] but confirmation or exclusion of positive cultures requires days, and more importantly, the sensitivity of the culture methods is sometimes low. These difficulties have prompted investigators to evaluate adjunctive diagnostic tests that may improve the accuracy of the identification of septic infants while awaiting culture results. Because sepsis is a life-threatening disease, the ideal test should have maximum sensitivity and negative predictive accuracy. Neonatologists want to ensure that every infected infant will have an abnormal test result (100% sensitivity) and that a normal test completely excludes sepsis (100% negative predictive value). The loss in specificity and positive predictive value is acceptable because the risks of overtreatment with antibiotics are much less than the risks of missing a septic neonate. Several hematologic data have been evaluated with these features in mind, but a reliable test that can confirm or refute the diagnosis of systemic infection at an early stage has not been found.

Polymerase chain reaction amplification of bacterial DNA has gained interest among investigators as an alternative to serologic tests for the early diagnosis of sepsis, because it might offer the advantages of directly identifying the presence of bacteria in the blood or other body fluids with a high sensitivity, specificity, speed, and economy.[3] Although promising, molecular triage has not proved to be an established approach, and serologic tests remain the most important diagnostic aid for the management of septic neonates.

LEUKOCYTE COUNTS

The utility of white blood cell counts for the diagnosis of neonatal sepsis has greatly improved since, in 1979, Manroe published her work on the total and immature neutrophil reference ranges in newborn infants.[4] Until then, the leukocyte count was felt to be of little value in the diagnosis of sepsis in newborn infants; normal at the time of initial evaluation in more than one third of infants with proven sepsis,[4–12] total leukocyte counts were particularly unreliable indicators of infection during the first several hours of early-onset sepsis.[12] Manroe and colleagues showed patterns of change sufficiently constant to establish limits of normal variation and suggested that the calculation of the absolute number of total or immature neutrophils and of immature to total neutrophil proportion might aid in the early recognition of neonatal infection. However, later studies only partly supported this premise. Most have shown abnormal neutrophil counts at the time of the onset of symptoms in only about two thirds of infants,[4–6, 13–16] although in some series, up to 80% to 90% of infected infants have had abnormal values.[17–19] However, the sensitivity and negative predictive value of the white blood cell count and differential cell count were considerably higher when a repeat evaluation was performed.[13, 20, 21] The neutrophil count, although slightly more sensitive than the total leukocyte count, is too often normal to be used as a guide for treatment.

In specific clinical situations, the neutrophil count can be of value. For instance, during the first days of life when the neutrophil counts are normally rising, low counts probably indicate infection except in those infants with a maternal history of severe pregnancy-induced hypertension.[4] In association with sepsis, low neutrophil counts may represent depletion of the neutrophil bone marrow storage pool, for which early diagnosis and aggressive therapy are critical for survival.[22]

Neutropenia may provide a marker for screening infants with respiratory distress in the first few hours of life and for separating early-onset sepsis from other causes of pulmonary disease. An example is the association between respiratory distress and early-onset sepsis caused by group B streptococci, for which neutropenia is a highly significant finding.[23–28] The diagnostic value of neutropenia for sepsis varies, however, in different studies. For example, Manroe and coworkers found that neutropenia was the best predictor of sepsis,[4] but Baley and associates, investigating the causes of neutropenia in neonates, found low neutrophil counts in a high percentage of infants, although less than one half of the episodes of neutropenia could be attributed to infection.[29]

Ureaplasma urealyticum pneumonia is another clinical condition for which the leukocyte count may be valuable for clinical diagnosis. An association between colonization of the respiratory tract and elevation in the leukocyte count caused by an increase in the number of mature and immature neutrophils has been reported, and in trials of interventions directed at eradication of *U. urealyticum*, it has been speculated that the leukocyte count may be a marker for *U. urealyticum* pneumonia.[30] In term newborn infants, evaluation of total and differential leukocyte counts may be useful for screening those delivered of mothers with premature rupture of membranes, a condition associated with a significantly increased incidence of positive blood cultures. In these cases, complete blood cell counts have a sensitivity of 86% and specificity of 66%.[31]

As high numbers of neutrophils are released from the bone marrow in response to infection, increasing numbers of immature cells enter the bloodstream and lead to a differential cell count with a "shift to the left." This response has been considered a marker for infection in the neonate. However, with few exceptions,[14, 32] the absolute band or immature (i.e., bands or metamyelocytes) neutrophil count has had little diagnostic value.[4, 8, 33, 34] In many infants, despite an increased proportion of immature cell types in the differential leukocyte count, exhaustion of the bone marrow reserves prevents a rise in the absolute number of band neutrophils in the circulation.[23] This is particularly common in the more seriously ill patients, for whom early diagnosis is most critical. Despite its relative insensitivity, the immature neutrophil count has had good positive predictive value; elevated values are unusual in uninfected infants, except in the early neonatal period, when perinatal events may sometimes explain elevated counts.

The unreliability of absolute band counts has led to the investigation of neutrophil ratios as an index of neonatal infection. These include the ratio of bands or all immature neutrophils (i.e., bands, metamyelocytes, and myelocytes) to segmented neutrophils or all neutrophils. Despite early enthusiasm of researchers, the clinical studies that include these determinations have failed to show a consistent correlation with the presence of serious bacterial disease. Low band counts caused by exhaustion of marrow can cause misleading low ratios in cases of serious or overwhelming infection.[14, 23, 26, 35–39] Initial studies in which the band to segmented neutrophil ratio was used have been disappointing, with normal values recorded in more than one third of infected infants. Band to total neutrophil ratios have been more extensively studied, but their diagnostic utility varies considerably among studies. For instance, Philip and Hewitt,[7] in evaluating infants younger than 7 days old, found that a band neutrophil to total neutrophil ratio of 0.2 or higher had a high sensitivity (90%).

Manroe and colleagues[26] were able to identify by an elevated immature to total neutrophil ratio, and an abnormal neutrophil count, 100% of the infants with respiratory distress and streptococcal disease. In contrast, Baley and associates[40] found that an elevated immature to total neutrophil ratio was of no value in the prediction of infection and a ratio of more than 0.8 was not predictive of neutrophil bone marrow storage pool depletion or outcome. DaSilva and Hammerberg[41] showed unreliability of leukocyte indices, including immature to total neutrophil ratios, in the clinical setting of late onset sepsis with coagulase-negative staphylococci.

The wide range of diagnostic accuracy may be explained by several factors. In some studies, infants with proven sepsis have been grouped with those with suspected sepsis. Differences in study populations may lead to variation, because clinical factors other than infection may cause hematologic changes in the newborn infant. Other causes of discrepancy include intraobserver variability in performance of differential cell counts,[42, 43] the type of sampling (i.e., white blood cell counts are higher in capillary than in arterial or venous specimens), and timing, because the white blood cell indices in the septic infant may be normal at the time of initial evaluation but abnormal several hours later.

Several investigators have shown that serious bacterial infection is associated with significant changes in neutrophil morphology, including the appearance of toxic granules, Dohle bodies, and vacuolization.[44, 45] These features have been considered as a means to improve diagnostic accuracy of neutrophil counts. However, their presence has at most a positive predictive value for sepsis of only slightly more than 50%.[4, 15, 44, 45] Identical morphologic findings can occur as artifacts in citrated blood samples stored for longer than 1 hour before smears are made.[47]

Differential leukocyte counts have also been extensively studied as markers for infectious disease in the newborn period. Increased percentages of lymphocytes have been described in association with congenital syphilis or sepsis.[48] Monocyte counts, normally higher in neonates than in older children, may further increase in some cases of congenital syphilis,[49] perinatal listeriosis,[50] and recovery from sepsis.[51] A dramatic fall in the absolute number of eosinophils frequently accompanies sepsis or serious infections.[44, 51, 52]

PLATELET COUNTS

Low platelet counts are commonly observed in infants who have intrauterine or acquired infections. A wide variety of intrauterine infections are associated with thrombocytopenia. The best known are those of the TORCH group (i.e., toxoplasmosis, other infections, rubella, cytomegalovirus infection, and herpes simplex)[53–54]; however, thrombocytopenia has also been associated with congenital syphilis,[55] mumps,[56] parvovirus B19 infection,[57, 58] and human immunodeficiency virus infection.[59, 60] In the neonatal period, thrombocytopenia is more frequent in infants with bacterial infection than in those with viral infection.[61, 62]

Although many would advise performing a work-up for sepsis on any thrombocytopenic infant, a reduction in the number of circulating platelets is an insensitive, nonspecific, and relatively late indicator of serious bacterial infection. Only 10% to 60% of neonates who have proven bacterial sepsis or meningitis have platelet counts of less than 100,000/mm^3.[4, 5–7, 11, 33, 46, 63] In these cases, the average duration of thrombocytopenia is about 1 week, but it can last 2 to 3 weeks.[15, 53, 64] The bacteria involved, whether gram positive or gram negative, do not seem to be a determining factor for thrombocytopenia, with the possible exception of *Acinetobacter calcoaceticus* and *Candida albicans*.[65, 66] Although platelet counts may begin to fall several days before the onset of clinical signs of infection, values in most cases remain elevated until 1 to 3 days after serious illness is already apparent.[11, 67] An elevated platelet count (up to three times the upper normal limit) in some instances may precede or follow infection in neonates.[68]

Thrombocytopenia accompanying bacterial infection has been thought to be caused by increased platelet destruction. This hypothesis is supported by the rapid fall in the platelet count observed in septic infants,[15] shortened platelet survival after transfusion of platelet concentrates in neonates,[15] shortened platelet survival,[69] and increased numbers of large (young) platelets, along with normal to increased numbers of megakaryocytes in the bone marrow. The mechanism of the increased platelet destruction may involve a direct effect of bacteria or bacterial products on platelets and vascular endothelium, leading to increased aggregation and adhesion, or increased platelet destruction caused by immune mechanisms.[4, 14, 70–73] Surprisingly, diminished platelet counts related to infections are not commonly caused by disseminated intravascular coagulopathy, which is generally limited to those with a more severe degree of thrombocytopenia (platelet counts $<50,000/mm^3$),[69] or accompanied by evidence of excessive bleeding. Although earlier studies suggested that decreased numbers of megakaryocytes are an unlikely mechanism of thrombocytopenia, later findings imply that a paucity of megakaryocytes may underlie or complicate thrombocytopenia associated with sepsis.[75]

Platelet volume measurements (mean platelet volume [MVP] and platelet distribution width [PDW]) have also been used for the prediction of bacteremia in neonates. In a sample of 156 infants, Patrick and associates[76] found a significantly increased presence of bacteremia in infants with MPV values greater than 10.8 fL, PDW values greater than 19.1%, or both. High MPV and PDW values showed high specificity for detecting late bacteremia, but neonates with blood cultures positive at birth (i.e., early infection) tended to have normal platelet volumes. O'Connor and colleagues[77] reviewed serial MPVs of 18 infants in whom coagulase-negative staphylococcal sepsis had developed and found a significant increase in the MPV values at the time of diagnosis and a return to baseline values after resolution of the infection. The increase in MPV occurred although thrombocytopenia developed in only two of the infants, and no difference was found in the mean platelet counts before and at the time of diagnosis of the infection.

ACUTE-PHASE REACTANTS

Acute phase refers to the complex of metabolic alterations that ensue immediately after the onset of infection, trauma, or other cellular destruction.[78–82] Fever, leukocytosis, and changes in the metabolism of many organs (mainly the liver) are important components of the clinical phenomenon.

Although the acute-phase response is preserved throughout vertebrate evolution and can be induced by numerous immunologic and nonimmunologic events, its functions are not well understood. Many investigators believe that the main functions of the acute-phase response are to prevent ongoing tissue damage, to neutralize the inflammatory agent, and to activate repair processes.[79]

The acute-phase reactants are a complex, multifunctional group, including complement components, coagulation proteins, protease inhibitors, metal-binding proteins, C-reactive protein (CRP), and others that increase in the serum in response to tissue injury or bacterial products.[83] Their exact role in the inflammatory process is largely unknown, but most appear to be part of a primitive, nonspecific defense mechanism. Synthesis of acute-phase proteins by hepatocytes is modulated by cytokines.[84] Interleukin (IL)-1β, IL-6, and tumor necrosis factor (TNF) are the most important regulators of acute-phase reactant synthesis. When released into the bloodstream, these cytokines mediate systemic changes such as fever or metabolic alterations, which explains the co-regulation of the appearance of acute-phase reactants and systemic involvement.

Acute-phase reactants are produced very early in fetal life, beginning in the fourth to fifth week of gestation.[85] Several acute-phase reactants have been extensively evaluated in neonatal sepsis, such as CRP, fibrinogen, haptoglobin, or orosomucoid.

C-Reactive Protein

In 1930, Tillett and Francis[86] showed that sera of acutely ill patients precipitated the polysaccharide fraction C of *Streptococcus pneumoniae*. This phenomenon quickly disappeared as patients recovered and was not detected in healthy individuals. When this substance was found to be a protein, the name *C-reactive protein* was assigned, and the term *acute phase* was introduced in reference to infected patients whose sera contained the C-reactive component.

CRP consists of five noncovalently bound, identical subunits, each containing 187 amino acids, with one intrachain disulfide bond and no carbohydrate modifications.[87] CRP binds to phosphocholine and galactose residues, other polysaccharides and peptidopolysaccharides found in bacteria, fungi, and parasites.[88, 89] After binding, CRP activates the classic pathway of complement and acts as an opsonin. CRP and complement components are the only acute-phase proteins directly involved in the elimination of microorganisms.[88] In vitro studies suggest that CRP activates neutrophils, inhibits platelet degranulation, enhances natural killer cell activity, potentially facilitates cell-mediated cytotoxic reactions against cells infected with microbes, and stimulates monocyte-macrophage tumoricidal activity.[88, 89] Binding of CRP to nucleic acids, heparin, histones, and myelin basic protein suggests that it has a direct role in clearing host tissue.

CRP has been detected in many disorders, including acute bacterial, viral, and other infections and noninfectious diseases such as acute myocardial infarction, rheumatic disorders, and malignancies.[88] Inflammation or tissue injury is the common theme that unites these entities of disparate origins. After inflammatory events or acute tissue injury, CRP synthesis increases within 4 to 6 hours, doubling every 8 hours thereafter, and peaks at 36 to 50 hours.[88–90] CRP levels remain elevated with ongoing inflammation and tissue destruction, but with resolution, they decline with time down to normal values because of a relatively short half-life of 19 hours.[91] The kinetics of CRP metabolism appear to closely parallel the degree of injury and repair, thereby supporting its value as a measure of disease activity.

Studies of paired sera from mothers and infants have shown that CRP crosses the placenta in exceedingly low quantities.[92, 93] Elevation in the neonate probably represents endogenous synthesis. Because infection is the most likely cause of inflammation in the newborn infant, elevation of CRP should be a useful marker for sepsis. In neonates with systemic infections, CRP can be elevated at the time of clinical signs.[7, 94–96] However, like the white blood cell count, the rise in CRP can be delayed for several hours after the onset of illness.[96, 97] CRP levels do not predict the severity of the disease, and neonates who fail to mount a CRP response may be at higher risk for death.[18] The use of CRP in the days after birth is complicated by a nonspecific 3-day rise related to the stress of delivery.[98] The specificity of CRP is also decreased when other inflammatory diseases are present. Increases of up to ten times normal values have been associated with neonatal or obstetric conditions such as meconium aspiration syndrome, respiratory distress syndrome, perinatal asphyxia, prolonged rupture of fetal membranes, tissue injury (e.g., bruises, cephalhematoma, ventriculoperitoneal shunt, chest tube), and shock that cause tissue destruction and inflammation.[93, 97, 99–101] Because these conditions are often associated with neonatal bacterial infection, such false-positive elevations greatly reduce the positive predictive value of CRP determinations with respect to sepsis. For these reasons, normal values for CRP are slightly higher in the first 2 days of life (<1.6 mg/dL on day 1 and 2 and <1 mg/dL thereafter).[102]

The sensitivity of CRP elevation in early detection of neonatal sepsis varies in different studies from 47% to 100%; specificity is 6% to 97%.[7, 94–96] Such wide ranges are the result of using different methods, timing of sampling, definition of infections, and test cutoff values. To overcome differences that may be caused by different diagnostic cutoff values, Russell and associates[103] compared serial neutrophil band cell counts with CRP measured by nephelometry. The gold standard was a positive culture, and the performance of the tests was compared using the technique of receiver operating characteristics (ROC) as well as sensitivity and specificity. ROC curves were constructed for all possible diagnostic cutoff values of the tests, and superior performance was demonstrated for CRP compared with band count and immature to total neutrophil ratio. CRP had the highest sensitivity and appeared to be a useful early indicator of infection in neonates.

Several investigators have shown that the sensitivity of CRP is lower for early-onset (<48 hours) sepsis, and a poor CRP response discriminates infants with group B streptococcal infection.[18, 104] In contrast, after the first days of postnatal life, CRP can be considered as a reliable diagnostic test for neonatal sepsis. When evaluating neonates with suspected infection, serial measurements of CRP are more accurate than a single determination.[7, 93, 94, 97, 104–107] A single negative CRP determination cannot exclude sepsis because of the possibility that the sampling preceded the rise in CRP. Normalization of an elevated CRP value has been proposed as a valuable criterion for determining an adequate response to antibiotics, although there are few follow-up data to support this hypothesis.[96]

The usefulness of CRP measurements in neonatal infections other than sepsis has been little explored. Superficial bacterial infections of the skin cause little or no response in the host, whereas cellulitis or abscesses provoke increased levels of CRP.[108] Serum levels are occasionally elevated in infants who have nonspecific acute diarrheal illness[109] and urinary tract infections,[97, 110] but no effort has been made to correlate these rises with the site of infection (e.g., bladder as opposed to kidney) or with the pathogenesis of the illness (e.g., secretory diarrhea as opposed to inflammatory ileocolitis). The response of CRP to nonbacterial infections is variable; elevated serum levels have been found in infants who have minor viral infections, whereas other infants with proven enteroviral meningitis,[111] congenital rubella, or congenital or perinatal herpes simplex virus infections[112] have had normal levels.

Methods for measuring CRP were originally based on the ability of serum to precipitate the C-fraction polysaccharide (i.e., Quellung reaction),[98] followed in later years by semiquantitative latex agglutination assays. After biochemical characterization of CRP in 1978 and the development of specific monoclonal antibodies, a wide array of sensitive quantitative immunologic methods for CRP measurement evolved. Currently, the most widely used technique for measuring CRP is nephelometry.[94] This method measures light scattering from aggregates of CRP with specific antibodies, providing accurate and reproducible results within 15 to 30 minutes and an analytic sensitivity of 0.04 mg/L.

Fibrinogen

Blood concentrations of fibrinogen increase during bacterial infections, and the erythrocyte sedimentation rate (ESR) increases. Normal fibrinogen values are less than 340 mg/dL during the first 2 days of life and rise to 400 to 500 mg/dL between days 3 and 12.[113–117] Clinical experience with the use of fibrinogen levels as a marker of sepsis is limited but generally disappointing. When neonates with various types of infection were evaluated, the median fibrinogen concentration, although higher in those who were infected, overlapped greatly with levels obtained from normal infants.[115–117] Low fibrinogen levels have been associated with disseminated intravascular coagulation,[15] respiratory distress syndrome,[114] and status after exchange transfusion. The blood concentration of fibrinogen is not affected by birth weight, gestational age, or gender.

Erythrocyte Sedimentation Rate

In the neonate, the ESR is performed by measuring the settling of erythrocytes in a vertically placed capillary tube in 1 hour (i.e., micro-ESR).[118] Normal values increase with postnatal age, probably as a result of increasing fibrinogen and falling hematocrit levels, and are equal to the day of life plus 3 mm/hr, up to a maximum of 14 mm/hr.[119] The micro-ESR seems to be less sensitive for the diagnosis of sepsis than the CRP or the immature to total neutrophil ratio, and, like the CRP, it increases slowly. In contrast, the micro-ESR is generally normal in noninfectious conditions, such as respiratory distress syndrome, aspiration pneumonia, or asphyxia. False-positive results can occur with hemolysis, whereas false-negative results may be caused by disseminated intravascular coagulation with consumption of fibrinogen.[94]

Orosomucoid

Orosomucoid is an α_2-acid glycoprotein produced by a number of cell types, including lymphocytes, monocytes, neutrophils, and hepatocytes.[120] Like other acute-phase reactants, orosomucoid is liberated into the plasma during the course of inflammatory processes. Its function is unknown, but it may have roles in forming collagen, binding steroid hormones, and modifying lymphocyte responsiveness.[121, 122]

Elevated orosomucoid levels usually accompany neonatal infection, and early studies suggested that orosomucoid might be a specific and sensitive indicator of neonatal bacterial infection.[123, 124] However, subsequent surveys failed to confirm that experience. Falsely low levels have been found in 15% to 50% of newborn infants at the time of onset of serious bacterial infection,[107, 125–127] and a poor response has been observed in cases of group B streptococcal infection.[101, 107] Because elevated orosomucoid concentrations usually occur with conditions such as asphyxia or respiratory distress syndrome, which are common in the early neonatal period, the specificity of orosomucoid assay for diagnosis of sepsis is considerably decreased in these circumstances.[124, 126]

In addition to poor predictive accuracy for the diagnosis of neonatal sepsis, orosomucoid is of limited value in monitoring the course of infection and the duration of antibiotic therapy because of its slower response and longer half-life[101] than those of other acute-phase reactants.

Haptoglobin

Haptoglobin is an α_2-glycoprotein produced by the liver during the acute-phase response. Although haptoglobin reacts with free hemoglobin to form a complex that is removed by the reticuloendothelial system, it does not seem to be an essential transport protein, because there is no serious disturbance in the catabolism of hemoglobin when it is absent from the circulation.[70]

The quantitative determination of haptoglobin has been suggested as a diagnostic aid to establish or exclude neonatal sepsis. Although the earliest study concluded that this determination was a highly specific and sensitive index of neonatal infection,[128] subsequent investigations have found the test to be extremely unreliable, with normal levels in a large proportion of infected infants.[101, 112]

Other Inflammatory Substances

Fibronectin

Plasma fibronectin is a high-molecular-weight, multifunctional glycoprotein that is found on many cell surfaces and in extracellular fluids. The soluble form of fibronectin, called plasma fibronectin, has binding sites for collagen, heparin, fibrin, fibrinogen, bacteria, and several other macromolecules. Fibronectin is thought to be a key modulator of the immune response, with important functions in neutrophil adhesion, bacterial opsonization, T cell activation, and vascular integrity.[129] Fibronectin levels increase with gestational age to a concentration at term of approximately one half of those of healthy adults.[130–132] Although plasma fibronectin is an acute-phase reactant, concentrations decrease significantly during the course of sepsis in neonates, probably as a result of clearance by the reticuloendothelial system.

There have been several attempts to evaluate the diagnostic utility of low plasma fibronectin in cases of neonatal sepsis. In a prospective study, Gerdes and Polin[8] found that a low plasma fibronectin concentration was a reasonably sensitive indicator of sepsis, but it provided little additional accuracy to a sepsis screen consisting of white blood cell count, immature to total neutrophil ratio, CRP, and micro-ESR. With the cutoff values of serum fibronectin concentrations set at 90 μg/mL for preterm and 100 μg/mL for term neonates, Kocak and associates[133] found a sensitivity of 100% and a specificity of 87.5% for diagnosing sepsis. As a predictor of mortality, they found that the sensitivity of low levels of fibronectin was 100% and the specificity was 88% to 95% for preterm and term infants. Notably, the diagnostic value of plasma fibronectin is diminished in the presence of clinical conditions such as respiratory distress syndrome, perinatal asphyxia, and intrauterine growth retardation, which cause a decrease in plasma fibronectin levels.[131]

Markers of Leukocyte Activity

Lactoferrin is an 80-kd, iron-binding glycoprotein originally isolated from milk.[134] Plasma lactoferrin is predominantly derived from neutrophils and therefore reflects neutrophil turnover rates. Elevated lactoferrin levels have been detected in neonates with bacterial sepsis,[112] and it has been speculated that the protein contributes to the protection against pathogens.

Elastase α_1-proteinase inhibitor is a neutrophil constituent released during cell activation from azurophilic granules. Neonatal studies comparing the diagnostic value of elastase α_1-proteinase inhibitor with other laboratory methods in relation to the onset and the course of the illness have shown high sensitivity in cases of early- and late-onset sepsis.[135, 136] However, little is known about the specificity of this test.

Procalcitonin

Procalcitonin, a propeptide of calcitonin, is a useful marker for diagnosing neonatal sepsis.[137, 138] The cellular sources and metabolic pathways of procalcitonin are unclear. It has been demonstrated in rabbits and humans that procalcitonin is released into the blood 3 to 6 hours after endotoxin injection and increases up to 24 hours[139]; the increase does not correlate with calcitonin levels and occurs even in subjects who have had thyroidectomy.[137]

The release of procalcitonin may depend on the cytokine response to microorganisms.[139] Gendrel and associates[138] demonstrated that very high serum procalcitonin levels are present in neonates with proven or clinically diagnosed bacterial infection, but neonates with viral infection, bacterial colonization, or respiratory distress have normal or slightly increased levels of procalcitonin. Monneret and colleagues[140] confirmed these observations, showing that elevated procalcitonin levels are associated with bacterial infection and that early decrease of these concentrations reflects appropriate antibiotic therapy. They also reported daily variations of procalcitonin levels in noninfected neonates, with a peak on day 1 of life followed by a regular decrease to normal levels.

Compared with CPR, procalcitonin has the advantage that it increases very rapidly, and because of its relatively long half-life (unlike that of cytokines), it is thought to be a reliable alternative in the prediction of sepsis in neonates. The procalcitonin test is simple and requires only 20μL of plasma, and results usually are available within 2 hours.

Calcitonin Gene-Related Peptide

Calcitonin gene-related peptide (CGRP) is a 37–amino acid neuropeptide that belongs to the calcitonin-CGRP family.[141] Like procalcitonin, CGRP is derived from the splicing of the calcitonin-CGRP gene, but these two peptides have distinct sources and functions.

CGRP is released at local sites after stimulation of sensory nerve endings. CGRP-containing nerve endings are present around blood vessels, in the skin and mucosal surfaces, and in the bone. CGRP has vasoregulatory, immunoregulatory, and inflammatory activities. Its overall role appears to be an integration of inflammatory and immune responses in local environments, like IL-10. In rodents, pigs, and humans, CGRP levels are elevated in blood during sepsis and shock.[142–144] Because of its potent vasodilatory actions, it has been hypothesized that CGRP contributes to the acute vascular collapse caused by endotoxin shock. In the newborn infant, CGRP levels increase in umbilical cord and infant blood in association with maternal complications (i.e., culture-positive chorioamnionitis and severe preeclampsia) and culture-positive sepsis or shock.[145] However, further work is needed to establish the clinical usefulness of CGRP measurements in the management of neonatal sepsis.

Intercellular Adhesion Molecule-1

The intercellular adhesion molecule-1 (ICAM-1) is an immunoglobulin-like molecule expressed by several cell types, including leukocytes and endothelial cells. It can be induced in a cell-specific manner by several cytokines, such as TNF, IL-1, and interferon-γ, and it can be inhibited by glucocorticoids. It functions as a costimulatory molecule on antigen-presenting cells to activate major histocompatibility complex (MHC) class II restricted T cells and on other cell types in association with MHC class I to activate cytotoxic T cells. ICAM-1 on endothelium plays an important role in the migration of activated leukocytes to sites of inflammation.

ICAM-1 is shed by the cell and detected in plasma as cICAM-1.[146] Increased serum cICAM-1 levels are present during states of inflammation.[147] The results of several studies indicate that high serum concentrations of cICAM-1 may be an early indicator of neonatal sepsis.[148–150] Elevated cICAM-1 concentrations have been found in the blood of neonates with sepsis, and the increase began an average of 2.2 days before clinical signs of sepsis appeared.[148]

L-Selectin

L-selectin is an adhesion molecule and a leukocyte surface glycoprotein involved in white blood cell migration from the bloodstream to the extravascular compartment. Its expression is rapidly down-regulated after leukocyte activation.[151] Buhrer and associates[152] showed that cord blood lymphocyte L-selectin expression is independent of gestational age, birth weight, white blood cell count, CRP level, or maternal fever before delivery. However, L-selectin expression on umbilical cord lymphocytes was decreased in neonates with bacterial infections acquired in utero compared with healthy newborn infants or those with noninflammatory disorders. A percentage of L-selectin lymphocytes of less than 42% has a sensitivity of 75% and a specificity of 82% in identifying infected newborn infants.[180]

CD45RO

The CD45RO antigen characterizes the primed or memory phenotype of T lymphocytes.[153] Up-regulation of CD45RO expression on umbilical cord lymphocytes may be a good indicator for intrauterine viral infections. Although highly specific (94.6%), CD45RO has low sensitivity, which does not support the use of this test for screening neonates to detect prenatally or early postnatally acquired infections.[154] Tezuka and colleagues[155] showed that the CD45RO expression on T lymphocytes is increased in the postnatal period in cases of viral and bacterial infections. Of clinical relevance, there was no overlap of CD45RO on CD34+ T lymphocytes expression between the group of infants with no infection and those with possible or definite infection.

CD14

CD14 functions as a receptor for lipopolysaccharide (LPS) complexes with LPS-binding protein on the surface of monocytes and macrophages.[156] The soluble form of CD14 (sCD14) in serum is increased in patients with clinical septicemia. The role of sCD14 in sepsis is being investigated. It seems that sCD14 works by activating cells lacking the cell membrane CD14 receptor, such as astrocytes, endothelial, and epithelial cells. Depletion of sCD14 from serum prevents responses to LPS.[157] Blanco and associates[158] found a definite sCD14 increase in newborns with sepsis and positive blood culture results. Although in this study sCD14 did not improve the diagnostic accuracy of other markers (i.e., CRP, IL-6, TNF-α, and fibronectin), there were significant differences in sCD14 levels between sepsis with gram-negative and gram-positive bacteria that were not observed with other markers.

Complement

The complement system consists of a series of more than 30 proteins that are essential components of host protection against an array of pathogenic organisms. The complement cascade is activated directly by bacteria and antigen-antibody complexes, and the degree of complement activation therefore may provide early and specific evidence for bacterial infection. Several studies have shown that the concentrations of C4d, Ba, and C3d are increased in the blood of neonates with proven sepsis.[159–161] However, as a marker for diagnosing neonatal sepsis, the measurements of complement levels have provided good specificity but exceedingly low sensitivity.

Cytokines

Cytokines such as IL-1β, IL-6, and TNF are endogenous mediators of the immune response to bacterial infections. Because cytokines play a critical role in the induction of CRP synthesis in the liver, it was hypothesized that during the course of bacterial infection these molecules could be detected earlier in blood than the acute-phase reactants. Studies support this hypothesis and suggest that elevated cytokine levels may provide an early and sensitive method for diagnosing neonatal infection. However, like other inflammatory markers, cytokine levels can be influenced by clinical complications of the perinatal period, which may be responsible for false-positive or false-negative results. For example, the concentration of IL-1β is increased in cord plasma specimens of infants born after induced vaginal or urgent cesarean deliveries.[162] The concentration of IL-6 is markedly elevated in infants with perinatal asphyxia,[163] and IL-6 and IL-8[164, 165] levels are increased in the cord blood of infants for whom there was histologic evidence but no culture evidence of chorioamnionitis.

Interleukin-1

IL-1, a soluble protein mainly produced by monocytes and macrophages, belongs to a group of cytokines (e.g., TNF, IL-6) with overlapping biologic properties. IL-1, IL-6, and TNF share the ability to stimulate T and B lymphocytes, augment cell proliferation, and initiate or suppress the gene expression of several proteins.[164, 166, 167] IL-1 increases dramatically in response to infection, microbial toxins, inflammatory agents, products of activated lymphocytes, complement, and clotting components. Its systemic effects are associated with the acute-phase response. These induce fever, the synthesis of hepatic acute-phase proteins, and the release of neutrophils. When produced in excessive amounts, IL-1 causes systemic hypotension.

Studies on the IL-1 levels of neonates with bacterial sepsis have produced conflicting results,[162, 168–170] with some reporting increased concentrations of IL-1 in septic neonates, others showing no difference between healthy and infected neonates, and others demonstrating decreased IL-1 production during severe septic episodes. These results suggest that IL-1β plays an important role in the pathophysiology of neonatal septicemia, but the importance of IL-1β determination as a diagnostic marker is not yet clear.

Interleukin-6

IL-6 is a pleiotropic cytokine involved in many aspects of the immune system. It is synthesized by a number of cells, such as monocytes, endothelial cells, and fibroblasts, after TNF and IL-1 stimulation.[171] IL-6 is the major inducer of hepatic acute-phase protein synthesis, including CRP, fibrinogen, and serum amyloid A protein.[172] In most cases of neonatal sepsis, IL-6 increases rapidly, several hours before the increase in the concentration of CRP, and decreases within 24 hours to undetectable levels. The short half-life of IL-6[173] is caused by binding to plasma proteins such as α_2-macroglobulin,[174] early clearance in the liver,[173] and inhibition by other cytokines.[175]

When used as a marker of infection, IL-6 has good sensitivity and good specificity.[176–180] In contrast to CRP, IL-6 is a very early marker, but levels can become normal even if infection continues, as shown by Hack and colleagues,[181] who reported falling levels of IL-6 in patients with persistent symptoms of endotoxic shock. This leads to an increasing proportion of false-negative findings when sampling is performed later in the course. The simultaneous determination of CRP can obviate this problem, because the rise in plasma CRP levels occurs 12 to 48 hours after the onset of infection, at a time when IL-6 levels probably would have fallen. When these two markers are combined, the sensitivity becomes 100% for infected infants at any postnatal age.[177]

Tumor Necrosis Factor-α

TNF-α is an important mediator of the pathophysiologic events that follow gram-negative bacterial sepsis or endotoxemia. Its primary biologic activities include endothelial cell activation, shock, and death. The intravenous injection of TNF-α in laboratory animals induces fever and leukopenia, increases hepatic acute-phase protein synthesis, decreases albumin levels, and causes anorexia, sleep loss, capillary leak, tissue damage, acidosis, hypotension, and, ultimately, death.[166, 182]

Several studies have compared TNF-α levels in septic and nonseptic neonates.[183–185] The serum concentrations of TNF-α are high in neonates with septicemia and even higher in those with septic shock. In these studies, increased levels of TNF-α were not a specific feature of gram-negative sepsis, and no differences were observed between sepsis caused by gram-negative bacteria and sepsis caused by gram-positive bacteria.[183]

Granulocyte Colony-Stimulating Factor

Granulocyte colony-stimulating factor (G-CSF) is a hematopoietic growth factor that plays a pivotal role in promoting the growth and differentiation of granulocyte precursors and increasing the functional activities of their mature progeny.[186] G-CSF production occurs in several types of cells, such as monocyte-macrophages, epithelial cells, endothelial cells, and fibroblasts. Because LPS is a major stimulus for G-CSF production, it was expected that G-CSF would increase in the blood of septic neonates.

Several studies evaluated G-CSF concentrations during the neonatal period, but their results were mixed. Ikeno,[187] measuring cord blood G-CSF levels in neonates with or without perinatal complications, found that G-CSF levels were higher in neonates with complications, such as infections, fetal distress, premature rupture of membranes, asphyxia, and meconium staining of amniotic fluid, and that they correlated with gestational age and cord blood leukocyte counts. Gessler and associates[188] also found increased G-CSF concentrations in infected neonates and a positive correlation between gestational age and G-CSF levels. In contrast, Kennon and colleagues did not observe such a correlation with gestational age and with neutrophil counts, although they found higher G-CSF concentrations in infected neonates, with a sensitivity of 95% for prediction of sepsis and a specificity of 73% for G-CSF levels of more than 200 pg/mL.[189]

Soluble Interleukin-2 Receptor

The cell-associated receptor for IL-2 is transiently expressed on lymphocytes on stimulation and mediates IL-2 signal transduction. After activation, a soluble form of the IL-2 receptor is shed from the cell surface, and its levels increase in serum.[190, 191] Soluble IL-2 receptor is unlikely to be useful as an initial screening test because of low sensitivity. However, its high specificity (100%) could allow the clinician to decrease the number of infants treated in the presence of a negative blood culture result.[192]

Immunoglobulins

IgM is the major immunoglobulin defense against gram-negative organisms. Its synthesis begins at about 11 weeks after conception. Because maternal IgM antibody does not cross the placenta, an increase in IgM levels probably is caused by intrauterine or neonatal bacterial or viral infection. Increased total IgM in umbilical cord sera was shown to be helpful in detecting infants with intrauterine infections, particularly those caused by rubella virus, cytomegalovirus, *Treponema pallidum*, or *Toxoplasma gondii*.[193] After these encouraging results, there were several attempts, especially in the late 1960s and early 1970s, to use IgM concentrations in the evaluation of infants suspected of having acute postnatal bacterial infections. These studies showed consistently low specificity and sensitivity, and the determination of IgM concentrations as an index of neonatal bacterial infection has largely been abandoned. Like IgM, total IgG or IgG subclasses have not been useful in differentiating septic from uninfected neonates.[194]

Metabolic Effects of Sepsis

The effects of sepsis on carbohydrate metabolism are well known. Infants with sepsis can be hypoglycemic or hyperglycemic.[195, 196] When normoglycemic, septic infants usually show an increased need for dextrose infusion.[197] The postulated mechanisms of sepsis-associated hypoglycemia include increased metabolic rate, altered glucose production, and increased insulin sensitivity.[198] Hyperglycemia is usually caused by insulin resistance.[199] Infants with sepsis also have significant elevations of plasma lactate concentrations.[197] The causes of lactic acidosis are largely unknown.

SCREENING PANELS

None of the adjunctive tests considered earlier is sufficiently sensitive and specific to exclude or confirm the diagnosis of neonatal sepsis. Clinicians have begun considering "screening panels" that combine data from several individual analyses. Such panels have included a combination of total leukocyte counts and differential cell counts, total neutrophil counts, total immature neutrophil counts, immature to total neutrophil ratio, platelet counts, and levels of alpha$_1$-acid glycoprotein, haptoglobin, cytokines, ESR, CRP, leukocyte enzyme activity, and blood glucose.[7, 8, 20, 200–203] At present, the best combination of markers for diagnosing late-onset sepsis consists of performing IL-6 and CRP on day 0 together with either TNF-α on day 1 or CRP on day 2.[179]

A hematologic scoring system may provide valuable diagnostic and prognostic information, which could be applied to the identification of possible candidates for treatment with hematopoietic growth factors, such as G-CSF. Overall, the results of these studies have shown little increase in positive predictive value compared with most of the individual screening tests, although negative predictive value is remarkably good, approaching 100% in some studies. Because of the high negative predictive value, screening panels may produce a significant decrease in the use of antimicrobial agents. With their use, fewer neonates would receive antimicrobial agents, and antibiotic treatment could be more confidently discontinued earlier.

References

1. Hammerschlag MR, Klein JO, Herschel M, et al: Patterns of use of antibiotics in two newborn nurseries. N Engl J Med 1977;296:1268.
2. Gerdes JS: Clinicopathologic approach to the diagnosis of neonatal sepsis. Clin Perinatol 1991;18:361.
3. Mc Cabe KM, Khan G, Zhang YH, et al: Amplification of bacterial DNA using highly conserved sequences: automated analysis and potential for molecular triage of sepsis. Pediatrics 1995;95:165.
4. Manroe BL, Weinberg AG, Rosenfeld CR, et al: The neonatal blood count in health and disease. I. Reference values for neutrophilic cells. J Pediatr 1979;95:89.
5. Spector SA, Ticknor W, Grossman M: Study of the usefulness of clinical and hematologic findings in the diagnosis of neonatal bacterial infections. Clin Pediatr 1981;20:385.
6. Kuchler H, Fricker H, Gugler E: La formule sanguine dans le diagnostic précoce de la septicémie du nouveauné. Helv Paediatr Acta 1976;31:33.
7. Philip AGS, Hewitt JR: Early diagnosis of neonatal sepsis. Pediatrics 1980;65:1036.
8. Gerdes JS, Polin RA: Sepsis screen in neonates with evaluation of plasma fibronectin. Pediatr Infect Dis J 1987;6:443.
9. King JC, Berman ED, Wright PF: Evaluation of fever in infants less than 8 weeks old. South Med J 1987;80:948.
10. Speer CH, Bruns A, Gahr M: Sequential determination of CRP, alpha-1 antitrypsin and haptoglobin in neonatal septicaemia. Acta Paediatr Scand 1983;72:679.
11. Moodley GP: The micro-erythrocyte sedimentation rate in black neonate and children. Part II. A comparative study of the micro-erythrocyte sedimentation rate, C-reactive protein test and total white blood cell count. S Afr Med J 1981;60:545.
12. Rozycki HJ, Stahl GE, Baumgart S: Impaired sensitivity of a single early leukocyte count in screening for neonatal sepsis. Pediatr Infect Dis J 1987;6:440.
13. Christensen RD, Rothstein G, Hill HR, et al: Fatal early onset group B streptococcal sepsis with normal leukocyte counts. Pediatr Infect Dis J 1985;4:242.
14. Zipursky A, Palko J, Milner R, et al: The hematology of bacterial infections in premature infants. Pediatrics 1976;57:839.
15. Zipursky A, Jaber HM: The haematology of bacterial infection in newborn infants. Clin Haematol 1978;7:175.
16. Akenzua GI, Hui YT, Milner R, et al: Neutrophil and band counts in the diagnosis of neonatal infections. Pediatrics 1974;54:38.
17. Benuck I, David RJ: Sensitivity of published neutrophil indexes in identifying newborn infants with sepsis. J Pediatr 1983;103:961.
18. Philip AGS: Response of C-reactive protein in neonatal group B streptococcal infection. Pediatr Infect Dis J 1985;4:145.
19. Gregory J, Hey E: Blood neutrophil response to bacterial infection in the first month of life. Arch Dis Child 1972;47:747.
20. Rodwell RL, Leslie AL, Tudehope DI: Early diagnosis of neonatal sepsis using a hematologic scoring system. J Pediatr 1988;112:761.
21. Greenberg DN, Yoder BA: Changes in the differential white blood cell count in screening for group B streptococcal sepsis. Pediatr Infect Dis J 1990;9:886.
22. Christensen RD, Rothstein G, Anstall HB, et al: Granulocyte transfusions in neonates with bacterial infection, neutropenia, and depletion of mature marrow neutrophils. Pediatrics 1982;70:1.
23. Christensen RD, Rothstein G: Exhaustion of mature marrow neutrophils in neonates with sepsis. J Pediatr 1980;96:316.
24. Menke JA, Giacoia GP, Jockin H: Group B beta hemolytic streptococcal sepsis and the idiopathic respiratory distress syndrome: a comparison. J Pediatr 1979; 94:467.
25. Leonidas JC, Hall RT, Beatty EC, et al: Radiographic findings in early onset neonatal group B streptococcal septicemia. Pediatrics 1977;59:1006.
26. Manroe BL, Rosenfeld CR, Weinberg AG, et al: The differential leukocyte count in the assessment and outcome of early-onset neonatal group B streptococcal disease. J Pediatr 1977;91:632.
27. Payne NR, Burke BA, Day DL, et al: Correlation of clinical and pathologic findings in early onset neonatal group B streptococcal infection with disease severity and prediction of outcome. Pediatr Infect Dis J 1988;7:836.
28. Neiburg PI: Prognostic/diagnostic factors in group B beta hemolytic streptococcal (GBBS) and other neonatal sepsis. Pediatr Res 1976;10:402.
29. Baley JE, Stork EK, Warkentin PI: Neonatal neutropenia: clinical manifestation, cause, and outcome. Am J Dis Child 1988;142:1161.
30. Ohlsson A, Wang E, Vearncombe M: Leukocyte counts and colonization with *Ureaplasma urealyticum* in preterm neonates. Clin Infect Dis 1993;17(Suppl 1):S144.
31. Marlowe SE, Greenwald J, Anwar M, et al: Prolonged rupture of membranes in the term newborn. Am J Perinatol 1997;14:483.
32. Christensen RD, Bradley PP, Rothstein G: The leukocyte left shift in clinical and experimental neonatal sepsis. J Pediatr 1981;98:101.
33. Engle WD, Rosenfeld CR: Neutropenia in high-risk neonates. J Pediatr 1984;982.

34. Speer CP, Hauptmann D, Stubbe P, et al: Neonatal septicemia and meningitis in Göttingen, West Germany. Pediatr Infect Dis J 1985;4:36.
35. Courtney SE, Hall RT: *Haemophilus influenzae* sepsis in the premature infant. Am J Dis Child 1978;132:1039.
36. Sherman MP, Goetzman BW, Ahlfors CE, et al: Tracheal aspiration and its clinical correlates in the diagnosis of congenital pneumonia. Pediatrics 1980; 65:258.
37. Wheeler JG, Chauvenet AR, Johnson CA, et al: Neutrophil storage pool depletion in septic neutropenic neonates. Pediatr Infect Dis 1984;3:407.
38. Christensen RD, Harper TE, Rothstein G: Granulocyte-macrophage progenitor cells in term and in preterm neonates. J Pediatr 1986;109:1047.
39. Alexander JB, Giacoia GP: Early-onset nonenterococcal group D streptococcal infection in the newborn infant. J Pediatr 1978;93:489.
40. Baley JE, Stork EK, Warkentin PI, et al: Buffy coat transfusions in neutropenic neonates with presumed sepsis: A prospective, randomized trial. Pediatrics 1987;80:712.
41. DaSilva O, Hammerberg O: Diagnostic value of leukocyte indices in late neonatal sepsis. Pediatr Infect Dis J 1994;5:409.
42. Schelonka RL, Yoder BA, Hall RB, et al: Differentiation of segmented and band neutrophils during the early newborn period. J Pediatr 1995;127:298.
43. Christensen RD, Rothstein G: Pitfalls in the interpretation of leukocyte counts of newborn infants. Am J Clin Pathol 1979;72:608.
44. Xanthou M: Leukocyte blood picture in ill newborn babies. Arch Dis Child 1972;47:741.
45. Amato M, Howald H, von Muralt G: Qualitative changes of white blood cells and perinatal diagnosis of infection in high-risk preterm infants. Padiatr Padol 1988;23:129.
46. Liu CH, Lehan C, Speer ME, et al: Degenerative changes in neutrophils: an indicator of bacterial infection. Pediatrics 1984;74:823.
47. Christensen RD: Morphology and concentration of circulating neutrophils in neonates with bacterial sepsis. Pediatr Infect Dis J 1987;6:429.
48. Cummer CL: Anemia and other blood changes in syphilis JAMA 1928;91:689.
49. Karayalcin G, Khanijou A, Kim KY, et al: Monocytosis in congenital syphilis. Am J Dis Child 1977;131:782.
50. Visintine AM, Oleske JM, Nahmias AJ: *Listeria monocytogenes* infection in infants and children. Am J Dis Child 1977;131:393.
51. Weinberg AG, Rosenfeld CR, Manroe BL, et al: Neonatal blood cell count in health and disease. II. Values for lymphocytes, monocytes, and eosinophils. J Pediatr 1985;106:462.
52. Gibson EL, Vaucher Y, Corrigan JJ Jr: Eosinophilia in premature infants: relationship to weight gain. J Pediatr 1979;95:99.
53. Modanlou HD, Ortiz OB: Thrombocytopenia in neonatal infection. Clin Pediatr 1981;20:402.
54. Boppana SB, Pass RF, Britt WJ, et al: Symptomatic congenital cytomegalovirus infection: neonatal morbidity and mortality. Pediatr Infect Dis J 1992;11:93.
55. Wendel GD Jr, Sanchez PJ, Peters MT, et al: Identification of *Treponema pallidum* in amniotic fluid and fetal blood from pregnancies complicated by congenital syphilis. Obstet Gynecol 1991;78:890.
56. Lacour M, Maherzi M, Vienny H, et al: Thrombocytopenia in a case of neonatal mumps infection: evidence for further clinical presentations. Eur J Pediatr 1993;152:739.
57. Vogel H, Kornman M, Ledet SC, et al: Congenital parvovirus infection. Pediatr Pathol Lab Med 1997; 17:903.
58. Wright IM, Williams ML, Cohen BJ: Congenital parvovirus infection. Arch Dis Child 1991;66:253.
59. Labrune P, Blanche S, Catherine N, et al: Human immunodeficiency virus-associated thrombocytopenia in infants. Acta Paediatr Scand 1989;78:811.
60. Beattie RM, Trounce JQ, Lyall EG, et al: Early thrombocytopenia in HIV infection. Arch Dis Child 1992;67:1093.
61. Modlin JF: Fatal echovirus 11 disease in premature neonates. Pediatrics 1980;66:775.
62. Ballard RA, Drew L, Hufnagle KG, et al: Acquired cytomegalovirus infection in preterm infants. Am J Dis Child 1979;133:482.
63. Dunham EC: Septicemia in the new-born. Am J Dis Child 1933;45:229.
64. Tchernia G, Subtil E, Dehan M, et al: Thrombopénies et infections bactériennes néo-natales. Nouv Rev Fr Hematol 1975:15:484.
65. Ng PC, Herrington RA, Beane CA, et al: An outbreak of *Acinetobacter* septicemia in a neonatal intensive care unit. J Hosp 1989;14:363.
66. Dyke MP, Ott K: Severe thrombocytopenia in extremely low birthweight infants with systemic candidiasis. J Paediatr Child Health 1993;29:298.
67. Töllner U, Pohlandt F: Septicemia in the newborn due to gram-negative bacilli: risk factors, clinical symptoms, and hematologic changes. Eur J Pediatr 1976;123:243.
68. Vora AJ, Lilleyman JS: Secondary thrombocytosis. Arch Dis Child 1993;68:88.
69. Neame PB, Kelton JG, Walker IR, et al. Thrombocytopenia in septicemia: the role of disseminated intravascular coagulation. Blood 1980;56:88.
70. Andrew M, Kelton J: Neonatal thrombocytopenia. Clin Perinatol 1984;11:359.
71. Tate DY, Karlton GT, Johnson D, et al: Immune thrombocytopenia in severe neonatal infections. J Pediatr 1981;98:449.
72. Kekomäki R, Kekomäki M, Elfving J: Platelet associated IgG in septicemia. N Engl J Med 1979;301:271.
73. Ellaurie M, Burns ER, Rubinstein A: Platelet-associated IgG in pediatric HIV infection. Pediatr Hematol Oncol 1991;8:179.
74. Kelton JG, Neame PB, Gauldie J, et al: Elevated platelet-associated IgG in the thrombocytopenia of septicemia. N Engl J Med 1979;300:760.
75. Sola MC, Juul SE, Li Y, et al: Thrombopoietin in preterm and term infants. Early Hum Develop 1999;53:239.
76. Patrick CH, Lazarchick J: The effect of bacteremia on automated platelet measurements in neonates. Am J Clin Pathol 1990;93:391.
77. O'Connor TA, Ringer KM, Gaddis ML: Mean platelet volume during coagulase-negative staphylococcal sepsis in neonates. Am J Clin Pathol 1993;99:69.
78. Stadnyc AW, Gauldie J: The acute phase protein response during parasitic infection. Immunol Today 1991;12:A7.
79. Baumann H and Gauldie J: The acute phase response. Immunol Today 1994;15:74.
80. Steel SM, and Whitehead AS: The major acute phase reactants: C-reactive protein, serum amyloid P component and serum amyloid A protein. Immunol Today 1994;15:81.
81. Redl H, Schlag G, Sciesser A, et al: Tumor necrosis factor is a mediator of phospholipase release during bacteremia in baboons. Am J Physiol 1993; 264:H2119.

82. Pruzasky W, Vadas P: Phospholipase A_2—a mediator between proximal and distal effectors of inflammation. Immunol Today 1991;12:143.
83. Pepys MB, Baltz ML: Acute phase proteins with special reference to C-reactive and related proteins (pentraxins) and serum amyloid A protein. Adv Immunol 1983;34:141.
84. Dinarello CA: Interleukin-1 and the pathogenesis of the acute-phase response. N Engl J Med 1984; 311:1413.
85. Gitlin D, Biasucci A: Development of IgG, IgA, IgM, β1C/β1A, C′1 esterase inhibitor, ceruloplasmin, transferrin, hemopexin, haptoglobin, fibrinogen, plasminogen, α1-antitrypsin, orosomucoid, β-lipoprotein, α-2-macroglobulin, and prealbumin in the human conceptus. J Clin Invest 1969;48:1433.
86. Tillet WS, Francis T: Serological reactions in pneumonia with a non-protein somatic fraction of pneumococcus. J Exp Med 1930;52:561.
87. Gewurz H, Zhang XH, Lint TF: Structure and function of the pentraxins. Curr Opin Immunol 1995;7:54.
88. Nudelman R, Kagan BM: C-reactive protein in pediatrics (Review). Adv Pediatr 1983;30:517.
89. Gewurz H: Biology of C-reactive protein and acute phase response. Hosp Pract 1982;6:67.
90. Steel DM, Whitehead AS: The major acute phase reactants: C-reactive protein, serum amyloid P component and serum amyloid A protein. Immunol Today 1994;15:81.
91. Vigushin D, Pepys M, Hawkins P: Metabolic and scintigraphic studies of radioiodinated human C-reactive protein in health and disease. J Clin Invest 1993;91:1351.
92. Kaapa P, Koistinen E: Maternal and neonatal C-reactive protein after interventions during delivery. Acta Obstet Gynecol Scand 1993;72:543.
93. Ainbender E, Cabatu E, Kuzman DN, et al: Serum C-reactive protein and problems of newborn infants. J Pediatr 1982;101:3438.
94. Powell KR, Marcy SM: Laboratory aids for diagnosis of neonatal sepsis. In Remington J, Klein J (eds): Infectious Diseases of the Fetus and Newborn Infant, 4th ed. Philadelphia: WB Saunders, 1995, p 1223.
95. Guttemberg TJ, Haneberg B, Jorgensen T: The latency of serum acute phase proteins in meningococcal septicemia, with special emphasis on lactoferrin. Clin Chim Acta 1984;136:173.
96. Maters NJ, Pohlandt F: Diagnostic audit of C-reactive protein in neonatal infection. Eur J Pediatr 1987;146:147.
97. Forest JC, Lariviere F, Dolce P, et al: C-reactive protein as biochemical indicator of bacterial infection in neonates. Clin Biochem 1986;19:192.
98. Jaye DJ, Waites KB: Clinical applications of C-reactive protein in pediatrics. Pediatr Infect Dis J 1997;16:735.
99. Schouten-VanMeeteren NYN, Rietveld A, Molenaar AJ, et al: Influence of perinatal conditions on C-reactive protein production. J Pediatr 1992;120:621.
100. Magny JF, Benattar C, Saby MA, et al: C-reactive proteine et diagnostic d'infection neonatale: etude rétrospecitve de 242 dossiers. Pediatrie 1986;41:105.
101. Pourcyrous M, Bada HS, Korones SB, et al: Acute phase reactants in neonatal bacterial infections. J Perinatol 1991;11:319.
102. Philip AGS: Neonatal Sepsis and Meningitis. Boston: GK Hall, 1985, p 76.
103. Russell GA, Smyth A, Cooke RW: Receiver operating characteristic curves for comparison of serial neutrophil band forms and C reactive protein in neonates at risk of infection. Arch Dis Child 1992;67:808.
104. Krediet T, Gerards L, Fleer A, et al: The predictive value of CRP and I/T-ratio in neonatal infection. J Perinat Med 1992;20:479.
105. Berger C, Uehlinger J, Ghelfi D, et al: Comparison of C-reactive protein and white blood cell count with differential in neonates at risk for septicemia. Eur J Pediatr 1995;154:138.
106. Kawamura M, Nishida H: The usefulness of serial C-reactive measurements in managing neonatal infection. Acta Pediatr 1995;84:10.
107. Sann L, Bienvenu F, Bienvenu J, et al: Evolution of serum prealbumin, C-reactive protein and orosomucoid in neonates with bacterial infection. J Pediatr 1984;105:977.
108. Felix NS, Nakayima H, Kagan BM: Serum C-reactive protein in infections during the first months of life. Pediatrics 1966;37:270.
109. Matesanz JL, Málaga S, Santos F, et al: Valor diagnóstico de la proteína reactiva en la sepsis neonatal. An Esp Pediatr 1980;13:671.
110. Sabel KG, Wadsworth CH: C-reactive protein (CRP) in early diagnosis of neonatal septicemia. Acta Pediatr Scand 1979;68:825.
111. Alt R, Willard D, Messer J, et al: Intéŕet de la C réactive protéine dans les infections bactériennes néonatales. Arch Fr Pediatr 1982;39:811.
112. Gutteberg TJ, Haneberg B, Jergensen T: Lactoferrin in relation to acute phase proteins in sera from newborn infants with severe infections. Eur J Pediatr 1984;142:37.
113. Sell EJ, Corrigan JJ Jr: Platelet counts, fibrinogen concentrations, and factor V and factor VIII levels in healthy infants according to gestational age. J Pediatr 1973;82:1028.
114. Jensen AH, Josso F, Zamet P, et al: Evolution of blood clotting factor levels in premature infants during the first 10 days of life: a study of 96 cases with comparison between clinical status and blood clotting factor. Pediatr Res 1973;7:638.
115. de Gamarra E, Savaglio N, Moriette, G, et al: Surveillance du taux de fibrinogène chez le nouveau-né: intéŕet au cours de l'évolution des infections bacter iériennes par contamination d'origine maternelle. Arch Fr Pediatr 1980;37:163.
116. Raichvarg D, Carre J, Relier JP, et al: Intéŕet de la détermination conjointe du fibrinogène et de l'orosomucoïde pour le diagnostic rapide de infections nèonatales. Ann Pediatr 1982;29:670.
117. Relier JP, de Gamarra E: Place du fibrinogène parmi les proteínes de l'inflammation dans les infections nèonatales. Pediatrie 1984;39:379.
118. Barrett BA, Hill PI: A micromethod for the erythrocyte sedimentation rate suitable for use on venous or capillary blood. J Clin Pathol 1980;33:1118.
119. Adler SM, Denton RL: The erythrocyte sedimentation rate in the newborn period. J Pediatr 1985;86:942.
120. Schmid K, Kaufman H, Isemura S, et al: Structure of alpha 1-acid glycoprotein. The complete amino-acid sequence, multiple amino-acid substitutions and homology with immunoglobulins. Biochemistry 1973;12:2711.
121. Philip AGS: Acute-phase proteins in neonatal infection. J Pediatr 1984;105:940.
122. Lee SK, Thibeault DW, Heiner DC: α_1-Antitrypsin and α_1-acid glycoprotein levels in the cord blood and amniotic fluid of infants with respiratory distress syndrome. Pediatr Res 1978;12:775.
123. Sann L, Krawiecki N, Bourgeois J, et al: Etude de l'orosomucoide chez le nouveau-né: intéŕet dans le diagnostic des infections bacteriennes. Arch Fr Pediatr 1976;33:961.

124. Goto H, Ishikawa N, Shioiri T, et al: Diagnostic significance of serum orosomucoid level in bacterial infections during neonatal period. Acta Paediatr Scand 1973;62:629.
125. Gill CW, Bush WS, Burleigh WM, et al: An evaluation of a C-reactive protein assay using a rate immunonephelometric procedure. Am J Clin Pathol 1981;75:50.
126. Bienvenu J, Sann L, Bienvenu F, et al: Laser nephelometry of orosomucoid in serum of newborns: reference interval and relation to bacterial infections. Clin Chem 1981;27:721.
127. Philip AGS, Hewitt JR: α_1-Acid glycoprotein in the neonate with and without infection. Biol Neonate 1983;43:118.
128. Salmi TT: Haptoglobin levels in the plasma of newborn infants with special reference to infections. Acta Paediatr Scand 1973;241:7.
129. Dyke MP, Forsyth KD: Decreased plasma fibronectin concentrations in preterm infants with septicaemia. Arch Dis Child 1993;68:557.
130. Gerdes JS, Yoder MC, Douglas SD, et al: Decreased plasma fibronectin in neonatal sepsis. Pediatrics 1983;72:877.
131. McCafferty MH, Lepow M, Saba TM, et al: Normal fibronectin levels as a function of age in pediatric population. Pediatr Res 1982;17:482.
132. Yoder MC, Douglas SD, Gerdes J, et al: Plasma fibronectin in healthy newborn infants: respiratory distress syndrome and perinatal asphyxia. J Pediatr 1983;102:777.
133. Kocak G, Ezer G, Vidinlisan S: Serum fibronectin in neonatal sepsis: is it valuable in early diagnosis and outcome prediction? Acta Pediatr Jpn 1997;39:428.
134. Lonnerdal B, Iyer S: Lactoferrin: molecular structure and biological function. Annu Rev Nutr 1995;15:93.
135. Speer CP, Ninjo A, Gahr M: Elastase α_1-Proteinase inhibitor in early diagnosis of neonatal septicemia. J Pediatr 1986;108:987.
136. Tegtmeyer FK, Horn C, Richter A, et al: Elastase α_1-proteinase inhibitor complex, granulocyte count, ratio of immature to total granulocyte count, and C-reactive protein in neonatal septicemia. Eur J Pediatr 1992;151:353.
137. Assicot M, Gendrel D, Carsin H, et al: High serum procalcitonin concentrations in patients with sepsis and infection. Lancet 1993;341:515.
138. Gendrel D, Assicot M, Raymond J, et al: Procalcitonin as a marker for the early diagnosis of neonatal infection. J Pediatr 1996;128:570.
139. Dandona P, Nix D, Wilson MF, et al: Procalcitonin increase after endotoxin injection in normal subjects. J Clin Endocrinol Metab 1994;79:1605.
140. Monneret G, Labaune JM, Isaac C, et al: Procalcitonin and C-reactive protein levels in neonatal infections. Acta Paediatr 1997;86:209.
141. McGillis JP, Mitsuhashi M, Pajan DG: Immunomodulation by tachykinin neuropeptides. Ann N Y Acad Sci 1990;594:85.
142. Joyce CD, Fiscus RR, Wang X, et al: Calcitonin gene-related peptide levels are elevated in patients with sepsis. Surgery 1990;108:1097.
143. Arden WE, Fiscus RR, Wang X, et al: Elevations in circulating calcitonin gene-related peptide correlate with hemodynamic deterioration during endotoxic shock in pigs. Circ Shock 1994;34:217.
144. Wang X, Han CD, Fiscus RR, et al: Hypotension- and endotoxin-induced alterations in calcitonin gene-related peptide: modulation by dexamethasone. Circ Shock 1991;34:217.
145. Parida AK, Schneider DB, Stoss TD, et al:. Elevated circulating calcitonin gene-related peptide in umbilical cord and infant blood associated with maternal and neonatal sepsis and shock. Pediatr Res 1998;43:276.
146. van de Stolpe A, van der Saag PT: Intercellular adhesion molecule-1. J Mol Med 1996;74:13.
147. Rothlein R, Minolfi EA, Czajkowsky M, et al: A form of circulating cICAM-1 in human serum. J Immunol 1991;147:4398.
148. Küster H, Degitz K: Circulating ICAM-1 in neonatal sepsis. Lancet 1993;341:506.
149. Edgar JD, Wilson DC, McMillan SA, et al: Predictive value of soluble immunological mediators in neonatal infection. Clin Sci 1994;87:165.
150. Lehrnbecher T, Schrod L, Rutsch, et al: Immunologic parameters in cord blood indicating early-onset sepsis. Biol Neonate 1996;70:206.
151. Buhrer C, Berlin C, Jablonski-Westrich D, et al: Lymphocyte activation and regulation of three adhesion molecules with supposed function in homing: LECAM-1 (MEL-14 antigen), LPAM-1/2 (α_4-integrin), and CD44 (Pgp-1). Scand J Immunol 1992;35:107.
152. Buhrer C, Luxenburger U, Metze B, et al: Diminished cord blood lymphocyte L-selectin expression in neonatal bacterial infection. Eur J Pediatr 1993;152:519.
153. Michael DR: Interleukin 2 induces the expression of CD45RO and the memory phenotype by $CD45RA^+$ peripheral blood lymphocytes. J Exp Med 1994;179:857.
154. Bruning T, Daiminger A, Enders G: Diagnostic value of CD45RO expression on circulating T lymphocytes of fetuses and newborn infants with pre-, peri- or early post-natal infections. Clin Exp Immunol 1997; 107:306.
155. Tezuka T, Sugita K, Mizobe N, et al: Transient increase in CD45RO expression on T Lymphocytes in infected newborns. Pediatr Res 1998;43:2:283.
156. Wright SD, Ramos RA, Tobias PS, et al: CD14, a receptor for complexes of lipopolysaccharide (LPS) and LPS binding protein. Science 1990;249:1431.
157. Frey EA, Miller DS, Jahar TG, et al: Soluble CD14 participates in the response of cells to lipopolysaccharide. J Exp Med 1992;176:1665.
158. Blanco A, Solis G, Arranz E, et al: Serum levels of CD14 in neonatal sepsis by gram-positive and gram-negative bacteria. Acta Pediatr 1996;85:728.
159. Peakman M, Senaldi G, Liossis G, et al: Complement activation in neonatal infection. Arch Dis Child 1992;67:802.
160. Kalayci AG, Adam B, Yilmazer F, et al: The value of immunoglobulin and complement levels in the early diagnosis of neonatal sepsis. Acta Paediatr 1997;86:999.
161. Drew JH, Arroyave CM: Complement activation: use in the diagnosis of infection in newborn infants. Acta Paediatr Scand 1981;70:255.
162. Miller LC, Isa S, Lo Preste G, et al: Neonatal interleukin-1β, interleukin-6 and tumor necrosis factor: cord blood levels and cellular production. J Pediatr 1990;117:961.
163. Yoon BH, Romero R, Yang SH, et al: Interleukin-6 concentrations in umbilical cord plasma are elevated in neonates with white matter lesions associated with periventricular leukomalacia. Am J Obstet Gynecol 1996;174:1433.
164. Sullivan JS, Kilpatrick L, Costarino AT Jr, et al: Correlation of plasma cytokine elevations with mortality rate in children with sepsis. J Pediatr 1992;120:510.
165. Singh B, Merchant P, Walker CR, et al: Interleukin-

6 expression in cord blood of patients with clinical chorioamnionitis. Pediatr Res 1996;39:976.
166. Dinarello CA: The proinflammatory cytokines interleukin-1 and tumor necrosis factor and treatment of the septic shock syndrome. J Infect Dis 1991;163:1177.
167. Dinarello CA: Interleukin-1 and interleukin-1 antagonism. Blood 1991;77:1627.
168. Atici A, Satar M, Alparslan: Serum interleukin-1β in neonatal sepsis. Acta Paediatr 1996;85:371.
169. Özdemir A, Oygür N, Gültekin M, et al: Neonatal tumor necrosis factor, interleukin-1β, and interleukin-6 response to infection. Am J Perinatol 1994;11:282.
170. de Bont ESJM, Martens A, van Raan J, et al: Tumor necrosis factor-alpha, interleukin-1 beta, and interleukin-6 plasma levels in neonatal sepsis. Pediatr Res 1993;33:380.
171. Kishimoto T: The biology of interleukin-6. Blood 1989;74:1.
172. Gauldie J, Richards C, Harnish D, et al: Interferon β2/B-cell stimulatory factor type 2 shares identity with monocyte-derived hepatocyte-stimulating factor and regulates the major acute phase protein response in liver cells. Proc Natl Acad Sci U S A 1987;84:7251.
173. Castell JV, Geiger T, Gross V, et al: Plasma clearance, organ distribution and target cells of interleukin-6/hepatocyte stimulating factor in the rat. Eur Biochem 1988;177:357.
174. Matsuda T, Hirano T, Nagasawa S, et al: Identification of α_2-macroglobulin as a carrier protein for IL-6. J Immunol 1989;142:148.
175. Lee JD, Swisher SG, Minehart EH, et al: Interleukin 4 down-regulates interleukin 6 production in human peripheral blood mononuclear cells. J Leukoc Biol 1990;47:475.
176. Buck C, Bundschu J, Gallati H, et al:. Interleukin-6: a sensitive parameter for the early diagnosis of neonatal bacterial infection. Pediatrics 1994;93:54.
177. Messer J, Eyer D, Donato L, et al: Evaluation of interleukin-6 and soluble receptors of tumor necrosis factor for early diagnosis of neonatal infection. J Pediatr 1996;129:574.
178. De Bont ESJM, Martens A, Van Raan J, et al: Diagnostic value of plasma levels of tumor necrosis factor α (TNFα) and interleukin-6 (IL-6) in newborn with sepsis. Acta Paediatr 1994;83:696.
179. Ng PC, Cheng SH, Chui KM, et al: Diagnosis of late onset neonatal sepsis with cytokines, adhesion molecule, and C-reactive protein in preterm very low birthweight infants. Arch Dis Child 1997;77:F221.
180. Smulian JC, Bhandari V, Campbell WA, et al: Value of umbilical artery and vein levels of interleukin-6 and soluble intracellular adhesion molecule-1 as predictors of neonatal hematologic indices and suspected early sepsis. J Matern Fetal Med 1997;6:254.
181. Hack CE, De Groot ER, Felt-Bersma RJ, et al: Increased plasma levels of interleukin-6 in sepsis. Blood 1989;74:1704.
182. Offenstadt G, Guidet B, Staikowsky F: Cytokines and severe infections. Pathol Biol (Paris) 1993;41:820.
183. Roman J, Fernandez F, Velasco F, et al: Serum TNF levels in neonatal sepsis and septic shock. Acta Paediatr 1993;82:352.
184. Girardin EP, Berner ME, Grau GE, et al: Serum tumor necrosis factor in newborns at risk for infections. Eur J Pediatr 1990;149:645.
185. Atici A, Satar M, Cetiner S, et al: Serum tumor necrosis factor-alpha in neonatal sepsis. Am J Perinatol 1997;14:401.
185. Demetri GD, Griffin JD: Granulocyte colony-stimulating factor and its receptor. Blood 1991;78:2791.
187. Ikeno K: Increased granulocyte colony stimulating factor (G-CSF) levels in neonates with perinatal complications. Acta Paediatr Jpn 1994;36:366.
188. Gessler P, Kirchmann N, Kientsch-Engel R, et al: Serum concentrations of granulocyte colony-stimulating factor in healthy term and preterm neonates and in those with various diseases including bacterial infections. Blood 1993;82:3177.
189. Kennon C, Overturf G, Bessman S, et al: Granulocyte colony-stimulating factor as a marker for bacterial infection in neonates. J Pediatr 1996;128:765.
190. Smith KA: The biomolecular structure of the interleukin-2 receptor. Immunol Today 1988;9:36.
191. Nelson DL, Kurman CC, Fritz ME, et al: The production of soluble and cellular interleukin-2 receptors by cord blood mononuclear cells following in vitro activation. Pediatr Res 1986;20:136.
192. Spear ML, Stefano JL, Fawcett P, et al: Soluble interleukin-2 receptor as a predictor of neonatal sepsis. J Pediatr 1995;126:982.
193. Aldorf CA Jr: Immunoglobulin determinations in the diagnosis of fetal infections. Pediatr Clin North Am 1971;18:99.
194. Kalayci AG, Adam B, Yilmazer F, et al: The value of immunoglobulin and complement levels in the early diagnosis of neonatal sepsis. Acta Paediatr 1997; 86:999.
195. Yeung CY: Hypoglycemia in neonatal sepsis. J Pediatr 1970;77:812.
196. James T III, Blessa M, Boggs TR Jr: Recurrent hyperglycemia associated with sepsis in a neonate. Am J Dis Child 1979;133:645.
197. Fitzgerald MJ, Goto M, Myers TF, et al: Early metabolic effects of sepsis in the preterm infant: lactic acidosis and increased glucose requirements. J Pediatr 1992;121:951.
198. Hill HR: Diagnosis and treatment of sepsis in the neonate. In Rool RK, Sande MA (eds): Septic Shock. New York: Churchill Livingstone, 1985, p 219.
199. Michie HR: Metabolism of sepsis and multiple organ failure. World J Surg 1996;20:460.
200. Rodwell RL, Taylor KMCD, Tudehope DI, et al: Hematologic scoring system in early diagnosis of sepsis in neutropenic newborns. Pediatr Infect Dis J 1993;12:372.
201. Philip AGS: Decreased use of antibiotics using a neonatal sepsis screening technique. J Pediatr 1981;98:795.
202. Kite P, Millar MR, Gorham P, et al: Comparison of five tests used in diagnosis of neonatal bacteraemia. Arch Dis Child 1988;63:639.
203. Misra PK, Kumar R, Malik GK, et al: Simple hematological tests for diagnosis of neonatal sepsis. Indian Pediatr 1989;26:156.

CHAPTER 18

Blood Banking and Transfusion Issues in Perinatal Medicine*

Ronald G. Strauss, M.D.

Extremely preterm neonates, particularly those with birth weights of less than 1.0 kg, usually require blood component transfusions. Transfusion practices for neonates are controversial, variable, and often based on logical assumptions rather than sound scientific information extracted from controlled clinical studies. Firm indications for blood component transfusions do not exist, and it is important to consider the underlying pathophysiology, goals of treatment, and all aspects of the benefit-risk ratio when making transfusion decisions. This chapter addresses all of these issues. Because many aspects of the pathophysiology of hematologic disorders are discussed extensively in other chapters, only a brief overview from the perspective of transfusion medicine is presented. Most of the discussion focuses on the rationale for blood component transfusions and on the best blood banking techniques to provide special components for neonatal transfusions.

NEONATAL BLOOD COMPONENT TRANSFUSIONS

Neonatal Anemia and Red Blood Cell Transfusions

Pathophysiology of Neonatal Anemia

All infants experience a decline in hemoglobin concentration, hematocrit, and circulating red blood cell (RBC) volume (mass) in the first weeks of life. This decline results from physiologic factors and, in sick preterm infants, from phlebotomy blood losses for monitoring. In healthy term infants, the nadir hemoglobin value rarely falls below 9 g/dL at an age of 10 to 12 weeks. This decline is more rapid (i.e., nadir at 4 to 6 weeks of age) and falls to lower levels in infants born prematurely. Without transfusion, the mean hemoglobin concentration falls from around 16 g/dL at birth to approximately 8 g/dL in infants with birth weights of 1.0 to 1.5 kg and to approximately 7 g/dL in infants with birth weights of less than 1 kg.[1–3] Because this postnatal drop in hemoglobin level is universal and well tolerated in term infants, it is commonly referred to as the *physiologic anemia of infancy*. However, the pronounced decline in hemoglobin concentration that occurs in many extremely preterm infants is associated with abnormal clinical signs and need for RBC transfusions, and acceptance of this anemia of prematurity as a normal, benign event has been questioned.[4, 5]

Many interacting physiologic factors are at play in neonatal anemia. A key reason that the hemoglobin nadir is lower in preterm than in term infants is the former group's diminished plasma erythropoietin (EPO) level in response to anemia.[3, 6–9] Although anemia provokes EPO production in premature infants, the plasma levels achieved in anemic infants at any given blood hemoglobin concentration are lower than those observed in comparably anemic older persons.[8] Erythroid progenitor cells in blood[10] and bone marrow[11] of preterm infants are quite re-

*Supported in part by NIH Program Project Grant P01 HL46925.

sponsive to EPO in vitro—a finding suggesting that inadequate production of EPO is the major cause of physiologic anemia, not marrow unresponsiveness.

The mechanisms responsible for the diminished EPO output by preterm neonates are only partially defined. One mechanism is that the primary site of EPO production in preterm infants is in the liver, rather than kidney.[12] This dependency on hepatic EPO is important, because the liver is less sensitive to anemia and tissue hypoxia, and relatively sluggish EPO secretion occurs in response to the falling RBC mass. The timing of the switch from liver to kidney is set at conception and is not accelerated by preterm birth. From a teleologic perspective, decreased hepatic production of EPO under in utero conditions of tissue hypoxia may be an advantage for the fetus. If this were not the case, normal levels of fetal hypoxia could trigger high levels of EPO and produce erythrocytosis and consequent hyperviscosity in utero. After birth, however, diminished EPO responsiveness to tissue hypoxia is disadvantageous and leads to anemia.

Diminished EPO production cannot entirely explain low plasma EPO levels in preterm infants. Extraordinarily high plasma levels of EPO have been reported for some fetuses, comparable to those of neonates treated in intensive care settings,[13, 14] and macrophages from human cord blood were found to produce normal quantities of EPO messenger RNA and protein.[15] These studies document intact synthetic capability under some circumstances. Additional mechanisms probably contribute to diminished EPO plasma levels. For example, plasma levels of EPO undoubtedly are influenced by metabolism (clearance) and by production. Data for human infants[16, 17] and neonatal monkeys[18] demonstrate that low plasma EPO levels may result from increased plasma clearance and volume of distribution and from shorter fractional elimination and mean residence times for EPO in neonates compared with adults. Accelerated catabolism may contribute to the low plasma levels, with the low plasma EPO concentration possibly resulting from decreased synthesis and increased metabolism.

Phlebotomy blood losses play a key role in the anemia of prematurity. Critically ill neonates must be monitored closely with serial cultures and laboratory studies of blood gases, electrolytes, and blood counts. Small preterm infants are the most critically ill, require the most frequent blood sampling, and suffer the greatest proportional loss of RBCs because their circulating RBC volumes are smallest. In the past, the mean volume of blood removed for sampling was 0.8 to 3.1 mL/kg per day during the first few weeks of life for preterm infants requiring intensive care.[19, 20] Promising in-line devices that withdraw blood, measure multiple analytes, and then reinfuse the sampled blood are being investigated. However, until these devices are proven effective and safe for infants, the replacement of blood losses from phlebotomy remains a key factor responsible for multiple RBC transfusions in critically ill neonates.

Need for Red Blood Cell Transfusions

Neonates, particularly when extremely preterm, are among the most heavily transfused of all patient groups. Only a few years ago, 80% of premature neonates with birth weights less than 1.5 kg required multiple RBC transfusions, and many infants were given cumulative transfusion volumes in excess of their total blood volumes at birth.[21] A smaller percentage receive other blood components such as fresh frozen plasma, cryoprecipitate, platelet, and neutrophil (i.e., granulocyte) concentrates.

As is true for patients of all ages, efforts have been made to reduce the number of transfusions given to neonates and to limit donor exposures. A study of blood use by neonates illustrated these changing practices by comparing RBC transfusions in the years 1982, 1989, and 1993.[22] The mean number of transfusions per infant (<1.5 kg birth weight) declined from 7.0 in 1982 to 5.0 in 1989 to 2.7 in 1993 (*P*<0.001). The percentage of relatively large preterm infants (birth weight of 1.0 to 1.5 kg) who were managed without transfusions increased from 17% in 1982 to 32% in 1989 to 64% in 1993. In contrast, nearly 100% of extremely preterm infants (birth weight<1.0 kg) required RBC transfusions in all years.[22] The need to effectively manage the early anemia of prematurity was emphasized because 70% of transfusions were given during the first month of life. As the survival of extremely preterm infants continues to increase, many of these tiny survivors will require blood component transfusions. Blood component transfusions provide a genuine benefit to many preterm infants and are indispensable to the neonatologist.

Guidelines for Red Blood Cell Transfusions

Guidelines for transfusing RBCs to neonates are controversial, and practices vary.[1, 23] The lack of a consistent approach stems from limited knowledge of the cellular and molecular biology of erythropoiesis during the perinatal period and from an incomplete understanding of the infant's response to anemia. Generally, RBC transfusions are given to maintain a level of hemoglobin or hematocrit believed to be most desirable for each neonate's clinical condition. Broad guidelines for RBC transfusions during early infancy are listed in Table 18-1.[24] These guidelines are general, and terms such as *severe* and *symptomatic* must be defined to fit local practices.

Table 18–1. **Guidelines for Neonatal Blood Component Transfusions**

Red Blood Cells
Hemoglobin <130 g/L (HCT <40%) with *severe** cardiopulmonary disease
Hemoglobin <100 g/L (HCT <30%) with *moderate* cardiopulmonary disease
Hemoglobin <100 g/L (HCT <30%) with *major* surgery
Hemoglobin <80 g/L (HCT <24%) with *symptomatic anemia*
Bleeding with >25% loss of circulating blood volume
Platelets
Platelets <100 × 10^9/L and bleeding
Platelets <50 × 10^9/L and invasive procedure
Platelets <20 × 10^9/L and no bleeding but clinically *stable*
Platelets <100 × 10^9/L and no bleeding but clinically *unstable*
Fresh Frozen Plasma
Severe clotting factor deficiency with bleeding
Severe clotting factor deficiency and invasive procedure
Vitamin K deficiency with bleeding
Dilutional coagulopathy with bleeding
Severe anticoagulant protein deficiency
Neutrophils
Neutrophils <3 × 10^9/L and *fulminant* sepsis during first week of life
Neutrophils <1 × 10^9/L and *fulminant* sepsis after first week

HCT, hematocrit.
*Words in italics must be defined according to local practices.

Most RBC transfusions given to neonatal patients are small in volume (10 to 15 mL/kg) and are repeated frequently to replace blood drawn for laboratory studies. There is no proven benefit to routinely replacing phlebotomy blood losses milliliter for milliliter. Instead, RBCs should be transfused to maintain a hematocrit level deemed appropriate for the clinical condition of each infant. In neonates with severe respiratory disease, such as those requiring high volumes of oxygen with ventilator support, it is customary to maintain the hematocrit above 40% (i.e., hemoglobin concentration >13 g/dL), particularly when blood is being drawn frequently for testing. This practice is based on the belief that transfused donor RBCs containing adult hemoglobin can provide optimal oxygen delivery throughout the period of diminished pulmonary function. Although this seemingly logical practice is widely recommended, little evidence is available to establish its efficacy.[1] Consistent with this rationale for ensuring optimal oxygen delivery in neonates with pulmonary failure, it seems logical to maintain the hematocrit above 40% in infants with congenital heart disease that is severe enough to cause cyanosis or congestive heart failure.

Definitive studies are not available to establish the optimal hemoglobin level for neonates facing major surgery. However, it seems reasonable to maintain the hemoglobin concentration higher than 10 g/dL (hematocrit >30%) because of the limited ability of the neonate's heart, lungs, and vasculature to compensate for anemia. Additional factors include inferior offloading of oxygen because of the diminished interaction between fetal hemoglobin and 2,3-diphosphoglycerate (2,3-DPG) and the developmental impairment of neonatal renal, hepatic, and neurologic function. This transfusion guideline is only a recommendation, and it should be applied with flexibility to individual infants facing surgical procedures.

The clinical indications for RBC transfusions in preterm infants who are not critically ill but nonetheless develop moderate anemia (hematocrit <24% or blood hemoglobin level <8 g/dL) are extremely variable. In general, infants who are clinically stable with modest anemia do not require RBC transfusions unless they exhibit significant problems ascribed to anemia or predicted to be corrected by RBC transfusions. For example, proponents of RBC transfusions to treat disturbances of cardiopulmonary rhythms believe that a low blood level of RBCs contributes to tachypnea, dyspnea, apnea, and tachycardia or bradycardia because of decreased oxygen delivery to the respiratory center of the brain.[25] Transfusions of RBCs may decrease the number of apneic spells by improving oxygen delivery to the central nervous system. To support this practice, RBC transfusions were shown in one study to diminish irregular breathing patterns and episodes of bradycardia in infants when the mean hematocrit was increased from 27% to 36%.[26] However, other investigators have reported no beneficial effects of RBC transfusions on breathing patterns.[27]

Another controversial clinical indication for RBC transfusions is to maintain a reasonable hematocrit level as treatment for unexplained growth failure. Some neonatologists consider poor weight gain to be an indication for RBC transfusion, particularly when the hematocrit is below 24% (hemoglobin level <8 g/dL) and other signs of distress are evident (e.g., tachycardia, respiratory difficulty, weak suck and cry, diminished activity). In this setting, growth failure is ascribed to the increase in metabolic expenditure required to support the work of labored breathing. In the past, a hematocrit below 30% was of concern, and Stockman and Clark[28] investigated the effects of RBC transfusion on weight gain in stable, but modestly anemic, low-birth-weight infants. Thirteen infants with birth weights less than 1.5 kg were studied for 1 week before and after RBC transfusions. Mean hemoglobin concentration was raised from 8.5 to 11.4 g/dL, mean daily weight gain increased from 20.8 to 28.0 g after the transfusions, and increased weight gain was associated with decreased metabolic rates. The researchers regarded anemia as only one of several possible causes for growth failure, and they recommended RBC transfusions for growth failure in symptomatic, anemic infants provided that nothing else could explain the poor weight gain.

To support the concept that RBC transfusions have little, or no, benefit in cases of asymptomatic anemia, Blank and associates[29] found no clinical advantages for prophylactic small-volume RBC transfusions in stable premature infants. Fifty-six premature infants were randomly assigned to a mandatory prophylactic transfusion group (i.e., hemoglobin level kept above 10 g/dL) or a control elective transfusion group in which RBCs were given only for marked clinical manifestations of anemia. At discharge, infants in the elective group exhibited significantly ($P<0.01$) lower hemoglobin levels and higher reticulocyte counts than those receiving prophylactic transfusions (hemoglobin level $= 9.10 \pm 1.67$ versus 11.75 ± 1.72 g/dL; reticulocytes $= 6 \pm 3\%$ versus $3 \pm 2\%$). Despite these hematologic differences, the two groups were comparable in the number of days required to regain birth weight, in weight at discharge, in the length and cost of hospitalization, and in the frequency and severity of clinical problems. On the basis of these findings, no apparent rationale exists to justify maintaining a given hematocrit level by prophylactic, small-volume RBC transfusions in stable, growing infants who seem to be otherwise healthy.

In practice, the decision about whether to transfuse RBCs is based on the desire to maintain the hematocrit or blood hemoglobin concentration at a level judged to be most beneficial for the infant's clinical condition. Investigators who believe this clinical approach is too imprecise have suggested the use of physiologic criteria such as RBC mass,[30] available oxygen,[31] mixed venous oxygen saturation, and measurements of oxygen delivery and use[32] to develop guidelines for transfusion decisions. Physiologic indications for RBC transfusion have shown promise in experimental studies,[33–37] and in one study of 10 human infants with severe (oxygen-dependent) bronchopulmonary dysplasia, improvement of physiologic end points (i.e., increased systemic oxygen transport and decreased oxygen use) was demonstrated as a consequence of small-volume RBC transfusions.[32] However, these promising but technically demanding methods are difficult to apply in the day-to-day practice of neonatology. The application of data obtained from studies of animals and adult humans that attempt to correlate tissue oxygenation with the clinical effects of anemia and the need for RBC transfusions is confounded by the differences between infants and adults in hemoglobin oxygen affinity, ability to increase cardiac output, and regional patterns of blood flow.

Another physiologic factor to be considered in the transfusion decision is use of the circulating RBC volume (mass) rather than the blood hematocrit or hemoglobin level.[5, 30, 38] Although circulating RBC volume is a potentially useful index of the blood's oxygen-carrying capacity, it cannot be predicted accurately from blood hemoglobin concentration or hematocrit in infants.[32] Low circulating RBC volume identifies, better than hemoglobin or hematocrit, infants who will respond to transfusion with a decrease in cardiac output.[39] Circulating RBC volume measurements are not widely available, but promising studies using a nonradioactive biotin label to tag RBCs may be adapted for infant studies.[38, 40]

Blood Banking Considerations for Red Blood Cell Transfusions

For small-volume (10 to 15 mL/kg) neonatal transfusions, many blood banks prefer RBCs collected from allogeneic donors, suspended in anticoagulant-preservative solution and concentrated by sedimentation or centrifugation before transfusion. Many physicians transfuse relatively fresh RBCs to preterm infants because of concerns about the increases in potassium and acidity of RBC suspensions and the decrease in RBC levels of 2,3-DPG during storage. The need to use fresh RBCs for small-volume transfusions has been questioned,[33] and four reports have documented that RBCs stored for extended periods could be safely transfused to neonates.[41–44] The findings of these reports indicated that the occurrence of donor exposure was decreased, without significant problems caused by hyperkalemia or acidosis. However, in three of the reports, relatively few transfusions with RBCs stored longer than 20 days were included.[41–43] These three reports did not address use of AS-1–extended storage (42 day) RBC preservative medium, which contains mannitol. Liu and colleagues[41] stored RBCs in citrate phosphate dextrose adenine-1 (CPDA1), a standard 35-day storage medium. Although the other two studies did not indicate which RBC storage solutions were used, AS-1 was probably not used, because mannitol was not listed as an ingredient.[42, 43] Because nearly all RBCs are routinely stored in a 42-day preservative medium, additional information is needed for neonates regarding the potential for toxicity associated with adenine (hepatic) and mannitol (renal) as constituents of extended storage RBC preservative media and for the possibility of a deficiency of 2,3-DPG caused by repeated transfusion of stored RBCs. Accordingly, the report in which AS-1 RBCs were transfused is described in more detail.[44]

In a two-arm, randomized, single-blinded study, the feasibility and safety of two techniques used to provide small-volume RBC transfusions to very-low-birth-weight infants (0.6 to 1.3 kg) were compared. In one arm, infants received AS-1 RBCs stored up to 42 days (stored AS-1 RBCs); in the other, infants received CPDA1 RBCs stored up to 7 days (fresh CPDA1 RBCs). The results have been reported elsewhere,[44] and only the safety aspects are summarized here. None of the CPDA1 RBCs was stored longer than 7 days, whereas 47% of AS-1 RBCs were stored 15 days or longer before transfusion. No clinical reactions occurred during 66 AS-1 RBC transfusions given to 15 infants or during 58 CPDA1 RBC transfusions given to 14 infants. Clinically significant changes in vital signs were infrequent and occurred similarly in infants in both groups. Before and after transfusion blood chemistry levels had no significant differences whether fresh CPDA1 or stored AS-1 RBCs were given. The hematocrit increased as expected. Changes in levels of glucose, lactate, pH, calcium, sodium, and potassium were very slight and not of clinical importance. No statistically significant differences in results of renal and hepatic chemistry levels were detected between infants who received fresh CPDA1 and those who received stored AS-1 RBCs. Levels of 2,3-DPG were similar, whether fresh CPDA1 or stored AS-1 RBCs. Levels of 2,3-DPG were similar, whether fresh CPDA1 or stored AS-1 RBCs were transfused. On the basis of these findings, AS-1 RBCs, collected from one donor and stored for up to 42 days, can safely provide all RBC transfusions needed by an individual infant.

Several studies have documented the feasibility and safety of transfusing stored RBCs to preterm infants.[41–44] At our center, newborn infants are assigned to long-term support with a fresh unit (stored <7 days) of RBCs in extended storage (42-day) media as follows. Infants with birth weights of less than 1.0 kg are assigned to a half unit (i.e., one half of the unit is reserved for the infant). Infants with birth weights of 1.0

to 1.3 kg are assigned to a quarter unit. Infants with birth weights of more than 1.3 kg are assigned to various volumes of RBC units, depending on transfusion needs estimated by the neonatal intensive care unit staff. One unit may be reserved for one 0.9-kg infant and two 1.2-kg infants. When RBC transfusions are ordered, aliquots are issued.[44] After a unit has been stored 14 days, it has become relatively aged, and no new neonates are assigned to it. When infants assigned to a unit no longer require RBC transfusions, the remainder of the unit is placed into the general inventory for transfusion to older children. Although several clinical studies have documented the safety of selecting stored RBCs for small-volume transfusions, this approach does not apply to large-volume (>25 mL/kg) transfusions, in which greater doses of extracellular constituents (e.g., potassium) may be harmful, especially if infused rapidly. Fresh or washed RBCs are preferred when large-volume transfusions are given to infants.

Alternatives to Red Blood Cell Transfusions

Recognition of the low plasma EPO levels in preterm infants provides a rational basis for the use of recombinant human EPO (rhEPO) as treatment for the anemia of prematurity. More than 20 controlled trials have tested several doses and treatment schedules in preterm infants, and results are mixed, making consensus on the optimal treatment with rhEPO impossible.[1, 45] Unquestionably, proper doses of rhEPO and iron are effective in stimulating erythropoiesis, as evidenced by increased marrow erythroid activity and blood reticulocyte counts. However, the efficacy of rhEPO to substantially diminish RBC transfusions, the major goal for which it is prescribed, has not been convincingly demonstrated.[46] In many trials, relatively large preterm infants or those in stable clinical condition were studied; these infants receive few RBC transfusions when given standard care (i.e., not given rhEPO).[22] Even without use of rhEPO, fewer than 50% of infants with birth weights of more than 1.0 kg receive RBC transfusions. Nearly all infants weighing less than 1.0 kg at birth are given RBCs, and most transfusions are given during the first 3 to 4 weeks of life. To illustrate the difficulty in avoiding transfusions, the multicenter, randomized American trial, in which infants received rhEPO or placebo during a 6-week study period, reported statistically significant but only modest success.[47] Although significantly fewer RBC transfusions were given to rhEPO-treated infants during the study phase (1.1 transfusions per infant versus 1.6 for placebo), all infants required multiple transfusions during the 3-week prestudy phase. Treatment with rhEPO exerted only a modest effect on total RBC transfusions given throughout the entire study (4.4 transfusions per infant for rhEPO versus 5.3 for placebo) and did not resolve the problem of severe neonatal anemia.[47]

Physicians wishing to prescribe rhEPO are in a dilemma. The relatively large or stable preterm infants who respond best to rhEPO plus iron are given relatively few RBC transfusions and have little need for rhEPO to avoid transfusions.[1, 22] Extremely preterm infants, who are sick and have the greatest need for RBC transfusions shortly after birth, have not consistently responded to rhEPO plus iron, questioning the efficacy of this approach.[46] However, extremely preterm infants are beginning to be evaluated in therapeutic trials of rhEPO and iron given intravenously shortly after birth.[48, 49] Although preliminary review of these promising studies suggests success in avoiding transfusions early in life, data are insufficient to clearly establish efficacy or to detect potential toxicity. Firm guidelines for the use of rhEPO in the treatment of the anemia of prematurity cannot be made at this time.

Another alternative to allogeneic RBC transfusions is the use of placental blood as a source of autologous RBCs.[50, 51] Although collection, storage, and transfusion of placental blood after delivery deserve careful consideration, at least three obstacles must be overcome before autologous transfusions of stored placental RBCs can be adopted for clinical use. One concern is that a sufficient number of RBCs cannot be obtained consistently from placental blood to avoid later allogeneic transfusions. The second issue is the sterility of placental blood. Because bacterial contamination of placental blood is a distinct possibility,[50] extensive testing is needed to ensure absolute safety. Third, acceptable quality of stored placental blood must be maintained.[51] Because of these concerns, collection and storage of placental blood has not been encouraged.[52] Instead, interest has been renewed in delayed clamping of the umbilical cord immediately after delivery. In a small pilot study, delayed cord clamping increased blood volume and circulating red cell mass and improved cardiovascular hemodynamics.[53] However, many questions regarding feasibility, efficacy, and possible risks remain to be answered.

Neonatal Bleeding and Transfusion Therapy

Pathophysiology of Neonatal Thrombocytopenia

Normal fetuses (≥17 weeks' gestation) and neonates have blood platelet counts greater than 150×10^9/L.[54–58] Lower platelet counts indicate potential problems, and high-risk infants—usually low-birth-weight, premature infants—commonly exhibit thrombocytopenia.[57–61] In one neonatal intensive care unit, 22% of infants had blood platelet counts lower than 150×10^9/L at some time during hospitalization.[60] Although multiple pathogenic mechanisms are involved in these sick neonates, the predominant one is accelerated platelet destruction, as shown by shortened platelet survival, increased mean platelet volume, normal number of megakaryocytes, and inadequate increment in blood platelets after platelet transfusion.[60, 62] In individual infants, the mechanism underlying accelerated platelet destruction cannot always be identified, but increased levels of platelet-associated immunoglobulin G and disseminated intravascular coagulation are commonly evident. Also contributing to neonatal thrombocytopenia is diminished platelet production, as evidenced by decreased numbers of clonogenic megakaryocyte progenitors[63] and relatively low levels of thrombopoietin[64] compared with levels in children and adults.

Thrombocytopenia is not the only hemorrhagic risk factor related to neonatal platelets. Extensive controversy exists regarding the function of fetal and neonatal platelets. As reviewed by Whaun,[65] fetal and neonatal platelets have diminished aggregation to collagen, adenosine diphosphate, thrombin, and epinephrine, the last of which is associated with diminished α-adrenergic binding sites of the platelet membrane. Not all investigators found diminished aggregation, and some have reported enhanced responses, particularly to ristocetin, a finding ascribed to increased plasma levels of von Willebrand factor.[66] Other reported abnormalities of neonatal platelets include decreased adhesion to glass, low platelet factor 3 levels, defective clot retraction, low serotonin levels, deficient cytoplasmic granulation, decreased release of adenine nucleotides, and abnormalities of arachidonic acid metabolism (i.e., relatively small quantities of cyclooxygenase metabolites compared with relatively large amounts of lipoxygenase products).[65]

Blood platelet counts lower than 100×10^9/L pose significant clinical risks for premature neonates. In one study, infants with birth weights less than 1.5 kg and a blood platelet count lower than 100×10^9/L were compared with nonthrombocytopenic control infants of similar size.[61] The bleeding time was prolonged when platelet counts were below 100×10^9/L, and in many infants, platelet dysfunction was suggested by bleeding times that were disproportionately long for the degree of thrombocytopenia. Hemorrhage was more likely in thrombocytopenic infants than in controls. The incidence of intracranial hemorrhage in thrombocytopenic infants with birth weights less than 1.5 kg was 78% for thrombocytopenic infants compared with 48% for nonthrombocytopenic infants of similar size. Moreover, the extent of hemorrhage and neurologic morbidity was greater in the group of thrombocytopenic infants.[61]

Thrombocytopenia occurs most commonly in sick preterm infants. When severe thrombocytopenia occurs in neonates who appear otherwise well, immune thrombocytopenia caused by placental transport of maternal antiplatelet antibodies should be suspected. The antibodies involved are autoimmune, with broad reactivity against platelets from all individuals, including the mother, or alloantibodies, with reactivity against an antigen inherited by the fetus from the father to which the mother has been immunized because her platelets lack the antigen. The diagnosis of passively acquired, autoimmune thrombocytopenia in a neonate usually is apparent because of a history of thrombocytopenia or presence of elevated platelet-associated immunoglobulin levels in the mother.[67] The diagnosis of neonatal alloimmune thrombocytopenia is less obvious, but it should be suspected whenever unexplained thrombocytopenia occurs in an infant whose mother has a normal platelet count without increased amounts of platelet-associated immunoglobulin.[68, 69]

Alloimmune thrombocytopenia can be extremely serious for the fetus and newborn. It requires careful management during gestation and the perinatal period. If platelet transfusions are needed for the fetus or neonate, the best blood banking approach is to collect a unit of platelets from the mother by plateletpheresis and to remove small aliquots sterilely as needed for each transfusion. Usually, maternal plasma (source of alloantibody) is removed by centrifugation or washing before transfusion. In contrast, autoimmune thrombocytopenia is almost never severe for the fetus and is only occasionally severe for the neonate. It is important to detect autoimmune thrombocytopenia during gestation, so that it can be distinguished from the more severe alloimmune thrombocytopenia. However, neonates born of women with autoimmune thrombocytopenia only occasionally require therapy during the postdelivery period. Mild or modest thrombocytopenia detected in women only during gestation does not pose a risk to the pregnant woman or to her fetus or newborn and needs no intervention.[70]

Guidelines for Platelet Transfusions

Although the use of prophylactic platelet transfusions to prevent bleeding in preterm neonates has been studied systematically,[58] no randomized clinical trials have been reported to establish the inefficacy as treatment for bleeding thrombocytopenic neonates. Even basic questions regarding the relative risks of different degrees of thrombocytopenia in various clinical settings during infancy remain unanswered. However, it seems logical to transfuse platelets to thrombocytopenic infants, and guidelines acceptable to many neonatologists are listed in Table 18-1. Two firm indications for neonatal platelet transfusions are to treat hemorrhage that has already occurred and to prevent it from complicating an invasive procedure. Little disagreement exists about using a blood platelet count of less than $50 \times 10^9/L$ as a "transfusion trigger" in these instances. However, platelet transfusions are given to infants by some physicians to treat bleeding that occurs at higher platelet counts (50 to $100 \times 10^9/L$) or to diminish the threat of intracranial hemorrhage in high-risk preterm infants when the count is less than $100 \times 10^9/L$.[61]

Prophylactic platelet transfusions can be given under two circumstances: to prevent bleeding when severe thrombocytopenia poses a risk of spontaneous hemorrhage or to maintain a normal platelet count to prevent the infant from slipping into high-risk situations. Regarding the first circumstance, most agree that it is reasonable to give platelets to any neonate whose count is less than $20 \times 10^9/L$. First, there is broadly accepted risk of spontaneous hemorrhage below this count.[71] Second, this risk is increased even in healthy neonates, who exhibit developmental abnormalities of platelets and of clotting proteins to compound the risk of bleeding. Almost any stress can accentuate these abnormalities to increase the potential for hemorrhage beyond that expected for the degree of thrombocytopenia alone. Third, severe thrombocytopenia occurs most commonly in sick infants who, because of their illnesses, receive medications that may further compromise platelet function. Because all of these factors are pronounced in extremely preterm infants, some neonatologists favor prophylactic platelet transfusion whenever the count falls below $50 \times 10^9/L$, or even below $100 \times 10^9/L$, in critically ill infants.[61]

Regarding the second circumstance, the need to maintain a normal platelet count in preterm infants without bleeding is unproven. Intracranial hemorrhage occurs commonly in sick preterm infants and, although the etiologic role of thrombocytopenia and the therapeutic benefit of platelet transfusions have not been conclusively established in this disorder,[56, 61] it seems logical to consider thrombocytopenia a risk factor.[72, 73] However, in a randomized trial designed to address this issue—transfusing platelets when the count fell below $150 \times 10^9/L$ and maintaining the average count above $200 \times 10^9/L$ versus transfusing platelets only when the count fell below $50 \times 10^9/L$—did not diminish the incidence of intracranial hemorrhage (28% versus 26%).[58] There is no documented benefit to transfusing prophylactic platelets to maintain a normal platelet count (i.e., at a level $\geq 250 \times 10^9/L$).

The goal of most platelet transfusions is to raise the count to above $100 \times 10^9/L$. This goal can be achieved consistently by the infusion of 5 to 10 mL/kg of standard platelet suspensions prepared from fresh units of whole blood or by automated platelet pheresis. Platelet suspensions should be transfused as rapidly as the baby's overall condition permits, certainly within 2 hours. Routinely reducing the volume of platelet concentrates by additional centrifugation steps is neither necessary nor wise.[58] Several calculations prove it is unnecessary. All units contain approximately 10×10^9 platelets per each 10 mL of suspension. Because the blood volume of an infant or child is about 70 mL/kg, a 1-kg neonate has 70 mL of circulating blood. When a 1-kg infant is given 10 mL/kg of a platelet suspension, the transfusion adds 10×10^9 platelets to 70 mL of blood, a number sufficient to increase the platelet count by $143 \times 10^9/L$. Acknowledging that post-transfusion platelet recovery generally is 50% to 60%, not 100%, this estimated increment is consistent with the actual increment reported in clinical studies.[58] Generally, 10 mL/kg is not an excessive transfusion volume, providing the intake of other intravenous fluids, medications, and nutrients is monitored and adjusted. Although proven methods exist to reduce the volume of platelet concentrates[74] when truly warranted (i.e., many group O platelet transfusions anticipated in which the quantity of passive anti-A or anti-B may lead to hemolysis in group A or B infants or failure to respond with acceptable increments to 10 mL/kg of unmodified platelet concentrate), additional processing should be performed with great care because of probable platelet loss, clumping, and dysfunction caused by the additional handling.

Pathophysiology of Neonatal Clotting Proteins

Hemostasis in the neonate is quantitatively and qualitatively different from that in the older child or adult, and the potential exists for serious hemorrhage or thrombosis. A comprehensive discussion of neonatal hemostasis is beyond the scope of this chapter, but because primary hemostasis (platelet plug formation) and fibrin clot formation are intimately intertwined, it is important to summarize a few important facts about neonatal clotting proteins before addressing issues of plasma transfusions.

Maternal clotting factors do not cross the placenta, and fetal levels depend on endogenous production. Clotting proteins are synthesized by the fetus beginning in the first trimester, with concentrations gradually increasing throughout gestation.[75] At birth, the mean levels of the contact factors (i.e., factors XII and XI, prekallikrein, and high-molecular-weight kininogen) are about 40% to 50% of adult values in term infants and about 30% to 40% of adult values in preterm infants. The vitamin K–dependent factors (i.e., II, VII, IX, and X) are about 40% to 50% of adult values in term infants and about 30% to 50% of adult values in preterm infants, with strikingly low levels seen in very immature neonates. Neonatal levels of factors VIII and XIII and fibrinogen are comparable to adult levels, although factor XIII can be quite low in some infants at birth. The natural anticoagulant proteins (i.e., antithrombin III and proteins C and S) are 30% to 50% of adult values. Fibrinolysis is less well studied but probably is diminished to a significant degree because of moderately low plasminogen levels.

Guidelines for Plasma Transfusions

Guidelines for neonatal fresh frozen plasma (FFP) transfusions are listed in Table 18-1. Clotting times are prolonged because of developmental deficiency of clotting proteins, and FFP should be transfused only after reference to normal values accepted for the birth weight and age of the infant. The indications for FFP in neonates include reconstitution of RBC concentrates to simulate whole blood for use in massive transfusions (e.g., exchange transfusions or cardiovascular surgery), hemorrhage from vitamin K deficiency, disseminated intravascular coagulation with bleeding, and bleeding in congenital coagulation factor deficiency when more specific treatment (i.e., a purified and viral inactivated factor concentrate) is unavailable or inappropriate. The use of prophylactic FFP transfusions to prevent intraventricular hemorrhage in premature infants is not recommended. Although still used occasionally as a suspending agent to adjust the hematocrit values of RBC concentrates before use for small-volume RBC transfusion to neonates, this practice should be discouraged because FFP offers no apparent medical benefit over the use of sterile solutions for this purpose. Similarly, the use of FFP in partial-exchange transfusion for the treatment of neonatal hyperviscosity syndrome (i.e., erythrocytosis) is unnecessary, because safer colloid solutions are available. When treating bleeding infants, cryoprecipitate is often considered as an alternative to FFP because of its small volume. However, cryoprecipitate contains only fibrinogen and factors VIII and XIII, and it is not effective for treating the more extensive clotting factor deficiencies that are commonly encountered, despite the desirability of a small infusion volume.

Neonatal Sepsis and Neutrophil Transfusions

Pathophysiology of Neonatal Neutropenia and Dysfunction

Neonates are unusually susceptible to severe bacterial infections, and several defects of neonatal body defenses have been reported as possible contributing factors. Polymorphonuclear neutrophils (PMNs) isolated from the blood of neonates exhibit quantitative and qualitative abnormalities that may be related to the increased incidence, morbidity, and mortality of bacterial infections. Abnormalities of neonatal PMNs include absolute and relative neutropenia, diminished chemotaxis, abnormal adhesion and aggregation, defective cellular orientation and receptor capping, decreased deformability, inability to alter membrane potential during stimulation, imbalances of oxidative metabolism, and a diminished ability to withstand oxidant stress.[76, 77] Only aspects particularly relevant to PMN transfusions and alternative therapies are reviewed in this chapter.

Neutropenia can occur during neonatal bacterial infections, particularly with fulminant sepsis. Because a physiologic neutrophilia occurs in normal neonates, it is considered abnormal for the absolute blood PMN count to fall below $3.0 \times 10^9/L$ in the first week of life. Although an abnormally low PMN count can occur in neonates with disorders as diverse as sepsis, asphyxia, and maternal hypertension, suspicion of severe bacterial infection must always be high when relative neutropenia (PMN count $<3.0 \times 10^9/L$) occurs. The mechanisms responsible are only partially defined, but abnormalities of neonatal granulopoiesis frequently are involved. First, the postmitotic marrow PMN storage pool (i.e., metamyelocytes and mature, segmented PMNs) is small. The PMN storage pool accounts for 26% to 60% of all nucleated cells in the bone marrow of normal neonates. Neonates with sepsis may exhibit a storage pool with less than 10% of nucleated marrow cells and are considered to have severely diminished marrow PMN reserves.[77, 78] Second, storage pool PMNs are released at an excessively rapid and apparently poorly regulated rate from the marrow during stress. Third, PMN production in response to infection is decreased. Numbers of committed (clonogenic) PMN precursors in marrow are lower in neonates than in older patients, and a high percentage of these cells are proliferating even when studied in an apparently basal state.[79, 80] Neonatal marrow is functioning at capacity and is unable to rapidly expand production to meet the increased demands of infection.[81] It is logical to consider PMN transfusions until the marrow recovers.

Guidelines for Neutrophil Transfusions

Because quantitative and qualitative abnormalities of neonatal PMNs have been reported, PMN transfusions have been used to treat neonatal sepsis whether or not neutropenia is present. Neonates exhibiting fulminat sepsis, relative neutropenia (PMN count $<3.0 \times 10^9/L$ during the first week of life or $<1.0 \times 10^9/L$ thereafter), and a severely diminished PMN marrow storage pool ($<10\%$ of nucleated marrow cells are postmitotic PMNs) are at increased risk of dying if treated only with antibiotics. Results of 11 studies on the use of PMN transfusions to treat infected neonates,[78, 82–91] six of which were designed as controlled studies,[78, 82–84, 89, 90] have been reported. Four of the six controlled studies found significant benefit from PMN transfusion.[78, 82–84] However, the controlled studies contain several experimental flaws. Although five professed to be randomized trials, two included nontransfused subjects who were deemed ineligible for randomization.[78, 90] In addition, two of the six reports dealt with the same study, which was reported first as a somewhat preliminary trial[83] and later after it was expanded and slightly modified.[84] The patients evaluated in all six studies were quite heterogeneous, with relatively few neonates exhibiting the complete clinical picture considered to be most indicative of poor prognosis (i.e., culture-proven sepsis, severe neutropenia for age, and a markedly depleted marrow PMN storage pool). The dosages and quality of the PMN concentrates transfused were quite variable, and in some instances they were almost certainly inadequate.[89–91]

Because of these scientific imperfections, firm recommendations for the role of PMN transfusions in treating neonatal sepsis cannot be made at this time. Guidelines for PMN transfusions are presented in Table 18-1. Although antibiotics are the key to successful treatment of neonatal sepsis, antibiotic therapy is not 100% successful, and attempts to bolster body defenses are warranted. Unfortunately, PMN transfusions have not provided a complete answer. Although efficacious for infants with neutropenia and fulminant sepsis,[92] only PMN transfusions obtained by automated leukapheresis have demonstrated effectiveness.[91, 92] Moreover, in many instances, standard supportive care with antibiotics seems adequate. Each institution must assess its own experience with neonatal sepsis. If nearly all infants survive without apparent long-term morbidity when treated only with antibiotics, PMN transfusions are unnecessary, and attention should be focused on prompt diagnosis and optimal antibiotic therapy. If the outcome of standard therapy is not optimal, alternative therapies such as PMN transfusions must be considered to improve the outlook.

If PMN transfusions are prescribed, they must be given effectively. The characteristics of an ideal PMN concentrate for neonatal transfusions are 1 to 2×10^9/kg of PMNs per infusion; 10 to 15 mL/kg per infusion; a donor seronegative for cytomegalovirus and for all required infectious disease tests; and RBC compatibility between donor and neonate. Local practices should be followed regarding γ-irradiation of cellular blood products for neonates. PMN concentrates must be infused promptly, certainly within a few hours of donation. Until more information becomes available, the only product of proven efficacy is a PMN concentrate prepared by automated leukapheresis.[91, 92]

Alternatives to Neutrophil Transfusions

Not all neonatologists prescribe PMN transfusions. Their proper role has not been irrefutably established by controlled clinical trials. Moreover, preparation of PMN concentrates by leukapheresis can be cumbersome and expensive, and the process of collecting and transfusing PMNs can pose risks for neonates and donors. Accordingly, alternative therapies have been suggested. However, their efficacy has not been clearly established, their risks are only partially defined, and they require extensive study before being widely accepted. Two modalities that have been suggested are intravenous immunoglobulin (IVIG) and myeloid cytokines or growth factors.

Use of IVIG to prevent or to treat neonatal sepsis has appeal, because it may correct abnormalities of humoral immunity and of PMN function. IVIG was found to be beneficial, particularly when given in combination with antibiotics, in treating experimental infections caused by a variety of microorganisms.[93–97] The expected increases in opsonic activity were observed with IVIG infusion, and PMN kinetics were also improved.[96, 97] Neither neutropenia nor depletion of the PMN storage pool occurred, and PMNs were released from marrow reserves to accumulate quickly at inflammatory sites. Although clinical trials in human infants have yielded conflicting results, IVIG has helped to prevent and to treat infections.

Most studies evaluating IVIG to prevent infections have found little or only modest benefit.[98–109] However, results are inconsistent, and only a few studies have suggested some prophylactic benefit.[98, 99, 101] In contrast, of the therapeutic studies reviewed,[110–116] several demonstrated a benefit from adding IVIG to antibiotics in the treatment of neonatal infections.[110–113, 116] Overall, data are insufficient to justify the use of IVIG routinely in all preterm neonates to prevent or treat sepsis. However, modest "physiologic" doses (0.3 to 0.4 mg/kg) may lessen the severity of bacterial sepsis in very-low-birth-weight newborns, who are likely to be hypogammaglobulinemic as a result of extreme premature birth (i.e., born before the major placental transport of IgG has taken place).

However, caution must be used when prescribing IVIG therapy to prevent or treat neonatal sepsis. IVIG therapy, particularly at high doses, may impair body defense mechanisms.[117–119] In leukopenic mice, IVIG at 0.8 g/kg impaired clearance of bacteria from the bloodstream and lowered the LD_{50}.[117] In neonatal rats, IVIG at a dose of 2.7 g/kg delayed bacterial clearance, whereas lower doses (0.15 g/kg) enhanced bacterial clearance and survival.[119] It has been suggested that infections in humans may be exacerbated by intravenous IgG.[117, 119] In a comparative study of infected human infants,[120] survival in the group receiving high-dose IVIG (1.0 g/kg/d on 3 consecutive days) plus antibiotics was 52%, compared with 97% in the group receiving PMN transfusions plus antibiotics ($P<0.004$ favoring PMN transfusions over IVIG).

Because of the ease with which IVIG can be prescribed for neonates, its apparent benefits to many body defense systems, and its safety in terms of only rarely transmitting donor infectious diseases, it is easy to become enthusiastic about its potential uses. However, it is crucial that the genuine benefits and risks of IVIG be examined carefully before it is used with impunity. For example, in a randomized study of 235 preterm infants, no significant reduction in certain or probable infections was observed in those given 500 mg of IVIG on days 0, 1, 2, 17, and 31 of life compared with controls given albumin. There was a suggestion of more frequent infections in the IVIG group, possibly because of the large quantity of IgG given.[121]

Myeloid cytokine therapy may be useful for preventing or treating neonatal sepsis in the future. A large number of cytokines—soluble molecules including growth factors and interleukins produced by a variety of cells—regulate the production of blood cells (i.e., hematopoiesis) and modulate their activities. The cytokine primarily responsible for PMN production and activation is granulocyte-colony stimulating factor (G-CSF). Studies of cytokine production in human neonates have yielded conflicting results, with investigators finding values that are higher than, equal to, and lower than adult values.[121–129] Although results are quite variable, G-CSF levels are generally lower in premature than in term neonates, and the ability of neonatal leukocytes to increase production when stimulated under many experimental conditions is diminished in preterm infants. Plasma levels of G-CSF are reported by some investigators to be markedly elevated in neonates with infection,[123, 124] but many investigators have found G-CSF mRNA expression and protein production to be decreased in neonatal leukocytes, particularly when attempts are made to increase production by activating the cells.[125–127] Similar findings have been reported for production of granulocyte-macrophage colony stimulating factor (GM-CSF) by neonatal leukocytes.[128, 129]

The mechanisms responsible for diminished G-CSF and GM-CSF production have not been defined. In one study, the decrease in mRNA expression was not caused by defective transcription, and abnormalities in post-transcriptional events, such as instability of mRNA, were suggested as possible mechanisms.[127] Although data are limited, studies of growth factor receptors and the growth of clonogenic myeloid progenitors in cultures stimulated with recombinant growth factors have not detected an impaired ability of neonatal myeloid progenitors to respond to exogenous myeloid growth factors.[125, 128, 129] It seems likely that human neonates can respond to the administration of recombinant G-CSF or GM-CSF.

In preclinical studies, administration of recombinant G-CSF and GM-CSF to neonatal animals with infections induced experimentally was beneficial.[128–134] Combination therapy with G-CSF plus stem cell factor or interleukin-6 was superior to therapy with G-CSF alone.[133, 134] Improvements in the resolution of infections and survival rates were accompanied by correction of neutropenia and abnormal PMN kinetics. G-CSF given to pregnant rats crossed the placenta and improved neonatal survival from experimentally induced infection.[135, 136]

When added to human neonatal leukocytes in vitro, recombinant GM-CSF enhances several PMN functions.[137, 138] Clinical studies of recombinant myeloid growth factors given to human neonates are limited. In a controlled study,[139] 42 neonates with presumed bacterial sepsis recognized within the first 3 days of life were randomly designated to receive three doses of G-CSF or a placebo. Although the outcome of sepsis was not reported, G-CSF induced a significant increase in the blood PMN count, an increase in the marrow PMN storage pool, and an increase in PMN membrane C3bi expression, an indication of enhanced functional capability.[139] In another study, G-CSF increased blood PMN counts of neutropenic neonates born to mothers with preeclampsia.[140]

In a controlled study of GM-CSF,[141] 20 premature neonates were designated within 72 hours of birth to receive GM-CSF or a placebo for 7 days. GM-CSF increased the blood PMN count, the marrow PMN storage pool, and C3bi receptor expression. Neonates receiving GM-CSF also exhibited an increase in blood monocyte and platelet counts. The study was not designed to assess efficacy in the prevention or treatment of infections, and additional clinical trials are needed to define the role and to identify possible adverse effects before myeloid should be routinely prescribed to human neonates.

RISKS OF NEONATAL BLOOD TRANSFUSIONS

General Risks of Allogeneic Blood

It seems inescapable that the need for multiple transfusions, especially when obtained from multiple blood donors, places infants at risk for transfusion-transmitted infections. Moreover, the severity of these acquired infections may be greater because of immaturity of neonatal immunity. In addition to blood banking measures employed to improve the safety of blood component collection and manufacturing, efforts by neonatologists to diminish the number of transfusions and donor exposures must continue.

In early studies, the percentage of infants and children with human immunodeficiency virus (HIV) infection acquired through transfusion rather than by other routes was disproportionately high compared with the percentage of adults with HIV who were infected by transfusions. In one survey, even when children with hemophilia were excluded, 15% of childhood cases of HIV infection were caused by blood transfusion, compared with 2% of adult cases.[142] Theses rates were determined before current methods of donor screening and testing and therefore overestimate the current rate of transfusion-transmitted HIV, which is about 1 case for every 680,000 donor exposures.[143] Once acquired, expression of HIV has been reported to be of greater[144] and of lesser[145] severity in infants compared with adults. Regardless of the controversy, efforts must continue to eliminate this rare complication of blood transfusions in infants.

The rate of transfusion-transmitted hepatitis has not been determined accurately for infants. Although the incidence of non-A, non-B hepatitis (most of which is hepatitis C) was believed to be low,[146] the rate caused by transfusions in difficult to establish accurately. There is no reason to think that the rate of transmission of infants is different from that in general (i.e., about 1 case per 100,000 donor exposures).[143] Disorders related to hepatitis C that lead to long-term morbidity (e.g., posthepatitic cirrhosis, hepatic cancer) are particularly alarming when hepatitis C is acquired during infancy because of the possibility of a costly period of extended treatment and disability.[147]

Transfusion-associated risks of a noninfectious nature that may occur in infants include fluid overload, graft-versus-host disease,[148, 149] electrolyte and acid-base imbalances, iron overload,[150] increased susceptibility to oxidant damage,[151] exposure to plasticizers,[152] hemolysis after plasma transfusions when T antigen activation of RBCs has occurred,[153] immunosuppression,[154] and alloimmunization, although alloimmunization to RBC and leukocyte antigens seems to be rare in infants.[155, 156] Some adverse effects are seen only in the setting of massive transfusions, such as exchange transfusions in which relatively large quantities of blood are needed, and occur rarely with the small-volume transfusions commonly given. The potential risks of all transfusions are not trivial, and blood components should be transfused only when indicated and with use of optimal blood banking techniques.

Leukocyte Reduction to Prevent Cytomegalovirus Infection

Certain infectious organisms are associated with white blood cells (WBCs), and the degree to which infection is transmitted by transfusion should be diminished by marked WBC reduction of cellular blood components. Examples of these organisms include the herpesviruses (e.g., cytomegalovirus [CMV], Epstein-Barr virus), retroviruses (e.g., human T cell lymphotropic virus), and certain bacteria (e.g., *Yersinia enterocolitica*). Primary infection with CMV, as with other herpesviruses, begins as an acute, transient, and often subclinical infection, which is followed by a latent state of chronic infection that is not well understood. CMV seems to be cell associated, but the WBC subpopulation infected with the virus has been debated. It is therefore reasonable to anticipate that removal of WBCs from a transfusion component obtained from a seropositive donor would decrease CMV exposure in the seronegative recipient.

The importance of transfusion-transmitted CMV in neonates is controversial. Studies conducted during the 1970s and early 1980s reported a disturbingly high incidence (25% to 50%) of CMV in infants transfused with cellular blood components.[157] This was particularly true in those most heavily transfused, some of whom died of severe CMV disease. Later studies suggested a diminishing, almost negligible risk of CMV.[157–159] However, these studies were criticized,[160] and the importance of transfusion-transmitted CMV during infancy remains somewhat controversial. Regardless of the controversy, after a personal decision or institutional policy has been made to transfuse blood components with low risk of transmitting CMV, cellular products transfused should be obtained from donors who are seronegative for antibody to CMV[157–163] or effectively leukocyte reduced.[156, 164] Frozen deglycerolized RBCs are used by some centers and appear to pose little, or no, risk of CMV.[161, 165] However, frozen RBCs are expensive, and RBC loss is unavoidable during deglycerolization, a situation that could lead to exposure to even greater numbers of donors. Similarly, frozen platelets do not transmit CMV, but this product is not available at most centers. As a more practical alternative, cellular blood components, consistently depleted of leukocytes to a level of less than 5×10^6 leukocytes per unit, offer safety comparable to that of blood products supplied by seronegative donors.[156, 164]

Prevention of CMV by WBC reduction has been extensively studied,[164] and it is clear that the risk of infection with this virus can be strikingly reduced by consistently depleting all cellular blood components of most WBCs. WBCs should be reduced in all cellular blood components (e.g., by filtration), not just RBCs. The precise dose of WBCs known to transmit CMV is unknown, but transfusions that contain less than 5×10^6 WBCs/unit are extremely unlikely to be infectious. Some experts prefer WBC reduction to less than 1×10^6 WBCs/unit. WBC-reduction filters provide a consistent means of removing several logs of contaminating WBCs.

Several reports have assessed the ability of WBC-reduction filters, sometimes used in conjunction with other methods of WBC removal, to eliminate transfusion-transmitted CMV.[166–171] All WBC-reduction filter studies have been strikingly successful. A few studies focused on the use of WBC reduction to prevent CMV infections specifically during infancy. In a study from Australia,[166] CMV infections were found in none of 30 infants who received filtered blood, compared with 9 of 42 (21%) infants who received unfiltered blood. Another study[169] included 26 infants who received blood depleted of WBCs by a spin-cool-filter technique and 22 infants who received filtered blood; none of these infants acquired CMV.

The inability to consistently achieve marked leukocyte reduction by some techniques is the probable reason for the occasional failure to prevent CMV by leukocyte reduction (e.g., washed blood products).[157–161] Leukocyte reduction is not an option when PMN (granulocyte) concentrates are to be transfused, and CMV antibody–negative donors must be used. Plasma products that have been frozen without cryoprotectants (e.g., FFP, cryoprecipitate) or pasteurized (e.g., albumin solutions) do not transmit CMV and do not have to be WBC reduced or obtained from donors seronegative for antibody to CMV.[172]

As an alternative to WBC reduction, the rate of transfusion-associated CMV has been reduced by selecting blood components collected from donors without antibodies to CMV. The recommendation has been made that seronegative infants receive only seronegative components for transfusion. Although this recommendation results in a significant reduction in the transmission rate of CMV, it is not perfect. A rate of 1% to 4% CMV infection, measured by CMV antibody seroconversion, viremia, or viruria, has been reported after transfusion of CMV-seronegative components.[164, 171, 173, 174] This finding can be attributed in part to the intrinsic false-negative rate of the test for antibody to CMV, a decrease in antibody titer over time in the blood donor to levels below detection, the possibility of transient viremia in seropositive patients that quenches circulating antibody, and a false-negative result for a donor in the antibody window phase of primary infection. It is therefore reasonable to conclude that WBC reduction by any method capable of achieving a residual WBC count of less than 1 to 5×10^6/unit allows reduction of CMV to a level at least equivalent to that of transfusion of CMV-seronegative components. Some experts believe data are too inconclusive to firmly declare WBC reduction and selection of blood components according to CMV antibody negativity to be equivalent in preventing transfusion-transmitted CMV. Neonatologists must choose the method they believe to be best. There are no data to document additive protection by the combined efforts of WBC reduction of blood components obtained from CMV-seronegative donors.

Gamma-irradiation to Prevent Graft-Versus-Host Disease

Neonates, particularly those who are extremely preterm, are considered to be at increased risk for transfusion-associated graft-versus-host disease (TA-GVHD). However, the exact degree to which they are at increased risk and the need, or lack thereof, to transfuse γ-irradiated cellular blood components are controversial issues for which no irrefutable, scientifically proved answers exist. Unquestionably, the immune system of neonates is abnormal, often with diminished function, compared with the immunity of older children and adults. The "immunomodulatory" effects of transfusion on the immune system of neonates is largely unknown, a situation that may be important because some infants receive multiple transfusions during the first few weeks of life.

In 1990, Sanders and Graeber[149] extensively reviewed infants in whom TA-GVHD developed within the first year of life. This earlier review was updated with a review of Japanese newborns.[148] Sixty-seven infants died of TA-GVHD during the first year of life (Table 18-2), and most were infants who had recognized risk factors for which γ-irradiated cellular blood components are recommended: underlying immunodeficiency disease, intrauterine or exchange transfusion for severe hemolytic disease, and transfusions from blood relatives. Only 5 of 67 infants who had TA-GVHD did not readily fit into a recognized high-risk group. One infant had severe aplastic anemia.[175] At some institutions, this infant would have received γ-irradiated blood products, because patients who have this disease, particularly if it is accompanied by lymphopenia, are sometimes considered to be at risk of TA-GVHD.[176] The other infants[148, 177] had no underlying disorders that clearly demonstrated an increased risk of TA-GVHD. Three infants were premature and had, respectively, birth weights and gestational ages of 720 g and 25 weeks,[148] 1528 g and 30 weeks,[148] and 855 g and 25 weeks.[177] Most infants who have a known propensity for the development of TA-GVHD already receive γ-irradiated cellular blood components at most institutions, and the scientific need for the routine practice of this technique can be debated.

In determining local policy, the decision of whether to transfuse γ-irradiated cellular blood components to neonates is based on three considerations: conviction that there is a scientifically proven need to do so, conformation to an

Table 18–2. **Fatal Transfusion-Associated Graft-Versus-Host Disease During the First Year of Life**

Underlying Medical Condition	Number Reported
Primary immunodeficiency disease	26
Intrauterine and exchange transfusion	5
Exchange transfusion only	6
Related blood donor	25
No apparent risk factor	5
Total	67

Data from Ohto H, Anderson KC: Posttranfusion graft-versus-host disease in Japanese newborns. Transfusion 1996;36:117, and from Sanders MR, Graeber JE: Posttransfusion graft-versus-host disease in infancy. J Pediatr 1990;117:159.

established standard of practice, and ability to provide γ-irradiated blood components to all neonates who need them in a safe and practical fashion. γ-Irradiated blood components to prevent TA-GVHD are probably needed only for neonates who are in the recognized high-risk groups of congenital immunodeficiency diseases with severe cellular immune defects, for those who are receiving intrauterine transfusions with or without subsequent exchange transfusions, and for those who are receiving blood components from blood relatives. A review of multiple case reports revealed only 4 of 67 episodes (excluding the patient who had aplastic anemia) that occurred outside these recognized settings, despite years of experience with thousands of preterm infants, many of whom received multiple transfusions. Because TA-GVHD during infancy is rarely reported, it is difficult to mandate use of irradiated cellular blood components for all neonates.

Some information is available to assess the standard of practice in the United States.[178] In 1989, a questionnaire was sent to 1790 members of the American Association of Blood Banks who might have been involved in the transfusion of blood to neonates; 1459 questionnaires were returned, for a response rate of 82%. Four hundred fifty-two respondents indicated that they were involved in such transfusions and provided sufficient data for analysis. Of 445 respondents who indicated institutional affiliations, 220 (49%) were from hospitals affiliated with a medical school (AMS), and 225 (51%) were from hospitals that were not affiliated with a medical school (NA). Among all hospitals, 13% routinely provided irradiated blood products for all neonates, 46% did for some neonates, and 41% did not routinely provide such products. Twenty percent of AMS hospitals routinely provided irradiated blood products for all neonates, 52% did for some neonates, and 28% did not routinely provide these products. Of the NA hospitals, only 10% routinely provided irradiated blood products for all neonates, 42% did for some neonates, and 48% did not routinely do so. The percentage of NA compared with AMS hospitals that did not routinely irradiate blood components was significantly different ($P = 0.002$). The type of hospital and the clinical status of the infants being treated must be considered when institutional policies are being made.

It is difficult to recognize all neonates who are in high-risk groups for TA-GVHD and should receive irradiated cellular blood components. An underlying primary immunodeficiency disorder may not be apparent shortly after birth when a transfusion is needed. To avoid the problem of overlooking neonates who truly are at risk of TA-GVHD, many centers caring for preterm infants provide γ-irradiated cellular blood products to all infants, rather than trying to distinguish high-risk neonates from those who probably are not. In a sense, this approach creates a standard of practice for other local institutions, and it must be recognized that the transfusion of γ-irradiated cellular blood components is sometimes based more on logistical and legal factors than on a proven scientific basis. It is a common practice among university hospitals to γ-irradiate all cellular blood components transfused to infants. Physicians must be aware of the standard of practice in their locality when establishing institutional practices.

References

1. Strauss RG: Red blood cell transfusion practices in the neonate. Clin Perinatol 1995;22:641.
2. Strauss RG, Sacher RA, Blazina JF, et al: Commentary on small-volume red cell transfusions for neonatal patients. Transfusion 1990;30:565.
3. Stockman JA: Anemia of prematurity: current concepts in the issue of when to transfuse. Pediatr Clin North Am 1986;33:111.
4. Wardrop CAJ, Holland BM, Beale KEA, et al: Nonphysical anaemia of prematurity. Arch Dis Child 1978;53:855.
5. Holland BM, Jones JG, Wardrop CAJ: Lessons from the anemia of prematurity. Hematol Oncol Clin North Am 1987;1:355.
6. Stockman JA III, Garcia JF, Oski FA: The anemia of prematurity: factors governing the erythropoietin response. N Engl J Med 1977;296:647.
7. Brown MS, Phibbs RH, Garcia JF, et al: Postnatal changes in erythropoietin levels in untransfused premature infants. J Pediatr 1983;103:612.
8. Stockman JA III, Graeber JE, Clark DA, et al: Anemia of prematurity: determinants of the erythropoietin response. J Pediatr 1984;105:786.
9. Brown MS, Garcia JF, Phibbs RH, et al: Decreased response of plasma immunoreactive erythropoietin to "available oxygen" in anemia of prematurity. J Pediatr 1984;105:793.
10. Shannon KM, Naylor GS, Tordildson JC, et al: Circulating erythroid progenitors in the anemia of prematurity. N Engl J Med 1987;317:728.
11. Rhondeau SM, Christensen RD, Ross MP, et al: Responsiveness to recombinant human erythropoietin of marrow erythroid progenitors from infants with the "anemia of prematurity." J Pediatr 1988;112:935.

12. Zanjani ED, Ascensao JL, McGlave PB, et al: Studies in the liver to kidney switch of erythropoietin production. J Clin Invest 1981;67:1183.
13. Widness JA, Susa JB, Garcia JF, et al: Increased erythropoiesis and elevated erythropoietin in infants born to diabetic mothers and in hyperinsulinemic rhesus fetuses J Clin Invest 1981;67:637.
14. Snijders RJM, Abbas A, Melby O, et al: Fetal plasma erythropoietin concentration in severe growth retardation. Am J Obstet Gynecol 1993;168:615.
15. Ohls RK, Yan LI, Trautman MS, et al: Erythropoietin production by macrophages from preterm infants: implications regarding the cause of the anemia in prematurity. Pediatr Res 1994;35:169.
16. Widness JA, Veng-Pedersen P, Peters C, et al: Erythropoietin pharmacokinetics in premature infants: developmental, nonlinearity, and treatment effects. J Appl Physiol 1996;80:140.
17. Ruth V, Widness JA, Raivio KO: Postnatal changes in serum Ep in relation to hypoxia before and after birth. J Pediatr 1990;116:950.
18. George JW, Bracco C, Shannon K, et al: Response of rhesus monkeys to recombinant human erythropoietin: comparison of adults and infants (Abstract). Pediatr Res 1989;25:269A.
19. Nexo E, Christensen NC, Olesen H: Volume of blood removed for analytical purposes during hospitalization of low-birthweight infants. Clin Chem 1981;27:759.
20. Obladen M, Sachsenweger M, Stahnke M: Blood sampling in very low birth weight infants receiving different levels of intensive care. Eur J Pediatr 1988; 147:399.
21. Sacher RA, Luban NLC, Strauss RG: Current practice and guidelines for the transfusion of cellular blood components in the newborn. Transfus Med Rev 1989;3:39.
22. Widness JA, Seward VJ, Kromer IJ, et al: Changing patterns of red blood cell transfusion in very low birth weight infants. J Pediatr 1996;129:680.
23. Ringer SA, Richardson DK, Sacher RA, et al: Variations in transfusion practice in neonatal intensive care. Pediatrics 1998;101:194.
24. Blanchette VS, Hume HA, Levy GJ, et al: Guidelines for auditing pediatric blood transfusion practices. Am J Dis Child 1991;145:787.
25. Kattwinkel J: Neonatal apnea: pathogenesis and therapy. J Pediatr 1977;90:342.
26. Joshi A, Gerhardt T, Shandloff P, et al: Blood transfusion effect on the respiratory pattern of preterm infants. Pediatrics 1987;80:79.
27. Keyes WG, Donohue PK, Spivak JL, et al: Assessing the need for transfusion of premature infants and role of hematocrit, clinical signs, and erythropoietin level. Pediatrics 1989;84:412.
28. Stockman JA, Clark DA: Weight gain: a response to transfusion in selected preterm infants. Am J Dis Child 1984;138:828.
29. Blank JP, Sheagren TG, Cajaria J, et al: The role of RBC transfusion in the premature infant. Am J Dis Child 1984;138:831.
30. Phillips HM, Holland BM, Abdel-Moiz A, et al: Determination of red cell mass in assessment and management of anaemia in babies needing blood transfusion. Lancet 1986;1:882.
31. Jones JG, Holland BM, Veale KEA, et al: "Available oxygen," a realistic expression of the ability of the blood to supply oxygen to tissues. Scand J Haematol 1979;22:77.
32. Alverson DC, Isken VH, Cohen RS: Effect of booster blood transfusions on oxygen utilization in infants with bronchopulmonary dysplasia. J Pediatr 1988; 113:722.
33. Gould SA, Rice CL, Moss GS: The physiologic basis of the use of blood and blood products. Surg Annu 1984;16:13.
34. Levine E, Rosen A, Sehgal L, et al: Physiologic effects of acute anemia: implications for a reduced transfusion trigger. Transfusion 1990;30:11.
35. McCormick M, Feustel PJ, Newell JC, et al: Effect of cardiac index and hematocrit changes on oxygen consumption in resuscitated patients. J Surg Res 1988;44:499.
36. Bland RD, Shoemaker WC, Abraham E, et al: Hemodynamic and oxygen transport patterns in surviving and nonsurviving postoperative patients. Crit Care Med 1985;13:85.
37. Weiskopf RB, Viele MK, Feiner J, et al: Human cardiovascular and metabolic response to acute, severe isovolemic anemia. JAMA 1998;279:217.
38. Hudson IR, Cavill IA, Cooke AD, et al: Biotin labeling of red cells in the measurement of red cell volume in preterm infants. Pediatr Res 1990;28:199.
39. Hudson I, Cooke A, Holland B, et al: Red cell volume and cardiac output in anaemic preterm infants. Arch Dis Child 1990;65:672.
40. Mock DM, Lankford GL, Widness JA, et al: Measurement of circulating red blood cell volume by a nonradioactive, biotin method: validation against ^{51}Cr. Transfusion 1999;39:149.
41. Liu EA, Mannino FL, Lane TA: Prospective, randomized trial of the safety and efficacy of a limited donor exposure transfusion program for premature neonates. J Pediatr 1994;125:92.
42. Lee DA, Slagle TA, Jackson TM, et al: Reducing blood donor exposures in low birth weight infants by the use of older, unwashed packed red blood cells. J Pediatr 1995;125:92.
43. Wood A, Wilson N, Skacl P, et al: Reducing donor exposure in preterm infants requiring blood transfusions. Arch Dis Child 1995;72:F29.
44. Strauss RG, Burmeister LF, Johnson K, et al: AS-1 red blood cells for neonatal transfusions: a randomized trial assessing donor exposure and safety. Transfusion 1996;36:873.
45. Strauss RG: Recombinant erythropoietin for the anemia of prematurity: still a promise, not a panacea. J Pediatr 1997;131:653.
46. Strauss RG: Erythropoietin in the pathogenesis and treatment of neonatal anemia. Transfusion 1995;35:68.
47. Sahnnon KM, Keith JF, Mentzer WC, et al: Recombinant human erythropoietin stimulates erythropoiesis and reduces erythrocyte transfusions in very-low-birth-weight preterm infants. Pediatrics 1995;95:1.
48. Ohls RK, Veerman MW, Christensen RD: Pharmacokinetics and effectiveness of recombinant erythropoietin administered to preterm infants by continuous infusion in total parenteral nutrition solution. J Pediatr 1996; 128:518.
49. Ohls RK, Harcum J, Schibler KR, et al: The effect of erythropoietin on the transfusion requirements of preterm infants weighing 750 grams or less: a randomized, double-blind, placebo-controlled study. J Pediatr 1997;131:661.
50. Anderson A, Fangman J, Wager G, et al: Retrieval of placental blood from the umbilical vein to determine volume, sterility, and presence of clot formation. Arch Pediatr Adolesc Med 1992;146:36.
51. Bifano EM, Dracker RA, Lorah K, et al: Collection and 28-day storage of human placental blood. Pediatr Res 1994;36:90.

52. Strauss RG: Autologous transfusions for neonates using placental blood: a cautionary note. Arch Pediatr Adolesc Med 1992; 146:21.
53. Kinmond S, Aitchison TC, Holand BM, et al: Umbilical cord clamping and preterm infants: a randomized trial. BMJ 1993;306:172.
54. Ludomirsk A, Weiner S, Ashmead CG, et al: Percutaneous fetal umbilical blood sampling: procedure safety and normal fetal hematologic indices. Am J Perinatol 1988;5:264.
55. Sell EJ, Corrigan JJ Jr: Platelet counts, fibrinogen concentrations, and factor V and factor VIII levels in healthy infants according to gestational age. J Pediatr 1973;82:1028.
56. Aballi AJ, Puapondh Y, Desposito F: Platelet counts in thriving premature infants. Pediatrics 1968;42:685.
57. Hemta P, Vasa R, Neumann L, et al: Thrombocytopenia in the high-risk infant. J Pediatr 1980;97:791.
58. Andrew M, Vegh P, Caco C, et al: A randomized trial of platelet transfusions in thrombocytopenic premature infants. J Pediatr 1993;123:285.
59. Scheifele DW, Olsen EM, Pendray MR: Endotoxinemia and thrombocytopenia during neonatal necrotizing enterocolitis. Am J Clin Pathol 1985;83:227.
60. Castle V, Andrew M, Kelton J, et al: Frequency and mechanism of neonatal thrombocytopenia. J Pediatr 1986;108:749.
61. Andrew M, Castle V, Saigal S, et al: Clinical impact of neonatal thrombocytopenia. J Pediatr 1987;110:457.
62. Castle V, Coates G, Kelton JG, et al: In-oxine platelet survivals in thrombocytopenic infants. Blood 1987;70:652.
63. Murray NA, Roberts, IAG: Circulating megakaryocytes and their progenitors in early thrombocytopenia in preterm neonates. Pediatr Res 1996;40:112.
64. Murray NA, Watts TL, Roberts IAG: Endogenous thrombopoietin levels and effect of recombinant human thrombopoietin on megakaryocyte precursors in term and preterm babies. Pediatr Res 1998;43:148.
65. Whaun JM: Platelet function in the neonate: including qualitative platelet abnormalities associated with bleeding. In Stockman JA, Pochedly C (eds): Developmental and Neonatal Hematology. New York: Raven Press, 1988, pp 131–144.
66. Ts'ao CH, Green D, Schultz K: Function and ultrastructure of platelets of neonates: enhanced ristocetin aggregation of neonatal platelets. Br J Haematol 1976;32:225.
67. Blanchette VS, Sacher RA, Ballem PJ, et al: Commentary on the management of autoimmune thrombocytopenia during pregnancy and in the neonatal period. Blut 1989;59:121.
68. Mueller-Eckhardt C, Kiefel V, Grubert A, et al: 348 Cases of suspected neonatal alloimmune thrombocytopenia. Lancet 1989;1:363.
69. Panzer S, Auerbach L, Cechova E, et al: Maternal alloimmunization against fetal platelet antigens: a prospective study. Br J Haematol 1995;90:655.
70. Burrows RF, Kelton JG: Fetal thrombocytopenia and its relation to maternal thrombocytopenia. N Engl J Med 1993;329:1463.
71. Strauss RG: The risks of thrombocytopenia and the standard uses of platelet transfusions. Plasma Ther Transfus Technol 1986;7:279.
72. Gibson B: Neonatal haemostasis. Arch Dis Child 1989;64:503.
73. Lupton BA, Hill A, Whitfield MR, et al: Reduced platelet count as a risk factor for intraventricular hemorrhage. Am J Dis Child 1988;142:1222.
74. Moroff G, Friendman A, Robkin-Kline L, et al: Reduction of the volume of stored platelet concentrates for use in neonatal patients. Transfusion 1984;24:144.
75. Reverdiau-Moalic P, Delahousse B, Body G, et al: Evolution of blood coagulation activators and inhibitors in the healthy human fetus. Blood 1996;88:900.
76. Strauss RG: Granulopoiesis and neutrophil function in the neonate: In Stockman JA, Pochedly C (eds): Developmental and Neonatal Hematology. New York: Raven Press, 1988, pp 88–101.
77. Rosenthal J, Cairo MS: Neonatal myelopoiesis and immunomodulation of host defenses. In Petz LD, Swisher SN, Kleinman S, Spence RK, Strauss RG (eds): Clinical Practice of Transfusion Medicine, 3rd ed. New York: Churchill Livingstone, 1995, pp 685–704.
78. Christensen D, Rothstein G, Anstall HB, et al: Granulocyte transfusions in neonates with bacterial infection, neutropenia and depletion of mature marrow neutrophils. Pediatrics 1982;70:1.
79. Christensen RD, McFarlane JL, Taylor NL, et al: Blood and marrow neutrophils during experimental group B streptococcal infection: quantification of the stem cell, proliferative, storage and circulating pools. Pediatr Res 1982;16:549.
80. Erdman SH, Christensen RD, Bradley PP, et al: Supply and release of storage neutrophils. Biol Neonate 1982;41:132.
81. Christensen RD, Harper TE, Rothstein G: Granulocyte-macrophage progenitor cells in term and preterm neonates. J Pediatr 1986;109:1047.
82. Laurenti F, Ferro R, Isacchi G, et al: Polymorphonuclear leukocyte transfusion for the treatment of sepsis in the newborn infants. J Pediatr 1981;98:118.
83. Cairo MS, Rucker R, Bennetts GA, et al: Improved survival of newborns receiving leukocyte transfusions for sepsis. Pediatrics 1984;74:887.
84. Cairo MS, Worcester C, Rucker R, et al: Role of circulating complement and polymorphonuclear leukocyte transfusion in treatment and outcome in critically ill neonates with sepsis. J Pediatr 1987;110:935.
85. DeCurtis M, Romano G, Scarpato N, et al: Transfusions of polymorphonuclear leukocytes (PMN) in an infant with necrotizing enterocolitis (NEC) and a defect of phagocytosis. J Pediatr 1981;99:665.
86. Christensen RD, Anstall H, Rothstein G: Neutrophil transfusion in septic neutropenic neonates. Transfusion 192;22:151.
87. Laing IA, Boulton FE, Hume R: Polymorphonuclear leukocyte transfusion in neonatal septicemia. Arch Dis Child 1983;58:1003.
88. Laurenti F, LaGreca G, Ferro R, et al: Transfusion of polymorphonuclear neutrophils in premature infant with *Klebsiella* sepsis. Lancet 1978;2:111.
89. Baley JE, Stork EK, Warkentin PI, et al: Buffy coat transfusions in neutropenic neonates with presumed sepsis: a prospective, randomized trial. Pediatrics 1987;80:712.
90. Wheeler JC, Chauvenet AR, Johnson CA, et al: Buffy coat transfusions in neonates with sepsis and neutrophil storage pool depletion. Pediatrics 1987;97:422.
91. Newman RS, Waffarn F, Simmons GE, et al: Questionable value of saline prepared granulocytes in the treatment of neonatal septicemia. Transfusion 1988;28:196.
92. Strauss RG: Current status of granulocyte transfusions to treat neonatal sepsis. J Clin Apheresis 1989;5:25.
93. Christensen RD, Rothstein G, Hill HR, et al: The effect of hybridoma antibody administration upon neutrophil kinetics during experimental type III group B stretococcal sepsis. Pediatr Res 1983;17:795.

94. Kim KS: Efficacy of human immunoglobulin and penicillin G in treatment of experimental group B streptococcal infection. Pediatr Res 1987;21:289.
95. Harper TE, Christensen RD, Rothstein G: The effect of administration of immunoglobulin to newborn rats with *Escherichia coli* sepsis and meningitis. Pediatr Res 1987;22:455.
96. Harper TE, Christensen RD, Rothstein G, et al: Effect of intravenous immunoglobulin G on neutrophil kinetics during experimental group B streptococcal infection in neonatal rats. Rev Infect Dis 1986;8:S401.
97. Redd H, Christensen RD, Fischer GW: Circulating and storage neutrophils in septic neonatal rats treated with immune globulin. J Infect Dis 1988;157:705.
98. Haque KN, Zaidi MN, Haque SK, et al: Intravenous immunoglobulin for prevention of sepsis in preterm and low birth weight infants. Pediatr Infect Dis 1986;5:622.
99. Chirico G, Rondini G, Plebani A, et al: Intravenous gammaglobulin therapy for prophylaxis of infection in high-risk neonates. J Pediatr 1987;110:437.
100. Clapp DW, Kliegman RM, Baley JE, et al: Use of intravenously administered immune globulin to prevent nosocomial sepsis to low birth weight infants: report of a pilot study. J Pediatr 1989;115:973.
101. Conway S, Ng P, Howel D, et al: Prophylactic intravenous immunoglobulin in preterm infants: a controlled trial. Vox Sang 1990;59:6.
102. Stabile A, Miceli Sopo S, Romanelli V, et al: Intravenous immunoglobulin for prophylaxis of neonatal sepsis in premature infants. Arch Dis Child 1988;63:441.
103. Magny JF, Bremard-Oury C, Brault D, et al: Intravenous immunoglobulin therapy for prevention in high-risk premature infants: report of a multicenter, double-blind study. Pediatrics 1991;88:437.
104. Baker CJ, Melish ME, Hall RT, et al: Intravenous immune globulin for the prevention of nosocomial infection in low-birth-weight neonates. N Engl J Med 1992;327:213.
105. Bussel JB: Intravenous gammaglobulin in the prophylaxis of late sepsis in very-low-birth-weight infants: preliminary results of a randomized, double-blind, placebo-controlled trial. Rev Infect Dis 1990;12:S457.
106. Fanaroff AA, Korones SB, Wright LL, et al: A controlled trial of intravenous immune globulin to reduce nosocomial infections in very-low-birth-weight infants. N Engl J Med 1994;330:1170.
107. van Overmeire B, Bleyaert S, van Reempts PJ, et al: The use of intravenously administered immunoglobulins in the prevention of severe infection in very low birth weight neonates. Biol Neonate 1993;64:110.
108. Weisman LE, Stoll BJ, Kueser TJ, et al: Intravenous immune globulin prophylaxis of late-onset sepsis in premature neonates. J Pediatr 1994;125:922.
109. Christensen RD, Hardman T, Thornton J, et al: A randomized, double-blind, placebo-controlled investigation of the safety of intravenous immune globulin administration to preterm neonates. J Perinatol 1988;9:126.
110. Sidiropoulos D, Boehme U, von Muralt G, et al: Immunoglobulin supplementation in prevention or treatment of neonatal sepsis. Pediatr Infect Dis J 1986;5:S193.
111. Haque KN, Zaidi MH, Bahakim H:lgM-enriched intravenous immunoglobulin therapy in neonatal sepsis. Am J Dis Child 1988;142:1293.
112. Friedman CA, Wender DG, Temple DM, et al: Intravenous gamma globulin as adjunct therapy for severe group B streptococcal disease in the newborn. Am J Perinatol 1989;6:453.
113. Weisman LE, Stoll BJ, Kueser TJ, et al: Intravenous immune globulin therapy for early-onset sepsis in premature neonates. J Pediatr 1992;121:434.
114. Christensen RD, Brown MS, Hall DC, et al: Effect on neutrophil kinetics and serum opsonic capacity of intravenous administration of immune globulin to neonates with clinical signs of early-onset sepsis. J Pediatr 1991;118:606.
115. Cairo MS, Worcester CC, Rucker RW, et al: Randomized trial of granulocyte transfusions versus intravenous immune globulin therapy for neonatal neutropenia and sepsis. J Pediatr 1992;120:281.
116. Haque KN, Remo C, Bahakim H: Comparison of two types of intravenous immunoglobulins in the treatment of neonatal sepsis. Clin Exp Immunol 1995;101:328.
117. Cross AS, Siegel G, Byrne WR, et al: Intravenous immune globulin impairs anti-bacterial defenses of a cyclophosphamide-treated host. Clin Exp Immunol 1989;76:159.
118. Weisman LE, Weisman E, Lorenzetti PM: High intravenous doses of human immune globulin suppress neonatal group B streptococcal immunity in rats. J Pediatr 1989;115:445.
119. Cross AS, Alving BM, Sadoff JC, et al: Intravenous immune globulin: a cautionary note. Lancet 1984; 1:912.
120. Cairo MS: The use of granulocyte transfusions in neonatal sepsis. Transfus Med Rev 1990;4:14.
121. Magny JF, Bremard-Oury C, Brault D, et al: Intravenous immunoglobulin therapy for prevention of infection in high-risk premature infants: report of a multicenter, double-blood study. Pediatrics 1991;88:437.
122. Bailie KEM, Irvine AE, Bridges JM, et al: Granulocyte and granulocyte-macrophage colony-stimulating factors in cord and maternal serum at delivery. Pediatr Res 1994;35:164.
123. Bedford Russel AR, Davies EG, McGuigan S, et al: Plasma granulocyte colony stimulating factor concentrations (G-CSF) in the early neonatal period. Br J Haematol 1994;86:642.
124. Gessler P, Kirchmann N, Kientsch-Engel R, et al: Serum concentrations of granulocyte colony-stimulating factor in healthy term and preterm neonates and in those with various diseases including bacterial infections. Blood 1993;82:3177.
125. Ohls RK, Li Y, Abdel-Mageed A, et al: Neutrophil pool sizes and granulocyte colony-stimulating factor production in human mid-trimester fetuses. Pediatr Res 1995;37:806.
126. Schibler KR, Liechty KW, White W, et al: Production of granulocyte colony-stimulating factor in vitro by monocytes from preterm and term neonates. Blood 1993;82:2478.
127. Lee S, Knoppel E, van de Ven C, et al: Transcriptional rates of granulocyte-macrophage colony-stimulating factor, granulocyte colony-stimulating factor, interleukin-3, and macrophage colony-stimulating factor genes in activated cord *versus* adult mononuclear cells: alteration in cytokine expression may be secondary to posttranscriptional instability. Pediatr Res 1993; 34:560.
128. English BK, Hammond WP, Lewis DB, et al: Decreased granulocyte-macrophage colony-stimulating factor production by human neonatal blood mononuclear cells and T cells. Pediatr Res 1992;31:211.
129. Cairo MS, Suen Y, Knoppel E, et al: Decreased stimulated GM-CSF production and GM-CSF gene expression but normal numbers of GM-CSF receptors in

human term newborns compared with adults. Pediatr Res 1991;30:362.
130. Frenck RW, Sarman G, Harper TE, et al: The ability of recombinant murine granulocyte-macrophage colony-stimulating factor to protect neonatal rats from septic death due to *Staphylococcus aureus*. J Infect Dis 1990;162:109.
131. Cairo MS, Mauss D, Kommareddy S, et al: Prophylactic or simultaneous administration of recombinant human granulocyte colony-stimulating factor in the treatment of group B streptococcal sepsis in neonatal rats. Pediatr Res 1990;27:612.
132. Cairo MS, Plunkett JM, Mauss D, et al: Seven-day administration of recombinant human granulocyte colony-stimulating factor to newborn rats: modulation of neonatal neutrophilia, myelopoiesis, and group B *Streptococcus* sepsis. Blood 1990;75:1788.
133. Cairo MS, Plunkett JM, Nguyen A, et al: Effect of stem cell factor with and without granulocyte colony-stimulating factor on neonatal hematopoiesis: in vivo induction of newborn myelopoiesis and reduction of mortality during experimental group B streptococcal sepsis. Blood 1992;80:96.
134. Cairo MS, Plunkett JM, Nguyen A, et al: Sequential administration of interleukin-6 and granulocyte colony-stimulating factor in newborn rats: modulation of newborn granulopoiesis and thrombopoiesis. Pediatr Res 1991;30:554.
135. Medlock ES, Kaplan DL, Cecchini M, et al: Granulocyte colony-stimulating factor crosses the placenta and stimulates fetal rat granulopoiesis. Blood 1993;81:916.
136. Novales JS, Salva AM, Modanlou HD, et al: Maternal administration of granulocyte colony-stimulating factor improves neonatal rat survival after a lethal group B streptococcal infection. Blood 1993;81:923.
137. Jaswon MS, Jones HM, Linch DC: The effects of recombinant human granulocyte-macrophage colony-stimulating factor on the neutrophil respiratory burst in the term and preterm infant when studied in whole blood. Pediatr Res 1994;36:623.
138. Frenck RW Jr, Buescher ES, Vandhan-Raj S: The effects of recombinant human granulocyte-macrophage colony-stimulating factor on in vitro cord blood granulocyte function. Pediatr Res 1989;26:43.
139. Gillan ER, Christensen RD, Suen Y, et al: A randomized, placebo-controlled trial of recombinant human granulocyte colony-stimulating factor administration in newborn infants with presumed sepsis: significant induction of peripheral and bone marrow neutrophilia. Blood 1994;84:1427.
140. Makhlouf RA, Doron MW, Bose CL, et al: Administration of granulocyte colony-stimulating factor to neutropenic low birth weight infants of mothers with preeclampsia. J Pediatr 1995;126:454.
141. Cairo MS, Christensen R, Sender LS, et al: Results of a phase I/II trial of recombinant human granulocyte-macrophage colony-stimulating factor in very low birthweight neonates: significant induction of circulatory neutrophils, monocytes, platelets, and bone marrow neutrophils. Blood 1995;86:2509.
142. Rogers MF, Thomas PA, Starcher ET, et al: Acquired immunodeficiency syndrome in children: report of the Centers for Disease Control national surveillance, 1982 to 1985. Pediatrics 1987;79:1008.
143. Aubuchon JP, Birkmeyer JD, Busch MP: Safety of the blood supply in the United States: opportunities and controversies. Ann Intern Med 1997;127:904.
144. Bertolli J, Caldwell B, Lindegren ML, et al: Epidemiology of HIV disease in children. Immunol Allergy Clin North Am 1995;15:193.
145. European Collaborative Study Group: Natural history of vertically acquired human immunodeficiency virus-1 infection. Pediatrics 1994;94:815.
146. Blajchman MA, Sheridan D, Rawls WE: Risks associated with blood transfusion in newborn infants. Clin Perinatol 1984;2:403.
147. Alter HJ, Purcell RH, Shih JW, et al: Detection of antibody to hepatitis C virus in prospectively following transfusion recipients with acute and chronic non-A, non-B hepatitis. N Engl J Med 1989;321:1494.
148. Ohto H, Anderson KC: Posttransfusion graft-versus-host disease in Japanese newborns. Transfusion 1996;36:117.
149. Sanders MR, Graeber JE: Posttransfusion graft-versus-host disease in infancy. J Pediatr 1990;117:159.
150. Inder TE, Clemett RS, Austin NC, et al: High iron status in very low birth weight infants is associated with an increased risk of retinopathy of prematurity. J Pediatr 1997;131:541.
151. Adamkin DH, Shott RJ, Cook LN, et al: Nonhyperoxic retrolental fibroplasia. Pediatrics 1977;60:828.
152. Sjoberg POJ, Bondesson UG, Sedin EG, et al: Exposure of newborn infants to plasticizers. Transfusion 1985;25:424.
153. Williams RA, Brown EF, Hurst D, et al: Transfusion of infants with activation of erythrocyte T antigen. J Pediatr 1989;115:949.
154. Pahwa S, Sia C, Harper R, et al: T lymphocyte subpopulations in high-risk infants: influence of age and blood transfusions. Pediatrics 1985;76:914.
155. Floss AM, Strauss RG, Goeken N, et al: Multiple transfusions fail to provoke antibodies against blood cell antigens in human infants. Transfusion 1986; 26:419.
156. Strauss RG: Selection of white cell-reduced blood components for transfusions during early infancy. Transfusion 1993;33:352.
157. Tegtmeier GE: The use of cytomegalovirus-screened blood in neonates. Transfusion 1988;28:201.
158. Preiksaitis JK, Brown L, McKenzie M: Transfusion-acquired cytomegalovirus infection in neonates: a prospective study. Transfusion 1988;28:205.
159. Griffin MP, O'Shea M, Brazy JE, et al: Cytomegalovirus infection in a neonatal intensive care unit. Am J Dis Child 1988;142:1188.
160. Adler SP: Transfusion-acquired CMV infection in premature infants (Letter). Transfusion 1989;29:278.
161. Hillyer CD, Snydman DR, Berkman EM: The risk of cytomegalovirus infection in solid organ and bone marrow transplant recipients: transfusion of blood products. Transfusion 1990;30:659.
162. Verdonck LF, deGraan-Hentzen YCE, Dekker AW, et al: Cytomegalovirus seronegative platelets and leukocyte-poor red blood cells from random donors can prevent primary cytomegalovirus infection after bone marrow transplantation. Bone Marrow Transplant 1987;2:73.
163. Mackinnon S, Burnett AK, Crawford RJ, et al: Seronegative blood products prevent primary cytomegalovirus infection after bone marrow transplantation. J Clin Pathol 1988;41:948.
164. American Association of Blood Banks Association: Leukocyte reduction to prevent transfusion-transmitted cytomegalovirus. Bulletin no. 97-2. Bethesda: AABB Press, 1997.
165. Brady MT, Milam JD, Anderson DC, et al: Use of deglycerolized red blood cells to prevent posttransfusion infection with cytomegalovirus in neonates. J Infect Dis 1984;150:334.
166. Gilbert GL, Hayes K, Hudson IL, et al: Prevention

of transfusion-acquired cytomegalovirus infection in infants by blood filtration to remove leukocytes. Lancet 1989;1:1228.

167. de Graan-Hentzen YCE, Gratama JW, Mudde GC, et al: Prevention of primary cytomegalovirus infection in patients with hematologic malignancies by intensive white cell depletion of blood products. Transfusion 1989;29:757.

168. Murphy MF, Grint PCA, Hardiman AE, et al: Use of leucocyte-poor blood components to prevent primary cytomegalovirus (CMV) infection in patients with acute leukaemia. Br J Haematol 1988;70:253.

169. Eisenfeld L, Silver H, McLaughlin J, et al: Prevention of transfusion-associated cytomegalovirus infection in neonatal patients by the removal of white cells from blood. Transfusion 1992;32:205.

170. Andreu G: Role of leukocyte depletion in the prevention of transfusion-induced cytomegalovirus infection. Semin Hematol 1991;28:26.

171. Bowden RA, Slichter SJ, Sayers M, et al: A comparison of filtered leukocyte-reduced and cytomegalovirus seronegative blood products for the prevention of transfusion-associated CMV infection after marrow transplant. Blood 1995;86:3598.

172. Bowden R, Sayers M: The risk of transmitting cytomegalovirus infection by fresh frozen plasma. Transfusion 1990;30:762.

173. Miller WJ, McCullough J, Balfour HH Jr, et al: Prevention of cytomegalovirus-infection following bone marrow transplantation: a randomized trial of blood product screening. Bone Marrow Transplant 1991; 7:227.

174. Lang DJ, Ebert PA, Rodgers BM, et al: Reduction of postperfusion cytomegalovirus infections following the use of leukocyte depleted blood. Transfusion 1977;17:391.

175. Jequier S, Azouz EM: Calculus cholecystitis in an infant with aplastic anemia and graft-versus-host reaction. J Clin Ultrasound 1985;13:424.

176. Strauss RG, Bove KE, Lake A, et al: Acquired immunodeficiency in hepatitis-associated aplastic anemia. 1975;86:910.

177. Funkhouser AW, Vogelsang G, Zehnbaur B, et al: Graft versus host disease after blood transfusion in a premature infant. Pediatrics 1991;87:247.

178. Strauss RG, Levy GJ, Sotelo-Avila C, et al: National survey of neonatal transfusion practices, II: blood component therapy. Pediatrics 1993;91:530.

Index

Note: Page numbers followed by *t* and *f* indicate tables and figures, respectively.

ISBN 0-7216-7727-4